Perioperative Nursing

Perioperative Nursing
An Introduction

3RD EDITION

EDITORS

SALLY SUTHERLAND-FRASER

MENNA DAVIES

BRIGID M. GILLESPIE

BEN LOCKWOOD

ELSEVIER

ELSEVIER

Elsevier Australia. ACN 001 002 357
(a division of Reed International Books Australia Pty Ltd)
Tower 1, 475 Victoria Avenue, Chatswood, NSW 2067

ISBN: 978-0-7295-4338-5

Notice

This publication has been carefully reviewed and checked to ensure that the content is as accurate and current as possible at time of publication. We would recommend, however, that the reader verify any procedures, treatments, drug dosages or legal content described in this book. Neither the author, the contributors, nor the publisher assume any liability for injury and/or damage to persons or property arising from any error in or omission from this publication.

National Library of Australia Cataloguing-in-Publication Data

 A catalogue record for this book is available from the National Library of Australia

---

Content Strategist: Libby Houston
Content Project Manager: Sukanthi Sukumar, Shravan Kumar
Edited by Chris Wyard
Proofread by Katie Millar
Permissions Processor: Prem Subash
Cover Designer: Alan Laver, Georgette Hall
Index by Innodata
Typeset by GWTech
Printed in Singapore by KHL Printing Co Pte Ltd

Last digit is the print number: 9 8 7 6 5 4 3 2

Contents

Foreword

It is a privilege to introduce this third edition of *Perioperative Nursing: an Introduction*, which continues to build upon the evolving models of care and technology available to perioperative nursing practice. The focus on safety and quality standards underpinning each chapter safeguards that patients will receive excellent care in operating and procedural suites.

The third edition again uses the considerable knowledge and expertise of Australian and New Zealand perioperative nurses practising in academic, management, education and clinical positions to bring together the most current contemporary and evidence based information. Chapters include the contributions of perioperative nurses from the Pacific island countries where, in 2019, the Pacific Island Operating Room Nursing Association (PIORNA) was formed.

The text remains broad and comprehensive to include all perioperative nursing roles and is aligned with the Australian College of Perioperative Nurses (ACORN) Standards for Perioperative Nurses, the New Zealand Perioperative Nursing College Standards, the Pacific Perioperative Practice Bundle, and the Australian National Safety and Quality Health Service (NSQHS) Standards.

The chapters logically follow the journey of the perioperative patient from pre-admission assessments through to day of surgery admission, anaesthetic care, intraoperative care, post-operative care and discharge to the surgical unit or home. The inclusion of the wide demographic of patients encountered and their diverse cultural and social needs contextualises the information presented to illustrate a holistic approach to perioperative care.

Patient scenarios are used throughout the book to link theory to practice, and clearly situate the information in the clinical context. Critical thinking questions linked to online resources allow a further assessment of practice. The final chapter uses a series of vignettes to allow readers to explore perioperative practice across a range of non-traditional settings that have developed as change and new opportunities arise.

This book remains a valuable source of evidence based information for beginner perioperative nurses, those undertaking post graduate studies in perioperative nursing and perioperative clinicians. The book is also an invaluable resource for educators, clinical support nurses and preceptors to guide the orientation of staff new to the perioperative environment.

I congratulate the editorial team and contributing authors in producing this update that is based on the contemporary perioperative nursing practices of Australasian nurses.

Carollyn Williams,
M Hlth Sc (Nur), FACORN, FACN
ACORN Excellence in Perioperative Nursing 2008
ACORN Board 2010 - 2014
ACORN Censor Panel
(Chair 2010 - 2016; Member 2018 - present)
Judith Cornell Orator 2016

Preface

This third edition of *Perioperative nursing: an introduction* bids farewell to two of the original editors, Dr Lois Hamlin and Marilyn Richardson-Tench, who with Menna Davies had the vision and passion to create this book for beginning perioperative nurses in 2009. More than a decade on, this third edition welcomes two new editors, Professor Brigid M. Gillespie from Queensland and Ben Lockwood from South Australia, who join Sally Sutherland-Fraser and Menna Davies. This new editorial team has an extensive working knowledge of the latest clinical practices as well as the underpinning research, evidence and practice trends in the nursing profession and the perioperative specialty. The team has curated a group of experienced and new contributors to provide this third edition with a broad international perspective and acknowledges the strengthening professional ties with perioperative nurses in the Asia-Pacific region.

The book continues to incorporate the national and international standards and guidelines current at the time of writing, including the World Health Organization (WHO) Surgical Safety Checklist, the Australian College of Perioperative Nurses (ACORN) and Perioperative Nurses College of the New Zealand Nurses Organisation (PNC NZNO) Standards and, in Australia, the National Safety and Quality in Health Service Standards. All of the chapters have been updated and many have been fully revised to reflect changes in perioperative practice and perioperative patient safety. The book continues to emphasise the concept of the patient journey. While most surgical patients travel an elective pathway, there is greater acknowledgement in this edition of those surgical patients who travel an emergency pathway.

The book is now structured in two parts, beginning with the principles of perioperative nursing practice. Chapters 1 and 2 set the scene for beginning nurses with a description of perioperative nursing roles, followed by an exploration of human factors and the implications for perioperative teams. A new sequence for the following chapters enhances the flow of content from medico-legal aspects (now Chapter 3), to patient safety and quality (now Chapter 4), while a description of the perioperative environment now lays the foundation for perioperative nurses' work health and safety (Chapter 5) and the practices of infection prevention and control including reprocessing of reusable medical devices (Chapter 6).

Part 2 focuses on the practical application of these principles and follows the sequence of a perioperative patient's journey. This begins with the patient's assessment and preparation for surgery (Chapter 7), through to their care during anaesthesia (Chapter 8), then follows intraoperative patient care (Chapter 9) and the surgical intervention (Chapter 10). Wound healing, haemostasis and wound closure are covered in Chapter 11, while postanaesthesia nursing care is located in Chapter 12. Chapter 13 now presents readers with insights into perioperative practice in non-traditional settings with some examples of professional roles that perioperative nurses may consider.

Most chapters include research boxes, where appropriate, and feature boxes that emphasise patient concerns in special populations. Four new patient scenarios are included in this third edition, which strengthen the links between chapters. These scenarios will test the readers' knowledge of perioperative nursing practice as they ask readers to consider and think critically about the care of these patients. A detailed description of these four patients is provided in the following Introduction to the book, while each chapter introduces new patient details as each of the relevant scenarios unfolds.

The nature of perioperative procedures, settings and models of care described here reflect the understanding and professional practice of our contributors. As perioperative care evolves continuously, readers are directed to use the resources provided in each chapter, as well as identifying and utilising other sources. The Evolve website continues to provide additional material for readers to test their knowledge by accessing the following online features:

- Answers for the Critical Thinking Questions that appear in every chapter
- Perioperative case studies and answer guide
- Self-assessment multiple choice and true/false questions and answers and rationales
- Further readings

- Web links
- Glossary
- Image collection.

Finally, this new edition acknowledges the extensive changes and significant developments in healthcare that have occurred over the last few years since publication of the second edition. During 2020, the historic international year of the nurse and midwife, the book was in its final production stages when the global population felt the significant impact of COVID-19 from the rapidly spreading SARS-CoV2 virus. Chapters were being finalised as governments and the international science and health communities launched their responses to this latest global pandemic. Wherever applicable, the editorial team introduced new content about these emerging practices in chapter feature boxes – for example, managing the risks during aerosol generating procedures appears in Chapter 8 Patient care during anaesthesia. The long-term impact of COVID-19 on the delivery of healthcare, much less perioperative patient care, is difficult to estimate at this time. We are more confident, however, about the positive impact of specialist education on perioperative nurses' perceived competence and the quality of care. This book will provide readers with the strong educational foundations they need to practice safely and to provide patients with holistic and culturally safe nursing care during their perioperative journey.

**Sally Sutherland-Fraser, Menna Davies,
Brigid M. Gillespie, Ben Lockwood**
July 2021

Editors

Menna Davies, RN, Cert (Sterilising Tech), GradCert (Periop Nsg), GradDip (Hlth Law), MHlthSc (Nsg), FACN, FACORN

Menna Davies is an independent Nurse Consultant, and was previously Director of *Health Education and Learning Partnerships Pty Ltd*, a consultancy and education company she founded with Sally Sutherland-Fraser, 2013–19. She previously held the position of Clinical Nurse Consultant at the Randwick Campus Operating Suite. She has worked as a perioperative Nurse Educator at Westmead Hospital and at the (then) NSW College of Nursing (now Australian College of Nursing (ACN)), during which time she assisted in the development of the first postgraduate distance education perioperative nursing course in Australia, coordinating the program for 10 years. She continues to work for ACN, most recently as a tutor/marker for a cohort of perioperative nurses from Pacific countries undertaking postgraduate studies at ACN.

Menna is Life Member of the NSW Operating Theatre Association (NSW OTA) and served two terms as President. She was a member of the surgical plume working party, assisting in the development of the 2015 NSW Health guidelines for the management of surgical plume in the perioperative environment. She was NSW representative on the Australian College of Perioperative Nurses (ACORN) Board and Conference Convener for the ACORN National Conference in 1995 in Sydney. Menna was a member of the ACORN competency working party and produced a number of educational videos on behalf of ACORN, including Scrubbing, Gowning and Gloving.

Menna has presented papers at state, national and international perioperative nursing conferences, published articles and contributed to perioperative nursing texts, received the inaugural ACORN Excellence in Perioperative Nursing Award in 2004 and is an Honorary Fellow of ACORN. In 2012 she presented the prestigious Judith Cornell Oration at the ACORN Conference in Darwin, NT.

Brigid M. Gillespie, RN, BHlth Sci (Hons), GradCert (Periop Nsg), PhD

Professor Brigid Gillespie is the conjoint Professor of Patient Safety in Nursing at the Gold Coast University Hospital and Griffith School of Nursing and Midwifery, Gold Coast campus. Her research focuses on two important areas of patient safety: compromised skin integrity, and teamwork and communication in surgery. She is recognised as a world leader in perioperative nursing and has authored over 170 peer-reviewed publications and 7 book chapters. She has won $10.4 million dollars in competitive research grants, including 5 National Health and Medical Research Council (NHMRC) grants. She has a sustained record as a funded keynote or plenary speaker at many international and interdisciplinary conferences or symposia. In recognition of her impact in the field of perioperative nursing and acute wound care, she was inducted into the Sigma Theta Tau Nurse Researcher Hall of Fame in 2020. She is a Fellow of ACORN, a Life Member of ACORN Queensland and in 2014 was awarded the ACORN Excellence in Perioperative Nursing Award.

Ben Lockwood, RN, Cert IV TAE, BNg (Hons), MACORN

Ben Lockwood has worked in perioperative services for the past 20 years, and since 2014 in the position of the Perioperative Advanced Nurse Educator for the Southern Adelaide Local Health Network (SALHN) – consisting of Flinders Medical Centre (a large tertiary trauma centre) and Noarlunga Hospital (a smaller regional facility). Working across a healthcare region with a large staff base, Ben oversees education and training for all roles of perioperative nurses, graduates, theatre orderlies, students (nursing and medical) and sterilisation services staff. Ben is an advanced life support trainer, who has a passion for simulation, eLearning and clinical skills training. Prior to this role, Ben was a Clinical Practice Consultant for SALHN perioperative services, undertaking a quality, safety and risk management portfolio, which successfully worked through the health network's first assessment against the National Standards in 2013. Ben is a member of the South Australian Perioperative Nurses Association (SAPNA), and has presented papers at state, national and international perioperative nursing conferences, and at the Sterilising Research and Advisory Council of Australia (SA) Inc. (SRACA). Ben has provided guest lectures in tertiary institutions, has published articles in the literature and has contributed to perioperative nursing texts.

Sally Sutherland-Fraser, RN, Cert IV TAE, BEd (Adult Ed), GradCert (Periop Nsg), MEd, MACN, FACORN

Sally is a facilitator and education consultant based in Sydney, Australia. She has more than 35 years' nursing experience in Australia and the United Kingdom, specialising in perioperative practice, education and mentorship. Sally was a partner and director of a small independent company she established in 2013 with Menna Davies, providing healthcare consultancy and education services. This partnership helped to produce the first Pacific Island standards for perioperative nurses and a suite of practice audit tools for ACORN.

Her early career included many years at the Royal Alexandra Hospital for Children, Camperdown and Westmead Children's Hospital. Sally eventually became the Area Clinical Nurse Consultant for a large public health district, based at St Vincent's Hospital, Sydney. During that decade, Sally conducted research into perioperative nurses' knowledge of pressure injury prevention and coordinated numerous area-wide clinical programs, including a perioperative education program for enrolled nurses (PEPEN). This unique workforce strategy to prepare enrolled nurses for the instrument nurse role formed the basis of education programs developed by the NSW Health Nursing and Midwifery Office (NaMO) and ACN. Sally has held executive positions in the NSW Operating Theatre Association (NSW OTA) and ACORN. In 2018, Sally delivered the Judith Cornell Oration and was the recipient of the ACORN Excellence in Perioperative Nursing Award in 2010.

Sally has provided education and mentorship programs for the Pacific Community, an international development organisation, and supports the Global Health Program of the Royal Australasian College of Surgeons (RACS) as the Nursing Specialty Coordinator. Sally continues to practise clinically at Sydney Hospital and Sydney Eye Hospital and finds time for regular remote travel in between writing projects.

Contributors

Amanda Adrian, RN, LLB, BA, FACN
Principal, Amanda Adrian and Associates,
New South Wales, Australia

Kristal Alken, RN, Cert IV TAE, MEd (Adult Ed)
Clinical Nurse Educator, Day Procedure Centre,
St Vincent's Hospital Sydney, New South Wales,
Australia

Tina Boric, RN, BN (Hons),
MN (Periop), MACORN
Nurse Educator, Perioperative, The Prince Charles
Hospital, Brisbane, Queensland, Australia;
Clinical Fellow of Australian Catholic University

Kim Bryant, RN, BN, GradCert (Adult Ed),
MEd, MACN
Principal Nursing and Midwifery Officer,
Nursing and Midwifery Council of New South Wales,
New South Wales, Australia

Deborah Burrows, RN, Cert III Sterilisation,
Cert IV TAE, BHlthSc (Nursing),
GradCert (Clinical Mgmt),
GradCert (Periop Nsg), MN, MACORN
District Clinical Nurse Consultant, Perioperative
Services, Southern NSW Local Health District,
New South Wales, Australia

Jannelle Carlile, RN, PGCert (ORNsg),
MInfecPrevCont, MACIPC, MACORN
Clinical Nurse Consultant, Infection Prevention and
Control, The Royal Hospital for Women, Randwick,
New South Wales, Australia

Tim Cole, Cert (Management),
Cert (Sterilising Tech)
Health Services Manager, Randwick Campus
Sterilising Services Department,
Prince of Wales Public Hospital, Randwick,
New South Wales, Australia

Menna Davies, RN, Cert (Sterilising Tech),
GradCert (Periop Nsg), GradDip (Hlth Law),
MHlthSc (Nsg), FACN, FACORN
Education Consultant, New South Wales, Australia

Paula Foran, RN, PhD, FACORN, FACPAN
Unit Coordinator, Masters by Coursework,
University of Tasmania, Victoria, Australia

Brigid M. Gillespie, RN, PhD, FACORN
Professor, NHMRC Centre for Research Excellence in
Wiser Wounds, Menzies Health Institute Qld (MHIQ),
Griffith University and Gold Coast University
Hospital, Gold Coast Health, Queensland, Australia

Meredith Gimblett, RN, BN,
GradCert (Periop Nsg), MACORN
Clinical Nurse Specialist/Surgical Clinical Reviewer,
Prince of Wales Hospital, New South Wales,
Australia

Melissa Hall, RN, BHlthSc (Nursing),
GradDip (Op Room Nsg), MN, MACORN
Clinical Nurse Specialist, Operating Suite,
The Tweed Hospital, New South Wales, Australia

Kathryn Johns, RN, GradDip (Perianaesthesia),
MProfEd&Trng
Acting Nurse Unit Manager, Elective Surgery Access
Unit, Barwon Health, Victoria, Australia

Tracey Lee, RN, MN (Hons)
HR Nurse Lead Workforce Development, Mater
Misericordiae University Hospital, County Dublin,
Ireland

Ben Lockwood, RN, Cert IV TAE,
BNg (Hons), MACORN
Perioperative Advanced Nurse Educator, Southern
Adelaide Local Health Network, South Australia,
Australia

Michelle Love, RN, BN, GradCert (Periop Nsg), GradDipN (Clin Nsg & Teaching), MACORN, MACPAN
Nurse Educator, Perioperative and Procedural Areas, The Prince Charles Hospital Chermside, Queensland, Australia

Sharon Minton, RN, Cert IV TAE, DipAppSc (Nsg), BAppSc (Nsg), GradDip Nsg (Op Suite), MN (Prof Studies Ed), MACORN
Clinical Nurse Educator, Perioperative Services, Hornsby Hospital, New South Wales, Australia

Sian Mitchell, RN, DipNsg, DipAppSci (Anaesthetic Technology), GradCert (Nsg)
National Clinical Nurse Consultant, Southern Cross Healthcare, Auckland, New Zealand

Fiona Newman, RN, Cert IV TAE, BN (Hons), BEd, GradCert (Admin), GradCert (Ed), GradCert (Anaes Nsg), MN(Clinical), FACPAN
Perioperative Introductory Program Coordinator, Princess Alexandra Hospital, Metro South Health, Brisbane, Queensland, Australia

Michelle Skrivanic, RN, Cert IV TAE, Cert IV (Project Mgmt), DipAppSc (Nsg), GradCert (Clin Teach), Cert (Periop Nsg), MACORN
Nurse Manager, Perioperative Services, Concord Repatriation General Hospital, New South Wales, Australia

Penny J. Smalley, RN, CMLSO, MACORN
Perioperative Nurse Consultant, Director, International Council on Surgical Plume, Chicago, Illinois, USA

Judy Smith, RN, BN, GradCert (Periop Nsg), MA Nursing, MACORN, MACN, MSTTI
Lecturer, Faculty of Health, University of Technology Sydney, New South Wales, Australia

Sally Sutherland-Fraser, RN, Cert IV TAE, BEd (Adult Ed), GradCert (Periop Nsg), MEd, MACN, FACORN
Facilitator and Education Consultant, New South Wales, Australia

Erin Wakefield, RN, GradCert (Clins Sim), GradCert (Periop Nsg), MN
Lecturer in Nursing, Monash University, Melbourne, Victoria, Australia

Julie Walters, RN, RM, Cert IV TAE, GradCert (Anaes & Rec Room Nsg), MACORN
Clinical Nurse Educator Anaesthetics, Randwick Campus Operating Suite, Prince of Wales Hospital, New South Wales, Australia

Louise Webber, RN, Nurse Practitioner, BA (Hons), MNsgSc
Wound Therapies (Director), Sunshine Coast, Queensland, Australia

Reviewers

Tarryn Armour, RN, BN, BaHealthProm,
GradCertHigherEd, GradDipAdvNrsgPrac (Periop),
MClinEd, FACORN
Lecturer in Nursing and Course Director,
Master of Nursing Practice (Perioperative),
Deakin University, Victoria, Australia

Karen Clark-Burg, RN, MBA (Exec), PhD
Professor and National Head of School,
School of Nursing, Midwifery,
Health Sciences and Physiotherapy,
Faculty of Medicine, Nursing and Midwifery and
Health Sciences, The University of Notre Dame,
Sydney, New South Wales, Australia

Mishelle Dehaini, RN, CCRN, GradCert HPE,
MACN-Perioperative
Teaching Associate, Post Graduate Perioperative
Program, Monash University, Melbourne, Australia;
Clinical Nurse Educator, Peninsula Private Hospital,
Ramsay Healthcare, Frankston, Victoria, Australia

Melanie Greenwood, RN, NeuroMed/Surg Cert,
Intensive Care Cert, BNurs, GradCert Uni L&T,
MNurs, PhD, FACCCN
Associate Professor, School of Nursing,
University of Tasmania, Tasmania, Australia

Sandra Leathwick, RN, Cert (OperatingRmNsg),
Cert (TropicalNsg), BHealth (Nursing), MEd
(Adult), PhD (Cand), MACORN, MHERDSA
Master of Clinical Nursing Course Coordinator,
Lecturer, Clinical Nursing and Postgraduate
Partnership Manager (Qld), Australian Catholic
University, Brisbane, Australia

Jo Perry, RN, CGRN, DipAppSc (Nurs), BSN, MSN,
MACORN
Specialty Coordinator, Perioperative Nursing,
Adelaide Nursing School, Faculty of Health and
Medical Sciences, Adelaide, Australia;
Education Specialist, Adelaide Education Academy,
Adelaide, Australia

ACKNOWLEDGMENTS

This revised edition would not have been possible without the dedication and combined efforts of our chapter contributors. We thank you for your patience and your commitment over the longer than expected period of revision, particularly with the impact of the global pandemic being felt in all quarters including our timelines. Despite all of these additional pressures, you have helped us to produce a new edition of this much-loved book with a number of new features while maintaining the depth and quality of content that is evidence based and relevant to contemporary practice within Australasia.

We recognise that our contributors balanced increased workloads during this revision, often requiring the understanding and support of managers and colleagues, as well as family and other loved ones. Astute readers will see evidence of this throughout the chapters, with facilities granting permission to reproduce resources and publish images of workplaces and staff. We are grateful for this collegial support and know that the book is all the better for it.

We also wish to acknowledge the work of our external reviewers, who provided insightful suggestions to improve the text. We are confident that nursing students and healthcare clinicians who use this book will benefit from the thorough approach that has been adopted in the preparation and completion of this book.

We are especially grateful to many people at Elsevier Australia for their constructive guidance and support throughout this project. In particular, we would like to thank Libby Houston, Senior Content Strategist, Nursing, Midwifery and Health Professions, for your leadership throughout the development of the third edition. Additionally, we extend our heartfelt thanks to Sukanthi Sukumar, Content Project Manager. Your patience, support and guidance steered us through the revision period and handover to Shravan Kumar, Content Project Manager, who continued with us on our journey through to publication. Chris Wyard (Copy Editor) and Graphic World (typesetter) deserve special mention, without their expert support and openness to welcome new ideas, we would have not reached here. Your combined contributions have ensured the production of a new edition of the highest quality that will engage new readers and surprise readers familiar with previous editions.

Finally, to our respective loved ones – Jenni Wilkins, Lorelle Kinsey, Joe Gillespie and Hamish Herd – thank you for your patience and support throughout the development of this book. Late nights, video-conference calls and seemingly endless emails, as well as hours of reading and editing, were powered by pots of tea, coffee and sometimes something stronger, always generously offered and sometimes accompanied by wise words about fresh eyes in the morning. We made it, together.

Sally Sutherland-Fraser, Menna Davies,
Brigid M. Gillespie and Ben Lockwood

Introduction: How to Use This Book

We recognise the potential diversity of our readers in terms of their knowledge and experience in healthcare and perioperative practice. We have written this new edition to meet the needs of all readers.

- Individual readers such as nursing students, new and experienced perioperative nurses, as well as perioperative support staff such as orderlies, can use this book to:
  - understand the underlying principles and rationales for perioperative nursing practices
  - identify standards for safe patient care during the perioperative patient journey
  - apply principles of perioperative practice to the clinical setting.
- Managers, educators and experienced perioperative nurse preceptors can use this book to:
  - examine workplace health and safety issues for perioperative nurses
  - develop orientation and education support programs for nursing and ancillary staff.
- Course coordinators can use this book to:
  - support courses/units relating to infection prevention and control, surgical nursing care and perioperative patient journeys
  - provide support materials for students to explore perioperative nursing roles and career pathways.

THE HEALTHCARE SETTING

The healthcare setting for these scenarios is a busy metropolitan public hospital with 20 commissioned operating rooms and a large postanaesthesia care unit (PACU). The hospital also has a large emergency department, a maternity service and an integrated day surgery ward, as well as a pre-admission clinic and several outpatient clinics providing pre- and postoperative services to surgical patients.

THE PERIOPERATIVE NURSES

The healthcare team in the operating suite provides a 24-hour service and includes perioperative nurses with different levels of experience and specialty skills. We present the nurses in alphabetical order by family name:

Nurses	Experience and Specialties
Student Nurse Rose Cheng	Third-year student nurse
RN Rob **Cohen**	Newly qualified nurse on the transition program in the instrument/circulating nurse role
RN Anne **Fuller**	Experienced rural/remote nurse
RN Ben **Lumby**	Part-time perioperative nurse surgical assistant (PNSA)
EN Marcus **Macedo**	Experienced in the anaesthetic nursing role
RN George **Markham**	Experienced surgical nurse
RN Margaret **McCormack**	Experienced in the anaesthetic nursing role
EN Pauline **Noakes**	Experienced in the instrument/circulating nurse role
RN Sandy **Pereira**	Experienced in the instrument/circulating nurse role
EN Sammy **Ravisi**	Experienced in all perioperative nursing roles
RN Jenny **Sang**	Experienced in anaesthetic and postanaesthetic nursing roles

PATIENT SCENARIO DETAILS

Throughout this book, we present four patient scenarios which demonstrate the diversity of the perioperative patient journey:

- **Mr James Collins** – a 78-year-old man admitted for an elective right total knee replacement (TKR)
- **Mrs Patricia Peterson** – a 42-year-old Indigenous woman admitted for an emergency laparoscopic cholecystectomy
- **Ms Janine Clark** – a 35-year-old pregnant woman admitted for an elective lower segment caesarean section (LSCS)
- **Master Thanh Nguyen** – a 3-year-old male child admitted as a day surgery patient for an elective left orchidopexy.

Each scenario includes a series of Critical Thinking Questions (CTQs) linked to one or more of these patients which asks readers to consider the patient's history and the information provided as the scenarios unfold. We have developed these scenarios to test readers' knowledge of perioperative nursing practice and prompt readers to think critically about the care of these patients. Many of CTQs are based on the perspective of the scenario's nurses who are working in different roles and have different experience levels. Other CTQs provide the opportunity for a more personal reflection by asking readers to consider their own perspective, their current workplace and recent clinical experiences. Readers may choose to answer the CTQs from different perspectives. We provide model answers for the CTQs, which readers can access online through the Elsevier Evolve site. A detailed medical history for each of our patients is provided here. More details will be introduced in the chapters as each of the relevant scenarios unfolds.

Mr James Collins is a 78-year-old man, who lives alone and independently in his own home. His presenting conditions are the chronic pain and reduced mobility from the bony degeneration of his right knee. He is being admitted for an elective right total knee replacement under a spinal anaesthetic with sedation. He will be administered a continuous nerve block for management of postoperative pain.

Mr Collins' medical history is:
- no known allergies
- healthcare-acquired methicillin-resistant *Staphylococcus aureus* (HA-MRSA)
- current smoker, with a 50-year smoking history of a pack of cigarettes per day
- severe chronic obstructive pulmonary disease (COPD), which is managed at home with oxygen of 2 L/min
- peripheral vascular disease
- hypertension
- body mass index (BMI) of 34 (weight 110 kg, height 180 cm), classifying him as obese

Mr Collins' surgical history is:
- bilateral inguinal hernia repair (20 years ago)
- three angioplasties (31 right leg, 32 left leg) to his legs over the past 5 years; the most recent procedure was about 1 year ago.

Mr Collins' current medications include:
- fentanyl 75 mg transdermal patch every 3 days (opioid analgesic prescribed for relief of pain from his arthritic knee)

- perindopril 4 mg BD (antihypertensive)
- atorvastatin 40 mg OD (cholesterol-lowering agent).
- clopidogrel 75 mg OD (anticoagulant).
- diclofenac 50 mg PRN (non-steroidal anti-inflammatory drug (NSAID)).

Mrs Patricia Peterson is a 42-year-old Indigenous woman who lives at home in a remote community with her husband and two teenage children. She was transferred to the emergency department of a metropolitan public hospital with increasing right upper quadrant pain, biliary cholic, nausea and vomiting. Mrs Peterson has been diagnosed with acute cholecystitis and is being admitted for an emergency laparoscopic cholecystectomy.

Mrs Peterson's medical history is:
- possible sensitivity to chlorhexidine
- hypertension
- type 2 diabetes
- BMI of 39.1 (weight 94 kg, height 155 cm), classifying her as obese

Mrs Peterson's surgical history is:
- endoscopic retrograde cholangiopancreatography (ERCP) 2 years ago for stone removal from cystic duct
- left knee arthroscopy 5 years ago.

Mrs Peterson's current medications include:
- telmisartan 40 mg OD (antihypertensive)
- metformin 500 mg BD (hypoglycaemic agent)
- simvastatin 20 mg OD (cholesterol-lowering agent).

Ms Janine Clark is a 35-year-old pregnant woman who lives at home with her partner and two young children. She is being admitted for an elective lower segment caesarean section (LSCS).

Ms Clark's medical history is:
- anaphylaxis to penicillin
- recurrent bouts of tonsillitis as a child.

Her surgical history includes:
- adenotonsillectomy at age 7
- two previous LSCSs (with difficult wound healing after her last LSCS).

Ms Clark takes no regular medications.

Master Thanh Nguyen is a 3-year-old male child who lives at home with his two parents and older sister. Thanh's father speaks Vietnamese, French and English, while his mother speaks Vietnamese. Thanh is being admitted as a day surgery patient for an elective orchidopexy of his undescended left testicle.

Thanh is a healthy child with no known allergies and no significant medical or surgical history.

CHAPTER 1

Perioperative Nursing

JUDY SMITH • KIM BRYANT • TRACEY LEE
EDITOR: SALLY SUTHERLAND-FRASER

LEARNING OUTCOMES

- Review key features of the regulatory environment for nurses working within Australasia
- Discuss the history and philosophy of perioperative nursing practice
- Examine cultural safety and the nurse's role as patient advocate within perioperative nursing practice
- Describe the patient journey and the overlap of perioperative nursing roles in the management of the patient
- Define the terms *scope of practice* and *advanced practice* in the context of perioperative nursing practice
- Outline the role of professional perioperative nursing organisations
- Discuss the need for professional development and the importance of research and an evidence-based approach to practice

KEY TERMS

accountability

advanced practice

advocacy

competence

continuing professional development

cultural safety

delegation

evidence-based practice

orientation programs

patient journey

perioperative

perioperative nursing roles

practice standards

professional associations

scope of practice

supervision

INTRODUCTION

This chapter introduces the beginning perioperative nurse to the key concepts and principles which inform perioperative practice within Australasia. We begin with a brief review of the regulatory environments for general nursing practice in Australia and New Zealand. We define key aspects of nursing regulation such as scope of practice and accountability and we explore the relationship between accountability, delegation and supervision. This chapter then turns to specialty nursing practice, beginning with a brief history of perioperative nursing and its underpinning philosophy of holistic patient care. We describe the perioperative patient journey and the importance of cultural safety. This sets the context for a description of each of the patient care roles that perioperative nurses perform, including advanced practice roles emerging in Australasian healthcare systems. The chapter then explores the ways in which education and professional associations support the development of specialty nursing expertise. In closing, we describe the value of professional practice standards, perioperative research and evidence-based practice (EBP). Throughout the chapter, we describe a series of patient scenarios to illuminate the chapter's key concepts, to prompt the reader to reflect on their experiences and to promote learning.

PATIENT SCENARIOS

Consider all four of the patient scenarios detailed at the front of the book as you read this chapter.

1. Mr James Collins is a 78-year-old man scheduled for a right total knee replacement – TKR.
2. Mrs Patricia Peterson is a 42-year-old Indigenous woman who requires an emergency laparoscopic cholecystectomy – lap chole.
3. Mrs Janine Clark is a 35-year-old woman scheduled for an elective lower segment caesarean section – LSCS.
4. Master Thanh Nguyen is a 3-year-old boy admitted as a day surgery patient for a left orchidopexy.

The following perioperative team members also appear in the patient scenarios:

Nursing team: EN Marcus Macedo (in the anaesthetic room), RN Sandy Pereira, RN Ben Lumby and RN Rob Cohen (in the operating room [OR]). Silvana Perez appears as the medical company representative (MCR).

THE REGULATORY ENVIRONMENT

The practice of health professionals is regulated to protect the public. Globally, nurses are the largest group of health professionals (International Council of Nurses [ICN], 2020a) while, in Australasia, nurses and midwives are collectively the largest group of regulated health professionals. In Australia, each state and territory has enacted a version of the Health Practitioner Regulation National Law (Australian Health Practitioner Regulation Agency [AHPRA], 2018), known simply as the National Law, while the Health Practitioner Competence Assurance Act 2003 regulates nursing practice in New Zealand (Ministry of Health, 2020). The Nursing and Midwifery Board of Australia (NMBA) is the statutory decision-making body under the National Law, responsible for registering nurses and ensuring that they are competent and fit to practise. In New Zealand, the equivalent decision-making body is the Nursing Council of New Zealand (NCNZ) (Fig. 1.1).

Nursing practice in Australasia is further informed by the international code of professional ethics (ICN, 2012; NCNZ, 2012a). There is also a range of position statements, policies and guidelines which regulatory bodies produce on issues such as protected titles, re-entry to practice (NMBA, 2019a), decision making about scopes of practice and delegations to others

Health Practitioner Regulation National Law 2009

- **Nursing and Midwifery Board of Australia (NMBA)** is responsible for registration, ensuring competence and fitness to practise, national codes of conduct and ethics, policies and guidelines
- **Australian College of Nursing (ACN)** is the peek national nursing organisation
- **Australian College of Perioperative Nurses (ACORN)** is the professional association for perioperative nurses which produces *ACORN Standards for perioperative nursing practice*
- **Australian College of Perianaesthesia Nurses (ACPAN)** is the professional association for anaesthesia care and postanaesthesia care nurses which produces *ACPAN Statements*
- **Australian Day Surgery Nurses Association (ADSNA)** is the professional association for healthcare professionals in day surgery settings which produces the *Australian best practice guidelines for day surgery*
- **Australian Nursing and Midwifery Federation (ANMF)** is the largest national professional nursing organisation and industrial body for nurses and midwives

Health Practitioner Competence Assurance Act 2003

- **Nursing Council of New Zealand (NCNZ)** is respponsible for registration, ensuring competence and fitness to practise, national codes of conduct and ethics, policies and guidelines
- **Perioperative Nurses College (PNC)** is the national professional organisation for perioperative nurses which produces the *PNC Standards*. New Zealand perioperative nursing practice is also informed by the Association of periOperative Registered Nurses *AORN Guidelines for practice*
- **New Zealand Nursing Organisation (NZNO)** is the national professional nursing organisation and industrial body

FIG. 1.1 Summary of Australasian regulatory and professional entities of relevance for perioperative nurses.

(NCNZ, 2012a; NMBA, 2020a), and the use of social media (NCNZ, 2012a; NMBA, 2019b). The medico-legal aspects of the regulatory environment which influence contemporary nursing practice are presented in Chapter 3.

Another aspect of regulation is the protection of health professional titles including those of 'nurse' and 'nurse practitioner' (NP) (NMBA, 2019c). This protects the public by ensuring that only those who possess the necessary qualifications and competence to practise are accepted to the register (NMBA, 2019c). Nursing **competence** is an essential element of safe patient care. It includes the nurse's knowledge, values and attitudes, as well as their technical and non-technical skills, and can be developed through education and clinical practice (Gillespie et al, 2018). In Australia, there are two divisions of nurse on the register: registered nurses (RNs), who are Division 1 nurses, and enrolled nurses (ENs), who are Division 2 nurses.

During their journey through the health system, the surgical patient will receive care from diverse multidisciplinary teams with the combined skills and capacities to provide holistic and individualised care. The perioperative team comprises regulated health professionals (e.g. RNs and ENs, NPs, doctors and allied health workers such as radiographers and anaesthetic technicians (a regulated role in NZ), as well as non-regulated staff in supporting and ancillary roles, working under the supervision of the perioperative RN (e.g. assistants-in-nursing [AINs], patient care assistants [PCAs], healthcare assistants [HCAs], orderlies, sterilisation technicians and medical company representatives [MCRs]). Students of nursing, medicine and/or allied health fields such as physiotherapy may also be present in the perioperative environment. The safe and effective performance of such a large and diverse team has its origins in a strong regulatory environment. The professional associations support this in their role as strong advocates for appropriate educational preparation, competence, scopes of practice and accountability of perioperative team members (Australian and New Zealand College of Anaesthetists [ANZCA], 2016; Australian College of Perioperative Nurses [ACORN], 2020a). Further information about the safe functioning of the perioperative team is provided in Chapter 2.

Scope of Practice

In regulatory terms, the NMBA describes **scope of practice** as the actions and activities for which nurses are educated and deemed competent to perform and which are permitted by law (2020a). All nurses must function within the profession's collective scope of practice and must meet the overarching requirements of the profession's national codes and standards of

practice (NCNZ, 2007, 2012b; NMBA, 2020a). This requirement applies equally to generalist and to specialist nurses. Individually, however, scopes of practice will differ between nurses. This is because a nurse's scope of practice is influenced by the specific health needs of the people in their care, the competence and confidence level of the nurse theirself as well as the needs and requirements of the service. Scope of practice is also influenced by the specific context of the practice setting. Perioperative nurses work in a unique environment and consequently have a more defined and specific scope of practice than the nursing profession as a whole. This is a theme that we will continue to explore throughout this chapter.

Accountability

In all of their activities, nurses remain accountable and responsible for their practice and, along with **advocacy**, these concepts are enshrined in an international code of ethics (ICN, 2012) and national codes of conduct (NCNZ, 2012a; NMBA, 2018a). The NCNZ simply defines **accountability** as answering for one's decisions and actions (2012a), a requirement that applies to all nurses equally, whether the nurse is an RN or an EN working under the supervision and direction of an RN (NMBA, 2021). Being accountable means that the nurse must be answerable to others (such as patients, colleagues, employers and regulatory bodies) for their actions and behaviours, as well as for any decisions they make during the performance of their role (NMBA, 2020a). For example, the RN has an additional level of accountability whenever they delegate activities to others, such as an EN, a less experienced RN or another member of the healthcare team from a different discipline (NMBA, 2020a). In this situation, the RN will also be held accountable for their decision to delegate.

Relationship Between Accountability, Delegation and Supervision

This brings us to the important relationship between accountability, **delegation** and **supervision**. Consider the example above, when delegation of patient care occurs in the perioperative setting. The national professional standards of ACORN require the perioperative RN to coordinate patient care activities and to do so by supervising, overseeing or directing the activities of ENs and other members in the team (ACORN, 2020b,c). In practice, this means that the delegating RN will need to consider not only the EN's scope of practice in the specific perioperative context, but must also provide the level of supervision required by the individual EN during the conduct of care and evaluate the outcomes of the EN's performance and the delegated activity (ACORN, 2020a,b; NMBA, 2021). By supervising the activity, the delegating RN can monitor whether the EN requires additional support or instruction in their performance of the activity. ACORN also stipulates that the perioperative RN must work in the circulating nurse role whenever an EN is working in the instrument nurse role (ACORN, 2020b,d), because the performance of the surgical count requires two nurses, one of whom must be an RN (see Chapter 9 for further information).

These perioperative examples demonstrate the 'delegation relationship' that exists when any nurse entrusts aspects of nursing practice to another person (NMBA, 2020a). Each delegation needs to be judged on the individual circumstances, and the actual outcomes of the delegation need to be assessed (NCNZ, 2012c; NMBA, 2020a). Regulatory bodies require that such delegations should be made only by RNs who are themselves competent to perform the activity and, therefore, capable of evaluating the outcomes of such delegations. This requirement ensures that the other person's performance (i.e. the EN in these examples) and the patient outcomes meet the expected professional standards.

A clearly structured and objective decision-making process can assist nurses to make these safe delegations. In Australia, the NMBA's decision-making framework (DMF) comprises a set of nationally agreed principles with the purpose of guiding nurses to make consistent and appropriate decisions about patient care and to determine who is best suited to provide that care (NMBA, 2020a). Box 1.1 outlines the DMF statements of principle that should guide nursing practice decisions, particularly in relation to allocation of care roles. The DMF is a particularly helpful tool when considering an expansion to the scope of practice of an individual nurse or group of nurses. The NCNZ has also produced two guidelines for RNs in New Zealand that highlight the important connection between accountability and the practice of delegation to ENs (NCNZ, 2012c) and healthcare assistants (NCNZ, 2012d). Specific examples of the perioperative RN's accountability for delegated decisions are provided in Box 1.2, while Box 1.3 provides a spotlight on scope of practice boundaries relating to medication administration.

THE HISTORY AND PHILOSOPHY OF PERIOPERATIVE NURSING

The term **perioperative** refers to the period of time encompassing preparation for an anaesthetic, surgery or other procedure and recovery from these interventions (Grocott, Plumb, Edwards, & Fecher, 2017). The

> **BOX 1.1**
> **Guide for Nursing Practice Decisions: Statements of Principle**
>
> 1. The primary motivation for any decision about a care activity is to meet people's health needs or to enhance health outcomes.
> 2. Nurses are responsible for making professional judgements about when an activity is beyond their scope of practice and for initiating consultation with, or referral to, other members of the healthcare team.
> 3. Expansion to scope of practice occurs when a nurse assumes responsibility for an activity that is currently outside the nurses's scope of practice, or where an employer seeks to initiate a change, because of evaluations of services and a desire to improve access to, or efficiency of, services to groups of people.
> 4. Registered nurses (the delegator) are accountable for making decisions about who is the most appropriate health professional or health worker to delegate to (delegatee) to perform an activity that is in the nursing plan of care.
> 5. Nursing practice decisions are best made in a collaborative context of planning, risk management and evaluation.

(Source: Nursing and Midwifery Board of Australia. (2020a). *Decision-making framework for nursing and midwifery* (pp. 5–6). Melbourne: Author.)

perioperative nurse is a skilled healthcare professional who provides care to patients during this period, in collaboration with other members of the healthcare team (ACORN, 2021a). The perioperative environment is one of the most complex work environments in healthcare. This complexity is evident in the diversity of surgical procedures performed, the specialised technology used and the number of staff required to ensure safe patient care. The nurse working in the perioperative environment may experience rapidly changing situations, requiring precision and coordination to manage patient care efficiently and effectively. The perioperative nurse also acts as a patient advocate during the perioperative journey, when patients may feel physically and psychologically vulnerable (Munday, Kynoch, & Hines, 2015). The philosophy of perioperative nursing encompasses a holistic, multidisciplinary approach that:

- acknowledges the dignity of persons with diverse physical, emotional and cultural backgrounds
- promotes the knowledge and skills of all multidisciplinary team members to deliver optimal patient outcomes and research-based healthcare
- ensures a safe physical environment for all.

BOX 1.2
Examples of the Perioperative RN's Accountability for Delegated Decisions

- The RN monitoring a nursing student's placement of a forced-air warming device on a patient in the anaesthetic bay
- The RN providing direct supervision and timely instructions for the EN instrument nurse who is learning a new surgical procedure
- The RN assessing a patient's skin integrity after the theatre orderly/health service assistant has removed the pneumatic tourniquet cuff from the patient's thigh
- The RN examining the functionality of the flexible scope after reprocessing by the sterilising technician before releasing it to the proceduralist
- The RN supervising the nursing student attending to the PACU patient's hygiene and comfort

See Chapter 3 for the legal and ethical implications of accountability, particularly in relation to the surgical count and with documentation.

(Source: Australian College of Perioperative Nurses. (2020a). *Standards for perioperative nursing in Australia* (16th ed., volume 2, Accountability for practice). Adelaide: Author.)

BOX 1.3
Spotlight on Scope of Practice Boundaries – Medication Administration

In Australia, registered nurses (RNs – Division 1) can administer medications to the patient via all routes. Enrolled nurses (ENs – Division 2), however, have a different scope of practice with medication administration. The following regulatory conditions apply:
- The EN must have completed a Board-approved EN medicine administration course.
- The EN's registration must be without notations restricting them from medication administration.
- The organisational policy must support and outline EN medication administration.
- The EN can only administer medication via intravenous (IV) injection after they have completed education in IV medication administration and only after they have demonstrated their competence in IV medication administration (NMBA, 2016c, 2016d, 2020b).

Differences in scope of practice, particularly with medication administration, will inform the allocation of perioperative roles. Pre-admission nurses, anaesthetic nurses and PACU nurses may be required to administer IV medications to patients during the preoperative or postoperative phases of their perioperative journey, while it is rare for circulating and instrument nurses to be required to administer IV medications during the intraoperative phase and surgical procedures. Differences between nurses' designations will also inform the allocation of perioperative roles. The management of restricted schedule medications is another area for consideration, while control of the keys to restricted medication rooms, secure cupboards and safes may be allocated to the RN but not the EN, regardless of their allocated perioperative role. In New Zealand, within the acute care setting, medicines should only be administered by regulated nurses/midwives who are competent to do so and aware of their accountability but otherwise medication administration is within an EN's scope of practice. The EN retains responsibility for their actions and remains accountable to the RN. It is recommended that access to controlled drugs, witnessing, administering and documentation of these medications is described in local workplace policies and guidelines (NZNO, 2012).

Perioperative nursing is one of the oldest nursing specialties, the foundations of which were laid by Florence Nightingale in the late 1800s when surgery was becoming more complex (Hamlin, 2020). Nurses were responsible not only for the care of surgical patients before and after surgery but also during surgery, when the nurses provided assistance to the surgeon (Hamlin, 2020). During the First World War, nurses continued to be recruited to the armed forces to be responsible for patients' perioperative care. During the Second World War, more advanced surgery was performed in field hospitals and required more technical equipment, which reinforced nurses' professional functions in the operating theatre (Blomberg, Bisholt, Nilsson, & Lindwall, 2015). Medical advancements and changes in healthcare delivery provide today's nurses with a choice of roles in the perioperative environment – an environment that is continually expanding its geographical boundaries and is no longer confined to the operating room. Furthermore, perioperative nurses have an accountability in their practice to explore strategies not only for professional development through continuing education and specialist postgraduate education, but also for practice development through engagement in research and evidence-based practice (ACORN, 2020e).

THE PERIOPERATIVE PATIENT JOURNEY

The patient's surgical pathway, also known as the perioperative **patient journey,** is underpinned by the six essential elements for comprehensive care delivery identified by the Australian Commission on Safety and Quality in Health Care (ACSQHC/the Commission) (Fig. 1.2). These elements inform the perioperative RN in their role

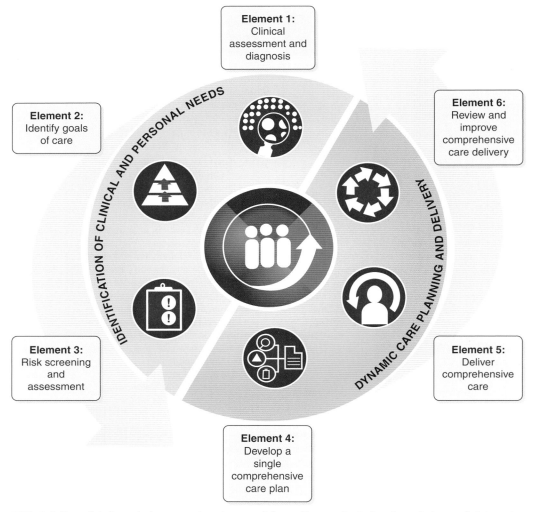

FIG. 1.2 Essential elements for comprehensive care delivery. (Source: Australian Commission on Safety and Quality in Health Care (ACSQHC/the Commission). (2018). Essential elements for comprehensive care delivery.)

as the coordinator of patient care and support the aim of delivering the best possible outcome for the patient. The first three elements focus on the preparation and information-gathering requirements for care delivery, while the remaining three elements address aspects of implementation and the delivery of care (ACSQHC/the Commission, 2018). During an elective admission to a health facility, the perioperative patient journey may begin as early as the pre-hospital onset of symptoms. It may include the surgeon's or the NP's assessment of symptoms and the decision to operate. It may include a period of in-patient management and continue through to a period of home recovery and rehabilitation in the

community (Fig. 1.3). The perioperative patient journey during a non-elective or emergency admission will be different and may begin with the patient's arrival in the emergency department of the health facility. The patient's personal details and medical history may be unknown. There may be minimal time to conduct diagnostic tests in preparation for the patient's interventional procedure or surgery, other than immediate resuscitation by the emergency service and first responders (Fig. 1.4).

Advances in surgical technology and procedures, improvements in anaesthetic techniques and changes in the healthcare environment have altered where and

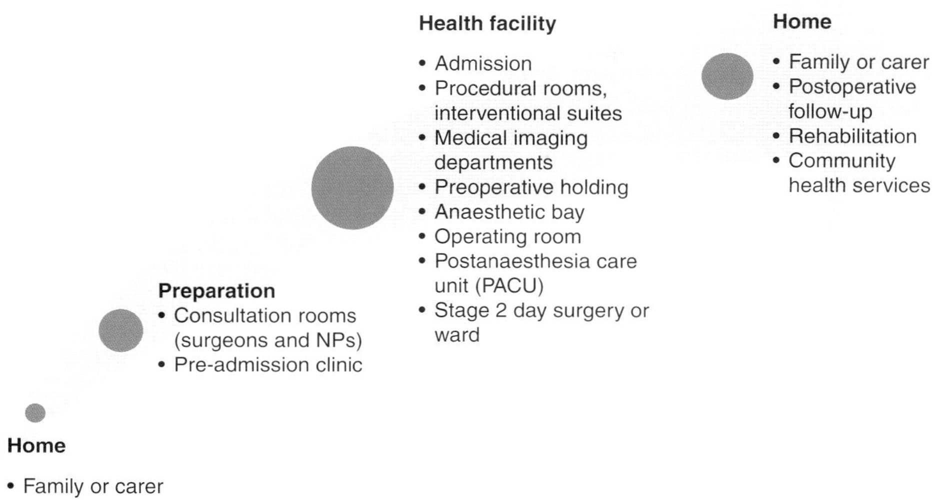

Health facility

- Admission
- Procedural rooms, interventional suites
- Medical imaging departments
- Preoperative holding
- Anaesthetic bay
- Operating room
- Postanaesthesia care unit (PACU)
- Stage 2 day surgery or ward

Home

- Family or carer
- Postoperative follow-up
- Rehabilitation
- Community health services

Preparation

- Consultation rooms (surgeons and NPs)
- Pre-admission clinic

Home

- Family or carer

FIG. 1.3 The perioperative patient journey: elective admission.

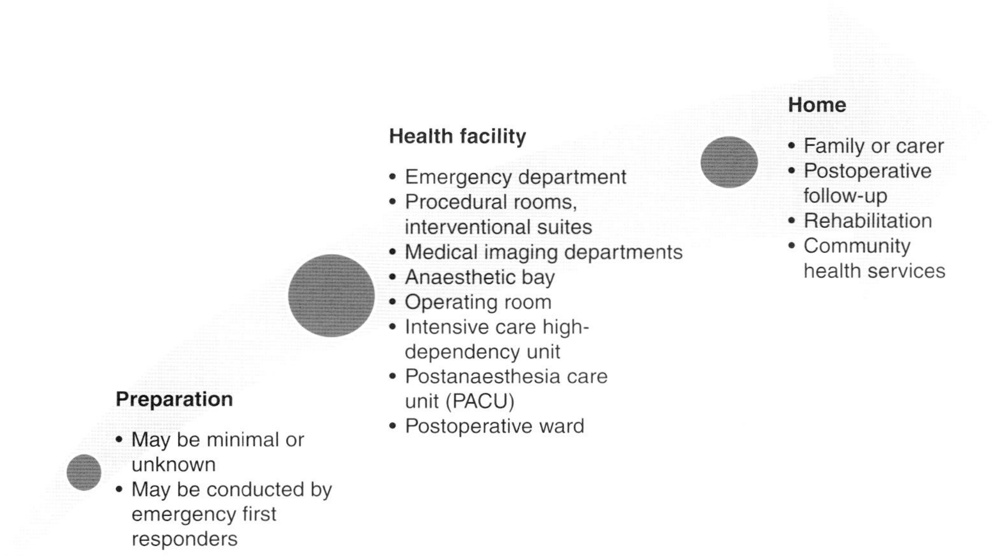

Health facility

- Emergency department
- Procedural rooms, interventional suites
- Medical imaging departments
- Anaesthetic bay
- Operating room
- Intensive care high-dependency unit
- Postanaesthesia care unit (PACU)
- Postoperative ward

Home

- Family or carer
- Postoperative follow-up
- Rehabilitation
- Community health services

Preparation

- May be minimal or unknown
- May be conducted by emergency first responders

FIG. 1.4 The perioperative patient journey: non-elective or emergency admission.

how surgery and invasive procedures are performed (these concepts are explored in following chapters). The journey of the patient undergoing surgery has expanded from the traditional boundaries of the OR to include broader perioperative environments, such as stand-alone day surgery facilities, ambulatory settings and endoscopy units, with over 53% of acute surgical procedures in Australia being performed in these settings (Australian Institute of Health and Welfare ([AIHW], 2019). The patient's surgical experience can also extend far beyond admission and discharge.

Regardless of when or where the surgical patient's experience takes place, the perioperative patient journey involves complex teamwork, requiring coordination and effective interpersonal communication between healthcare professionals (Kaptain, Ulsoe, & Dreyer, 2019). Teamwork, collaboration and safety-minded work processes that focus on error prevention have been found to minimise patient risks and maximise safety (Gillespie et al., 2017) during the perioperative patient journey. These issues are addressed in more detail in Chapter 2. Perioperative nurses contribute to a safe patient journey and ensure better patient outcomes not only through their role as patient advocate, but also by the application of their specialist knowledge and skills, which must be underpinned by a culturally safe and ethically caring approach.

CULTURAL SAFETY

Healthcare professionals work in richly multicultural environments, and rising levels of immigration from other countries means there is increasing cultural diversity in Australia and New Zealand (Australian Human Rights Commission [AHRC], 2018). Culture is largely underpinned by values, which are the sets of rules by which individuals and communities live. Values form the principles and standards for beliefs, attitudes and behaviours. Although all cultures have values, the way these values are expressed differs widely (Jacob, 2016). The Nursing Council of New Zealand (NCNZ, 2011a, p. 7) defines **cultural safety** as:

> *The effective nursing practice of a person or family from another culture, and is determined by that person or family. Culture includes, but is not restricted to, age or generation; gender; sexual orientation; occupation and socioeconomic status; ethnic origin or migrant experience; religious or spiritual belief; and disability.*

In Australia, the principles of person-centred practice, cultural practice and respectful relationships are recognised in the national Code of conduct for nurses (NMBA, 2018a). In complying with the code, nurses are expected to demonstrate cultural safety through the delivery of holistic and inclusive patient care. Such patient care acknowledges, without bias or racism, the cultural needs and values of Aboriginal and/or Torres Strait Islander peoples (NMBA, 2018a). Nurses have a duty of care to ensure that the needs of their patients are met by the provision of nursing care that is not only technically competent but is also culturally safe and individually appropriate. An understanding of the patient's beliefs and cultural background, which are not always aligned to ethnicity, is fundamental to meeting these differing needs. In the New Zealand nursing context, cultural safety relates directly to the individual's experience. The nurse practises cultural safety by empowering their patients to comment on the planned care and their expectations for the care outcomes (NCNZ, 2011a). The origins of cultural safety are described further in Feature box 1.1.

For perioperative nurses, the implications of cultural safety apply not only to the patients in their care, but also to their colleagues working within culturally diverse healthcare teams (ACORN, 2020f; Hughes, 2018). Cultural competence aims to decrease the inequities and barriers that place people from culturally diverse backgrounds at risk of culturally unsafe experiences, which may make patients reluctant to seek care in the future and may even cause harm (Muise, 2019). Cox and Simpson (2015) suggest that these power imbalances can be perpetuated by the actions (and/or inactions) of healthcare professionals. Patients are stripped of the vestiges of their personal and social identities through the donning of a hospital gown, and by an environment where medical technology is omnipresent and where healthcare professionals use the impersonal language of surgery. Culturally competent healthcare services move from discrimination to cultural sensitivity, with the final goal of cultural safety, which restores the balance of power back to the patient (Muise, 2019).

Religious Considerations

Spirituality and religion play critical roles in how some patients cope with illness and with their decision-making processes. Integrating a patient's religion and spirituality into clinical practice has been found to improve empathy, build trust and increase understanding of the patient's behaviour (Zaidi, 2018). The ICN's code of ethics (2012, p. 2) stipulates that *'nurses promote an environment in which the human rights, values, customs and spiritual beliefs of the individual, family and community are respected'*. While it is

The term 'cultural safety' has its origins in New Zealand, where nursing leaders recognised that the national nursing curriculum of the 1980s did not adequately reflect the perspectives of Māori peoples. Cultural safety was formally adopted by the Nursing Council of New Zealand in 1992, after it became a state examination requirement (Papps & Ramsden, 1996). While the terminology has continued to be refined, cultural safety in New Zealand remains focused on the improvement of the health status of all peoples. It acknowledges the unequal power relationship that may exist between caregivers (including nurses and midwives) and those peoples in their care. Cultural safety recognises other inequities and differences in such relationships including age, ethnicity, belief systems, gender and sexual orientation. Caregivers who might harbour negative attitudes about those who are different from them are unable to provide truly patient-focused care (Papps & Ramsden, 1996).

The writings of Indigenous scholar Irihapeti Ramsden have been pivotal to the formation of cultural safety, not only in New Zealand but also in Australia (AHRC, 2018). The value of a cultural safety framework has been recognised in Australia, especially by organisations that represent and/or provide services to Aboriginal and Torres Strait Islander peoples. The Congress of Aboriginal and Torres Strait Islander Nurses and Midwives (CATSINaM), a national peak body founded in 1997, identifies cultural safety *'as the final step on a continuum of nursing and/or midwifery care that includes cultural awareness, cultural sensitivity, cultural knowledge, cultural respect and cultural competence'* (CATSINaM, 2014, p. 1). CATSINaM supports the provision of cultural safety training for all healthcare professionals and has called for it to be embedded in national nursing and midwifery curricula (CATSINaM, 2017).

not possible for perioperative nurses to understand the nuances and impact of each religion on the perioperative patient journey, they can support differing patients' religious beliefs by knowing where and how to access information and appropriate resources, such as hospital chaplains. Patients' cultural backgrounds and religious beliefs should be documented at the start of the patient's perioperative journey during the admission processes (see Chapter 7). This information supports perioperative nurses to deliver holistic, patient-centred care throughout the rest of that journey.

PATIENT ADVOCACY

Advocacy is a complex process which has been described as supporting patients emotionally and preserving their dignity (Goodman, 2012; Sundqvist, Nilsson, Holmefur, & Anderzén-Carlsson, 2016). Advocacy is an important perioperative nursing role when implemented judiciously. An advocate is a person who puts forward a case on someone else's behalf or publicly supports a cause or policy (Oxford Dictionaries, 2019). Acting as the patient's advocate has legal and ethical implications. Due to their work environment, perioperative nurses have the added responsibility to advocate for patients who are sedated or are unconscious and unable to look after themselves or communicate their needs or wishes during surgery or other invasive procedures. Whether it is their first surgical experience or a return to theatre, patients may feel vulnerable, fearful or insecure during the perioperative patient journey (Cousley, 2015). As patient advocate, the perioperative nurse works to ensure that the patient's physical and emotional needs are met and must be ready to intervene to protect the patient's safety. This may include speaking up when potential exists for injury or if correct standards of perioperative practice or local policies are not being followed.

Advocating for patients is not without its challenges (Sundqvist et al., 2016). To be an effective advocate, the perioperative nurse must understand and anticipate individual patient needs. However, the professional relationship between the patient and the perioperative nurse is brief. Unlike colleagues in other units, the perioperative nurse has a short timeframe to assess, plan and implement individualised care. Assessment tools assist the perioperative nurse to efficiently gather relevant data including contact details for next of kin and languages spoken, as well as cultural and religious information. The perioperative nurse must spend sufficient time communicating with patients and conducting the necessary assessments then, in response, must spend sufficient time providing culturally safe and appropriate care. The perioperative nurse must also ensure that all of the patient's relevant information is brought to the attention of the perioperative team during subsequent clinical handovers or reviews.

Protecting the patient is one of the key factors of patient advocacy, and nurses, as the patient advocate, are responsible for protecting the patient from harm such as inadequate care provided by other healthcare team members (Davoodvand, Abbaszadeh, & Ahmadi, 2016). This can be challenging, especially if acting on behalf of the patient brings the perioperative nurse into conflict with colleagues, some of whom may be friends or more experienced senior colleagues. However, failure to speak up may compound the harm to the patient. It is also in conflict with codes of conduct and ethics (ICN, 2012; NCNZ, 2012a; NMBA, 2018a) and may place the perioperative nurse at risk of legal proceedings and professional scrutiny. If faced with this type of situation, the nurse must take the initiative and speak up on behalf of the patient, which is not only a vital part of patient safety, it is also an important contribution to effective teamwork (Ingvarsdottir & Halldorsdottir, 2018). The perioperative nurse may also seek advice from more senior colleagues to confirm the appropriate course of action, which may include escalation to the unit manager. See Chapter 3 for further information on the legal and ethical implications of advocacy.

PERIOPERATIVE NURSING ROLES

Perioperative nursing is a highly skilled specialty, incorporating a number of subspecialties. Within each environment, there are clearly defined **perioperative nursing roles** providing patient care within a large multidisciplinary team whose combined goal is patient safety (Table 1.1). Perioperative patient care focuses on the core elements of the perioperative patient journey, including partnering with the patient for shared decision making, pre-procedure preparation, which supports management of the patient's perioperative risks, and a multidisciplinary team approach to

ensure the patient's individual perioperative pathway is followed (Agency for Clinical Innovation [ACI], 2016). This requires perioperative nurses to be educated in nursing theory and the health sciences and to have highly developed non-technical skills in interpersonal communication, teamwork, situation awareness and coping with stress (Bezemer, Korkiakanagas, Weldon, Kress, & Kneebone, 2016; Levada et al., 2018) and to practise cultural safety (NMBA, 2018a). The perioperative nurse's knowledge of the relevant professional standards and current sources of evidence informing perioperative practice are also essential for all nursing roles. This body of knowledge encompasses national nursing codes and standards, and national quality and safety standards as well as current guidelines and position statements issued by professional bodies and colleges. Perioperative nurses may function as clinicians in principally hands-on roles, or as managers and consultants, educators or researchers, while some nurses skilfully combine these functions. The scope of perioperative nursing practice reflects the numerous discrete clinical settings along the patient's entire perioperative journey, with roles including pre-admission nurse, anaesthetic nurse, circulating nurse, instrument nurse, PACU nurse and the advanced practice role of perioperative NP, as well as roles requiring advanced nursing practice (surgical assistant, nurse sedationist and nurse endoscopist).

TABLE 1.1 Where Perioperative Nurses Work Across the Perioperative Continuum			
Role	Preoperative	Intraoperative	Postoperative
Surgical outpatient clinic nurse	✓	✓	✓
Pre-admissions nurse	✓		
Enhanced recovery after surgery nurse (ERAS)	✓		✓
Day stay nurse (depending on workplace requirements)	✓	✓	✓
Nurse assistant to the anaesthetist	✓	✓	✓
Circulating/scout nurse	✓	✓	
Instrument/scrub nurse		✓	
Surgical assistant nurse		✓	
Registered nurse first surgical assistant (RNSFA)	✓	✓	✓
Medical imaging nurse	✓	✓	✓
Post anaesthetic care unit (PACU) nurse			✓
Surgical ward nurse	✓		✓
Perioperative nurse practitioner	✓	✓	✓

(Source: New Zealand Nurses Organisation. (2016). *New Zealand perioperative nursing knowledge and skills framework*. Wellington: Author.)

PATIENT SCENARIOS

SCENARIO 1.1: CULTURAL SAFETY

EN Marcus Macedo is receiving patients into the department. His patient is Mrs Patricia Peterson, a 42-year-old Indigenous woman, who lives at home in a remote community with her husband and two teenage children. She has just been transferred into the holding bay from the emergency department. Refer to the Introduction at front of the book to read Mrs Peterson's complete history.

At clinical handover, EN Macedo learns that Mrs Peterson is unhappy about being admitted into the hospital overnight. She is most anxious about being away from her family.

Critical Thinking Question
• Based on Mrs Peterson's history and your reading so far, identify at least three aspects of cultural safety that EN Macedo will need to consider when caring for Mrs Peterson and her family.

SCENARIO 1.2: PATIENT ADVOCACY

Since her arrival in the holding bay, Mrs Peterson's pain has started to ease. She is not convinced that she needs the surgery now and she asks EN Macedo if it is too late to change her mind.

Critical Thinking Question
• Thinking about the nurse's role as patient advocate, list the actions EN Macedo can take to address Mrs Peterson's concerns about the need for surgery. Provide rationales for these actions.

Preoperative Patient Assessment and Education Nurse

The perioperative environment is information intensive and requires the efficient flow of information between phases, locations and providers. Effective patient assessment and preparation for surgery requires the coordinated and combined efforts of the perioperative team. The information identified during such processes assists by defining patients' vulnerabilities or risk factors for poor surgical outcomes and contributes to patient/family satisfaction (Delaney, Bayley, Olszewsky, & Gallagher, 2015; Malley, Kenner, Kim, & Blakeney, 2015). Due to their specialised experience and practice settings, perioperative nurses can develop the combination of knowledge and skills required to conduct effective patient assessments and to provide patient education during the preoperative period (ACORN, 2020g; NZNO, 2016). While this nursing role may have different titles and settings, such nurses work in collaboration with the anaesthetic and surgical team to optimise patients' health in preparation for the surgical episode. This includes communicating with patients about the required preoperative tests and providing patient education and resources about the planned procedure or surgery, as well as completing assessments and planning for patients' discharge arrangements and follow-up (ACORN, 2020g). Box 1.4

summarises the responsibilities associated with the role. See Chapter 7 for further information about preoperative patient assessment and preparation for surgery.

BOX 1.4 Role Responsibilities of the Preoperative Patient Assessment and Education Nurse
• Inform and educate patients about the perioperative journey for the planned procedure or surgery
• Provide supportive educational material about patients' preoperative preparation and postoperative care
• Communicate with patients about preoperative tests and postoperative expectations
• Conduct patient assessments, including baseline vital signs and risk assessments such as pressure injury risk, fall risks, etc.
• Discuss and assess patients' postoperative needs and plan for patients' discharge
• Ensure that documentation of admission demographics such as patient identification, allergies and next of kin is accurate and all fields are complete for paper and electronic health records
• Facilitate coordination and communication between other healthcare providers (ACORN, 2020g; NZNO, 2014a)

SCENARIO 1.3: DELEGATION IN THE OR

RN Sandy Pereira has delegated the intraoperative care of Mrs Patricia Peterson to EN Pauline Noakes, the instrument nurse. During the procedure, EN Macedo, the anaesthetic nurse, returns to the theatre to relieve RN Pereira for her meal break.

Critical Thinking Questions

- What aspects of delegation must RN Pereira take into account as the delegator?
- What aspects of delegation must EN Noakes take into account as the recipient of this delegation?

Include rationales for your answers. You may benefit from reviewing the DMF (NMBA, 2020a) and your relevant professional nursing standards when considering your response.

Anaesthetic Nurse

The anaesthetic nurse is integral to the care of the perioperative patient and cares for the patient in the immediate time period prior to, during and after surgery. Specifically, the anaesthetic nurse provides nursing care to the patient and procedural support to the anaesthetic team during the preparation for and induction of anaesthesia, throughout maintenance of anaesthesia and during emergence from anaesthesia. The presence of an appropriately educated assistant to the anaesthetist – with the requisite knowledge, skills and competence – is integral for the safe and efficient administration of anaesthesia (ANZCA, 2015, 2016). Both ACORN (2020h) and the Perioperative Nurses College within the NZNO support the RN undertaking the anaesthetic nurse role (NZNO, 2014a). While in some facilities the role of assistant to the anaesthetist may be performed by an EN or anaesthetic technician, the predominant professional group providing assistance to the anaesthetist in New Zealand is anaesthetic technicians, who are diploma trained and regulated (Medical Sciences Council of New Zealand (MSCNZ), 2018, 2021). Whichever healthcare worker is allocated to assist the anaesthetist, each must work within their own defined scope of practice under appropriate supervision as determined by the relevant regulatory board authority (ACORN, 2020h; ANZCA, 2016; MSCNZ, 2018, 2021; NZNO, 2014a). Box 1.5 outlines the role responsibilities of the anaesthetic nurse.

Circulating Nurse

The circulating nurse (also known as the scout nurse in Australia) is critical to the patient's surgical outcome and the patient and family's experience. With the prime aims of identifying risk and maximising safety, the circulating nurse serves as patient advocate while patients are least able to care for themselves. The focus of patient assessment before, during and after the operation or procedure is based on the patient's physiological, psychosocial and emotional needs. Both ACORN (2020d) and the Perioperative Nurses College (NZNO, 2016) support the RN

BOX 1.5
Role Responsibilities of the Anaesthetic Nurse

- Participate in patient identification and other processes during clinical handover with the preoperative nurse
- Participate in all processes outlined in the Surgical Safety Checklist (SSC), focusing on the stages of 'Sign In' with the anaesthetic team and team 'Time Out' with the intraoperative team
- Advocate for the patient throughout the anaesthetic episode, particularly:
  - when the patient is awake during local and/or regional anaesthesia
  - during induction and emergence phases of general anaesthesia
- Collaborate with and assist the anaesthetist throughout the anaesthetic episode to maintain the patient's airway, provide intravenous access and monitor haemodynamic status
- Anticipate and provide equipment/supplies for routine (and emergency) anaesthetic procedures
- Provide a comprehensive clinical handover to the intraoperative nurses
- Assist with patient transfer and positioning before and after surgery
- Evaluate the effectiveness of planned care such as patient transfer and positioning
- Ensure that documentation of anaesthetic nursing care is accurate and complete, including monitoring data, fluid balance records and patient outcomes
- Collaborate with postanaesthesia care unit staff to provide patient care (ACORN, 2020h; NZNO, 2014a)

BOX 1.6
Role Responsibilities of the Circulating Nurse

- Participate in all processes outlined in the Surgical Safety Checklist (SSC), focusing on the stages of team 'Time Out' and 'Sign Out'
- Adhere to and maintain aseptic technique throughout the procedure
- Anticipate the needs of the instrument nurse before and during the surgical procedure
- Work directly with the instrument nurse to support the surgical team
- Collaborate with the instrument nurse to:
  - advocate for the patient, in particular during the surgical procedure
  - prepare the instruments and equipment needed for the surgical procedure
  - monitor any breach in aseptic technique and initiate corrective action
  - perform the surgical count at prescribed stages
  - ensure correct handling of surgically removed human tissue and explanted items
  - ensure that documentation of intraoperative nursing care is accurate and complete, including patient outcomes
  - provide a comprehensive clinical handover to the nurse caring for the patient in the PACU (ACORN, 2020d)

BOX 1.7
Role Responsibilities of the Instrument Nurse

- Participate in all processes outlined in the Surgical Safety Checklist (SSC), focusing on the stages of team 'Time Out' and 'Sign Out'
- Adhere to and maintain aseptic technique throughout the procedure
- Work directly with the surgical team
- Collaborate with the circulating nurse to:
  - advocate for the patient, in particular during the surgical procedure
  - anticipate the needs of the surgical team before and during the surgical procedure
  - prepare the instruments and equipment needed for the surgical procedure
  - monitor any breach in aseptic technique and initiate corrective action
  - perform the surgical count at prescribed stages
  - ensure correct handling of surgically removed human tissue and explanted items
  - ensure that documentation of intraoperative nursing care is accurate and complete, including patient outcomes
  - provide a comprehensive clinical handover to the nurse caring for the patient in the PACU (ACORN, 2020i)

undertaking this role. The circulating nurse's role is complex, encompassing management of nursing care of the patient within the OR and coordination of the needs of the surgical team and other care providers necessary for the completion of surgery. During the procedure, the circulating nurse needs to be mobile and remains outside of the aseptic field. This ensures the circulating nurse is always well positioned to observe the surgery and the surgical team from a broad perspective and to assist the team in creating and maintaining a safe and comfortable environment for the patient. The circulating nurse often has only a short timeframe in which to establish rapport and a therapeutic bond with the patient and their family or carers. However, the circulating nurse's ability to form relationships during their time with the patient has a positive influence on the patient, resulting in them feeling safe and secure (Kaptain et al., 2019). Box 1.6 outlines the responsibilities associated with the circulating nurse role.

Instrument Nurse

The instrument nurse (also known as the scrub nurse) works directly with the surgeon within the aseptic field, managing the instruments and other items needed during the procedure. The circulating nurse and the instrument nurse have a dual role in checking to ensure that all appropriate sterile instrumentation and surgical supplies are available and functional before the scheduled theatre list commences (ACORN, 2020i; NZNO, 2016). The responsibilities of the circulating and instrument nurses may overlap with those of the anaesthetic nurse, depending on local policy, the competency and scope of practice of the individual nurses within the team and the structure of the surgical team. For instance, in some facilities it is the responsibility of the anaesthetic nurse to check the patient's details (e.g. correct identity/surgical site, consent, allergies and so forth) on admission to the department, whereas this duty may be incorporated into the role of the circulating or instrument nurse in other facilities. During surgery, the instrument nurse's role should be distinct from, and not overlap with, the role of the first surgical assistant – that is, the person assisting the surgeon. While there may be times when these roles overlap to ensure patient safety (e.g. managing patient haemorrhage, difficult access to the operative site), this should not occur routinely. The instrument nurse role, together with the roles of circulating nurse and anaesthetic nurse, forms the core of the nursing team during the intraoperative phase of the

- Receive the patient into the PACU and ensure the clinical handover is comprehensive, including confirmation of postoperative orders and required documentation
- Conduct a thorough patient assessment and monitor vital signs at prescribed times
- Manage the patient's postoperative position and comfort, wound dressings and drains, acute pain, nausea and vomiting
- Monitor and manage the patient's haemodynamic status
- Document nursing care and patient outcomes
- Respond promptly to and report any aberrant changes in the patient's condition to the anaesthetist and/or surgeon
- Recognise deterioration and respond to emergencies by initiating resuscitation or by contributing to a team resuscitation response
- Provide a comprehensive clinical handover to the nurse caring for the patient in the receiving postoperative unit (ACORN, 2020j; NZNO, 2016)

patient's perioperative journey. Box 1.7 outlines the responsibilities associated with the instrument nurse role. The next phase of the patient's perioperative journey begins when a member of the intraoperative nursing team (commonly the instrument nurse or circulating nurse) conducts the patient's clinical handover with the postanaesthesia care unit nurse.

Postanaesthesia Care Unit (PACU) Nurse

The PACU nurse (also known as the recovery room nurse) is an important member of the perioperative team, providing patient care immediately following a surgical or other procedure, and usually including recovery from anaesthesia (ACORN, 2020j; NZNO, 2016). The role of the PACU nurse is to ensure patient safety following clinical handover and transfer of care from the nursing and medical teams in the OR to the PACU. Vigilance is crucial in achieving this intended outcome as the patient is at increased risk during the immediate postoperative phase of the journey, when many serious physiological changes can occur rapidly in the patient and there are great demands on both delivering and receiving staff for a smooth transfer (Randmaa, Martensson, Swenne, & Engstrom, 2015). In some healthcare facilities, the PACU and anaesthetic nurse roles are interchangeable, with nurses working across both subspecialties. Enrolled nurses may be included in the PACU nursing team, working under the supervision of the experienced PACU nurse to provide safe patient care (ACORN, 2020j). Box 1.8 outlines the responsibilities associated with the PACU nurse role.

Evolving and Advanced Roles for Perioperative Registered Nurses

A range of roles within the nursing profession purport to be **advanced practice** roles (Carryer, Wilkinson, Towers, & Gardner, 2018; Gardner, Duffield, Doubrovsky, & Adams, 2016). In Australia and New Zealand, the only advanced practice role formally recognised by the national regulatory authority is the NP (Australian Nursing and Midwifery Federation [ANMF], 2017; NMBA, 2016a), which is a protected title in Australia under the National Law (NMBA, 2019c). The NMBA (2016a) defines the concept of advanced nursing practice (ANP) as:

> *a continuum along which nurses develop their professional knowledge, clinical reasoning and judgement, skills and behaviours to higher levels of capability (that is recognisable). Nurses practising at an advanced level incorporate professional leadership, education and research into their clinically based practice. Their practice is effective and safe. They work within a generalist or specialist context and they are responsible and accountable in managing people who have complex health care requirements.*

Changes in healthcare delivery have precipitated the recognition of advanced and extended practice roles for RNs generally (Carryer et al., 2018; Gardner et al., 2016) and also specifically for RNs working in the perioperative setting (ACORN, 2020k; Lynn & Brownie, 2015). Perioperative RNs practising at advanced levels in this specialist context have included surgical assistants, nurse endoscopists and nurse sedationists. ACORN supports RNs working in roles at these levels of advanced practice. Furthermore, ACORN recognises the regulatory requirements and educational pathway for the NP role and actively promotes the transition of such nurses towards perioperative NP roles (ACORN, 2020k). These roles are described in the following sections.

Perioperative Nurse Practitioner

The NP in Australia is an advanced practice role with a protected title, regulated by legislation and professional standards (NMBA, 2014, 2019c). These requirements include Master's level educational, a minimum of 3 years advanced nursing practice experience and extensive continuing professional development (NMBA, 2016b). The perioperative NP is an RN with extensive experience of perioperative practice at an advanced level who is Master's prepared and has acquired the expert knowledge base, complex decision-making skills and clinical competencies to provide direct patient care throughout any,

> **BOX 1.9**
> **Role Responsibilities of the NP**
>
> - Conduct comprehensive health assessments and make decisions using diagnostic capability
> - Order and interpret diagnostic and laboratory tests
> - Plan care in partnership with patients and families
> - Collaborate with the patient, surgeon and other healthcare team members to develop and implement therapeutic surgical interventions
> - Refer to other healthcare professionals for management of issues which fall outside the perioperative NP scope of practice
> - Evaluate postoperative patient outcomes including pain management, wound management and education needs (ACORN, 2020k; NCNZ, 2017; NMBA, 2014; 2016a)

> **BOX 1.10**
> **Role Responsibilities of Surgical Assistant Nurses (e.g. PNSA/NMSA)**
>
> - Assist with skin preparation and surgical draping
> - Assist with haemostasis, cutting sutures/ligatures, retracting organs and skin closure
> - Provide postoperative care in wound management
> - Develop education programs for patients and staff (AANSA, 2012; ACORN, 2020l; NZNO, 2015)

or all, phases of a patient's perioperative period (ACORN, 2020k; NZNO, 2016; Yang & Hains, 2017). Legislation also provides the NP with rights for ordering diagnostic tests, prescribing medications and making referrals to other members of the healthcare team (NMBA, 2014). NPs practising at an advanced level in a specific area of practice were first introduced in New Zealand in 2000. In 2017, the NCNZ made changes to NP education programs, the endorsed scope of practice was broadened and the requirement to restrict New Zealand NPs to a specific area of practice was removed (NCNZ, 2020). Box 1.9 outlines the responsibilities which may be associated with the perioperative NP role.

Surgical Assistant Nursing Roles

Surgical assistant nursing roles are known as the perioperative nurse surgeon's assistant (PNSA) in Australia and the registered nurse first surgical assistant (RNFSA) in New Zealand (NZNO, 2016). Collectively, these roles have also been named as the non-medical surgical assistant (NMSA), with orthopaedics and general surgery being reported as the most common areas of practice (Hains, Turner, & Strand, 2016). Both ACORN and the Australian Association of Nurse Surgical Assistants (AANSA) stipulate that the PNSA is an advanced nursing practice role for the RN, with a minimum of 3 years perioperative nursing experience, postgraduate perioperative qualifications and requisite hours of practical supervision (ACORN, 2020l; AANSA, 2012). In New Zealand the role is also recognised as expanded nursing practice with specialised knowledge and skills required, and therefore should meet expanded practice guidelines as outlined by the NZNO (2015). As such, these roles do not function at the same level as NPs. The specific scope

of clinical practice for these roles should be determined by the local facility and this may include local credentialling criteria (ACORN, 2020l). Despite these stipulations, a small Australian survey of perioperative nurses found that perioperative RNs and ENs without the requisite training or qualifications were required on an ad hoc basis to assist during surgery or to assist while also acting as the instrument nurse (Hains, Turner, & Strand, 2017). Ultimately, these NMSA roles remain constrained by the lack of recognition by national regulatory authorities (Hains, Turner & Strand, 2018; Lynn & Brownie, 2015). Box 1.10 outlines the responsibilities which may be associated with these RN roles.

Nurse Endoscopist

Perioperative RNs working in the nurse endoscopist role undertake advanced patient assessment, interpret diagnostic interventions and pathology, including performing flexible sigmoidoscopy, colonoscopy and upper gastrointestinal endoscopy, and establish differential diagnoses and management plans, including selection and prescription of appropriate medication and direct referrals to other healthcare professionals (Gastroenterological Nurses College of Australia [GENCA], 2015; NCNZ, 2011b; South Australia Health, 2018). Feature box 1.2 provides an overview of the development of the nurse endoscopist role and summarises the differing positions about the educational preparation and regulation of the role.

Nurse Cystoscopist

The role of the nurse cystoscopist is one in which the RN is practising at an advanced level of skill and is defined as a role for *'appropriately trained registered nurses who are credentialled to perform a flexible cystoscopy'* (State of Victoria, 2015). Nurse-led flexible cystoscopy developed in the UK over the past decade; however, in the Australian public health system, traditionally it has been the role of junior medical officer to perform flexible cystoscopies. Between 2008 and 2010, the Department of Health funded Melbourne Health and Monash Health to develop and

---

FEATURE BOX 1.2
Development and Regulation of the Nurse Endoscopist Role

The nurse endoscopist (NE) is a long-established nursing role in the UK, US and Europe. While the role was established more recently in Australia, its origins were driven by the same clinical needs: to curb the growing trend in bowel cancer deaths within the population (South Australia Health, 2018). Additional driving forces within Australia, such as a shortage of medical staff and an increasing demand for endoscopy services, produced training pathways and models of care for the NE role in a number of Australian states, including an NP model in Queensland and advanced practice models in Victoria and South Australia (Duffield, Chapman, & Rowbotham, 2017; Duncan, Bonney, Au, & Bennett, 2017; South Australia Health, 2018).

Although national nursing organisations in Australia and New Zealand generally welcome the NE role, there is ongoing debate about regulation of the role. Whether the NE role should meet the nationally legislated requirements and protected title of the NP or remain as an advanced practice nursing role, it is accepted that the first step for perioperative RNs who wish to undertake this role is to complete an appropriate training program and then to demonstrate a capacity to practise at a higher level than RNs across a range of domains, including clinical care, research and leadership (Duffield et al., 2017). The Gastroenterological Nurses College of Australia (GENCA) maintains that RNs, educated and trained in the techniques of flexible endoscopy, may assume the responsibility of performing flexible endoscopy in an acute hospital setting within a collaborative multidisciplinary team environment. The education provided, however, must be of a level and depth required to support clinical care during the procedure, as well as general patient management, and endoscopic skills training should be equivalent to that of gastroenterology medical trainees (GENCA, 2015). In Victoria, training for the role of advanced practice nurse endoscopist has been provided through the Victorian Nurse Endoscopy Program at a number of facilities (Austin Health, 2015). The New Zealand Society of Gastroenterology (NZSG) also supports the NE role, working within an agreed practice framework with established training, supervision, safety, quality, competency and practice standards (NZSG, 2012).

---

evaluate a nurse-led bladder cancer surveillance model. The model provided nurses with additional skills and training to perform flexible cystoscopies to detect recurrence of bladder cancer. The model has seen a reduction in waiting times for diagnostic cystoscopy by up to 70% (State of Victoria, 2015). The role is evolving to encompass a wider range of procedures that complement the delivery of modern urological services in a safe and effective manner to ensure that patients can access screening services as quickly as possible (State of Victoria, 2015).

Nurse Sedationist

The role of the nurse in anaesthetics has a wide-ranging scope of practice around the world: certified nurse anaesthetist is the common role in the US while assistant to the anaesthetist (be it technician or nurse) is the common role in Australia and New Zealand (ANZCA, 2016). Similar to the nurse endoscopist and nurse cystoscopist roles, the nurse sedationist role emerged in Australia in response to increased demand for services and a shortfall in the medical workforce (Jones, Long, & Zeitz, 2011). A trial in South Australia found positive patient satisfaction from the nurse sedation service and reported no adverse events (Jones et al., 2011), while key stakeholders perceived the role as needed, valued and making an impact on patient outcomes. The nurse sedationist works under the supervision of a medical officer to provide procedural sedation for minor procedures or investigations and requires additional training in the administration of intravenous sedation and monitoring of the patient's response to sedation (ACI, 2015). There is evidence to suggest that procedural sedation administered by non-anaesthetists, including nurse sedationists, produces low rates of adverse events (Gouda et al., 2017). Despite this, the role has met with concern from professional colleges such as the ANZCA, which recommends a national standard be developed if this model is to be pursued in Australia (and/or New Zealand) (ANZCA, 2014). In New South Wales, the ACI initiated a state-wide, multidisciplinary project on safe procedural sedation (ACI, 2015). The project produced a set of minimum standards for care provided pre-, intra- and post-procedure, to support non-anaesthetists who provide procedural sedation in NSW facilities (ACI, 2015).

Cosmetic Nurse

Cosmetic nursing is a rapidly evolving practice area in Australia and New Zealand, with ENs, RNs and NPs practising as cosmetic nurses (also known as aesthetic nurses). The scope of practice for cosmetic nurses will vary between facilities and private practices, influencing the context of nursing care. For example, cosmetic nurses might be practising in collaboration with medical colleagues such as dermatologists in private or public healthcare settings, or with cosmetic physicians or surgeons, or plastic surgeons. They might also work in nurse-led clinics or independently in private practice (Australasian College of Cosmetic

Surgery [ACCS], 2015). The scope of practice for cosmetic nurses may include cosmetic injections, chemical peels, intense pulsed laser therapy, removal of tattoos and unwanted hair, minor surgery (such as removal of skin tags) or schlerotherapy (Australian College of Nursing [ACN], 2020a). The regulation of the cosmetic industry, however, has been problematic. For example, a parliamentary inquiry into complaints about providers of cosmetic health services in New South Wales reported instances where unregistered and untrained staff were providing treatments and instances of improper use of protected titles and nurses working beyond their scope of practice (NSW Parliament, 2018). To practise safely in such diverse settings and remain within their individual scope of practice, cosmetic nurses must follow all relevant policies, standards and guidelines that apply, including infection prevention and control and the quality use of medicines, and must also be competent in emergency procedures (ACN, 2020a; NMBA, 2018b). Feature box 1.3 provides more information about the regulation and educational preparation of cosmetic nurses.

INFORMAL AND CONTINUING PROFESSIONAL DEVELOPMENT

All RNs and ENs commit to developing their professional and personal qualities throughout their career (Maloney & Harper, 2017; NMBA, 2016e, 2020c). This commitment is even more important in specialty areas such as perioperative nursing, where patient safety depends on nurses' knowledge of technology, health policy and nursing practice (ACORN, 2020e). As part of the national registration process for all health professionals, nurses must meet a number of requirements to maintain their annual authority to practise (NMBA, 2020c). This includes the need to demonstrate recency of practice and meet a prescribed level of **continuing professional development** (CPD). In Australia, under the National Law, nurses are required to participate in a minimum of 20 hours CPD each year. Set by the NZNC under the Health Practitioners Competence Assurance Act 2003, nurses in New Zealand are required to complete 60 hours of professional development over 3 years (Ministry of Health, 2020). Nurses are responsible for planning and recording their CPD activities, which may include:

- formal education programs or certified courses
- workplace learning, including mandatory education activities
- online learning and courses
- self-directed activities such as journal reading, which should be relevant to the nurse's area of practice and matched to individual learning goals. In New Zealand, journal clubs must take place within a formal framework (NMBA, 2020c; NCNZ, n.d.).

Neither the NMBA nor the NZNC mandates the process or the tool for recording CPD activities, but each stipulates that nurses should describe how the activity has contributed to their professional development (NCNZ, n.d.; NMBA, 2020c). Table 1.2 depicts the use

---

FEATURE BOX 1.3
Regulation Affecting Healthcare Workers Providing Cosmetic Services

In 2015, three separate incidents were referred for investigation by the Health Care Complaints Commission (HCCC) New South Wales. Each incident occurred in a small private clinic during an invasive procedure performed by cosmetic surgeons, with two of the patients requiring admission to intensive care units for resuscitation and further treatment (Patty, 2015, p. 3). In 2018, the NSW Parliament held an inquiry into cosmetic health service complaints at the request of the Committee on the Health Care Complaints Commission (NSW Parliament, 2018). The inquiry received 25 submissions which identified a number of serious patient incidents and practice issues, including an EN who was referred to the Nursing and Midwifery Council of NSW (NMC) in 2012 and eventually suspended in 2018 for unsupervised and unsatisfactory professional performance (NMC, 2018). Significant patient incidents such as these have prompted calls from the professions and the public for wider scrutiny and regulation of cosmetic doctors and nurses (also known as

aesthetic nurses) working in these settings (ACN, 2020a). In 2015, the ACCS published *The professional practice standards and scope of practice for aesthetic nursing practice in Australia*, the first description of standards of professional practice for cosmetic nurses in the Australian context (ACCS, 2015). In 2020, the NMBA reissued its *Position statement on nurses and cosmetic procedures*, which states that cosmetic nurses require additional education to attain the desired level of competence in the specific procedures they wish to perform (NMBA, 2018b). They are also required to comply with relevant state and territory drugs and poisons legislation regarding using, obtaining, selling, storing, prescribing, administering and supplying scheduled medicines (NMBA, 2018b). There is a range of educational programs available for cosmetic nurses, including vocational level courses for ENs and postgraduate level programs. The ACCS proposes that cosmetic nurses be educated to the level of NP (ACCS, 2015).

TABLE 1.2
CPD Records in the Operating Suite

Date	Source or Provider Details	Identified Learning Needs	Action Plan	Type of Activity	Description of Topic/s Covered During Activity and Outcome	Reflection on Activity and Specification to Practice	Evidence Provided	CPD Hours
A. CPD RECORDS FOR RN TEAM LEADER IN THE OPERATING SUITE								
April 2020	NMBA	RN Standard 2: Engages in therapeutic & professional relationships. 2.7 fosters a culture of safety and learning	Need to clarify responsibility for aspects of care with other members of the health team. Unsure of my delegation responsibilities in the workplace. Plan: Access and review NMBA decision-making framework (DMF)	Self-directed Review DMF from the National Board website: <https://www.nursingmidwiferyboard.gov.au/Codes-Guidelines-Statements/Frameworks.aspx>	Reviewed the scope of practice for my profession and that of me as an individual. Gained an appreciation of the principles I need to apply when making decisions about my nursing practice and when and how I decide to delegate activities to other RNs and ENs.	As a team leader working in the operating room I will be able to apply the nursing decision-making framework when I allocate staff to patient care and delegate tasks as they arise during a shift.	Refer to portfolio	2 hours
B. CPD RECORDS FOR A NEWLY QUALIFIED NURSE DURING ORIENTATION TO THE OPERATING SUITE								
April 2020	Perioperative educator	Orientation to perioperative suite Principles of perioperative nursing	Department orientation folder Copy of timetable and objectives in portfolio	Mixed workshop, clinical instruction, self-directed learning and reading	Clinical handover Scrubbing, gowning and gloving . . .	I will use ISBAR when receiving patients into the suite and when taking patients into PACU I learnt a new technique for 'open-gloving' and will practise this at home	Program objectives and certificate in portfolio	2 hours 3 hours

(Source: Adapted from the NMBA sample template for documenting CPD: Nursing and Midwifery Board of Australia. (2020c). Continuing professional development [fact sheet]. Melbourne: Author.)

BOX 1.11
ACORN's Essential Values for Perioperative Nurses' Professional Development

- There should be an emphasis on continuous learning, which is the foundation for the overall approach to staff development
- Nurses are accountable for providing quality care through safe, ethical and effective practice and maintaining competence for practice
- Professional development assists nurses to maintain the highest standard of clinical practice
- Professional development is also facilitated by nurses acting as preceptors and mentors for less experienced colleagues
- Nurses should become self-directed learners to ensure personal and professional growth through:
  - self-assessment of learning gaps
  - evaluation of self and others
  - critical thinking
  - critical appraisal

(Source: Australian College of Perioperative Nurses. (2020e). *Standards for perioperative nursing in Australia* (16th ed., volume 2 - Professional standards, Professional development). Adelaide: Author.)

of the NMBA template for documenting CPD activities by perioperative nurses with different experience levels (NMBA, 2020c). Other professional organisations and nursing colleges provide members with resources for documenting CPD; for example, the NCNZ provides a downloadable template for recording evidence of CPD activities (NCNZ, 2011c). Professional portfolios can also be used to record CPD activities and will, more importantly, provide an effective mechanism for the nurse to reflect on practice. ACORN (2020e) standards identify the essential values that underpin CPD for perioperative nurses (see Box 1.11).

FORMAL EDUCATION

While nurses may gain entry to the perioperative workforce without specialist qualifications, formal education provides the theoretical basis for the specialist clinician and enables the delivery of safe patient care (ACORN, 2020e; ANMF, 2016). Professional associations may advocate for postgraduate studies and some will provide incentives for their members to acquire specialist qualifications. For example, ACORN provides education and research grants for its members, and encourages graduates to consider research activities as a means of advancing perioperative nursing practice.

RNs seeking to enhance their perioperative knowledge and clinical skills can choose from a number of postgraduate studies, including graduate certificates and diplomas up to Master's and Doctoral level. While courses for advanced practice roles and NP roles begin at Master's level, there are many postgraduate certificates in Australia providing specialisation in the circulating and instrument nurse roles, anaesthetics, postanaesthesia care, pain management and critical care nursing. Other areas, such as health management, safety and quality, infection prevention, or teams and communication, may also be relevant to the perioperative clinician or the aspiring nurse academic.

There are many providers of tertiary qualifications in Australia, including universities in every state as well as the Australian College of Nursing, which offers fully online postgraduate certificate programs (ACN, 2018). Latrobe University offers an Advanced Clinical Nursing in Perioperative Nurse Surgical Assistant as part of the Master of Nursing program, the first postgraduate program of its kind in Australia (La Trobe University, 2018). Postgraduate nursing programs are provided by a range of universities in New Zealand, as well as polytechnics and institutes of technology, including one institution providing a certificate in RNFSA with the potential to progress into the nursing Diploma and Master's program. The NCNZ accredits and monitors postgraduate courses, including those that contribute to a program of study towards registration as an NP (NCNZ, 2020).

For ENs, the entry-level qualification is the Diploma of Nursing, having evolved from Certificate and then Certificate IV on the Australian Qualification Framework (AQF). The next level on the AQF is the Advanced Diploma of Nursing, which enables the EN to specialise in perioperative nursing practice (ACN, 2019a). ENs in New Zealand must pass assessments and exams and complete an 18-month program at Level 5 as accredited by the NCNZ (2017). ENs may also choose to complete an RN conversion program to access a more diverse education pathway leading to postgraduate qualifications.

Nursing Specialisation

For undergraduate nurses in Australia and New Zealand, entry to the perioperative environment may be possible as a specialist clinical placement lasting several days or weeks, or as a single visit to complement a ward-based clinical placement. Such placements can enhance the student's understanding of the patient's surgical experience (ACORN, 2020m). While specialist clinical placements are desirable for all nursing students, even a short visit accompanying the surgical patient on their perioperative journey can have many benefits for the nursing student. These include the opportunity for direct observation of the specialist activities provided by each of the nursing care roles as they interact with the patient and with each other during clinical handover. The student nurse will also be able to observe the ways in which members of the multidisciplinary team care for the perioperative patient and can enquire about anaesthetic and surgical techniques, communication and teamwork.

The educational benefits of a guided clinical placement may also extend the nursing student's knowledge beyond the walls of the perioperative environment and prepare them for pre- and postoperative surgical patient care (see Research box 1.1; Foran, 2016) and can influence the student's future career choice in perioperative nursing (ACORN, 2020m). In 2015 the Sax Institute published a report on the benefits of providing undergraduate student clinical placements. The report suggested that a quality clinical placement has positive outcomes including:

- Students on clinical placements provided a positive addition to the service provision of the health service provider.
- Students on clinical placements made a real contribution to the health service organisation.
- Students on clinical placements added value to the service by interacting with patients in a number of roles.

- Successful clinical placements saw a rise in graduates pursuing a career in the area placed (Sax Institute, 2015).

Educators and staff developing **orientation programs** should have regard for these elements as they apply equally for graduate nurses and other new staff entering the perioperative environment. Table 1.3 outlines potential content for an orientation program for new perioperative nurses, from a 1-week clinical placement to part of an extended transition-to-practice program. This content can be tailored depending on the supernumerary time allocated, the clinical demands of the department and the individual's goals and prior learning.

THE ROLE OF PROFESSIONAL ASSOCIATIONS

The primary purpose of **professional associations** is to protect, enhance and advance the common interests of the organisation and its professional and non-professional members (Hamlin, 2012). Professional associations in nursing are essential in maintaining a profession that advocates for the needs of nurses and their patients and which upholds the public's trust. Professional associations operate at local, state, national and international levels and perform a number of functions, including gaining support through political lobbying, providing education

---

RESEARCH BOX 1.1
The Impact of a Guided Operating Theatre Experience on Undergraduate Nursing Students' Surgical Nursing Care

It can be challenging for faculty staff to prioritise and refine the educational content of their undergraduate nursing core curriculum. Consequently, only a small proportion of undergraduate nurses have the opportunity to undertake a clinical placement in the perioperative environment. An Australian perioperative nurse researcher set out to explore the impact of a guided operating theatre experience on the practical experience of undergraduate nursing students in surgical wards. The research was designed first to identify the different models of operating suite education offered to Australian undergraduate nursing students and then to explore which of these models yielded the best educational outcomes. These investigations ultimately formed the following research question:

- Do undergraduate nurses need to be involved in guided operating suite practical experience in order to achieve skills and knowledge that support a high

standard of nursing care in the pre- and postoperative surgical wards?

A total of 332 undergraduate nurses were tested on their knowledge of pre- and postoperative nursing. Test scores were statistically higher in undergraduate nurses who had completed a guided experience in the operating theatre compared with ward experience alone. These findings support the merits of a guided operating theatre experience, and the researcher recommended that a guided operating theatre experience should be included in the undergraduate core curricula for all nursing students.

This research is interesting because it demonstrated the value of a guided operating theatre experience for undergraduate nurses not only in working effectively outside the perioperative environment but also in the preparation of undergraduate nurses for surgical ward nursing.

(Source: Foran, P. (2016). Undergraduate surgical nursing preparation and guided operating room experience: a quantitative analysis. *Nurse Education in Practice*, *16*(1), 217–224.)

TABLE 1.3
Sample Content of an Orientation Program

Weeks	Modules	Overview of Content
1	1. Orientation to the environment 2. Infection prevention and aseptic technique	• Nursing roles • Pathways (patient, equipment, staff) • Theatre etiquette and perioperative attire • WH&S and PPE • Aseptic technique and the aseptic field • Validating, opening and dispensing sterile items • Specimen management • Cleaning practices
2 to 4	3. Perioperative patient safety 4. Patient positioning 5. Patient-centred care 6. Perioperative clinical handover	• Patient advocacy • Communication and the multidisciplinary team • Airway safety and emergency management • Surgical safety • Operating tables and positioning equipment • The surgical count • Perioperative documentation and information systems • Clinical handover using ISBAR
4 to 8	Commence specialty program modules	Consolidating practice and working independently • Circulating and instrument nurse • Anaesthetic nurse • Postanaesthetic care unit nurse
By week 6	Informal appraisal of goal achievements Learning and development goal setting for perioperative specialty roles	
9 to 24	Continue specialty program modules	Working independently, managing different specialties and emergencies • Circulating and instrument nurse • Anaesthetic nurse • Postanaesthetic care unit nurse

(Source: Southern Adelaide Local Health Network (SALHN) (2019a). New/Junior OTS Nurse or TPPP OTS Role Progression Plan (6 months) V3.1: 2019; SALHN. (2019b). New/Junior Anaesthetic Nurse or TPPP Anaesthetics Role Progression Plan (6 months); SALHN. (2019c). New/Junior PACU Nurse or TPPP PACU Role Progression Plan (6 months). Adelaide: Author.)

and resources for members and the public and developing standards for professional practice (Hamlin, 2012). While professional associations have a key role in developing standards for professional practice (Nerland & Karseth, 2015), they also provide some or all of the following opportunities for their members:

• development of standards for use within their sphere of practice
• educational activities, such as conferences, public seminars and ongoing professional education
• scholarships for study and grants for research
• networking and mentoring opportunities
• credentialling, accreditation or recognition of the contribution of members to the specialty

• accreditation of independent provider education programs
• consultation with government on policy issues
• political lobbying on behalf of members and opportunities to contribute to policy making.

Professional Nursing Associations

The International Council of Nurses (ICN) is a federation of more than 130 national nurse associations, representing more than 16 million nurses worldwide. Founded in 1899, the ICN is the world's first and widest-reaching international organisation for health professionals. The ICN is led by nurses and works to ensure that they are included in policy and decision making of high-level bodies such as the World Health Organization (WHO) (ICN, 2020b). In Australia and New Zealand, more than 70 professional nursing organisations represent clinical, managerial, educational, research-based and industrial interests. In Australia, the Australian College of Nursing (ACN) is the key national professional nursing organisation which aims to advance nursing leadership (ACN, 2020b). The ACN advocates for nurses and has a strong focus on influencing health policy nationally. It is also an accredited education provider, offering graduate Certificates for RNs and advanced Diplomas for ENs in perioperative nursing as well as other specialty areas (ACN, 2020c). The Australian Nursing and Midwifery Federation (ANMF) is both a trade union and a professional organisation for nurses as well as midwives and AINs (ANMF, 2014). It uses this integrated role to promote the nursing and midwifery professions' contributions to the health and aged care systems in Australia.

In New Zealand, there is one coalition of nurses' organisations: the New Zealand Nurses Organisation (NZNO). It serves the professional and industrial needs of more than 46,000 nurses and health workers and embraces Te Tiriti O Waitangi, '[seeking] to improve the health status of all peoples of Aotearoa/New Zealand through participation in health and social policy development' (NZNO, 2014b, para. 3). The NZNO has a number of sections or colleges, made up of groups of members with a focus on a specific field or subspecialty of nursing (e.g. the Perioperative Nursing College – see Fig. 1.1). Both the ACN and the NZNO are members of the ICN.

Perioperative Nursing Associations – Australasia

Perioperative nursing associations (PNAs) have a much shorter history but otherwise have the same remit as the professional associations mentioned above. Initially, Australian PNAs functioned at local, state and then national levels, but a more recent development has been the formation of international entities whose membership comprises national PNAs (Hamlin, 2012).

Australian College of Perioperative Nurses (ACORN)

State- and territory-based PNAs began to emerge in Australia during the 1950s and 1960s. The concept of a national body representing perioperative nurses was envisaged in 1975, when a group of nurses from around the country gathered in Melbourne (ACORN, 2021b). Two milestone decisions came out of that initial meeting: to hold a national conference and to establish a national body with responsibility for developing

and monitoring standards of practice. In 1977, both outcomes were achieved with the first national conference for Australian perioperative nurses and the founding of the (then) Australian Confederation of Operating Room Nurses. ACORN became the Australian College of Operating Room Nurses in 2000 and the Australian College of Perioperative Nurses in 2016.

Perioperative nurses become members of ACORN through membership of their individual state- and territory-based organisation. ACORN's mission is to advance safe, quality perioperative nursing care for Australians (ACORN, 2021c). The college provides national leadership in perioperative nursing care through standard setting and by supporting nursing research through annual scholarships. ACORN also fosters continuing professional development through a range of educational activities (e.g. conferences, leadership summits and publication of a national journal).

Australian College of Perianaesthesia Nurses (ACPAN)

The Australian College of Perianaesthesia Nurses (ACPAN) was founded in 1994 as the Victorian Society of Post Anaesthetic and Anaesthetic Nurses group (VSPAAN), to provide education for perianaesthesia nurses, as other special interest groups were not addressing their perianaesthesia needs. In 2016, VSPAAN became a national college (ACPAN), with more than 700 members Australia wide. ACPAN's focus is on the professional development of anaesthesia and postanaesthesia nurses through regular meetings, education, scholarships, conferences and publications. ACPAN works closely with ACORN and ANZCA to promote best practice in perianaesthesia nursing through development of professional practice (ACPAN, 2019). ACPAN is an affiliated member of the International Collaboration of PeriAnaesthesia Nurses (ICPAN), which supports perianaesthesia nursing organisations and advocates for global networking groups and international perianaesthesia nursing collaborations (ICPAN, 2019).

Australian Day Surgery Nurses Association (ADSNA)

The Australian Day Surgery Nurses Association (ADSNA) is a national body formed in 1996 which works with state-based day surgery groups to promote the role of nurses working in day surgery units and ambulatory care settings. The ADSNA produces the Day surgery best practice guidelines and disseminates information through networking events, seminars and conferences in collaboration with the state-based groups. As a national body, the ADSNA also seeks to inform government and relevant bodies on matters which influence the safety of patients, such as clinical indicators for day surgery patients (ADSNA, 2017a). The ADSNA is also a member of the International Association for Ambulatory Surgery (IAAS) (ADSNA, 2017b).

Perioperative Nurses College of the New Zealand Nurses Organisation (PNC NZNO)

The Perioperative Nurses College (PNC) is the professional organisation of perioperative nurses in New Zealand and is legally affiliated with the NZNO. The mission of the PNC is to support safe and optimal care of patients undergoing operative and other invasive procedures and it achieves this by promoting high standards of nursing practice through education and research (NZNO, 2014c). Specific functions of the PNC include:

- providing strategic direction and leadership for perioperative nursing
- developing professional standards for perioperative nursing
- providing leadership and perioperative nursing representation
- promoting New Zealand perioperative nursing nationally and internationally
- developing and coordinating education programs and resources
- providing a mechanism for communicating with members on perioperative trends and issues via a journal and newsletters and organisation of national and international conferences (NZNO, 2014c).

The PNC has a core set of six standards as well as a number of guidance statements and service guidelines. Perioperative nurses use these documents in conjunction with the NCNZ *Competencies for registered nurses* (NCNZ, 2007). Members of the PNC NZNO are also guided in their perioperative practice by the Association of periOperative Registered Nurses (AORN) *Guidelines for perioperative practice* (2020b), which the association makes available for its members.

Professional Nursing Associations – International

The AORN and the Association for Perioperative Practice (AfPP) are two of the oldest international PNAs. Both are well known in Australasia by individual membership or attendance at their conferences, as well as through their publication of journals, standards of practice and guidelines. A number of other international PNAs have emerged in the past two decades, including the European Operating Room Nurses Association (EORNA, est. 1992), the Nordic Operating Room Nurses Association (NORNA, est. 1993) and the Asian Perioperative Nurses Association (ASIORNA, est. 2009). These PNAs have national organisations as their members and function within largely geographical regions. Representing perioperative nursing interests at the global level is the International Federation of Perioperative Nurses (IFPN), also structured with a membership base of national organisations. In the Asia Pacific region, the Papua New Guinea Perioperative Nurses Society (PNGPNS) and the Pacific Islands Operating Theatre Nurses Association (PIORNA) are two new PNAs which have emerged in recent years. The following section describes a selection of these PNAs in more detail.

The International Federation of Perioperative Nurses (IFPN)

The International Federation of Perioperative Nurses (IFPN), launched in 1999, is the only international specialty organisation representing perioperative nurses at a global level, through its affiliation with the ICN. In this capacity, the IFPN is involved in international activities, strategic engagement and formation of policies on nursing issues, exercising influence in relation to perioperative nursing activity, with a number of affiliate specialty groups within the ICN and WHO agendas. The IFPN represents more than 450,000 perioperative nurses in 15 national organisations worldwide including the AfPP (UK), ACORN (Australia), AORN (US), CORN (China), EORNA (25 European countries), SPN (India), IPNA (Israel), GORNA (Greece), KAORN (South Korea), JONA (Japan), ORNAC (Canada), PIORNA (Pacific Islands), PNCNZ (New Zealand), PNGPNS (Papua New Guinea), SOBECC (Brazil) and TSORA (Turkey) (IFPN, 2020).

The IFPN's mission is to *'support perioperative nurses working towards improving patient care globally; by promoting a safe surgical experience for patients, through evidence-based best researched practice standards and education, together with member organisations and other relevant collaborators'* (IFPN, 2020). The IFPN is particularly committed to improving standards of patient care in developing countries and its activities are focused on providing universally applicable guidelines for practice. There are IFPN 'ambassadors' for Africa, South America and the Asia Pacific to support perioperative nursing in these regions (Melville, 2019) and the IFPN provides open access via its website to position statements and educational tools, including many from other global professional associations.

The Association of Perioperative Registered Nurses (AORN)

The Association of Perioperative Registered Nurses (AORN) is based in the US and was founded in 1949, making it one of the oldest PNAs globally (AORN, 2020a). AORN offers membership plus a wide range of educational and other services including online resources, a core curriculum for delivery by health facilities and a number of perioperative journals. It articulates nursing practices for surgical patients by researching and distributing evidence-based recommendations in a similar way to other PNAs. AORN's *Guidelines for perioperative practice* (AORN, 2020b) are used in many countries outside the US including New Zealand, to inform perioperative practices and support local standards (NZNO, 2014d). AORN is also politically active with a structured and planned approach to influencing health policy. One example of AORN successfully engaging its members to achieve an organisational goal is its lobbying for the enactment of legislation in all US states to ensure that every OR has an RN circulator (Hamlin, 2012).

The Association for Perioperative Practice (AfPP)

The Association for Perioperative Practice (AfPP) is based in the United Kingdom (UK). It was founded in 1964 as the National Association of Theatre Nurses (NATN). Its name was changed in 2005 to reflect the growing membership and inclusion of support worker roles and operating department practitioners (AfPP, n.d.). The AfPP's *Standards and recommendations for safe perioperative practice* provide guidance for local policies governing staff within UK perioperative settings and associated sterilisation services. It also publishes a journal of perioperative practice and produces a number of educational resources.

The Papua New Guinea Perioperative Nurses Society (PNGPNS)

Established in 2004, the Papua New Guinea Perioperative Nurses Society (PNGPNS) has aimed to provide advice to the government on health department policy and functions as a perioperative education forum (Woodhead, 2006). The PNGPNS has grown steadily across many of the country's provinces with a membership base of 350 nurses, including those employed in operating theatres as well as surgical wards, intensive care units and emergency departments (Laim, 2019). The society holds an annual conference to bring colleagues together for discussion and sharing of new knowledge on care of the surgical patient.

The Pacific Islands Operating Room Nurses Association (PIORNA)

The Pacific Islands Operating Room Nurses Association (PIORNA) was formally established in 2019 to promote the practice and ethical principles of OR nurses across the Pacific region (Mamea, 2019) (Feature box 1.4). PIORNA is the sole professional association within the Pacific region specifically for operating room nurses, with its membership base representing 14 individual Pacific Island countries (PICs). Geographically, PIORNA membership stretches from the northern and western PICs (Palau, Federated States of Micronesia, Republic of Marshall Islands, Kiribati and Nauru) to the central and southern PICs (Solomon Islands, Vanuatu, Fiji, Tuvalu, Tokelau, Samoa, Tonga, Niue and Cook Islands). PIORNA aims to promote activities that provide for the exchange of information as well as continuing education, peer review and research in OR nursing. On a practical level, PIORNA also functions as a forum for OR nurses in PICs to discuss matters affecting their practice (PIORNA, 2019). PIORNA gained pre-membership status with the IFPN during its formation and continues to build upon its membership base within PICs and Australasia (ACORN, n.d.).

Professional Practice Standards

As the national regulatory bodies for nursing, the NMBA and the NCNZ produce a number of professional standards as well as the codes of conduct and ethics. While these national documents relate to all nurses in general and are by nature overarching, they are none the less important because they inform specialty nursing practice for NPs, RNs and ENs in their respective countries.

Specialty professional **practice standards** define perioperative nurses as a community and function as a reminder for professional practice, assisting perioperative nurses when advocating for consistency in quality patient care. Standards are often used to ensure the quality of professional work and make principles of practice more transparent for user groups, consumers and other stakeholders. Standards provide minimum requirements for practice and are regarded as generally accepted principles of patient care and perioperative management. In healthcare, standards provide a common language and set of expectations that enable healthcare professionals, systems and organisations to work together for the best patient outcomes. Standards and guidelines for practice are also dynamic because there is an imperative for continual, rigorous review and updating in response to changes in healthcare

---

FEATURE BOX 1.4
Perioperative Nursing Standards in Pacific Island Countries (PICs)

The Pacific Islands Operating Room Nurses Association (PIORNA) is the professional association for OR nurses in 14 Pacific Island countries (PICs). PIORNA's origins date back to 2015, when reports from Royal Australasian College of Surgeons (RACS) visiting surgical teams in these countries noted regional discrepancies in OR nursing practices (Davies, Sutherland-Fraser, Taoi, & Williams, 2016). In response, a Pacific-based organisation (Strengthening Specialised Clinical Services in the Pacific [SSCSiP]) assembled a small working group of OR nurse representatives to devise solutions to the issue. The group initiated an international project to identify and develop the first benchmark in nursing standards for Pacific perioperative nurses. The project included perioperative nurse consultants from Australia (Health Education & Learning Partnerships [HE&LP]) and was supported by ACORN and the IFPN, who shared their perioperative standards as reference documents.

The Pacific Perioperative Practice Bundle (PPPB) project was funded by governmental agencies (AusAID and the Pacific Community SPC) and, within a year, the group developed the first bundle of standards. The following year, the group held its first regional implementation workshop with the addition of financial support from ACORN (Davies, Sutherland-Fraser, Mamea, Raddie, & Taoi, et al., 2017). The group subsequently produced the second bundle of standards and held two further regional implementation workshops. The third bundle of standards was completed in 2021. The project has produced sixteen perioperative practice standards in total, grouped into three bundles: infection control, patient safety and safe environment. A matching bundle of audit tools was developed to measure OR nurses' and facility compliance with these standards. Audit results, implementation success stories and lessons learned have been shared within the PICs, presented at conferences both regionally and internationally and published in journals (Isaia et al., 2018; Mamea & Nofoaiga, 2019; Mamea et al., 2018; Raddie, 2019; Sutherland-Fraser & Davies, 2017; Taoi & Sutherland-Fraser, 2016).

Since coming together in 2015, the group has continued to pursue bigger dreams for Pacific perioperative nurses and a better future. An interim committee was established in 2018 with the PIORNA constitution ratified in 2019, guided by foundation documents used to establish professional associations in Papua New Guinea and Africa (Davis & Woodhead, 2005; Woodhead, 2006). At the start of 2019, PIORNA successfully registered its pre-membership of the IFPN. A more significant milestone was achieved later in 2019, when PIORNA was formally registered in Samoa as the professional body for perioperative nursing across the Pacific. A small setback was the deferment of PIORNA's 2020 inaugural conference due to the COVID-19 pandemic.

The geographical spread of PIORNA's membership base, the diversity of healthcare systems and unpredictable supply lines are ongoing challenges for this newborn association. Despite such challenges, the success of PIORNA's journey so far has been demonstrated by recognition of the PPPB as the minimum standards for perioperative nursing in the Pacific and the uptake of PPPB audit programs to measure compliance across the PICs. Furthermore, reports by RACS visiting surgical teams to these countries since the project's inception have verified the improvements in OR nursing practices.

(Sources: Nerrie Raddie, PIORNA Interim Secretary (Solomon Islands); Natasha Mamea, PIORNA Interim President (Samoa); Mabel Hazelman Taoi, The Pacific Community.)

---

practice, policy and legislation, and the emergence of new research, technologies and trends in surgery (ACORN, 2019b; Halcomb, Stephens, Bryce, Foley, & Ashley, 2017; Schmidt & McArthur, 2018). In Australia, their standing has been clearly demonstrated in the law courts; this is further explored in Chapter 3.

RESEARCH AND EVIDENCE-BASED PRACTICE

The field of implementation science promotes the uptake of research findings and, as such, it is becoming an increasingly important skill for healthcare professionals (Wensing & Grol, 2019). Before new research findings make their way into practice, they need to be synthesised, understood and shared through a dynamic process known as knowledge translation (KT) (Curtis, Fry, Shaban, & Considine, 2016). This process may also be useful in identifying long-standing practices which lack an evidence base (Wensing & Grol, 2019). Perioperative nurses use research findings in a variety of ways in practice and on a daily basis. For example, the World Health Organization Surgical Safety Checklist (WHO SSC) has been shown to decrease patient morbidity and mortality (Shear et al., 2018). Where possible, evidence-based research findings underpin the ACORN (2020n) standards and AORN's *Guidelines for perioperative practice* (AORN, 2020b, 2020c). Perioperative nurse clinicians also conduct research into their own practice, often in collaboration with others. Research boxes 1.1 and 1.2 present the findings of research projects that should be of interest to all perioperative nurses regardless of their experience.

RESEARCH BOX 1.2
Surgical Hand Antisepsis to Reduce Surgical Site Infection

Medical professionals routinely carry out surgical hand antisepsis before undertaking invasive procedures to destroy transient microorganisms and inhibit the growth of resident microorganisms. Antisepsis may reduce the risk of surgical site infections (SSIs) in patients. A Cochrane review assessed the effects of surgical hand antisepsis on the numbers of colony-forming units (CFUs) of bacteria on the hands of the surgical team. The review concluded that, although there was no firm evidence that one type of hand antisepsis is better than another in reducing SSIs, chlorhexidine gluconate scrubs may reduce the number of CFUs on hands compared with povidone iodine scrubs. Alcohol rubs with additional antiseptic ingredients may reduce CFUs compared with aqueous scrubs alone. With regard to duration of hand antisepsis, the review concluded that a 3-minute initial scrub reduced CFUs on the hand compared with a 2-minute scrub.

(Source: Tanner, J., Dumville, J., Norman, G., & Fortnam, M. (2016). Surgical hand antisepsis to reduce surgical site infection. *Cochrane Database of Systematic Reviews*, 1. CD004288.)

An Evidence-based Approach to Practice

Duff and colleagues (2014) identify the commitment to **evidence-based practice** (EBP) as a defining difference between the nursing profession and technicians, or non-nurses. The perioperative nurse's engagement with the latest EBP enables them to critically appraise the evidence and determine its application to practice (Hunt, 2018). The perioperative nurse's ability to justify department policies or aspects of patient care is demonstrated most effectively when the nurse can articulate the rationales for their practice. While there will always be a requirement to follow departmental policies, this does not equate with a rationale for practice. If told that 'the policy says we should do it this way', the new perioperative nurse should enquire about the rationale beyond this explanation. For example, perioperative staff completely cover their hair not because it is a policy requirement but because of the rationale that human hair harbours bacteria and other microorganisms that may contribute to patients' surgical site infections (SSIs) and staff must minimise the dispersal of such microorganisms by wearing hats or scarves that completely cover and contain their hair (Spruce, 2017).

The perioperative nurse can seek rationales for practice from organisations that promote and support the synthesis, transfer and utilisation of evidence. The Cochrane Collaboration is a global independent network of researchers, professionals, patients and carers that publishes systematic reviews of the effects of healthcare interventions and summaries of the latest research findings. These are accessible resources for nurses seeking to support and justify changes to practice. The Joanna Briggs Institute (JBI) is an international agency, collaborating internationally with more than 70 entities worldwide and incorporating nursing, midwifery and allied health research findings. Systematic reviews that inform perioperative nursing practice include:

- Cochrane reviews
  - Surgical hand antisepsis to reduce surgical site infections (Tanner et al., 2016) (see Research box 1.2)
  - Supplemental perioperative intravenous crystalloids for postoperative nausea and vomiting (Jewer et al., 2019)
- JBI systematic reviews
  - Pediatric postanaesthesia care unit discharge criteria: a scoping review protocol (Ryals & Palokas, 2017)
  - Effectiveness of teaching strategies to improve critical thinking in nurses in clinical practice: a systematic review protocol (da Costa Carbogim et al., 2017).

Although nurses should foster evidence-based practice, there is a significant delay in the transfer of research results to their practice (Camargo et al., 2018). To improve patient outcomes, however, perioperative nurses have a responsibility to seek ways to implement research into their practice. Skills developed in EBP not only enable perioperative nurses to justify department policies, but also enhance their ability to explain the care they are providing for their patients (Spruce, 2015).

PATIENT SCENARIOS

SCENARIO 1.4: EVIDENCE-BASED PRACTICE

Now consider EBP from the perspective of EN Macedo, the anaesthetic nurse caring for Mrs Patricia Peterson. EN Macedo will need to explain to Mrs Peterson that he is covering her with a blanket filled with warmed air not only for her comfort but also because her temperature is lower than 36°C. When Mrs Peterson asks why her temperature is so important, he will be able to explain that her low temperature may increase her recovery time and may also increase her risk of developing a postoperative wound infection (Duff et al., 2017). It should be noted that, when explaining the reason behind any care activity or intervention, the perioperative nurse must always consider each patient's capacity and individual desire to be informed before making a clinical judgement about how much information is appropriate to provide.

THE FUTURE OF PERIOPERATIVE NURSING

The safe and efficient delivery of health services is reliant on a highly educated workforce and IS adaptable to change. Workforce innovation is therefore an important consideration for the healthcare sector, particularly the development of nursing roles, including roles that may challenge professional boundaries. Influences for change in nursing practice arise for several reasons, not the least of which may be work practice changes, such as the introduction of new models of care initiated by organisations or professional groups, changes in other health professions or emergence of new healthcare roles (NMBA, 2020a).

The development of advanced practice roles for RNs which were explored earlier in this chapter, such as the NP, PNSA or RNFSA roles, are examples of how these influences for change have shaped perioperative nursing practice in Australia and New Zealand during the past decade. The journey towards advanced practice roles for ENs in Australia has been slower than in New Zealand, where the EN instrument nurse role has been a constant feature of the perioperative workforce. Once considered an advanced practice role for ENs in Australia, the piloting of state-wide education programs and policy to articulate the scope of practice has seen the EN instrument nurse role accepted as part of the perioperative nursing model in Australia. It should be noted that appropriate allocation of the instrument nurse role (and indeed all nursing roles) remains dependent on the specific patient's needs and the knowledge, skills and scope of practice of the individual nurse, whether the allocation is to an RN or an EN (ACORN, 2020i).

Ancillary and Unregulated Worker Roles

In Australia, ancillary workers represent a small but important part of the perioperative workforce (ACN, 2019b). Earlier in this chapter, we acknowledged the varying levels of education and skills sets of the ancillary workers who provide care to surgical patients during their perioperative journey. This mix includes roles which fall outside the remit of regulatory bodies, such as AINs, PCAs, HCAs, orderlies and sterilisation technicians, as well as regulated roles such as nursing, medical and/or allied health students. It is important to note that the long-standing ancillary role of the anaesthetic technician is regulated in New Zealand, with a national accreditation process for the qualifications and training providers (MSCNZ, 2021). The Australian Anaesthesia Allied Health Practitioners (AAAHP) is a professional body which supports the interests of anaesthesia technicians and continues to work towards national registration of the role in Australia (AAAHP, 2015). The New Zealand Anaesthetic Technicians' Society (NZATS) is the equivalent professional body representing anaesthetic technicians in New Zealand (NZATS, n.d.).

RNs and midwives are expected to be flexible to meet the changing demands of healthcare and to make safe decisions about when and if certain aspects of patient care can be delegated to ancillary and unregulated workers (NMBA, 2020a) (see Table 1.2). The NMBA and the NCNZ both publish national decision-making guidelines and frameworks to assist RNs and midwives not only to understand the limits of their own scope of practice, but also to support them to make safe delegations of patient care to these other healthcare workers (NCNZ, 2010, 2012b, 2012c; NMBA, 2020a).

ACORN's position on ancillary workers is that they must work under the supervision and management of appropriately educated and experienced RNs at all times (ACORN, 2020c), providing indirect patient care only. In the UK, the RN also works in a multidisciplinary team. This may include diploma-prepared, non-nurse, operating department practitioners (ODPs), who are regulated and who undertake activities traditionally completed by nurses. In the US, the non-nursing role of the scrub technologist is supervised by the RN circulating nurse. Legislation has been enacted in many US states to ensure that there is at least one RN present in the OR, working as the circulating nurse (AORN, 2019) to oversee nursing care and supervise workers such as the scrub technologist.

While discussions about professional roles and responsibilities in the perioperative environment are at times controversial, nursing practice and nurses need to be flexible and able to adjust to changes in the healthcare environment, especially in ways that are beneficial for perioperative patients (NMBA, 2020a).

PATIENT SCENARIOS

SCENARIO 1.5: DELEGATION IN THE OR

RN Sandy Pereira is in the tea-room at lunch and meets up with an old colleague, RN Ben Lumby, who now works part-time as a PNSA with one of the orthopaedic surgeons in the private sector. RN Lumby tells RN Pereira that he has had a very enjoyable morning circulating in the orthopaedic list because he knows Silvana Perez, the medical company representative (MCR). RN

Lumby tells RN Pereira that Silvana has been helpful and has been opening the sterile stock while he has been completing the documentation on the computer. Silvana has also been opening the prostheses, which RN Pereira knows is not an appropriate role or delegation for Silvana (MCRs are visitors to the facility and are non-regulated members of the perioperative team).

Critical Thinking Question

- Outline RN Lumby's responsibilities as circulating nurse when working with visitors such as Silvana and other MCRs. Include rationales for your answers. You may benefit from reviewing your local policy or the relevant professional standards about delegation to unregulated workers and/or visitors to the perioperative environment (ACORN, 2020o; NCNZ, 2012d; NMBA, 2020a) and your relevant professional nursing standards when considering your response.

SCENARIO 1.6: PERIOPERATIVE PRACTICE

One of RN Rob Cohen's friends who is now working in the oncology ward of your hospital challenges him with this question: 'When are you going to take up real nursing again?'

Critical Thinking Questions

- Has this happened to you or one of your colleagues? What two examples of perioperative patient care from your own experience would you describe as 'real nursing' in response to this question?
- Provide rationales that explain how these two examples of your practice as a 'real nurse' reflect the philosophy of perioperative nursing and patient-centred care. You may prefer to answer this question using your patient scenario in this chapter: Mrs Patricia Peterson.

CONCLUSION

In this introductory chapter, we have outlined the regulatory environment in Australia and New Zealand and defined key aspects of nursing regulation such as scope of practice, accountability and responsibility. A brief history of perioperative nursing and its underpinning philosophy of culturally safe and holistic patient care set the context for descriptions of the perioperative patient journey and the patient care roles performed by perioperative nurses. We have explored the role of professional nursing associations and highlighted the importance of practice standards and the role of evidence-based practice for perioperative nursing. In closing, we have considered the future of perioperative nursing practice and established the need for the specialty to adjust to changes in the healthcare environment that improve the delivery of perioperative patient care. Throughout the chapter, we have asked you, the reader, to reflect on patient scenarios relating to clinical care and perioperative nursing roles. These scenarios will continue to unfold in coming chapters.

RESOURCES

Agency for Clinical Innovation (ACI)
https://aci.health.nsw.gov.au
Anaesthesia Perioperative Care Network
https://aci.health.nsw.gov.au/networks/anaesthesia-perioperative-care
Association of periOperative Registered Nurses (AORN)
https://www.aorn.org

Austin Hospital Victoria, State Endoscopy Training Centre
https://www.austin.org.au/StateEndoscopyTrainingCentre/
Australian Anaesthesia Allied Health Practitioners (AAAHP)
    https://www.aaahp.org.au/
Australian Association of Nurse Surgical Assistants (AANSA)
https://www.aansa.org.au
Australian College of Nursing (ACN)
https://www.acn.edu.au
Australian College of Perianaesthesia Nurses (ACPAN)
https://acpan.edu.au
Australian College of Perioperative Nurses (ACORN)
https://www.acorn.org.au
Australian Education Network
https://www.australianuniversities.com.au
Australian Health Practitioner Regulation Agency (AHPRA)
https://www.ahpra.gov.au
https://www.ahpra.gov.au/About-AHPRA/What-We-Do/
    Legislation.aspx
Cochrane Library
https://www.cochranelibrary.com
College of Nurses Aotearoa New Zealand
https://www.nurse.org.nz
International Federation of Perioperative Nurses (IFPN)
https://www.ifpn.org.uk
https://www.ifpn.world/resources/education-tools
Joanna Briggs Institute
https://joannabriggs.org
New Zealand Health Workforce Statistics
https://www.health.govt.nz/nz-health-statistics/health-statistics-
    and-data-sets/workforce-data-and-stats
New Zealand Nurses Organisation (NZNO)
https://www.nzno.org.nz
Nursing and Midwifery Board of Australia (NMBA)
https://www.nursingmidwiferyboard.gov.au

Nursing Council of New Zealand (NCNZ)
https://www.nursingcouncil.org.nz
https://www.nursingcouncil.org.nz/Public/Nursing/Standards_ and_guidelines/NCNZ/nursing-section/Standards_and_ guidelines_for_nurses.aspx?hkey=9fc06ae7-a853-4d10-b5fe-992cd44ba3de
Perioperative Nurses College (PNC) of NZNO
https://www.nzno.org.nz/groups/colleges/perioperative_ nurses_college
Professional Development and Recognition Programmes (PDRP)
https://www.nzno.org.nz/support/professional_development
Queensland Health
https://www.health.qld.gov.au/nmoq/optimisingnursing/ endoscopy.asp

REFERENCES

Agency for Clinical Innovation (ACI). (2015). *Minimum standards for safe procedural sedation. Anaesthesia Perioperative Care Network and Surgical Services Taskforce.* Retrieved from <https://www.aci.health.nsw.gov.au/resources/anaesthesia-perioperative-care/sedation/safe-sedation-resources>.

Agency for Clinical Innovation (ACI). (2016). *The perioperative toolkit webpage [webpage]. Anaesthesia Perioperative Care Network and Surgical Services Taskforce.* Retrieved from <https://www.aci.health.nsw.gov.au/resources/anaesthesia-perioperative-care/the-perioperative-toolkit/the-perioperative-toolkit-webpage>.

Association for Perioperative Practice (AfPP). (n.d.). *About AfPP* [webpage]. Retrieved from <https://www.afpp.org.uk/about-AfPP>.

Association of periOperative Registered Nurses (AORN). (2019). AORN position statement on perioperative registered nurse circulator dedicated to every patient undergoing an operative or other invasive procedure. *AORN Journal, 110*(1), 82–85. https://dx.doi.org/10.1002/aorn.12741

Association of periOperative Registered Nurses (AORN). (2020a). *About AORN* [webpage]. Retrieved from <https://www.a.org/about-aorn>.

Association of periOperative Registered Nurses (AORN). (2020b). *Guidelines for perioperative practice.* Retrieved from <https://aornguidelines.org/guidelines?bookid=2260>.

Association of periOperative Registered Nurses (AORN). (2020c). *Evidence-based practice* [online]. Retrieved from https://www.aorn.org/guidelines/clinical-resources/evidence-based-practice.

Austin Health. (2015). *State endoscopy training centre.* Retrieved from <https://www.austin.org.au/StateEndoscopyTrainingCentre>.

Australian Anaesthesia Allied Health Practitioners (AAAHP). (2016). *AAAHP Code of conduct.* Retrieved from <https://www.aaahp.org.au/resources/Documents/pdf/conduct2016.pdf>.

Australian Anaesthesia Allied Health Practitioners (AAAHP). (2018). *AAAHP Constitution.* Retrieved from <https://www.aaahp.org.au/resources/Documents/pdf/constitution2018.pdf>.

Australasian College of Cosmetic Surgery (ACCS). (2015). *Professional practice standards and scope of practice for aesthetic nursing practice in Australia.* Retrieved from <https://www.accs.org.au/images/uploads/images/final-professional-practice-standards-scope-practice-aesthetic-nursing-practice-in-australia-20150709.pdf>.

Australian and New Zealand College of Anaesthetists (ANZCA). (2014). *PS09 guidelines on sedation and/or analgesia for diagnostic and interventional medical, dental or surgical procedures.* Canberra: Author. Retrieved from <https://www.anzca.edu.au/resources/professional-documents>.

Australian and New Zealand College of Anaesthetists (ANZCA). (2015). *PS08 BP 2015 statement on the assistant for the anaesthetic* [Background paper]. Canberra: Author. Retrieved from <https://www.anzca.edu.au/resources/professional-documents>.

Australian and New Zealand College of Anaesthetists (ANZCA). (2016). *PS08 statement on the assistant for the anaesthetist.* Canberra: Author. Retrieved from <https://www.anzca.edu.au/resources/professional-documents>.

Australian Association of Nurse Surgical Assistants (AANSA). (2012). *AANSA position description – perioperative nurse surgical assistant.* Retrieved from <http://www.aansa.org.au/about/scope-of-practice.aspx>.

Australian College of Nursing (ACN). (2018). *Graduate certificates.* Retrieved from <https://www.acn.edu.au/postgraduate>.

Australian College of Nursing (ACN). (2019a). *HLT64115 Advanced Diploma of Nursing.* Retrieved from <https://www.acn.edu.au/education/vet-courses>.

Australian College of Nursing (ACN). (2019b). *Regulation of the unregulated health care workforce across the health care system – a White Paper by ACN 2019.* Canberra: Author. Retrieved from <https://www.acn.edu.au/wp-content/uploads/white-paper-regulation-unregulated-health-care-workforce-across-health-care-system.pdf>.

Australian College of Nursing (ACN). (2020a). *Nurse administering cosmetic treatment and cosmetic procedures* [Information sheet]. Retrieved from <https://www.acn.edu.au/wp-content/uploads/info-sheet-nurses-administering-cosmetic-treatment-procedures.pdf>.

Australian College of Nursing (ACN). (2020b). *About us* [webpage]. Retrieved from <https://www.acn.edu.au/about-us/who-we-are-what-we-do>.

Australian College of Nursing (ACN). (2020c). *Education* [webpage]. Retrieved from <https://www.acn.edu.au/education>.

Australian College of Perianaesthesia Nurses (ACPAN). (2019). *History and mission.* Retrieved from <https://acpan.edu.au/about/>.

Australian College of Perioperative Nurses (ACORN). (2020a). *ACORN standards for perioperative nursing in Australia* (16th ed., Vol. 2). Accountability for practice, Adelaide: Author. Retrieved from <https://www.acorn.org.au/standards>.

Australian College of Perioperative Nurses (ACORN). (2020b). *ACORN standards for perioperative nursing in Australia.* (16th ed., Vol. 2). Enrolled nurse. Adelaide: Author. Retrieved from <https://www.acorn.org.au/standards>.

Australian College of Perioperative Nurses (ACORN). (2020c). *ACORN standards for perioperative nursing in Australia.* (16th ed., Vol. 2). Ancillary workers. Adelaide: Author. Retrieved from <https://www.acorn.org.au/standards>.

Australian College of Perioperative Nurses (ACORN). (2020d). *ACORN standards for perioperative nursing in Australia.* (16th ed., Vol. 2). Circulating nurse. Adelaide: Author. Retrieved from <https://www.acorn.org.au/standards>.

Australian College of Perioperative Nurses (ACORN). (2020e). *ACORN standards for perioperative nursing in Australia.* (16th ed., Vol. 2). Professional development. Adelaide: Author. Retrieved from <https://www.acorn.org.au/standards>.

Australian College of Perioperative Nurses (ACORN). (2020f). *ACORN standards for perioperative nursing in Australia.* (16th ed., Vol. 2). Cultural diversity. Adelaide: Author. Retrieved from <https://www.acorn.org.au/standards>.

Australian College of Perioperative Nurses (ACORN). (2020g). *ACORN standards for perioperative nursing in Australia.* (16th ed., Vol. 2). Preoperative patient assessments and education nurse. Adelaide: Author. Retrieved from <https://www.acorn.org.au/standards>.

Australian College of Perioperative Nurses (ACORN). (2020h). *ACORN standards for perioperative nursing in Australia.* (16th ed., Vol. 2). Anaesthetic nurse. Adelaide: Author. Retrieved from <https://www.acorn.org.au/standards>.

Australian College of Perioperative Nurses (ACORN). (2020i). *ACORN standards for perioperative nursing in Australia.* (16th ed., Vol. 2). Instrument nurse. Adelaide: Author. Retrieved from <https://www.acorn.org.au/standards>.

Australian College of Perioperative Nurses (ACORN). (2020j). *ACORN standards for perioperative nursing in Australia.* (16th ed., Vol. 2). Post anaesthesia care unit nurse. Adelaide: Author. Retrieved from <https://www.acorn.org.au/standards>.

Australian College of Perioperative Nurses (ACORN). (2020k). *ACORN standards for perioperative nursing in Australia.* (16th ed., Vol. 2). Advanced practice nursing and nurse practitioner roles. Adelaide: Author. Retrieved from <https://www.acorn.org.au/standards>.

Australian College of Perioperative Nurses (ACORN). (2020l). *ACORN standards for perioperative nursing in Australia.* (16th ed., Vol. 2). Perioperative nurse surgeon's assistant. Adelaide: Author. Retrieved from <https://www.acorn.org.au/standards>.

Australian College of Perioperative Nurses (ACORN). (2020m). *ACORN standards for perioperative nursing in Australia.* (16th ed., Vol. 2). Undergraduate nursing students. Adelaide: Author. Retrieved from <https://www.acorn.org.au/standards>.

Australian College of Perioperative Nurses (ACORN). (2020n). *ACORN standards for perioperative nursing in Australia.* (16th ed., Vol. 2). Introduction. Adelaide: Author. Retrieved from <https://www.acorn.org.au/standards>.

Australian College of Perioperative Nurses (ACORN). (2020o). *ACORN standards for perioperative nursing in Australia.* (16th ed., Vol. 2). Visitors. Adelaide: Author. Retrieved from <https://www.acorn.org.au/standards>.

Australian College of Perioperative Nurses (ACORN). (2021a). *Perioperative nursing career pathways.* Retrieved from <https://www.acorn.org.au/perioperative-careers>.

Australian College of Perioperative Nurses (ACORN). (2021b). *ACORN history.* Retrieved from <https://www.acorn.org.au/acorn-history>.

Australian College of Perioperative Nurses (ACORN). (2021c). *Strategy and implementation plan 2019–2022.* Retrieved from <https://www.acorn.org.au/strategic-plan>.

Australian College of Perioperative Nurses (ACORN). (n.d.). *Pacific Islands Operating Room Nurses Association (PIORNA).* Retrieved from <https://www.acorn.org.au/piorna>.

Australian Commission on Safety and Quality in Health Care (ACSQHC/the Commission). (2018). *Essential elements for comprehensive care delivery.* Retrieved from <https://www.safetyandquality.gov.au/our-work/comprehensive-care/essential-elements-comprehensive-care>.

Australian Day Surgery Nurses Association (ADSNA). (2017a). *About day surgery* [webpage]. Retrieved from <http://adsna.info/abdaysurgery.php>.

Australian Day Surgery Nurses Association (ADSNA). (2017b). *History* [webpage]. Retrieved from <http://adsna.info/history.php>.

Australian Health Practitioner Regulation Agency (AHPRA). (2018). *What we do/Legislation.* Canberra: Author. Retrieved from <http://www.ahpra.gov.au/About-AHPRA/What-We-Do/Legislation.aspx>.

Australian Human Rights Commission (AHRC). (2018). *Cultural safety for Aboriginal and Torres Strait Islander children and young people: a background paper to inform work on child safe organisations.* Retrieved from <https://www.humanrights.gov.au/our-work/childrens-rights/child-safe-organisations-and-cultural-safety>.

Australian Institute of Health and Welfare (AIHW). (2019). *Hospitals at a glance 2017–18.* Retrieved from <https://www.aihw.gov.au/reports/hospitals/hospitals-at-a-glance-2017-18>.

Australian Nursing and Midwifery Federation (ANMF). (2014). *About the ANMF.* Canberra: Author. Retrieved from <http://anmf.org.au/pages/about-landing>.

Australian Nursing and Midwifery Federation (ANMF). (2016). *Policy: Nursing specialty.* Canberra: Author. Retrieved from <http://anmf.org.au/documents/policies/P_Nursing_specialty.pdf>.

Australian Nursing and Midwifery Federation (ANMF). (2017). *Policy: nurse practitioners.* Canberra: Author. Retrieved from <http://anmf.org.au/documents/policies/P_Nurse_Practitioners.pdf>.

Bezemer, J., Korkiakanagas, T., Weldon, S., Kress, G., & Kneebone, R. (2016). Unsettled teamwork: communication and learning in the operating theatres of an urban hospital. *Journal of Advanced Nursing, 72*(2), 361–372.

Blomberg, A., Bisholt, B., Nilsson, J., & Lindwall, L. (2015). Making the invisible visible – operating theatre nurses' perception of caring in perioperative practice. *Scandinavian Journal of Caring Sciences, 29,* 361–368.

Camargo, F., Iwamoto, H., Galvao, C., Pereira, G., Andrade, R., & Masso, G. (2018). Competences and barriers for the evidence-based practice in nursing: an integrative review. *Revista Brasileira de Enfermagem, 71*(4), 2030–2038.

Carryer, J., Wilkinson, J., Towers, A., & Gardner, G. (2018). Delineating advanced practice nursing in New Zealand: a national survey. *International Nursing Review, 65*(1), 24–32. https://dx.doi.org/10.1111/inr.12427

Congress of Aboriginal and Torres Strait Islander Nurses and Midwives (CATSINaM). (2014). *Cultural safety position statement.* Retrieved from <https://www.catsinam.org.au/communications/publications>.

Congress of Aboriginal and Torres Strait Islander Nurses and Midwives (CATSINaM). (2017). *Position statement: embedding cultural safety across Australian nursing and midwifery.* Retrieved from <https://www.catsinam.org.au/static/uploads/files/embedding-cultural-safety-across-australian-nursing-and-midwifery-may-2017-wfca.pdf>.

Cousley, A. (2015). Vulnerability in perioperative patients: a qualitative study. *Journal of Perioperative Practice, 25*(12), 246–256.

Cox, L. G., & Simpson, A. (2015). Cultural safety, diversity and the servicer user and carer movement in mental health research. *Nursing Inquiry, 22*(4), 306–316. https://dx.doi.org/10.1111/nin.12096

Curtis, K., Fry, M., Shaban R. Z., & Considine, J. (2016). Translating research findings to clinical nursing practice. *Journal of Clinical Nursing, 26*, 862–872. https://dx.doi.org/10.1111/jocn.13586

da Costa Carbogim, F., de Oliveria, L., Campos, G., Araujo Nunes, E., Alves, K., & Puschel, V. (2017). Effectiveness of teaching strategies to improve critical thinking in nurses in clinical practice: a systematic review protocol. *JBI Database of Systematic Reviews and Implementation Reports, 15*(6), 1602–1611.

Davies, M., Sutherland-Fraser, S., Mamea, N., Raddie, N., & Taoi, M. H. (2017). Implementing standards in Pacific Island countries: the Pacific perioperative practice bundle (Part 2). *Journal of Perioperative Nursing in Australia, 30*(1), 41–48.

Davies, M., Sutherland-Fraser, S., Taoi, M. H., & Williams, C. (2016). Developing standards in Pacific Island countries: the Pacific perioperative practice bundle (Part 1). *Journal of Perioperative Nursing in Australia, 29*(2), 42–47.

Davis, P., & Woodhead, K. (2005). *Toolkit for Start-up Specialist Nursing Organisations (revised 2016)* [unpublished resource provided by authors].

Davis and Woodhead, 2018 revision for ICN is available from <https://www.ifpn.world/resources/education-tools.

Davoodvand, S., Abbaszadeh, A., & Ahmadi, F. (2016). Patient advocacy from the clinical nurses' viewpoint: a qualitative study, *Journal of Medical Ethics and History of Medicine, 9*(5), 1–9e.

Delaney, D., Bayley, E., Olszewsky, P., & Gallagher, J. (2015). Parental satisfaction with paediatric preoperative assessment and education in a pre-surgical care centre, *Journal of PeriAnaesthesia Nursing, 30*(4), 290–300.

Duff, J., Butler, M., Davies, M., Williams, R., & Carlile, J. (2014). Perioperative nurses' knowledge, practice attitude and perceived barriers to evidence use: a multisite, cross-sectional survey. *ACORN Journal, 27*(4), 28–35.

Duff, J., Walker, K., Edward, K., Ralph, N., Giandianato, J., Alexander, K., Gow, J., & Stephenson, J. (2017). Effect of a thermal care bundle on the prevention, detection and treatment of perioperative inadvertent hypothermia, *Journal of Clinical Nursing, 27*(5–6), 1239–1249.

Duffield, C., Chapman, S., & Rowbotham, S. (2017). Nurse-performed endoscopy: implications for the nursing profession in Australia, *Policy, Politics, and Nursing Practice, 18*(1), 36–43.

Duncan, N., Bonney, D., Au, C., & Bennett, P. (2017). Introduction of the nurse endoscopist role in one Australian health service. *Gastroenterology Nursing, 40*(5), 350–356.

Foran, P. (2016). Undergraduate surgical nursing preparation and guided operating room experience: a quantitative analysis. *Nurse Education in Practice, 16*(1), 217–224. https://dx.doi.org/10.1016/j.nepr.2015.08.005

Gardner, G., Duffield, C., Doubrovsky, A., & Adams, M. (2016). Identifying advanced practice: a national survey of a nursing workforce. *International Journal of Nursing Studies, 55*, 60–70.

Gastroenterological Nurses College of Australia (GENCA). (2015). *Position statement: nurse endoscopist.* Beaumarice: Author. Retrieved from <https://www.gesa.org.au/resources/position-statements/>.

Gillespie, B. M., Harbeck, E., Kang, E., Steel, C., Fairweather, N., & Chaboyer, W. (2017). Correlates of non-technical skills in surgery: a prospective study. *British Medical Journal Open, 7*, 1–9.

Gillespie, B. M., Harbeck, E. B., Falk-Brynhildsen, K., Nilsson, U., & Jaensson, M. (2018). Perceptions of perioperative nursing competence: A cross-country comparison. *BMC Nursing, 17*, 12. https://doi.org/10.1186/s12912-018-0284-0

Goodman, T. (Ed.). (2012). *Advocacy, an issue of perioperative nursing clinics* [E-book], vol. 7(4), The Clinics: Nursing. St. Louis, MO: Saunders/Elsevier Health Sciences.

Gouda, B., Gouda, G., Borle, A., Singh, A., Sinha, A., & Singh, P. M. (2017). Safety of non-anesthesia provider administered propofol sedation in non-advanced gastrointestinal endoscopic procedures: a meta-analysis. *Saudi Journal of Gastroenterology, 23*, 133–143.

Grocott, M. P. W., Plumb, J. O., Edwards, M., & Fecher, I. (2017). Re-designing the pathway to surgery: better care and added value. *Perioperative Medicine, 6*, 9. https://dx.doi.org/10.1186/s13741-017-0065-4

Hains, T., Turner, C., & Strand, H. (2016). Practice audit of the role of the non-medical surgical assistant in Australia, an online survey. *International Journal of Nursing Practice, 22*, 546–555. https://dx.doi.org/10.1111/ijn.12462

Hains, T., Turner, C., & Strand, H. (2017). Knowledge and perceptions of the NMSA role in Australia: a perioperative staff survey. *Journal of Perioperative Nursing, 30*(3), 39–45. https://dx.doi.org/10.26550/2209-1092.1017

Hains, T., Turner, C., & Strand, H. (2018). The non-medical surgical assistant in Australia: who should contribute to governance? *Australian Journal of Advanced Nursing, 35*(2), 51–57.

Halcomb, E., Stephens, M., Bryce, J., Foley, E., & Ashley, C. (2017). The development of professional practice standards for Australian general practice nurses. *Journal of Advanced Nursing, 73*(8), 1958–1969. https://dx.doi.org/10.1111/jan.13274

Hamlin, L. (2020). From theatre to perioperative: A brief history of early surgical nursing. *Journal of Perioperative*

Nursing, 33(4), e-19-24. https://doi.org/10.26550/2209-1092.1107.

Hamlin, L. (2012). International perioperative organizations: diversity, development, divergence. *AORN Journal, 96*(6), 647–651.

Harper, M., & Maloney, P. (2017). The Updated Nursing Professional Development Scope and Standards of Practice. *Journal of continuing education in nursing, 48*(1), 5–7. https://doi.org.acs.hcn.com.au/10.3928/00220124-20170110-02.

Hughes, M. (2018). Cultural safety requires cultural intelligence. *Kai Tiaki Nursing New Zealand, 24*(6), 24–25.

Hunt, D, (2018). Evidence-based, best practice professional standards for perioperative nursing. *ACORN Journal of Perioperative Nursing, 31*(3), 53–54.

Ingvarsdottir, E., & Halldorsdottir, S. (2018). Enhancing patient safety in the operating theatre: from the perspective of experienced operating theatre nurses. *Scandinavian Journal of Caring Sciences, 32*(2), 951–960.

International Collaboration of PeriAnaesthesia Nurses (ICPAN). (2019). *About ICPAN* [webpage]. Retrieved from <https://www.icpan.org/about-us.html>.

International Council of Nurses (ICN). (2012). *The ICN code of ethics for nurses.* Geneva: Author. Retrieved from <https://www.icn.ch/sites/default/files/inline-files/2012_ICN_Codeofethicsfornurses_%20eng.pdf>.

International Council of Nurses (ICN). (2020a). *President's message* [webpage]. Retrieved from <https://www.icn.ch/who-we-are/presidents-message>.

International Council of Nurses (ICN). (2020b). *ICN strategic priorities* [webpage]. Retrieved from <https://www.icn.ch/nursing-policy/icn-strategic-priorities>.

International Federation of Perioperative Nurses. (IFPN). (2020). *International partnerships –IFPN* [webpage]. Retrieved from <https://www.ifpn.world>.

Isaia, H., Raddie, N., Mamea, N., Bio, T., Naitini, A., Kumar, S., & Taraare, R. (2018). *Advancement and innovations in Pacific perioperative nursing practice (conference paper).* Presented by Heaven Isaia and Nerrie Raddie at the 19th South Pacific Nurses Forum, Rarotonga, Cook Islands, 15th–19th October, 2018. Retrieved from <http://www.spnf.org.au>.

Jacob, S. (2016). Chapter 10: Cultural competence and social issues in nursing and health care. In B. Cherry & S. Jacob (Eds.), *Contemporary nursing: issues, trends and management* (7th ed., pp. 179–201). St. Louis, MO: Elsevier.

Jewer, J. K., Wong, M. J., Bird, S. J., Habib, A. S., Parker, R., & George, R. B. (2019). Supplemental perioperative intravenous crystalloids for postoperative nausea and vomiting. *Cochrane Database of Systematic Reviews, 3*, CD012212. https://dx.doi.org/10.1002/14651858.CD012212.pub2

Jones, N., Long, L., & Zeitz, K. (2011). The role of the nurse sedationist. *Collegian, 18*(3), 115–123. https://dx.doi.org/10.1016/j.colegn.2011.04.001

Kaptain, K., Ulsoe, M. L., & Dryer, P. (2019). Surgical perioperative pathways – patient experiences of unmet needs show that a person-centered approach is needed. *Journal of*

Clinical Nursing, 28, 2214–2224. https://dx.doi.org/10.1111/jocn.14817

La Trobe University. (2018). Perioperative nurse surgical assistant (PSNA). Retrieved from <http://latrobe.custhelp.com/app/answers/detail/a_id/2349/~/perioperative-nurse-surgical-assistant-%28pnsa%29>.

Laim, E. (2019). Nurses discuss work ideas. *The National,* 22 November. Retrieved from <https://www.thenational.com.pg/nurses-discuss-work-ideas/>.

Levada, L., Dang-Iw, K., Kuck, E., O'Connor, M., Ravell, V., Whitehouse, N., & Osborne, S. (2018). Above and beyond: enhancing instrument nurses' non-technical skills. *ACORN: The Journal of Perioperative Nursing in Australia, 31*(2), 57–59.

Lynn, A., & Brownie, S. (2015). The perioperative nurse surgeon's assistant: issues and challenges associated with this emerging advanced practice nursing role in Australia. *Collegian, 22*, 109–115. https://dx.doi.org/10.1016/j.clegn.2013.12.004

Malley, A., Kenner, C., Kim, T., & Blakeney, B. (2015). The role of the nurse and the preoperative assessment in patient transition. *AORN Journal, 102*(2), 181.e1–181.e9.

Mamea, N. (2019). *Pacific Islands Operating Room Nurses Association (PIORNA) IFPN Report IFPN Board meeting, York, August 2019.* Retrieved from <https://www.ifpn.world/news/member-country-editorials>.

Mamea, N., & Nofoaiga, M. (2019). *Nursing education and learning: preceptorship in connecting practice and education – the current perspective in Samoa Hospital [unpublished conference paper].* Presented at the 120th International Council of Nurses Congress, Marina Bay Sands, Singapore, June–July 2019.

Mamea, N., Raddie, N., Bio, T., Isaia, H., Naitini, A., & Kumar, S. (2018). *Coming of age of the Pacific perioperative nurses (unpublished conference paper, awarded novice paper prize).* Presented by Natasha Mamea and Nerrie Raddie at the inaugural ACORN & ASIORNA international conference, Adelaide, Australia, 23–26th May 2018.

Medical Sciences Council of New Zealand. (MSCNZ). (2021). *Policy and guidelines: Registration. May 2021.* Retrieved from <https://www.mscouncil.org.nz/resources-2/>.

Medical Sciences Council of New Zealand. (MSCNZ). (2018). *Competence Standards for Anaesthetic Technicians in Aotearoa New Zealand Revised November 2018.* Retrieved from <https://www.mscouncil.org.nz/assets_mlsb/Uploads/RP-MSC003-V3-AT-Competence-Standards-Nov2018.pdf>.

Melville, R. (2019). *IFPN Pacific Islands, PNG and Asia Ambassador report, August 2019.* Retrieved from <https://www.ifpn.world/application/files/9215/6531/1538/IFPN_Ambassador_Report_201916096.pdf>.

Ministry of Health. (2020). New Zealand Legislation (reprinted 1 December 2020). *Health Practitioner Competence Assurance Act 2003.* Retrieved from <www.legislation.govt.nz/act/public/2003/0048/latest/DLM203312.html>.

Muise, G. (2019). Enabling cultural safety in indigenous primary healthcare. *Healthcare Management Forum, 32*(1), 25–31.

Munday, J., Kynoch, K., & Hines, S. (2015). Nurses' experiences of advocacy in the perioperative department: a systematic review. *JBI Database of Systematic Reviews and Implementation Reports, 13*(8), 146–189. Adelaide: JBI Library. https://dx.doi.org/10.11124/jbisrir-2015-2141

Nerland, M., & Karseth, B. (2015). The knowledge work of professional associations: approaches to standardisation and forms of legitimisation. *Journal of Education and Work, 28*(1), 1–23. https://dx.doi.org/10.1080/13639080.2013.802833

New South Wales Parliament. (2018). *Inquiry into cosmetic health service complaints/Parliament of New South Wales, Committee on the Health Care Complaints Commission.* (Report no. 4/56) [online resource]. Retrieved from <https://www.parliament.nsw.gov.au/committees/inquiries/Pages/inquiry-details.aspx?pk=2476>.

New Zealand Anaesthetic Technicians' Society (NZATS). (n.d.). *Membership* [webpage]. Retrieved from <https://www.nzats.co.nz/membership/>.

New Zealand Nurses Organisation (NZNO). (2012). *Guidelines for nurses on the administration of medicines.* Wellington: Author.

New Zealand Nurses Organisation (NZNO). (2014a). *Knowledge and skills framework for registered nurse assistant to the anaesthetist for operating theatre in New Zealand.* Wellington: Author. Retrieved from <https://www.nzno.org.nz/Portals/0/Files/Documents/Groups/Perioperative%20Nurses/Registered%20Nurse%20Assistant%20to%20the%20Anaesthetist.pdf>.

New Zealand Nurses Organisation (NZNO). (2014b). *About us* [webpage]. Retrieved from <https://www.nzno.org.nz/about_us>.

New Zealand Nurses Organisation (NZNO). (2014c). *Welcome to the Perioperative Nurses College of NZNO* [webpage]. Retrieved from <https://www.nzno.org.nz/groups/colleges_sections/colleges/perioperative_nurses_college>.

New Zealand Nurses Organisation (NZNO). (2014d). *Standards* [webpage]. Retrieved from <https://www.nzno.org.nz/groups/colleges_sections/colleges/perioperative_nurses_college/resources/standards_and_documents>.

New Zealand Nurses Organisation (NZNO). (2015). *Registered nurse first surgical assistant for operating theatres in New Zealand service policy guidelines.* Wellington: Author. Retrieved from <https://www.nzno.org.nz/Portals/0/Files/Documents/Groups/Perioperative%20Nurses/RNFSA%20Service%20Guidelines%202014.pdf>.

New Zealand Nurses Organisation (NZNO). (2016). *New Zealand perioperative nursing knowledge and skills framework.* Wellington: Author. Retrieved from <https://www.nzno.org.nz/Portals/0/Files/Documents/Groups/Perioperative%20Nurses/PNC%20KSF%20Book%20Final.pdf>.

New Zealand Society of Gastroenterology (NZSG). (2012). *New Zealand Society of Gastroenterology position statement on nurse endoscopy.* Retrieved from <https://nzsg.org.nz/assets/Uploads/NZSG-Position-Statement-on-Nurse-Endoscopy-151112-Final.pdf>.

Nursing and Midwifery Board of Australia (NMBA). (2014). *Nurse practitioner standards for practice* [updated 2018]. Melbourne: Author. Retrieved from <https://www.nursingmidwiferyboard.gov.au/Codes-Guidelines-Statements/Professional-standards/nurse-practitioner-standards-of-practice.aspx>.

Nursing and Midwifery Board of Australia (NMBA). (2016a). *Advanced nursing practice and specialty areas within nursing* [fact sheet.] Melbourne: Author. Retrieved from <https://www.nursingmidwiferyboard.gov.au/Codes-Guidelines-Statements/FAQ/fact-sheet-advanced-nursing-practice-and-specialty-areas.aspx>.

Nursing and Midwifery Board of Australia (NMBA). (2016b). *Registration standard: Endorsement as a nurse practitioner.* Melbourne: Author. Retrieved from <https://www.nursingmidwiferyboard.gov.au/registration-and-endorsement/endorsements-notations.aspx>.

Nursing and Midwifery Board of Australia (NMBA). (2016c). *Registered nurse standards for practice.* Melbourne: Author. Retrieved from <https://www.nursingmidwiferyboard.gov.au/codes-guidelines-statements/professional-standards.aspx>.

Nursing and Midwifery Board of Australia (NMBA). (2016d). *Enrolled nurse standards for practice.* Melbourne: Author. Retrieved from <https://www.nursingmidwiferyboard.gov.au/codes-guidelines-statements/professional-standards.aspx>.

Nursing and Midwifery Board of Australia (NMBA). (2016e). *Registration standard: Continuing professional development.* Melbourne: Author. Retrieved from <https://www.nursingmidwiferyboard.gov.au/Registration-Standards/Continuing-professional-development.aspx>.

Nursing and Midwifery Board of Australia (NMBA). (2018a). *Code of conduct for nurses.* Melbourne: Author. Retrieved from <http://www.nursingmidwiferyboard.gov.au/Codes-Guidelines-Statements/Professional-standards.aspx>.

Nursing and Midwifery Board of Australia (NMBA). (2018b). *Position on nurses providing cosmetic procedures* [updated 2020]. Melbourne: Author. Retrieved from <https://www.nursingmidwiferyboard.gov.au/codes-guidelines-statements/position-statements/nurses-and-cosmetic-procedures.aspx>.

Nursing and Midwifery Board of Australia (NMBA). (2019a). *Re-entry to practice for nurses and midwives* [fact sheet]. Melbourne: Author. Retrieved from <https://www.nursingmidwiferyboard.gov.au/Codes-Guidelines-Statements/FAQ/fact-sheet-reentry-to-practice.aspx>.

Nursing and Midwifery Board of Australia (NMBA). (2019b). *Social media: how to meet your obligations under the National Law* [Guideline]. Melbourne: Author. Retrieved from

<https://www.nursingmidwiferyboard.gov.au/Codes-Guidelines-Statements/Codes-Guidelines/Social-media-guidance.aspx>.

Nursing and Midwifery Board of Australia (NMBA). (2019c). *The use of health practitioner protected titles* [fact sheet]. Melbourne: Author. Retrieved from <https://www.nursingmidwiferyboard.gov.au/codes-guidelines-statements/faq/the-use-of-health-practitioner-protected-titles.aspx>.

Nursing and Midwifery Board of Australia (NMBA). (2020a). *Decision-making framework for nursing and midwifery.* Melbourne: Author. Retrieved from <https://www.nursingmidwiferyboard.gov.au/Codes-Guidelines-Statements/Frameworks.aspx>.

Nursing and Midwifery Board of Australia (NMBA). (2020b). *Enrolled nurses and medicine administration* [fact sheet]. Melbourne: Author. Retrieved from <https://www.nursingmidwiferyboard.gov.au/codes-guidelines-statements/faq/enrolled-nurses-and-medicine-administration.aspx>.

Nursing and Midwifery Board of Australia (NMBA). (2020c). *Continuing professional development* [fact sheet]. Melbourne: Author. Retrieved from <https://www.nursingmidwiferyboard.gov.au/codes-guidelines-statements/faq/cpd-faq-for-nurses-and-midwives.aspx>.

Nursing and Midwifery Board of Australia (NMBA). (2021). *Supervision guidelines for nursing and midwifery.* Melbourne: Author. Retrieved from <https://www.nursingmidwiferyboard.gov.au/Registration-and-Endorsement/Supervised-practice.aspx>.

Nursing and Midwifery Council of NSW (NMC). (2018). *Submission No. 16. Cosmetic health service complaints in New South Wales.* Retrieved from <https://www.parliament.nsw.gov.au/committees/Pages/inquiryprofile/cosmetic-health-service-complaints-in-nsw.aspx#tab-submissions>.

Nursing Council of New Zealand (NCNZ). (2007). *Competencies for registered nurses.* Wellington: Author. Retrieved from <https://www.nursingcouncil.org.nz/Public/Nursing/Standards_and_guidelines/NCNZ/nursing-section/Standards_and_guidelines_for_nurses.aspx?hkey=9fc06ae7-a853-4d10-b5fe-992cd44ba3de>.

Nursing Council of New Zealand (NCNZ). (2010). *Decision-making process for expanding scope of registered nursing practice.* Wellington: Author. Retrieved from <https://www.nursingcouncil.org.nz/Public/Nursing/Scopes_of_practice/Registered_Nurse/NCNZ/nursing-section/Registered_nurse.aspx?hkey=57ae602c-4d67-4234-a21e-2568d0350214>.

Nursing Council of New Zealand (NCNZ). (2011a). *Guidelines for cultural safety, the Treaty of Waitangi, and Māori health in nursing education and practice.* Wellington: Author. Retrieved from <https://www.nursingcouncil.org.nz/Public/Nursing/Standards_and_guidelines/NCNZ/nursing-section/Standards_and_guidelines_for_nurses.aspx?hkey=9fc06ae7-a853-4d10-b5fe-992cd44ba3de>.

Nursing Council of New Zealand (NCNZ). (2011b). *Expanded practice for registered nurses* [guideline]. Wellington: Author. Retrieved from <https://www.nursingcouncil.org.nz/Public/Nursing/Standards_and_guidelines/NCNZ/nursing-section/Standards_and_guidelines_for_nurses.aspx?hkey=9fc06ae7-a853-4d10-b5fe-992cd44ba3de> .

Nursing Council of New Zealand (NCNZ). (2011c). *Professional development activities template.* Wellington: Author. Retrieved from <https://www.nursingcouncil.org.nz/Public/Nursing/Continuing_competence/NCNZ/nursing-section/Continuing_Competence.aspx?hkey=6542ac27-9b56-4e89-b7ae-db445c5cb952>.

Nursing Council of New Zealand (NCNZ). (2012a). *Code of conduct for nurses.* Wellington: Author. Retrieved from https://www.nursingcouncil.org.nz/Public/Nursing/Code_of_Conduct/NCNZ/nursing-section/Code_of_Conduct.aspx?hkey=7fe9d496-9c08-4004-8397-d98bd774ef1b.

Nursing Council of New Zealand (NCNZ). (2012b). *Competencies for enrolled nurses.* Wellington: Author. Retrieved from <https://www.nursingcouncil.org.nz/Public/Nursing/Standards_and_guidelines/NCNZ/nursing-section/Standards_and_guidelines_for_nurses.aspx?hkey=9fc06ae7-a853-4d10-b5fe-992cd44ba3de>.

Nursing Council of New Zealand (NCNZ). (2012c). *Responsibilities for direction and delegation of care to enrolled nurses* [guideline]. Wellington: Author. Retrieved from <https://www.nursingcouncil.org.nz/Public/Nursing/Standards_and_guidelines/NCNZ/nursing-section/Standards_and_guidelines_for_nurses.aspx?hkey=9fc06ae7-a853-4d10-b5fe-992cd44ba3de>.

Nursing Council of New Zealand (NCNZ). (2012d). *Delegation of care by a registered nurse to a health care assistant* [guideline]. Wellington: Author. Retrieved from <https://www.nursingcouncil.org.nz/Public/Nursing/Standards_and_guidelines/NCNZ/nursing-section/Standards_and_guidelines_for_nurses.aspx?hkey=9fc06ae7-a853-4d10-b5fe-992cd44ba3de>.

Nursing Council of New Zealand (NCNZ). (2017). *Competencies for the mātanga tapuhi nurse practitioner scope of practice.* Retrieved from <https://www.nursingcouncil.org.nz/Public/Nursing/Scopes_of_practice/Nurse_practitioner/NCNZ/nursing-section/Nurse_practitioner.aspx>.

Nursing Council of New Zealand (NCNZ). (2017). *Appendix 9. Requirements for registration as an enrolled nurse – information for students.* Wellington: Author. Retrieved from <https://www.nursingcouncil.org.nz/Public/Nursing/How_to_become_a_nurse/NCNZ/nursing-section/How_to_become_a_nurse.aspx?hkey=de5efbe7-eca4-4d52-ba87-f155f655784f>.

Nursing Council of New Zealand (NCNZ). (2020). *Mātanga tapuh nurse practitioner scope of practice guidelines for applicants.* Retrieved from <https://www.nursingcouncil.org.nz/Public/Nursing/Scopes_of_practice/Nurse_practitioner/NCNZ/nursing-section/Nurse_practitioner.aspx?hkey=1493d86e-e4a5-45a5-8104-64607cf103c6>.

Nursing Council of New Zealand (NCNZ). (n.d.). *Continuing competence* [webpage]. Retrieved from <https://www.nursingcouncil.org.nz/Public/Nursing/Continuing_competence/NCNZ/nursing-section/Continuing_Competence.aspx?hkey=6542ac27-9b56-4e89-b7ae-db445c5cb952>.

Oxford Dictionaries. (2019). *Advocate.* Retrieved from <https://en.oxforddictionaries.com/definition/advocate>.

Pacific Islands Operating Room Nurses Association (PIORNA). (2019). *Constitution*. Samoa: Author. Retrieved from <https://phd.spc.int/programmes/clinical-services/pacific-clinical-organisations-networks>.

Papps, E., & Ramsden, I. (1996). Cultural safety in nursing: the New Zealand experience. *International Journal for Quality in Health Care, 8*(5), 491–497.

Patty, A. (2015). Cardiac arrest during cosmetic surgery: overdose of local anaesthetic likely. *Sydney Morning Herald*, 28 July, p. 3.

Raddie, N. (2019). *Standards implementation leading to practice improvements by audit data: agents of change in the Solomon Islands* [unpublished conference paper]. Presented at the inaugural ACORN Queensland State Conference 'Agents of Change', 2–4 May 2019.

Randmaa, M., Martensson, G., Swenne, C. L., & Engstrom, M. (2015). An observational study of postoperative handover in anesthetic clinics: the content of verbal information and factors influencing receiver memory. *Journal of Perianesthesia Nursing, 30*(2), 105–115.

Ryals, M., & Palokas, M. (2017). Pediatric post-anesthesia care unit discharge criteria: a scoping review protocol, *JBI Database of Systematic Reviews and Implementation Reports, 15*(8), 2033–2039. https://dx.doi.org/10.11124/JBISRIR-2016-003325

Sax Institute. (2015). *The costs and benefits of providing undergraduate student clinical placements*. Retrieved from <https://www.saxinstitute.org.au/publications/evidence-check-library/the-costs-and-benefits-of-providing-undergraduate-student-clinical-placements/>.

Schmidt, B. J., & McArthur, E.C. (2018). Professional nursing values: a concept analysis. *Nursing Forum, 53*(1), 69–75. https://dx.doi.org/10.1111/nuf.12211

Shear, T., Deshur, M., Avram, M., Greenberg, S., Murphy, G., Ujiki, M., . . . Wijas, B. (2018). Procedural timeout compliance is improved with real-time clinical decision making. *Journal of Patient Safety, 14*(3), 148–152.

South Australia Health. (2018). *Evaluating nurse endoscopist advanced practice roles in a South Australia metropolitan health service. Final evaluation report*. Adelaide: Author. Retrieved from <https://www.sahealth.sa.gov.au/wps/wcm/connect/7dde8be1-7676-4605-893a-fe86183906a2/Evaluating+nurse+Endoscopist+advanced+practice+roles+in+SA+metropolitan+health+service+Final+Evaluation+Report+2018.pdf?MOD=AJPERES>.

Southern Adelaide Local Health Network (SALHN). (2019a). *New/Junior OTS Nurse or TPPP OTS Role Progression Plan (6 months) V3.1: 2019*. Adelaide: Author.

Southern Adelaide Local Health Network (SALHN). (2019b). *New/Junior Anaesthetic Nurse or TPPP Anaesthetics Role Progression Plan (6 months)*. Adelaide: Author.

Southern Adelaide Local Health Network (SALHN). (2019c). *New/Junior PACU Nurse or TPPP PACU Role Progression Plan (6 months)*. Adelaide: Author.

Spruce, L. (2015). Back to basics: implementing evidence-based practice. *AORN Journal, 101*(1), 106–112. https://dx.doi.org/10.1016/j.aorn.2014.08.009

Spruce, L. (2017). Surgical head coverings: a literature review. *AORN Journal, 106*(4), 306–316.

State of Victoria. (2015). *Implementing a nurse cystoscopy service: a guide for public health services*. Retrieved from <https://www2.health.vic.gov.au/about/publications/policiesandguidelines/implementing-a-nurse-cystoscopy-service>.

Sundqvist, A. S., Nilsson, U., Holmefur, M., & Anderzén-Carlsson, A. (2016). Perioperative patient advocacy: an integrative review. *Journal of Perianethesia Nursing, 31*(5), 422–433.

Sutherland-Fraser, S., & Davies, M. (2017). *Collaboration leads to successful change in Pacific Island countries* [conference poster]. Presented at the National Nursing Forum, Sydney, August, 2017.

Tanner, J., Dumville, J., Norman, G., & Fortnam, M. (2016). Surgical hand antisepsis to reduce surgical site infection. *Cochrane Database of Systematic Reviews, 1*, CD004288. https://dx.doi.org/10.1002/14651858.CD004288.pub3.

Taoi, M. H., & Sutherland-Fraser, S. (2016). *Collaboration leads to successful change in Pacific Island countries* [conference paper]. Presented at the 18th South Pacific Nurses' Forum, Honiara Solomon Islands, November, 2016.

Wensing, M., Grol, R. (2019). Knowledge translation in health: how implementation science could contribute more. *BMC Medicine, 17*, 88. https://dx.doi.org/10.1186/s12916-019-1322-9

Woodhead, K. (2006). Developing a new perioperative organisation in Papua New Guinea. *Journal of Perioperative Practice, 16*(8), 389–392.

Yang, L., & Hains, T. (2017). The plight of the perioperative nurse practitioner in Australia. *Australian Nursing and Midwifery Journal, 24*(10), 36–37.

Zaidi, D. (2018). Religion and spirituality in health care practice. *AMA Journal of Ethics, 20*(7), 607–674.

FURTHER READING

Martin, J. A. (2016). *Procedural sedation: policy, practice and knowledge. Doctor of Nursing Practice (DNP) Final Clinical Projects*. 2. Retrieved from <https://commons.lib.jmu.edu/dnp201019/2>.

Nursing and Midwifery Board of Australia (NMBA). (2021). *Supervision guidelines for nursing and midwifery*. Melbourne: Author. Retrieved from <https://www.nursingmidwiferyboard.gov.au/Codes-Guidelines-Statements/Frameworks.aspx>.

Sundqvist, A. S. (2017). *Perioperative patient advocacy – having the patient's best interests at heart*. Örebro Studies in Care Sciences 71. Örebro University, Sweden. Retrieved from <https://oru.diva-portal.org/smash/get/diva2:1077898/FULLTEXT01.pdf>.

CHAPTER 2

Human Factors and the Perioperative Team

BRIGID M. GILLESPIE • MENNA DAVIES
EDITOR: BRIGID M. GILLESPIE

LEARNING OUTCOMES

- Explore the prominent features of perioperative culture and describe its influence on team dynamics
- Discuss the components of human factors and their importance to patient safety
- Explain the importance of clinical leadership and emotional intelligence in shaping the culture of the perioperative department
- Apply the principles of communication and graded assertiveness to effective teamwork

---

KEY TERMS

communication	**professional hierarchy**
emotional intelligence	**shared mental model**
graded assertiveness	**situation awareness**
human factors	**teamwork**

INTRODUCTION

Chapter 1 introduced the framework in which perioperative nursing is practised and identified the individual nursing roles that form part of the perioperative team. Chapter 2 examines perioperative team dynamics and how team members function as effective providers of patient care within a unique culture. The factors that underpin team dynamics and how the surgical team members relate to each other and interact with their environment are discussed under the umbrella term *human factors*. This encompasses non-technical skills such as communication, teamwork and situation awareness, and environmental elements such as ergonomics, noise and task management – all of which can have a positive, but potentially a negative, impact on patient safety. Consider the patient scenarios detailed in the Introduction to this book as you read this chapter. Revisit the critical thinking questions throughout the chapter based on your knowledge, experience and new understandings you develop as you read this chapter.

PATIENT SCENARIOS

SCENARIO 2.1: TEAM BUILDING

In a busy metropolitan public hospital with 20 commissioned operating rooms, the interdisciplinary team of 3 nurses, 2 surgeons and 2 anaesthetists are allocated to an all-day orthopaedic list. Surgical team members include:
- RN Ben Lumby, RN Rob Cohen and EN Pauline Noakes

- Dr Patrick Slattery and Dr Ivy West (orthopaedic surgeon and registrar)
- Dr Marion Thomas and Dr Vince De Silva (anaesthetic consultant and registrar)
- RN Margaret McCormack, anaesthetic nurse
- Theatre orderly Jimmy Montano.

Members of the team have not worked together as a team before now.

The first patient is Mr James Collins, a 78-year-old man, who has been admitted for an elective right total knee replacement (TKR). Mr Collins' full history and a brief description of the healthcare setting appear at the front of the book for readers to review when answering the questions in this unfolding scenario.

Critical Thinking Questions

- As team members in this team have not worked with each other before, what simple strategies would you use as 'ice-breakers' to ensure the team is 'on the same page'?
- What strategies could you use to manage the potential for hierarchical relations among team members from different disciplines/professional backgrounds and variable levels of clinical experience?

THE INTERDISCIPLINARY TEAM

The anaesthetic, instrument, circulating and postanaesthesia care unit (PACU) nurse roles described in Chapter 1 combine with the following medical team roles to create the interdisciplinary team responsible for the patient's safety and well-being:

- The consultant anaesthetist administers anaesthesia and closely monitors the patient's physiological status during the surgery/procedure. The consultant anaesthetist is often assisted by a second (trainee) anaesthetist. Anaesthetic technicians may also be part of the team and are responsible for the maintenance of anaesthetic equipment. In some facilities, they may also act as the anaesthetic assistant and participate in patient care.
- The consultant surgeon/proceduralist performs the surgery/procedure, generally assisted by other surgeons at various levels of specialty training.

In addition, ancillary staff such as radiographers, orderlies, sterilising technicians, store keepers, cleaners and administrative staff perform important roles, assisting the surgical team in the smooth running of the perioperative environment.

A successful surgical outcome for the patient and smooth operational management of the patient's admission and scheduling of surgery are the culmination of complex administrative processes that are managed by administration staff. Although these ancillary staff members are not involved in direct patient care, their role responsibilities involve a large component of the pre-admission preparation of the patient, liaising with nursing staff to structure the operating theatre lists, admission and preoperative management prior to the patient's transfer to the operating suite.

Operating suite nurse managers undertake a coordinating role in the wider hospital environment, being closely involved with administrative processes related to issues such as patient flow, waiting lists and availability of postoperative beds. They are responsible for ensuring the availability of operating rooms for both elective and emergency surgery and for rostering appropriately skilled staff in each operating room (Australian College of Perioperative Nurses [ACORN], 2020a).

THE PERIOPERATIVE TEAM AND PROFESSIONAL HIERARCHY

The operating suite is a fast-paced, busy and diverse environment and the perioperative team is likewise diverse, made up of an interdisciplinary group of highly skilled medical and nursing professionals with differing clinical backgrounds and expertise. These team members must work together effectively to provide a safe outcome for patients. For patients, this is an anxious period of their hospitalisation when they are at their most vulnerable, as they are anaesthetised or heavily sedated with no control over their surroundings or what is happening to them (Cousley, Martin, & Hoy, 2014). The perioperative team therefore has total responsibility for the patient's safety and well-being.

Although most teams work effectively together and produce safe outcomes for patients, sometimes teams are not cohesive and this can contribute to adverse outcomes for patients or be the cause of near misses (Green, Oeppen, Smith, & Brennan, 2017). The reasons why some surgical teams fail to function effectively are complex and may partly be historical. Traditionally, the consultant surgeon, due to their skills and perceived elevated position in society, was placed at the top of the surgical team hierarchy, with team members, including nurses, adopting 'subordinate' roles and being often fearful or reluctant to question the consultant's authority. Such a 'pecking order' with its power imbalance discourages effective teamwork and communication, and evidence shows that poor communication and dysfunctional teams contribute to adverse events (Green et al., 2017). Although anecdotally remnants of this type of hierarchy still exist in some perioperative environments, positive steps to improve communication and teamwork by participating in human factors training are slowly changing the traditional hierarchy and socialisation practice in the perioperative environment (Chen, Fu, & Zhao, 2015).

Exploring how **professional hierarchy** and socialisation are negotiated between nurses and other disciplines in the perioperative setting often highlights differing perceptions of professional roles, abilities and responsibilities. Status differentials between nurses, doctors and other health professionals affect social relations. The effect of professional hierarchy and socialisation has been studied in many different clinical contexts.

Stein's (1978) influential paper on the 'doctor–nurse game' identified the pressures exerted on medical and nursing students and demonstrated the differences in their role socialisation and occupational orientations. Tanner and Timmons (2000), in their early work on perioperative team dynamics, labelled the perioperative environment, with its restricted access away from public gaze, as the surgeon's 'backstage' where relaxed behaviours are evident. Practices still seen today include a level of familiarity towards other staff not normally seen outside the perioperative environment, as well as colleagues engaging in conversations that would be viewed as unprofessional if they occurred in full view of the public. Examples include joking, teasing, gossiping and discussing social events – activities undertaken freely without fear of being heard by the anaesthetised patients. For nurses, however, the perioperative environment is their 'front stage' where they work each day and their professional behaviour is in direct contrast to the relaxed behaviours of their medical colleagues, blurring professional boundaries and sometimes leading to tensions between the two groups.

In addition, staff identities, and therefore the status of members, are often concealed because of the uniformity of dress (i.e. wearing of scrubs), resulting in suspension of the visual hierarchy; the professional hierarchy, however, is still strong enough to be exerted when required (Tanner & Timmons, 2000). Staff in the perioperative environment often adopt an informal code of dress, such as wearing brightly coloured socks or a coloured headscarf, or carrying a pager in order to inject a sense of individuality.

THE CULTURE AND CONTEXT OF THE PERIOPERATIVE ENVIRONMENT

It can be confusing for a novice nurse entering the complex perioperative environment to learn the subtleties of the work culture, yet these 'social mores' are frequently influential in forming the novice's developing sense of work and role identity (Chen et al., 2015). As part of the socialisation process, individuals are not only expected to master particular skills and adapt to a specific group climate, they must also learn to work within the existing hierarchal structures of the subculture of which they are nominal members (Chen et al., 2015).

'Culture' symbolises the 'glue' that binds a workplace together through shared meanings, expressed through language, and the effects of culture pervade all workplaces and impact on all types of employees (Chen et al., 2015). A good workplace culture enables its employees to thrive, whereas a negative workplace culture can cause disharmony, uncertainty and unrest – leading to staff attrition. Understanding workplace culture is an important part of both providing a successful one and coexisting within one. Workplace culture is influenced by the norms and expectations that guide the thinking and behaviours of employees. Furthermore, workplace stability depends on the extent to which individuals are accepted as team members and the socialisation practices within the particular workplace and specialty (Chen et al., 2015).

Every workplace has its own culture and the perioperative environment is no different, with its necessary separation from other departments and restricted access contributing to a unique culture. The defining features of the perioperative culture are born out of being an intense, time-pressured environment where the organisational arrangement of reward systems, social ranking, and specialty knowledge and judgement are highly valued. 'Survival' in the perioperative setting depends on how well individuals are socialised into this secluded and often geographically isolated environment.

Novices need to learn about the culture in which they work, as well as mastering an array of highly technical skills. Technology is evident in nearly every facet of the patient's journey (e.g. automatic blood pressure machine, monitoring devices, anaesthetic machine, microscopes). However, the technical expertise that the perioperative team must possess will not always be enough to guarantee a good patient outcome. There are also a number of non-technical factors the team must master in order to ensure patient safety and these are discussed under the term *human factors*.

HUMAN FACTORS

Human factors are the interrelationships between people and their environment and each other that need to be considered so as to optimise performance

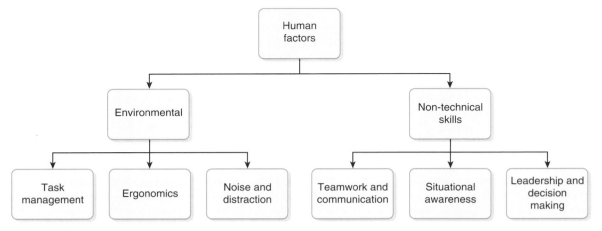

FIG. 2.1 Components of human factors. (Source: Adapted from Flin, R., & O'Connor. (2017). *Safety at the sharp end: a guide to non-technical skills*. Baton Rouge, FL: CRC Press.)

and ensure safety. In healthcare, these range from the design of tools such as medical devices to services and systems, as well as the working environment and working practices such as tasks, roles and team behaviours. Failure to apply the principles of human factors in healthcare settings has the potential to lead to errors (Flin & O'Connor, 2017).

Subsumed within the broad concept of human factors is the notion of 'non-technical skills' and interpersonal skills associated with technical skills that contribute to safe and efficient clinical performance (Flin, 2013; Flin & O'Connor, 2017). Non-technical skills describe a set of social and cognitive abilities encompassing situational awareness, risk assessment, clinical decision making, leadership, communication skills and teamwork (Gordon, Baker, Catchpole, Darbyshire, & Schocken, 2015). Human factors can be divided into two distinct streams: individual non-technical skills and environmental considerations (see the discussion below and Fig. 2.1).

Non-technical Skills

The early work of Flin, O'Connor and Crichton (2008) identified the specific intraoperative non-technical skills for scrub practitioners as communication, teamwork, situation awareness and task management. The results of later research with anaesthetists (Flin & Patey, 2011; Zwaan et al., 2016) and surgeons (Fecso, Kuzulugil, Babaoglu, Bener, & Grantcharov, 2018) identified the additional non-technical skills of leadership and decision making to these medical specialists. Mitchell, Chung, Williamson and Molesworth (2011) found that a lack of non-technical skills was the main contributing

factor in 48 unexpected health-related patient deaths that were the subject of coronial inquests in Australia.

During orientation to the perioperative environment, considerable time is spent teaching new staff members technical skills such as how to operate the many pieces of equipment found in the operating room. While knowledge of equipment is important for patient safety, technical knowledge alone does not guarantee patient safety. In the complex and often stressful perioperative environment, it is essential that the surgical team combine their individual technical skills with these non-technical skills to provide safe and effective care of the patient (Alken et al., 2018; Fecso et al., 2018).

Lessons learnt from aviation

The aviation industry has provided valuable information about the effectiveness of non-technical skills in promoting good communication and teamwork as being essential in the safety of passengers. In examining the circumstances surrounding a series of air disasters in the 1970s, investigators found that in many cases the cause was not mechanical failure or pilot error, but rather failures of interpersonal skills, communication, decision making and leadership. Within the cockpit crew, a steep cockpit hierarchical structure existed that discouraged questioning of the captain's decisions in critical situations, even when the crew knew that these decisions were incorrect and would contribute to the subsequent disaster (Brennan & Davidson, 2019).

Following the 1978 Portland air crash (see Feature box 2.1) and in attempt to avert further disasters, the US

FEATURE BOX 2.1
The Crash of United Airlines Flight 173

In December 1978, United Airlines Flight 173 crashed into a wooded, populated area of suburban Portland, Oregon, during an approach to Portland International Airport. The aircraft had delayed landing for about an hour while the flight crew coped with a landing gear malfunction and prepared the passengers for a possible emergency landing. The plane crashed about 10 km southeast of the airport, destroying the aircraft and killing 10 passengers and crew from the total of 189 passengers and crew on board.

The National Transportation Safety Board (1978) determined that the probable cause of the accident was the failure of the captain to properly monitor and respond to the aircraft's low fuel supply despite a crew member's advice that fuel was running low. The captain's inattention resulted from his preoccupation with a landing gear malfunction and preparations for a possible landing emergency.

Contributing to the accident was the failure of the other two flight crew to either fully comprehend the critical state of the fuel supply or successfully communicate their concern to the captain.

(Source: Adapted from https://ivypanda.com/essays/united-airlines-flight-173-accident/.)

RESEARCH BOX 2.1
Surgical Safety Checklist

Australian researchers performed a systematic review of seven independent, previously published studies testing the effectiveness of surgical safety checklists on post-operative (PO) complications. In all of the studies, WHO's Surgical Safety Checklist or a modified version was used. A meta-analysis was performed in which the results of the studies, representing 37,339 patients, were integrated. All patients had either elective surgery or emergency surgery.

Pooled results of the meta-analysis suggested that using a checklist in surgery significantly reduced overall PO complications, wound infections and blood loss. According to the review, there were 3.7% fewer PO complications overall, 2.9% fewer wound infections and a 3.8% reduction in patients who had blood loss greater than 500 mL. The use of a checklist, however, did not significantly reduce mortality rates, pneumonia or unplanned return to surgery.

(Source: Gillespie, B. M., Chaboyer, W., Thalib, L., John, M., Fairweather, N., & Slater, K. (2014). Effect of using a safety checklist in surgery on patient complications: a systematic review and meta-analysis. *Anaesthesiology, 120*, 1380–1389.)

---

aviation industry instigated a new training program known as Crew Resource Management (CRM), incorporating human factors (teamwork, communication, situation awareness, leadership, decision making). CRM was designed to promote team cohesiveness and reduce the effects of the hierarchal structure within the flight-deck crew. This successful strategy has been universally adopted by the aviation industry with pilots and flight-deck crews undergoing mandatory annual CRM training. Similar training programs are used across other high-risk industries including nuclear power plants, shipping and the military (Flin & O'Connor, 2017; Lin, Wernick, Tolentino, & Stawicki, 2018).

There are parallels between the captain and cockpit crew and the surgeon and surgical team in relation to the previous discussion on hierarchical structures and the reluctance to challenge the captain/surgeon's authority. Recognition of the importance of non-technical skills has seen the adoption in surgery of many of the tools used in CRM training (Salas & Rosen, 2013). These tools include the use of surgical safety checklists for correct patient identification ('Time Out') and patient handover, interdisciplinary simulation training and greater contributions from the surgical team to intraoperative patient planning and care through preoperative briefings (Alken et al., 2018; Martin & Langell, 2017).

In 2004, the World Health Organization (WHO) developed the Surgical Safety Checklist (see Research box 2.1) as a global initiative to promote safer surgery. This checklist has been adopted and adapted in many countries including Australia and New Zealand (Gillespie et al., 2014, 2018). Practical application of the checklist is discussed in Chapter 9 on intraoperative patient care, but its relevance to human factors comes from the information in the checklist that communicates key facts about the patient and anticipated critical events; it also identifies key personnel involved in the patient's care. The checklist focuses team members' attention on key aspects of the patient's care and standardising team communications using the checklist to ensure that everyone is on the same page or sharing the same mental model (see later in this chapter). Possessing the same knowledge of the patient's status assists each member of the surgical team to prepare for events that may occur during surgery. Using a checklist also provides an opportunity for all team members, regardless of professional experience or discipline, to raise any concerns they may have about the procedure (Gillespie, Withers, Lavin, Gardiner, & Marshall, 2016). While the Surgical Safety Checklist cannot be directly linked to improved patient outcomes, its use emphasises the need for discussion and therefore enhances teamwork and communication between members of the surgical team.

Teamwork

Teamwork is defined as a group of individuals who work together to achieve a common goal, working interdependently to perform tasks and managing their relationships and clinical roles across professional boundaries. Effective teamwork relies on commitment, collaboration, competence, a supportive culture and communication. Teamwork and communication are fundamental interrelated non-technical skills that contribute to the delivery of safe surgical care and are enshrined in perioperative culture (Salas, Shuffler, Thayer, Bedwell, & Lazzara, 2015). The results of 84 root cause analysis reports suggested that 44 (52%) errors stemmed from miscommunications. Of these, 35 (86%) included handover errors, 19 (43%) included miscommunications between different staff groups, 10 (23%) were because of hesitancy in speaking up and 8 (18%) were from miscommunications during teamwork (Rabøl et al., 2011).

As members of an interdisciplinary team, individuals do not work in 'splendid isolation' of others. An important feature that distinguishes perioperative teams is that each member brings different levels of expertise and knowledge to the task, termed *distributed expertise*. Surgical teams work together interdependently – that is, members are mutually dependent on each other in relation to performing a specified task and must adapt to one another to achieve team goals (Gillespie et al., 2018).

The interdependency of the surgical team required to function effectively can be adversely affected by workplace bullying and harassment. Despite the zero tolerance reflected in the policies of many Australian and New Zealand healthcare organisations, horizontal violence in the form of workplace bullying and harassment remains an unfortunate reality (Llewellyn, Karageorge, Nash, Li, & Neuen, 2018; Worksafe NZ, 2014) . Workplace bullying appears to flourish in environments where there is a strict hierarchical order and where a high value is placed on the skills required to perform work roles competently (Budden, Birks, Cant, Bagley, & Park, 2017). It could be argued that the perioperative environment is one such workplace. Workplace bullying has been described in relation to decreased job satisfaction, diminished work performance, burnout and nurse attrition (Budden et al., 2017), although in many cases it still goes unreported. Examples of workplace bullying include:

- behaving aggressively
- pressuring someone to act inappropriately

- making belittling comments
- practising social exclusion
- making unreasonable work demands (Australian Government, 2014).

The prevalence of workplace bullying compounds the existing difficulties experienced by nursing specialties in terms of their ability not only to retain nurses, but also to recruit nurses in the future. As a result, emphasis is placed on preventing workplace bullying and, in many healthcare institutions, primary prevention is underpinned by education and training of staff. The ACORN and the Australian College of Nursing (ACN) have each published a position statement that details the obligations of individuals and organisations in relation to the prevention and management of workplace bullying and the imperative to promote 'a culture of zero tolerance' in perioperative environments (ACN, 2018; ACORN, 2020b).

Highlighted in Research box 2.2 is an example of workplace bullying and harassment involving undergraduate nurses on clinical placement. This research highlights the challenges faced by undergraduate nurses undertaking clinical experience while being subjected to inappropriate behaviours from other nurses. In addition, it shows the difficulties in speaking out against colleagues who have acted inappropriately and unprofessionally. Courage is required to report inappropriate and bullying behaviours and nurses should seek out colleagues who can be supportive and advise on the appropriate reporting process.

Communication

Communication between the multidisciplinary team may be based on previous professional and social relationships and may have the potential to hinder team effectiveness. This is particularly true when team members are transitory and there is a significant reliance on casual or agency staff. Teams who consistently work together develop an understanding of each other's work capabilities and communicate more effectively, which reduces the risk of adverse events occurring. It is often easy to spot a team that regularly works together and has a deep understanding of the practical steps of the procedure. The instrument nurse anticipates the surgeon's move, so that verbal communication related to the procedure is minimal, but purposeful and deliberate. Similarly, the circulating nurse anticipates the team's need for additional supplies and equipment so that the procedure is smooth and coordinated. In contrast, surgeons who work with a different instrument nurse for each procedure have more difficulty in establishing a coordinated team (Gillespie, Gwinner, Fairweather, &

RESEARCH BOX 2.2
Example of Workplace Harassment

Budden and colleagues (2017) surveyed 888 Australian nursing students to determine their experiences of bullying and harassment while on clinical placement. Half the students surveyed indicated they had experienced such behaviours, with the perpetrators being mainly registered nurses (56.6%), followed by patients (37.4%) and enrolled nurses (36.4%). Clinical facilitators (25.9%), preceptors (24.6%) and managers (22.8%) were also implicated. The behaviour was generally non-violent, with a low incidence of gender-based, sexual orientation and racist remarks, together with unfair treatment in relation to rostering and work allocation. Of the students surveyed, 60 to 80% reported being harshly criticised and neglected, ignored or denied opportunities for learning. Approximately 11.6% of students reported sexual harassment of various types and there was low incidence of reported physical abuse, which included being shoved, pushed, slapped or punched, although it was not reported who was responsible for these behaviours.

When asked if they had reported incidents, 71.3% responded that they had not for reasons that included fear of being victimised and that nothing would be done, conceding it was 'part of the job' or 'rite of passage'. The impact of being bullied/harassed for 60% of the nurses was feelings of anger, anxiety and inadequacy, leading to half of them considering whether they should leave nursing. Budden and colleagues concluded that the findings have a far-reaching economic and workforce impact on the nursing workforce.

(Source: Budden, L., Birks, M., Cant, R., Bagley, T., & Park, T. (2017). Australian nursing students' experience of bullying and/or harassment during clinical placement. *Collegian, 24*, 125–133.)

Chaboyer, 2013). In addition, nurses and doctors are socialised into different communities of practice and therefore have different foci and communication styles. For example, doctors tend to approach a clinical situation using a diagnosis-and-treatment model, whereas nurses operate using a provision-of-care model (Gessler, Rosenstein, & Ferron, 2012). Hence, there is a danger that miscommunication may occur between team members.

Miscommunication reduces team effectiveness and may also contribute to adverse patient outcomes. Brindley and Reynolds (2011) support the use of 'fly-by-voice' commands as a method of confirming the completion of a task. The term is taken from aviation when pilots are deliberately taught to vocalise routine actions as a double-check of tasks completed. In the perioperative environment, examples might include team members communicating to the rest of the team that they have completed certain tasks – for example, 'diathermy is on coagulation 30', 'penicillin administered', 'aortic clamp applied at 1430'.

While the benefits of teamwork in enhancing patient care have been emphasised in many studies, there are a growing number of retrospective and observational studies that highlight the negative consequences of communication breakdown in surgery (Gillespie, Chaboyer, & Fairweather, 2012; Lin et al., 2018; Manias, Geddes, Watson, Jones, & Della, 2015; Shubeck, Kanters, & Dimick, 2019). Retained sponges, wrong-site surgery, incomplete clinical handover and mismatched blood transfusions can be the result of interpersonal dynamics, where communication breakdowns occur between team members. The hierarchical structure can also contribute to such communication breakdowns when junior team members are afraid to speak up, even if they note an adverse event is about to happen. Similar to the human factors training undertaken by pilots, the development of 'horizontal communication', which empowers junior members of the team to speak up, is becoming incorporated into medical and nursing training (Brindley & Reynolds, 2011).

The provision of high-quality and safe patient care linked to effective communication and the ability to work in a multidisciplinary team can be enhanced via informal 'team briefings' or 'team huddle' (Jones & Ritzman, 2018). This involves the surgical team meeting just prior to commencement of the surgical list each day to discuss the procedures, possible complications, equipment and supplies required. This briefing is over and above the requirement to complete the Surgical Safety Checklist. Research findings (Brindle et al., 2018; Gillespie et al., 2018) suggest that briefings and debriefings by surgical teams improved communication and brought to light defects in equipment and lack of availability of supplies. Identifying these issues prior to surgery allows time for them to be rectified, reducing delays and thereby contributing to patient safety.

Team training and the use of interdisciplinary simulation exercises have also been beneficial in improving teamwork. Simulation exercises may involve, for example, an emergency case scenario where the team members must work together to identify and manage the emergency. Debriefing following the exercise provides opportunities for the team members to discuss and evaluate their performance (Wacker & Kolbe, 2014).

Most surgical teams experience high-pressure situations, where the outcomes are high stakes. Stressful situations include a difficult intubation, excessive bleeding

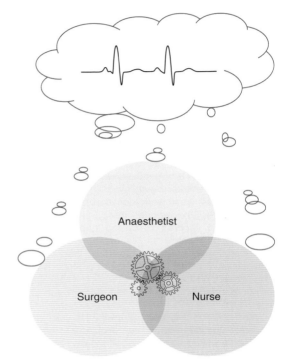

FIG. 2.2 Depiction of a shared mental model between the anaesthetist, the nurse and the surgeon. (Source: Adapted from Department of Defense. (2006). TeamSTEPPS Multimedia Resource Kit. [TeamSTEPPS: Team strategies & tools to enhance performance and patient safety. USA: Agency for Healthcare Research & Quality.)

FEATURE BOX 2.2
Key Human Factors Messages When Working Under Pressure

Nine tips for better teamwork when working under pressure:
1. Brief the whole team, even if rapid and short
2. Take deliberate action when under stress
3. Lead by being open and inclusive for rapidly changing scenarios
4. Help staff unfamiliar with the work
5. Use checklists and aides-memoire to support tasks
6. Encourage staff to speak up
7. Recognise performance-limiting factors
8. Debrief as a team to learn from experiences
9. Think about the wider healthcare team

(Source: Clinical Human Factors Group 2020 Version 1.2.)

---

on the operating table and resuscitating a COVID-19 patient when PPE is not within arms' reach. The Clinical Human Factors Group has developed a guideline for working under pressure for frontline staff. Feature box 2.2 presents some strategies teams can use to build a shared mental model.

Shared mental models

It is essential to consider the patient holistically across the continuum of care, as opposed to being task oriented. The more effective teamwork and communication are between individuals in the surgical team, the more likely the members are to build an accurate **shared mental model** of the situation. A *mental model* is the term applied to understanding a particular situation and all of the factors that influence the situation. The concept of a shared mental model is defined by McComb and Simpson (2014) as 'individually held knowledge structures' that enable team members to function collaboratively within their environment and assist them in predicting what each member is going to do and what they are going to need in order to do it. In its simplest form, a shared mental model is established when all the team members are thinking as one, or colloquially 'being on the same page', as can be seen in Fig. 2.2 where the anaesthetist, the surgeon and the nurse have a shared mental model in relation to the monitoring that is required. As mentioned previously, the Surgical Safety Checklist provides an opportunity to share information consistent with developing a shared mental model – for example, the section on the checklist in which the surgeon shares critical or

unexpected events with all team members (Gillespie et al., 2018). Consequently, team members are then able to strategise their actions and behaviours should an unexpected event occur.

Critical Thinking Question

- What strategies could you use to optimise team communication to ensure team members are 'on the same page' while caring for Mr Collins?

Situation awareness

Situation awareness is a non-technical skill that refers to an ability to identify and process many pieces of information from within the operating room environment and act accordingly. It requires the ability to watch, listen and understand cues, anticipating what might happen next (Lin et al., 2018). Team members

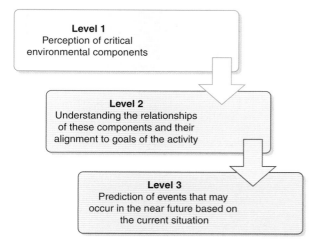

FIG. 2.3 Levels of situation awareness.

need to be aware of the big picture rather than focusing on a particular task. To achieve this, an individual takes in data from their senses, interprets the data and finally makes predictions of what will happen in the future (Flin & O'Connor, 2017). Situation awareness relies on good teamwork and communication and, as described by Ensley (1995), has been viewed in relation to three levels of processes, as illustrated in Fig. 2.3.

The first level is where sensory data from our senses are extracted from the environment. The second level is where the sensory data are interpreted, such as identifying decreases in blood pressure or a surgical instrument request. In the third and final level of situation, a person is able to extrapolate how events will unfold or what actions are best taken to achieve a set objective (Ensley, 1995). For example, the circulating nurse may attend to level 1 information that shows a mean arterial blood pressure reading of 53 mmHg. The interpretation made at level 2 indicates an increased risk. The instrument nurse may predict (level 3) that additional clamps may be required.

Good situation awareness alerts staff to a sudden change in the surgeon's tone of voice, a comment about blood loss or an intraoperative complication for which urgent action may be required. Recognition of these vital cues can initiate immediate and possibly life-saving actions, whereas a lack of situation awareness may mean delays in obtaining equipment, causing the patient's condition to be compromised. It can be easy as a novice perioperative nurse to become focused on one task or element of care but oblivious to what else is happening within the operating room (Flin &

O'Connor, 2017). Research box 2.3 highlights research findings about situation awareness. Feature box 2.3 is a real-life clinical example demonstrating the aspect of 'overhearing' described by Gillespie and colleagues (2013) and illustrates how novice nurses may need prompting and guidance in developing their non-technical skills.

RESEARCH BOX 2.3
Research Findings About Situation Awareness

In a qualitative study using observations and interviews, Gillespie and colleagues (2013) found that instrument nurses used strategies such as 'overhearing' and 'thinking ahead' to increase their situation awareness during surgical procedures. The deliberate act of listening at the operating table during surgery enables instrument nurses to coordinate their activities, anticipate unexpected events and plan contingency responses. By gathering cues presented in the environment and integrating information from different sources, nurses used situation awareness to build a mental model which is based on their familiarity and experience with the surgeon and the procedure.

(Source: Gillespie, B. M., Gwinner, K., Fairweather, N., & Chaboyer, W. (2013). Building shared situational awareness in surgery through distributed dialog. *Journal of Multidisciplinary Healthcare, 6*, 109-118.)

FEATURE BOX 2.3
Situation Awareness in Clinical Practice

It was a routine laparoscopic cholecystectomy on a fit, healthy 45-year-old woman and Mary, the Clinical Nurse Educator, Anaesthetics, was working with a newly graduated nurse, Josh, who had just commenced a 3-month rotation into anaesthetics. They had assisted the anaesthetist in the patient's induction of anaesthesia and all seemed to be progressing well with the surgery. The doors from the operating room into the anaesthetic bay were open and Mary was showing Josh how to set up for the next patient.

Suddenly, the surgeon commented: 'I've got a bit of bleeding here.' Mary immediately returned to the operating room to see whether the anaesthetist required any additional fluids or equipment. She noticed that Josh was still focusing on priming an intravenous line in the anaesthetic bay, seemingly oblivious of what was happening in the operating room. On returning to the anaesthetic bay, Mary asked Josh whether he had heard the surgeon's comment. He had not and Mary made a joke about having 'to grow your third ear' – in other words, the ability to 'overhear' other conversations between team members and act on them appropriately.

Leadership and a multigenerational workforce

In the perioperative setting, there are at least four diverse generations: Baby Boomers, Generation X, Generation Y and Millennials (Graystone, 2019). Each generation brings vastly different core values, beliefs and expectations to the workplace. They also have different priorities, attitudes, communication styles and ways to engage with peers and work design that influence organisational culture and performance. Therefore, understanding these underlying core values and beliefs has important implications for those who are tasked with leading intergenerational teams. Leaders who capitalise on the inherent differences between generations can create a dynamic and engaged workforce, giving them a competitive edge in attracting and retaining staff. Having a multigenerational workforce is not new, though traditionally the age groups were separated by a clear chain of command: the older workers were generally the managers, while the younger workers were junior staff. The new reality is a much more flattened organisational structure in which nurses of different ages and generations work more closely together and junior staff are less afraid to vocalise opinions and requests (Graystone, 2019; Green et al., 2017; Stewart, Manges, & Ward, 2015).

Leadership is the ability to motivate and direct others to achieve shared goals to attain the best outcomes for perioperative patients. Leadership skills are developed through experience, role modelling and critical reflection (Kaye, Fox, & Urman, 2012). Enabling people to connect and collaborate and finding the appropriate style and content of communication are challenging but essential tasks for perioperative leaders. Just because a person holds a leadership role does not necessarily mean that they are an effective leader. In fact, there are very few natural leaders. Leadership skills need to be learned. Importantly, there is growing acknowledgement that emotional intelligence is an essential quality of effective leadership (Edelman & van Knippenberg, 2018).

Emotional intelligence is defined as the 'ability to understand and manage our emotions and those around us (Edelman & van Knippenberg, 2018). This quality gives individuals a variety of skills, such as the ability to manage relationships, navigate social networks, influence and inspire others' (Fletcher, 2012, para. 2). The ability to lead and bring out the best in others is especially applicable when considering how closely perioperative nurses work with others as part of an interdisciplinary team. In managing relationships, individuals need to show empathy and use social awareness when communicating with others

> ### Critical Thinking Questions
>
> - Identify a colleague you consider to be a clinical leader or role model. This person does not have to hold a position of designated authority (e.g. nurse unit manager), but should demonstrate leadership qualities.
>   - What are the qualities that you especially admire, and why?
>   - What is their leadership style?
>   - What strategies do they use to motivate or 'get the best' out of others in the team?
>   - What strategies do they use to ensure that team members are included in the decision-making process?
>   - What strategies do they use to build team trust?

(Edelman & van Knippenberg, 2018). Leaders with good emotional intelligence understand the importance of workplace relationships and realise that positive outcomes can be achieved only as a result of a team effort. Goleman (2011) identifies four domains of emotional intelligence: social awareness, relationship management, self-management and self-awareness. Fig. 2.4 illustrates the interrelationships between these domains.

Environmental Factors

The environmental elements of human factors comprise task management, ergonomics and noise and distraction. Each of these has the potential to impact on team performance.

Task management

Task management refers to the organisation of resources necessary to provide smooth, safe and effective patient care. It is also concerned with maintaining standards of care and dealing with stressful situations that occur in the perioperative environment (Flin & O'Connor, 2017). There are many physical and mental demands present when working in an operating room that can affect the safe and effective performance of the surgical team. For the nursing staff, there is a great deal of detail to remember when setting up the operating room for surgery, prioritising tasks and managing the environment when surgery is in progress. Managing this process effectively is important for patient safety and missing a step (e.g. forgetting to set up a piece of equipment) can result in procedural delays and errors that can compromise patient safety. Rather than relying

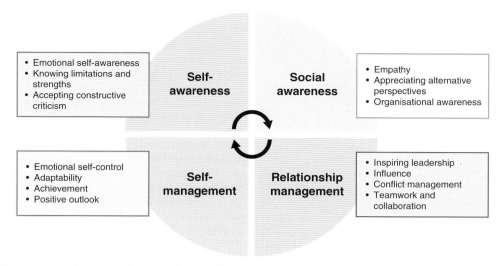

FIG. 2.4 Domains of emotional intelligence. (Source: Adapted from Goleman, D. (2011). *Leadership: The power of emotional intelligence.* Northampton, UK: More Than Sound.)

on memory alone, the nursing team can be assisted by following standardised policies and processes and by using effective checklists (Gillespie et al., 2018; Hardy et al., 2018).

Some helpful resources may include:

- surgeon's preference cards – so that all equipment required by each surgeon can be obtained ready for use
- diagrams showing where specific equipment is located within the operating room
- a checklist for setting up each piece of equipment
- tray lists to check each instrument tray prior to and following surgery
- team 'Time Out' checklist for correct identification of the patient
- algorithms for managing adverse events (e.g. loss of a sponge intraoperatively, or a difficult airway).

Task management also refers to the ability of staff to maintain correct standards of practice and to withstand the pressures of time or requests from other staff members to cut corners in practice. This is not easy to manage, especially for new staff members (Mitchell L. et al., 2011). The hierarchical structure of the surgical team may contribute to the pressure to disregard established protocols. It requires courage and good communication skills to resist such pressures. Agreeing to undertake an inappropriate practice not only puts the patient at risk, but can also call into question staff members' professional practice. Graded assertiveness, discussed later in the chapter, provides strategies to manage such challenging situations.

Ergonomics

Closely aligned to task management is ergonomics, which is defined as 'the scientific discipline concerned with the understanding of the interactions between humans and other elements of a system' (Hallbeck & Paquet, 2019; Human Factors & Ergonomics Society of Australia [HFESA], 2015, para. 1). In the context of the perioperative environment, ergonomics is concerned with the positioning of equipment, room layout, safe access and unimpeded movement for staff (Hallbeck & Paquet, 2019). The amount of equipment used during a procedure varies and can be significant. As well as correctly setting up individual pieces of equipment (discussed under task management), positioning the equipment is equally important to allow all staff members to access and view video screens and monitors. If the surgeon or anaesthetist is unable to view monitoring devices clearly, or if nurses cannot quickly access equipment controls to change settings, patient safety may be compromised (Hallbeck & Paquet, 2019). There is increasing evidence emerging about the impact that technology has on surgical teams' communications during surgery. The findings of a systematic review are summarised in Research box 2.4.

Another element of ergonomics is workplace health and safety – for example, manual handling and the trip hazards involved in moving equipment and positioning electrical cords. Many operating rooms have overhead pendant systems into which electrical cords and suction tubing can be connected, reducing trip hazards. However, pendants often add to inflexibility in the layout of the operating room as they are either fixed or have limited

---

RESEARCH BOX 2.4
Impact of Robotic Technologies on Team Communications in Surgery

A systematic mixed studies review by Gillespie and colleagues (2020) described the impact of surgical robots on team performance. In all, 19 research articles, 16 quantitative and 3 qualitative, were included. Robotic-assisted surgeries (RAS) were undertaken in the specialties of cardiology, general surgery, urology and gynaecology. Review findings suggest that:

- The presence of the robot changes the way information is distributed among team members.
- There is a need for increased and deliberate communication, especially when there is limited visual access to clinical information.
- An experienced surgeon at the console who controls the flow of information can compensate for an inexperienced team.
- Standardising surgical steps can help minimise disruptions caused by equipment changes.

(Source: Gillespie, B. M., Gillespie, J., Boorman, R. J., Granqvist, K., Stranne, J., & Erichsen-Andersson, A. (2020). The impact of robotic-assisted surgery on team performance: a systematic mixed studies review. *Human Factors*. https://doi.org/10.1177/0018720820928624.)

---

movement. In the future, Bluetooth technology will make the environment 'wireless', enabling monitoring and audiovisual equipment to be positioned with greater flexibility, as well as reducing trip hazards by eliminating electrical cords (ElBardissi & Sundt, 2012). (See Chapter 5 for further information about the perioperative environment.) Strategies designed to enhance the ergonomics of the operating room include standardising the placement of commonly used equipment and items to improve staff efficiency and reduce time wastage and potentially life-threatening errors (Carayon, Xie & Kianfar, 2014).

Ergonomics extends to the design of medical devices (e.g. infusion pumps, monitors, defibrillators). Designing the interface between the user and the device must take into consideration features that will reduce the risk of misuse, inappropriate actions and the possibility that data may be incorrectly interpreted, all of which could lead to patient safety being compromised. Design features should include, for example, functional grouping of controls, size, colour and brightness of displays, unambiguous labels, easy-to-operate keys, clear instructions and audible warning alarms (Clinical Human Factors Group, 2013).

Noise and distraction

The amount of noise in the operating room can contribute to adverse events and requires monitoring and managing. Noise can come from music, mobile phones and pagers, drills, electronic equipment, alerts on monitors and general conversation. Many surgeons enjoy background music playing while they operate and music does have soothing qualities. However, noise can be a danger by distracting staff, hindering effective communication and interfering with the surgeon's ability to concentrate. If music is played, the volume should be at a level that does not affect requests for equipment from being heard or mask monitor alarms. In addition, staff should not use personal electronic devices during surgery for texting or accessing social media, as this reduces situation awareness and distracts staff from critical events occurring during surgery. Such activities should take place during breaks away from the clinical area.

All of these distractions can compromise patient safety if they are not properly managed. Some operating rooms have policies on the use of mobile phones and pagers indicating that they must be on silent mode, or left in staff lockers or at reception for messages to be taken (Clark, 2013; Putnam, 2015). See Chapter 5 for further information about noise in the perioperative environment.

Most conversations between surgical team members are a necessary part of exchanging information about the procedure or requesting equipment, but at times the conversation may be informal 'chatter' unrelated to surgery. Such chatter during critical moments of surgery can distract team members (just like the plane's cockpit crew mentioned below) and compromise patient safety. As a result, some operating rooms follow another lesson learned from aviation: the concept of the 'sterile cockpit' (ElBardissi & Sundt, 2012).

The 'sterile cockpit' and 'below 10,000 feet'

The 'sterile cockpit' has nothing to do with a clean physical operating room environment, but rather refers to a clean mental environment, free from distractions that could compromise patient safety (Broom, Capek, Carachi, Akeroyd, & Hilditch, 2011). Evidence gathered from cockpit voice recorders (black boxes) following air disasters in the 1970s showed that, just prior to a plane crashing, the flight crew were frequently engaged in non-essential activities or conversations with colleagues in the cockpit or with flight attendants – tasks unrelated to their role of flying the plane. This distracting 'chatter' took their focus away from essential tasks, especially during the critical periods of the flight, and resulted in a number of adverse events including plane crashes. In an attempt to promote safety, the aviation industry invoked the 'sterile cockpit' or 'below 10,000 feet' rule stating that during critical phases of flying (e.g. landing, take-off, taxiing), no members of the flight crew were to engage in any activities other than those duties required to fly the plane safely. This also included banning interruptions from flight attendants unless there was a life-threatening event (Broom et al., 2011; Clark, 2013).

A parallel may be drawn between critical activities in the cockpit and those in an operating room. A 'sterile cockpit' rule could be invoked during one of the many critical periods that occur during surgery such as induction and reversal of anaesthesia, counting swabs and sponges, ligating vessels and so forth. It is imperative that during these types of activities the team does not become distracted or interrupted by informal conversations, music or mobile phones, which may erode their situation awareness and place the patient at risk. Perioperative nurses may find themselves in the position of managing noise and other distractions in the operating room and this requires a level of assertiveness, which is discussed in the next section (ElBardissi & Sundt, 2012; Clark, 2013). Feature box 2.4 provides an example of how two motivated perioperative nurses implemented the 'below 10,000' concept in their practice setting.

FEATURE BOX 2.4
Clinical Example of Below 10,000

In 2013, two anaesthetic nurses, John Gibbs and Pete Smith, at the University Hospital in Geelong introduced the 'below 10,000' concept. The impetus to reduce noise and distraction was based on colleagues' shared experiences where up to five separate conversations in an operating room made the anaesthetic work environment less safe while navigating critical stages of anaesthesia.

Gibbs and Smith reasoned that the anaesthetic phases of induction and emergence can be likened to aviation's 'sterile cockpit' rule, which prohibits non-essential activity that distracts from the task during 'critical phases of flight'. The metaphor of 'below 10,000' was selected as a powerful mental image and is supported by a body of evidence describing high-risk, high-safety team behaviours and performance.

Gibbs and Smith's strategies for implementing 'below 10,000' included inviting colleagues to discuss examples of noise and distraction and seeking clinician engagement for the implementation of the trigger phrase in their clinical setting. Gibbs and Smith also produced engaging merchandise to advertise and promote the concept throughout their operating theatre. The trigger phrase 'below 10,000' was introduced into the operating room vocabulary and could be voiced by any staff member in the room as a conflict-free tool to heighten situational awareness and team communication and improve task focus by the cessation of extraneous noise and distraction. In addition to its use during anaesthetic activities, the use of 'below 10,000' was expanded into other critical intraoperative activities including the surgical count and completion of the surgical safety checklist.

Since its introduction in Geelong, the initiative has been adopted by a number of operating suites worldwide, including Mercy Hospital, Dunedin, and East Lancashire Hospital Trust in the UK.

(Sources: Adapted from P. Smith (personal communication, April 19, 2019) and Gibbs, J., & Smith, P. (2016). Below ten thousand: an effective behavioural noise reduction strategy. *Journal of Perioperative Nursing in Australia, 29*(3), 29–32.)

PATIENT SCENARIOS

SCENARIO 2.2: A CACOPHONY OF SOUND

There is a significant amount of noise pollution as Mr Collins' total knee replacement progresses. The sounds of hammers, drills, saws, necessary discussion among surgical team members and mobile phones can impede the timely transfer of important case-related information.

Critical Thinking Questions

- Identify the sources of noise and distraction within your operating theatre.
- Consider how these affect the ability of the team to function safely and effectively.
- What strategies can you use to reduce the noise/distraction?

Graded Assertiveness

Assertiveness is a form of communication in which a person's needs or wishes are stated clearly with respect for the individual and the other person in the interaction. It differs from aggressive communication, where the needs or wishes are stated in a hostile or demanding manner (Zeigler-Hill & Shackelford, 2017). It can be difficult for nurses new to the perioperative environment to speak up when faced with situations where patient or staff safety is compromised. The hierarchical structure within the surgical team may discourage questioning or challenging senior staff. This situation may be exacerbated if the staff member's traditional cultural background discourages questioning of any authority.

Providing an environment in which staff members feel supported if the need to speak up arises is important; additionally, the use of **graded assertiveness** may assist in promoting effective dialogue. There are several different models of graded assertiveness that can be used and, as with all elements of good communication, they require practice for the team member to feel comfortable using them. Two models commonly used are explored in Feature boxes 2.5 and 2.6. At the start, neither strategy will be easy to initiate, but with practice the ability to speak up and question colleagues about practice issues becomes easier to achieve. The perioperative nurse is an advocate for the patient and in some situations for the safety of colleagues. Courage to act and to speak up using graded assertiveness is a necessary communication skill that perioperative nurses must practise and master.

PATIENT SCENARIOS

SCENARIO 2.3: GRADED ASSERTIVENESS

RN Jenny Sang is caring for Mr James Collins in the PACU following his TKR. RN Sang is concerned that Mr Collins is experiencing apnoeic episodes. RN Sang contacts the anaesthetist, Dr Marion Thomas, to outline the details of Mr Collins' condition. However, Dr Thomas does not offer to come to review Mr Collins herself.

Critical Thinking Question

- Using the STEP advocacy model, how should RN Sang respond to Dr Thomas?

Feature box 2.7 illustrates the significant part played by human factors in the adverse outcome for one patient, Elaine Bromiley, who underwent 'just a routine

---

FEATURE BOX 2.5
PACE Model of Graded Assertiveness

Probe: 'Doctor, do you know that this patient is allergic to latex?'

Alert: 'Can we reassess the situation before proceeding with surgery?'

Challenge: 'Please stop what you are doing while we obtain latex-free gloves.'

Emergency: 'STOP what you are doing!'

The final step might be confronting for nurses to undertake, but it may be necessary only to state the 'Probe' and 'Alert' steps: these two statements may be sufficient to halt the person proceeding any further and for remedial action to be taken (i.e. in this example obtaining the latex-free gloves).

(Source: Brindley, P. G., & Reynolds, S. F. (2011). Improving verbal communication in critical care medicine. *Journal of Critical Care, 26*, 155–159.)

FEATURE BOX 2.6
STEP Advocacy Approach to Graded Assertiveness

- Attention getter: 'Excuse me, Doctor Bob.'
- State your concern: 'I believe you have just contaminated your sterile gloves.'
- State the problem as you see it: 'The instruments are now contaminated and the aseptic field has been compromised.'
- State a solution: 'You will need to change your gloves.'
- Obtain an agreement: 'I have a pair of gloves ready for you here; is that OK with you?'

Again, by the time the concern has been stated, Dr Bob should have stopped his actions and proceeded to change his gloves without the need to work through the other steps.

(Source: Brindley, P. G., & Reynolds, S. F. (2011). Improving verbal communication in critical care medicine. *Journal of Critical Care, 26*, 155–159.)

FEATURE BOX 2.7
'Just a Routine Operation'

Elaine Bromiley was a fit and healthy young woman who was admitted to hospital for routine sinus surgery. During induction of anaesthetic, she experienced breathing problems and the anaesthetist was unable to insert a breathing tube to secure her airway. After 10 minutes it was a situation of 'can't intubate, can't ventilate' – a recognised anaesthetic emergency for which guidelines exist. For a further 15 minutes, three highly experienced consultants made numerous unsuccessful attempts to secure Elaine's airway and she suffered prolonged periods with dangerously low levels of oxygen in her bloodstream.

Early on, the nurses informed the team that they had brought emergency equipment to the room (instrumentation to perform a tracheostomy) and booked a bed in intensive care, but neither option was utilised.

Thirty-five minutes after starting the anaesthetic it was decided that Elaine should be allowed to wake up naturally and she was transferred to the recovery unit. When she failed to wake up she was transferred to ICU. Elaine never regained consciousness and after 13 days the decision was made to withdraw life support.

(Sources: Bromiley, M., & Mitchell, L. (2009a). Just a routine operation. https://elearning.rcog.org.uk/new-human-factors/teachingresources/case-study-just-routine-operation; Bromiley, M., & Mitchell, L. (2009b). Would you speak up if the consultant got it wrong? . . . and would you listen if someone said you'd got it wrong? *Journal of Perioperative Practice, 19*(10), 326–329.)

operation'. In reviewing the incident from a human factors perspective, it is clear that the team caring for Elaine failed in a number of areas:

- **Situation awareness** – the stress of the situation caused the medical team to become fixated on repeated attempts to secure the airway and lose sight of the bigger picture: that of Elaine's overall condition. They had no sense of the time that was passing and the increasing severity of the situation.
- **Decision making** – there was no clear leader who could step back from the situation, review actions and make appropriate decisions. Although very experienced, the three consultants were not communicating with each other.
- **Teamwork** – with no clear team leader, there was no shared mental model communicated between the team members. Each team member provided their own strategies for managing Elaine's airway. This resulted in uncoordinated actions that were not in line with the 'can't intubate, can't ventilate' emergency protocol.
- **Culture** – the nurses present recognised the seriousness of the situation very early and tried to make suggestions and bring in the appropriate emergency equipment. However, the hierarchy of the three consultants present affected the nurses' ability to intervene and effectively communicate their concerns and suggestions with the team.

Following Elaine Bromiley's death, her husband, Martin, an airline pilot, dedicated himself to promoting greater understanding about human factors within healthcare, particularly for surgical teams. He founded the Clinical Human Factors Group in the UK, which has produced some excellent resources – these are included in the Resources section at the end of the chapter.

Feature box 2.2 identifies nine strategies that surgical teams can use when working under pressure.

CONCLUSION

Patients are at their most vulnerable when they enter the confines of the perioperative environment for surgery. There is little doubt that human factors play a pivotal role in promoting patient safety. This chapter has examined several ways in which effective interdisciplinary teamwork and communication, including assertiveness, can contribute to safe patient outcomes in the perioperative environment. As patient advocates, it is important that perioperative nurses develop their skills in human factors to enable them to effectively advocate for patients and contribute to the team and patient safety.

RESOURCES

Below Ten Thousand Medical
https://www.belowtenthousand.com
Below 10,000 – Patient Safety Initiative, Mercy Hospital, Dunedin
https://youtu.be/ijrtOs1_t-A
Clinical Human Factors Group
https://www.chfg.org//
Human Factors & Ergonomics Society of Australia (HFESA)
https://www.ergonomics.org.au/resource_library/definitions
https://www.ergonomics.org.au/
'Just a Routine Operation' (UK)
https://patientsafety.health.org.uk/resources/just-routine-operation-human-factors-patient-safety
New Zealand Nursing Organisation
https://www.nzno.org.nz/support/workplace_rights/workplace_bullying
The Council on Surgical and Perioperative Safety
https://www.cspsteam.org
The Elaine Bromiley Case (Australian context)
https://vimeo.com/103516601
The Human Factor: Learning from Gina's Story
https://www.youtube.com/watch?v=IJfoLvLLoFo&app=desktop
The Patient Safety Initiative
https://www.thepatientsafetyinitiative.com
US Government
https://www.ntsb.gov/investigations/AccidentReports/Reports/AAR7907.pdf
What if? Teamwork in emergency airway management – the vortex approach
https://vimeo.com/112524096

REFERENCES

Alken, A., Luursema, J.-M., Weenk, M., Yauw, S., Fluit, C., & van Goor, H. (2018). Integrating technical and non-technical skills coaching in an acute trauma surgery team training: is it too much? *American Journal of Surgery*, *216*(2), 369–374. https://dx.doi.org/10.1016/j.amjsurg.2017.08.011

Australian College of Nursing (ACN). (2018). *Bullying in the workplace: position statement* (p. 3). Canberra: ACN.

Australian College of Perioperative Nurses (ACORN). (2020a). *ACORN standards for perioperative nursing in Australia.* (16th ed., Vol. 2). Managing the perioperative environment. Adelaide: Author.

Australian College of Perioperative Nurses (ACORN). (2020b). *ACORN standards for perioperative nursing in Australia.* (16th ed., Vol. 2). Bullying and harassment. Adelaide: Author.

Australian Government. (2014). *Fairwork Commission antibullying guide*. Canberra: Author.

Brennan, P., & Davidson, M. (2019). Improving patient safety: we need to reduce hierarchy and empower junior doctors to speak up. The BMJ opinion. Retrieved from <https://blogs.bmj.com/bmj/2019/05/03/improving-patient-safety-we-need-to-reduce-hierarchy-and-empower-junior-doctors-to-speak-up/#_ftn1>.

Brindle, M. E., Henrich, N., Foster, A., Marks, S., Rose, M., Welsh, R., & Berry, W. (2018). Implementation of surgical debriefing programs in large health systems: an exploratory qualitative analysis. *BMC Health Services Research, 18*(1), 210.

Brindley, P. G., & Reynolds, S. F. (2011). Improving verbal communication in critical care medicine. *Journal of Critical Care, 26*(2), 155–159.

Bromiley, M., & Mitchell, L. (2009a). Just a routine operation. Retrieved from https://elearning.rcog.org.uk/new-human-factors/teachingresources/case-study-just-routine-operation.

Bromiley, M., & Mitchell, L. (2009b). Would you speak up if the consultant got it wrong? . . . and would you listen if someone said you'd got it wrong? *Journal of Perioperative Practice, 19*(10), 326–329. https://dx.doi.org/10.1177/175045890901901004

Broom, M. A., Capek, A. L., Carachi, P., Akeroyd, M. A., & Hilditch, G. (2011). Critical phase distractions in anaesthesia and the sterile cockpit concept. *Anaesthesia, 66*(3), 175–179. https://dx.doi.org/10.1111/j.1365-2044.2011.06623.x

Budden, L., Birks, M., Cant, R., Bagley, T., & Park, T. (2017). Australian nursing students' experience of bullying and/or harassment during clinical placement. *Collegian, 24*, 125–133.

Carayon, P., Xie, A., & Kianfar, S. (2014). Human factors and ergonomics as a patient safety practice. *British Medical Journal Quality and Safety, 23*(3), 196–205. https://dx.doi.org/10.1136/bmjqs-2013-001812

Chen, X., Fu, R., & Zhao, S. (2015). Culture and socialization. In J. Grusec (Ed.), *Handbook of socialization: theory and research* (2nd ed., pp. 451–471). New York: Guilford Publications.

Clark, G. J. (2013). Strategies for preventing distractions and interruptions in the OR. *AORN Journal, 97*(6), 702–707. https://dx.doi.org/10.1016/j.aorn.2013.01.018

Clinical Human Factors Group. (2013). *Getting to grips with the human factor: strategic actions for safer care. a learning resource for boards.* Retrieved from <https://chfg.org/getting-to-grips-with-the-human-factor-boards-resource/>.

Cousley, A., Martin, D., & Hoy, L. (2014). Vulnerability in the perioperative patient: a concept analysis. *Journal of Perioperative Practice, 24*(7-8), 164–171.

Department of Defense. (2006). TeamSTEPPS Multimedia Resource Kit. AHRQ Publication No. 06-0020-3. Rockville MD: Agency for Healthcare Research and Quality.

Edelman, P., & van Knippenberg, D. (2018). Emotional intelligence, management of subordinate's emotions, and leadership effectiveness. *Leadership & Organization Development Journal, 39*(5), 592–607.

ElBardissi, A. W., & Sundt, T. M. (2012). Human factors and operating room safety. *Surgical Clinics of North America, 92*(1), 21–35. https://dx.doi.org/10.1016/j.suc.2011.11.007

Ensley, M. (1995). Toward a theory of situational awareness in dynamic systems. *Human Factors, 37*(1), 37–64.

Fecso, A. B., Kuzulugil, S. S., Babaoglu, C., Bener, A. B., & Grantcharov, T. P. (2018). Relationship between intraoperative non-technical performance and technical events in bariatric surgery. *British Journal of Surgery, 105*(8), 1044–1050. https://dx.doi.org/10.1002/bjs.10811

Fletcher, S. (2012). Five reasons why emotional intelligence is critical for leaders. Retrieved from <https://leadchangegroup.com/5-reasons-why-emotional-intelligence-is-critical-for-leaders>.

Flin, R. (2013). Non-technical skills for anaesthetists, surgeons and scrub practitioners (ANTS, NOTSS and SPLINTS). Aberdeen: The Health Foundation, 1-9. Retrieved from <https://improve.bmj.com/sites/default/files/resources/non_technical_skills_for_anaesthetists_surgeons_and_scrub_practitioners.pdf>.

Flin, R., & O'Connor, P. (2017). *Safety at the sharp end: a guide to non-technical skills* (2nd ed.). Baton Rouge, FL: CRC Press.

Flin, R., O'Connor, P., & Crichton, M. (2008). *Safety at the sharp end: a guide to non-technical skills.* Baton Rouge, FL: CRC Press.

Flin, R., & Patey, R. (2011). Non-technical skills for anaesthetists: developing and applying ANTS. *Best Practice & Research Clinical Anaesthesiology, 25*(2), 215–227.

Gessler, R., Rosenstein, A., & Ferron, L. (2012). How to handle disruptive physician behavior. *American Nurse Today, 7*(11), 8–10.

Gibbs, J., & Smith, P. (2016). Below ten thousand: an effective behavioural noise reduction strategy. *Journal of Perioperative Nursing in Australia, 29*(3), 29–32.

Gillespie, B. M., Chaboyer, W., & Fairweather, N. (2012). Factors that influence the expected length of operation: results of a prospective study. *British Medical Journal Quality and Safety, 21*(1), 3–12.

Gillespie, B. M., Chaboyer, W., Thalib, L., John, M., Fairweather, N., & Slater, K. (2014). Effect of using a safety checklist on patient complications after surgery: a systematic review and meta-analysis. *Anesthesiology, 120*(6), 1380–1389.

Gillespie, B. M., Gillespie, J., Boorman, R. J., Granqvist, K., Stranne, J., & Erichsen-Andersson, A. (2020). The impact of robotic-assisted surgery on team performance: a systematic mixed studies review. *Human Factors.* Retrieved from <https://doi.org/10.1177/0018720820928624>.

Gillespie, B. M., Gwinner, K., Fairweather, N., & Chaboyer, W. (2013). Building shared situational awareness in surgery through distributed dialog. *Journal of Multidisciplinary Healthcare, 6*, 109–118. https://dx.doi.org/10.2147/JMDH.S40710

Gillespie, B. M., Harbeck, E., Lavin, J., Hamilton, K., Gardiner, T., Withers, T., & Marshall, A. (2018). Evaluation of a patient safety programme on Surgical Safety Checklist compliance: a prospective longitudinal study. *British Medical Journal Quality, 7*, 1–9.

Gillespie, B. M., Withers, T. K., Lavin, J., Gardiner, T., & Marshall, A. P. (2016). Factors that drive team participation in surgical safety checks: a prospective study. *Patient Safety in Surgery, 10*, 3. https://dx.doi.org/10.1186/s13037-015-0090-5

Goleman, D. (2011). *Leadership: the power of emotional intelligence.* Northampton, UK: More Than Sound.

Gordon, M., Baker, P., Catchpole, K., Darbyshire, D., & Schocken, D. (2015). Devising a consensus definition and framework for non-technical skills in healthcare to support educational design: a modified Delphi study. *Medical Teacher, 37*(6), 572–577. https://dx.doi.org/10.3109/0142159X.2014.959910

Graystone, R. (2019). How to build a positive, multigenerational workforce. *Journal of Nursing Administration, 49*(1), 4–5.

Green, B., Oeppen, R. S., Smith, D. W., & Brennan, P. A. (2017). Challenging hierarchy in healthcare teams – ways to flatten gradients to improve teamwork and patient care. *British Journal of Oral and Maxillofacial Surgery, 55*(5), 449–453. https://dx.doi.org/10.1016/j.bjoms.2017.02.010

Hallbeck, M. S., & Paquet, V. (2019). Human factors and ergonomics in the operating room: contributions that advance surgical practice: preface. *Applied Ergonomics, 78,* 248–250. https://dx.doi.org/10.1016/j.apergo.2019.04.007

Hardy, J.-B., Gouin, A., Damm, C., Compère, V., Veber, B., & Dureuil, B. (2018). The use of a checklist improves anaesthesiologists' technical and non-technical performance for simulated malignant hyperthermia management. *Anaesthesia Critical Care and Pain Medicine, 37*(1), 17–23. https://dx.doi.org/10.1016/j.accpm.2017.07.009

Human Factors & Ergonomics Society of Australia (HFESA). (2015). Retrieved from <https://www.ergonomics.org.au/>.

Jones, K., & Ritzman, T. (2018). Perioperative safety. *Orthopedic Clinics of North America, 49*(4), 465–476.

Kaye, A. D., Fox III, C. J., & Urman, R. D. (2012). *Operating room leadership and management.* Cambridge, UK: Cambridge University Press.

Lin, A., Wernick, B., Tolentino, J. C., & Stawicki, S. P. (2018). *Wrong-site procedures: preventable never events that continue to happen. Vignettes in patient safety – Vol. 2.* London: IntechOpen.

Llewellyn, A., Karageorge, A., Nash, L., Li, W., & Neuen, D. (2018). Bullying and sexual harassment of junior doctors in New South Wales, Australia: rate and reporting outcomes. *Australian Health Review, 43*(3) 328–334. https://dx.doi.org/10.1071/AH17224

Manias, E., Geddes, F., Watson, B., Jones, D., & Della, P. (2015). Communication failures during clinical handovers lead to a poor patient outcome: lessons from a case report. *SAGE Open Medical Case Reports, 3,* 2050313X15584859.

Martin, L., & Langell, J. (2017). Improving on-time surgical starts: the impact of implementing pre-OR timeouts and performance pay. *Journal of Surgical Research, 219,* 222–225.

McComb, S., & Simpson, V. (2014). The concept of shared mental models in healthcare collaboration. *Journal of Advanced Nursing, 70* (7), 1479–1488.

Mitchell, L., Flin, R., Yule, S., Mitchell, J., Coutts, K., & Youngson, G. (2011). Thinking ahead of the surgeon. An interview study to identify scrub practitioners' nontechnical skills. *International Journal of Nursing Studies, 48,* 818–828.

Mitchell, R., Chung, A., Williamson, A., & Molesworth, B. (2011). Human factors and healthcare-related deaths: review of coronial findings using a human factors classification framework. *Ergonomics Australia–Human Factors & Ergonomics Society of Australasia (HFESA) Conference Edition, 11*(18), 1–6.

National Transportation Safety Board. (1978). *Aircraft incident report.* Retrieved from <https://www.ntsb.gov/investigations/AccidentReports/Reports/AAR7907.pdf>.

Putnam, K. (2015). Minimizing electronic distractions in the OR. *AORN Journal, 102*(1), 7–9. https://dx.doi.org/10.1016/S0001-2092(15)00530-X

Rabøl, L. I., Lehmann Andersen, M., Østergaard, D., Bjørn, B., Lilja, B., & Mogensen, T. (2011). Descriptions of verbal communication errors between staff. An analysis of 84 root cause analysis-reports from Danish hospitals. *British Medical Journal Quality and Safety, 20,* 268–274.

Salas, E., & Rosen, M. A. (2013). Building high reliability teams: progress and some reflections on teamwork training. *British Medical Journal Quality and Safety, 22*(5), 369–373. https://dx.doi.org/10.1136/bmjqs-2013-002015

Salas, E., Shuffler, M. L., Thayer, A. L., Bedwell, W. L., & Lazzara, E. H. (2015). Understanding and improving teamwork in organizations: a scientifically based practical guide. *Human Resource Management, 54*(4), 599–622. https://dx.doi.org/10.1002/hrm.21628

Shubeck, S. P., Kanters, A. E., & Dimick, J. B. (2019). Surgeon leadership style and risk-adjusted patient outcomes. *Surgical Endoscopy, 33*(2), 471–474. https://dx.doi.org/10.1007/s00464-018-6320-z

Stein, L. (1978). The doctor–nurse game. In R. Dingwall & J. Mcintosh (Eds.), *Readings in the sociology of nursing* (pp. 108–117). Edinburgh: Longman.

Stewart, G. L., Manges, K. A., & Ward, M. M. (2015). Empowering sustained patient safety: the benefits of combining top-down and bottom-up approaches. *Journal of Nursing Care Quality, 30*(3), 240–246. https://dx.doi.org/10.1097/ncq.0000000000000103

Tanner, J., & Timmons, S. (2000). Backstage in the theatre. *Journal of Advanced Nursing, 32*(4), 975–980. https://dx.doi.org/10.1046/j.1365-2648.2000.01564.x

Wacker, J., & Kolbe, M. (2014). Leadership and teamwork in anesthesia: making use of human factors to improve clinical performance. *Trends in Anaesthesia and Critical Care, 4,* 200–205.

Worksafe New Zealand. (2014). Bullying prevention toolbox. Retrieved from <https://www.worksafe.govt.nz/topic-and-industry/bullying/>.

Zeigler-Hill, V., & Shackelford, T. (2017). Foundations of assertiveness. In *Encyclopedia of personality and individual differences* (Living ed.). Retrieved from <https://link.springer.com/referenceworkentry/10.1007%2F978-3-319-28099-8_1044-1>.

Zwaan, L., Len, L. T. S., Wagner, C., van Groeningen, D., Kolenbrander, M., & Krage, R. (2016). The reliability and usability of the Anesthesiologists' Non-Technical Skills (ANTS) system in simulation research. *Advances in Simulation, 1*(1), 18.

FURTHER READING

Broom, M., Capek, A., Carachi, P., Akeroyd, M., & Hilditch, G. (2011). Critical phase distractions in anaesthesia and the sterile cockpit concept. *Anaesthesia, 66*(3), 175–179.

Ford, D. (2015). Speaking up to reduce noise in the OR. *AORN Journal 102*, (1), 85–89.

Gillespie, B. M., Gillespie, J., Boorman, R., Granqvist, K., Stranne, J., & Erichsen-Andersson, A. (2020). The impact of robotic assisted surgery on team performance: an systematic mixed studies review. *Human Factors, Jul 2*, 18720820928624. https://dx.doi.org/10.1177/0018 7208 20928624 [Online ahead of print]

Gillespie, B. M., Harbeck, H., Kang E., Steel, C., Fairweather, N., Panuwatwanich, K., & Chaboyer, W. (2017). Effect of a brief team-training program on surgical teams' non-technical skills: an interrupted time-series study. *Journal of Patient Safety*, April 27, 1–7. https://dx.doi.org/10.1097/PTS.0000000000000361 [Epub ahead of print]

Gillespie, B. M., Harbeck, H., Kang E., Steel, C., Fairweather, N., Panuwatwanich, K., & Chaboyer, W. (2017). Correlates of non-technical skills in surgery: a prospective study. *British Medical Journal Open, 7*, e014480.

Hay, G. (2020). *Ladies and gentlemen, this is your surgeon speaking: exploring the human factor in aviation and surgery.* Kima Beach: Publicious.

Kang, E., Gillespie, B. M., & Massey, D. (2014). What are the non-technical skills used by scrub nurses? An integrated review. *ACORN Journal, 27*(4), 16–25.

Kang, E., Massey, D., & Gillespie, B. M. (2015). Factors that influence the non-technical skills performance of scrub nurses: a prospective study. *Journal of Advanced Nursing, 71*(12), 2846–2857. https://dx.doi.org/10.1111/jan.12743

Lin, Y., Scott, J. W., Yi, S., Taylor, K. K., Ntakiyiruta, G., Ntirenganya, F., . . . Riviello, R. (2018). Improving surgical safety and nontechnical skills in variable-resource contexts: a novel educational curriculum. *Journal of Surgical Education, 75*(4), 1014–1021.

Maran, N., Edgar, S., & May, A. (2013). Non-technical skills. In K. Forrest, J. McKimm, & S. Edgar (Eds.), *Essential simulation in clinical education* (pp. 131–145). London: John Wiley & Sons.

Weigl, M., Weber, J., Hallett, E., Pfandler, M., Schlenker, B., Becker, A., & Catchpole, K. (2018). Associations of intraoperative flow disruptions and operating room teamwork during robotic-assisted radical prostatectomy. *Urology, 114*(1), 105–113.

CHAPTER 3

Medico-legal Aspects of Perioperative Nursing Practice

AMANDA ADRIAN • MENNA DAVIES
EDITOR: MENNA DAVIES

LEARNING OUTCOMES

- Discuss the statutes and common law cases that guide nursing practice
- Apply statutes and common law cases in relation to negligence, consent to care and treatment, and documentation
- Examine the management of complaints against nurses and the conduct of disciplinary hearings
- Understand and differentiate between privacy and confidentiality
- Explore the use of social media as it relates to patient privacy and professional nursing practice

KEY TERMS

advance health directive

consent to treatment

coroners' courts

disciplinary hearings

documentation

negligence

privacy and confidentiality

professional conduct

professional misconduct

professional standards

social media

unprofessional conduct

INTRODUCTION

This chapter focuses on medico-legal and ethical topics as they relate to the delivery of patient care in the perioperative setting. In addition to the regulatory framework, codes of conduct and professional standards discussed in Chapter 1, nursing practice is also informed by legislation and common law decisions, and by state and federal health department or national ministry of health policies. In particular, this chapter explores consent to treatment, negligence, patient confidentiality and individual as well as organisational privacy. It also examines pitfalls when using social media in healthcare settings. At a time of strong public and professional scrutiny of patient safety, perioperative nurses require an understanding of the processes contained within the regulatory framework associated with managing adverse patient outcomes and complaints made about nursing care.

PATIENT SCENARIOS

SCENARIO 3.1

Mr James Collins is a 78-year-old man who has been admitted for an elective right total knee replacement (TKR). His full history and a brief description of the healthcare setting is provided in the Introduction at the front of the book for readers to review when answering the questions in this unfolding scenario.

Following anaesthetic assessment and discussion with Mr Collins, it has been decided to undertake the procedure under spinal anaesthesia combined with sedation and a femoral nerve block.

Mr Collins has arrived in the receiving area of the operating suite. The handover from the ward nurse, RN George Markham, to anaesthetic nurse, RN Margaret McCormack, takes place. When Mr Collins is asked to confirm the nature of the operation, his response indicates that he is unsure of the operation he is about to undergo.

Critical Thinking Question

- What are RN McCormack's responsibilities as Mr Collins's advocate in this situation, and what action should she take? Provide rationales for your answer.

Accountability and Advocacy

In all of their activities, perioperative nurses remain accountable for their practice and, as necessary, advocate on behalf of their patients (see Chapter 1). These roles are enshrined in the Nursing and Midwifery Board of Australia (NMBA) *Code of professional conduct for nurses in Australia* (NMBA, 2018), the International Council of Nurses (ICN) *The ICN code of ethics for nurses* (ICN, 2012) (adopted by the NMBA) and the New Zealand Code of Health and Disability Services Consumers' Rights (Code of Rights) (New Zealand Health and Disability Commissioner, 1996). Indeed, being a patient advocate is fundamental to the nurse's role and is reflected in definitions of nursing (Feature box 3.1). In its simplest form, as reflected in Virginia Henderson's words, advocacy can be defined as intervening or speaking up on behalf of patients when they are unable to do so due to their physical or mental condition. The concept of advocacy (addressed in Chapter 1) has three basic assumptions:

- being an advocate is proactive rather than passive
- the nurse is prepared to speak up and act on behalf of the patient
- some difficulty or challenge exists that requires action as an advocate (Kerridge, Lowe, & Stewart, 2013).

There are few better examples of acting on behalf of the patient than doing so in the perioperative environment, where patients are, for the most part, either sedated or anaesthetised and unable to look after themselves. As patient advocate, the perioperative nurse has an obligation to ensure the patient's physical, emotional and ethical needs are met, and must be ready to intervene to protect the patient's safety. This may include speaking up if correct policies or procedures are not being adhered to or when potential exists for injury without intervention.

Acting as the patient's advocate has legal and ethical implications that the perioperative nurse must consider, and the role is not without its challenges. This is especially so if acting on behalf of the patient brings the perioperative nurse into conflict with others, some of whom may be close colleagues. If faced with this situation, the nurse may need to confront the person concerned. This is best done after seeking advice from more senior colleagues who can advise on an appropriate course of action.

Some situations, however, may require a more serious response. Turning a blind eye to incorrect or inappropriate behaviour may result in harm to the patient and is in conflict with the NMBA codes of ethics and professional conduct and the New Zealand code of rights. In addition, under Section 140 of the National Law 2009, registered health practitioners and employers have a legal obligation to make a mandatory notification if they have formed a reasonable belief that a health practitioner has behaved in a way that constitutes notifiable conduct in relation to the practice of their profession (Australian Health Practitioner Regulation Agency [AHPRA], 2013). This places great responsibility on the nurse to act, and consulting with a senior colleague can clarify the course of action to be taken. Documentation of the facts of the situation is essential when proceeding with mandatory reporting of a colleague and will be used in any subsequent investigation. The case of *Nursing and Midwifery Board of Australia v George* [2015] VCAT 1878 (25 November 2015) specifically deals with a nurse's failure to advocate for a patient in a perioperative setting (Feature box 3.2). The ACORN competency standards (ACORN,

---

FEATURE BOX 3.1
Definition of Nursing

The unique function of a nurse is to assist the individual, sick or well, in the performance of those activities contributing to health or its recovery (or to peaceful death) that he would perform unaided if he had the necessary strength, will or knowledge, and to do this in such a way as to help him gain independence as rapidly as possible.

(Source: Henderson, V. (1964). The nature of nursing. *American Journal of Nursing, 64*(8), p. 66.)

FEATURE BOX 3.2
EN's Failure to Act as Patient Advocate

In 2011, a patient underwent a late-stage termination of pregnancy at a Victorian private hospital and was discharged home. The following day, relatives reported the patient as being drowsy and unable to be roused. She returned to the hospital for treatment of complications including a septic uterus and possible organ failure. The patient, who had limited command of English, was admitted to the operating theatre by an experienced anaesthetic EN, placed on the operating table and given oxygen. The EN had noted on admission that the patient was drowsy, but responsive.

However, the anaesthetist and surgical team determined that the patient was unconscious and proceeded with an evacuation of the uterus without providing any anaesthesia or pain relief. Despite being aware that the patient was conscious, though drowsy, just prior to the commencement of the procedure, the EN failed to alert the medical and nursing teams of her observations or concerns. The patient's condition deteriorated in the postoperative period, requiring urgent transfer to a tertiary hospital for further treatment.

The EN was charged with 'unprofessional conduct' for failing to state her observations concerning the patient's state of consciousness and to question whether it was appropriate to continue the procedure in light of those observations. In addition, it was alleged that the EN failed to adequately document the care of the patient.

The EN was reprimanded by the Victorian Civil and Administrative Tribunal for her failure to advocate for her patient and her failure to make adequate notes in the patient record. She was ordered to complete further education in law and ethics.

(Source: *Nursing and Midwifery Board of Australia v George* (Review and Regulation) [2015] VCAT 1878 (25 November 2015).)

2012–13) were reviewed as part of the case, clearly demonstrating the professional responsibilities.

LEGISLATION AND CASE LAW

Various statutes (legislation) and common law (case law) precedents impact on perioperative nursing practice in Australasia. The relevant legislation is outlined in Table 3.1. In addition, in New Zealand the Health and Disability Commissioner Act 1994 and the Health and Disability Commissioner Amendment Act 2003 incorporate the code of rights, which extends to any person or organisation providing a health service to the public. The code of rights covers all health professionals, and one obligation is to take reasonable action in the circumstances to give effect to the rights and comply with the duties. Furthermore, in July 2008, Australian health ministers endorsed the Australian charter of healthcare rights (Australian Commission on Safety and Quality in Health Care [ACSQHC/the Commission], 2008), describing the rights of patients and others using the Australian health system. These rights are essential to make sure that, wherever and whenever care is provided, it is of high quality and safe.

Case Law or Common Law

Common law decisions also have a direct bearing on practice in the perioperative area, such as those related to negligence (see discussion below), which is a civil wrong (or tort), and to consent to treatment (see later in this chapter). Failure to gain consent from patients before treating them constitutes the civil wrong of trespass to the person, specifically assault and battery. This should not be confused with the civil wrong of negligence. The underpinning legal principles associated

TABLE 3.1
Statute Law

Subject Area	Australia	New Zealand
Regulation of nursing practice	Health Practitioner Regulation National Law Act 2009 (the National Law) as in force in each state and territory	Health Practitioners Competence Assurance Act 2003
Privacy and confidentiality	Privacy Act 1988 (Cth) Health Records and Information Privacy Act 2002 (NSW) Health Records Act 2001 (Vic) Information Act 2003 (NT)	Privacy Act 1993
Poisons and drugs	Therapeutic Goods Act 1989 (Cth) Health (Drugs and Poisons) Regulation 1996 (Qld) Medicines, Poisons and Therapeutic Goods Act 2008 (ACT)	Misuse of Drugs Act 1975

with all civil wrongs are well-established common law principles developed by the courts over several centuries (thereby establishing precedents) and sometimes referred to as case law. Some of the principles addressing the law of civil wrongs or torts have been extended by national, state or territory legislation, all of which vary somewhat (Staunton & Chiarella, 2020). In each Australian state and territory and in New Zealand, legislation applies to adults who are not competent to give consent (Government of Western Australia, Department of Health, 2016; Medical Council of New Zealand, 2019).

Health Policies and Professional Practice Standards

Various state, territory and national health department/ministry policies have a direct bearing on perioperative practice; for example, New South Wales (NSW) Health has a policy related to the conduct of the surgical count, which is mandatory in public hospitals (NSW Health, 2013). In addition, New Zealand, the Commonwealth and all Australian states and territories have infection control policies that have a significant impact on perioperative nursing practice – for example, the *Australian guidelines for the prevention and control of infection in healthcare* (National Health and Medical Research Council [NHMRC], 2019) and the Surgical Site Infection Improvement Programme (New Zealand Health Quality and Safety Commission, 2018).

There are perioperative nursing practice standards that are not mandatory; however, they can and have been influential when used in cases of negligence or hearings relating to professional practice and conduct. Both the Australian College of Perioperative Nurses (ACORN, 2020) and the Perioperative Nurses College of the New Zealand Nurses Organisation (PNC NZNO) (2016) have standards (howsoever titled) that have been developed by specialty nurses to guide practice in perioperative settings. Failure to adhere to these standards can have adverse consequences for patients. Additionally, such actions may result in the practice of individual nurses being examined by regulatory authorities (see Chapter 1 for further information).

Negligence

Negligence is the most widely known civil wrong or tort. Although there is no one accepted definition of negligence, the cardinal principle is that the party complaining (the plaintiff) is owed a duty of care by the party complained of (the defendant), this duty of care has been breached and, as a consequence of that breach, the party complaining has suffered damage (Staunton & Chiarella, 2020).

The roles that perioperative nurses undertake while caring for surgical patients require diligence and discipline because the incidence of perioperative-related adverse events (such as death or serious injury) is greater than occurs in other settings. This is due to the vulnerability of individuals undergoing surgical intervention and the nature of the surgical environment itself. Some examples of incidents that surgical patients may experience and that could lead to adverse outcomes include:

- incorrect positioning
- inadvertently retained surgical items
- lost tissue specimens
- incorrect operation or operative site
- medication error
- equipment failure.

(See Chapter 4 for further information on adverse events.)

When entering the operating suite, patients are at one of the most vulnerable periods of their hospitalisation. They place their trust in the surgical team to ensure that no harm will come to them. Unfortunately, sometimes incidents do occur that result in patients being injured. Patients who experience injury may decide to bring a civil case for negligence against the health service and/or those health professionals who they believe are responsible. The plaintiff (or the person's family, if the patient has died or is no longer competent to bring the action themself) can allege that the patient was injured as a result of the health professional's care falling below the required or accepted standard of care – that is, the acts (or omissions) were not those expected of a reasonable health professional with the necessary skills, knowledge, experience and judgement. Nurses can and do become involved in legal proceedings, resulting in their practice being examined. However, it should be noted that it is rare for nurses to have an action brought against them directly (i.e. to be sued individually).

Vicarious liability

As the majority of nurses are employees in most jurisdictions, the doctrine of vicarious liability is likely to apply. *Vicarious liability* means that an employer is deemed liable for the acts of its employees if an action arises while an employee is acting in good faith as part of their employment. It is only when the employee is found to be 'on a frolic of their own' (acting totally outside the recognised policies and procedures of the employer) that the doctrine will not apply (Staunton & Chiarella, 2020).

PATIENT SCENARIOS

SCENARIO 3.2: PROFESSIONAL PRACTICE

RN Rob Cohen and RN Ben Lumby are the circulating nurses for Mr Collins' procedure and are working with an experienced instrument nurse, EN Pauline Noakes. During the course of the initial count, RN Cohen notes that EN Noakes is not counting items according to practices set out in the operating suite's policy manual, which are based on contemporary professional standards.

Critical Thinking Questions

- How should RN Cohen handle this situation? Provide rationale(s) for your response.
- What are the circulating nurse's professional responsibilities in relation to conducting the count of accountable items?

Pursuing cases of negligence in civil courts

Pursuing an action for negligence through the courts in Australia can be a complex (and expensive) process. Legislation has been enacted by each Australian state and territory (e.g. the Civil Law Act 2002 [NSW]) in response to increased litigation and the subsequent rise in the cost of public liability and medical indemnity insurance, which has become unsustainable. The legislation seeks to balance the costs involved with insurance premiums, settling negligence claims and the rights of individuals to be compensated for harm resulting from health professionals' negligence (Kerridge et al., 2013; Staunton & Chiarella, 2020).

The legal situation in relation to medical negligence is very different in New Zealand, where a 'no fault' accident compensation scheme was established as early as 1974. Although this has evolved over time, the Injury Prevention, Rehabilitation and Compensation Amendment Act (No. 2) 2005 provides cover for unintended injuries to patients caused by treatment provided by health professionals (Barnett-Davidson, 2013).

In Australia, when a negligence action against a nurse goes before a court, the patient or plaintiff has to prove a number of elements to establish that, on the balance of probabilities, there was negligence on the part of the nurse. These elements include establishing that:

- the nurse owed the patient a duty of care – this is usually unequivocal
- there was a breach of the duty of care (i.e. the nurse failed to act according to accepted practice standards – for example, the *Registered nurse standards for practice* (NMBA, 2016) or *Standards for perioperative nursing* (ACORN, 2020)
- there was damage to the patient, which can be physical or psychological
- there was a direct link between the breach of the duty of care and the damage suffered by the patient (Staunton & Chiarella, 2020).

All of these elements are exemplified in the Australian negligence case, *Langley & Another v Glandore Pty Ltd (in Liq) & Another* (1997) outlined in Feature box 3.3. The elements of negligence from this case were as follows:

- the surgical team owed a duty of care to the patient during surgery
- the nurses breached their duty of care by failing to follow accepted standards in relation to counting. This was determined by reference to the ACORN (1996) *Standards, guidelines and policy statements: Standard A6: Managing accountable items*, which was current at the time of the incident
- the sponge left inside the patient caused damage, pain and suffering.

FEATURE BOX 3.3
Langley & Another v Glandore Pty Ltd (in Liq) & Another (1997)

A patient underwent a hysterectomy in a Queensland hospital. After suffering adverse symptoms over a period of months following the surgery, investigations revealed that a surgical sponge had been inadvertently left in her abdomen. This was removed in a second operation 10 months after the first procedure. The patient sued the surgeons and the hospital, as the latter was vicariously responsible for the perioperative nurses. The judge found the surgeons negligent for leaving the sponge inside the patient, but the nurses were found not to be negligent. The surgeons appealed the judgment on the basis that the circulating and instrument nurses played a crucial role in accounting for the sponges used in the procedure. At the appeal hearing, the judge agreed with the surgeons and, in a significant judgment for perioperative nurses, made it clear that both of the nurses were 'primarily responsible' for the count. Neither nurse could provide an explanation as to how a counting error occurred or why the count sheet from the original operation was shown to be complete (Staunton & Chiarella, 2020).

- The sponge inadvertently left inside the patient's abdomen was the direct cause of the damage to the patient.

Significant points highlighted by this case include the use of the ACORN standards in court in order to establish the standard of care expected when handling accountable items and the point made by the judge in the appeal hearing placing 'primary responsibility' for the count in the hands of the circulating and instrument nurses. It should be noted that the count sheet produced in evidence in this case was complete, with no indication of a counting error evident. This case and others that have since arisen (e.g. *Elliot v Bickerstaff* [1999]) highlight the need for vigilance when conducting and recording counts and handling accountable items intraoperatively (Staunton & Chiarella, 2020).

Open disclosure

Where an adverse event results in patient harm, it is considered best practice to explain to the patient what has happened. This is not necessarily considered an admission of fault or liability, which may have prevented open disclosure occurring in the past. Open disclosure is supported by the National Safety and Quality Health Service (NSQHS) Standards (ACSQHC/ the Commission, 2017a). The elements of *open disclosure* are:

- an apology or expression of regret, which should include the words 'I am sorry' or 'we are sorry'
- a factual explanation of what happened
- an opportunity for the patient, family and carers to relate their experience
- a discussion of the potential consequences of the adverse event
- an explanation of the steps being taken to manage the adverse event and prevent recurrence (ACSQHC/ the Commission, 2017b).

In Australia the Commission has published the *Open disclosure framework* (ACSQHC/ the Commission, 2017b) and state/territory health departments have also published policies in relation to this – for example, South Australia (Government of South Australia, 2016). In New Zealand, the code of rights supports the right of the consumer to open disclosure (New Zealand Health and Disability Commissioner, 1996).

Consent to Treatment

All adult patients undergoing surgery must understand the nature and risks of the surgery and give informed consent to the procedure. This is the same for any healthcare treatment, which patients may accept or decline (Staunton & Chiarella, 2020). Health department and local policies set out the requirements for obtaining valid consent. In Australia, these are largely based on common law decisions, and policies (e.g. Queensland Health, 2017) vary across the eight jurisdictions. In some cases they are also enshrined in legislation; for example, in New Zealand the code of rights (New Zealand Health and Disability Commissioner, 1996) outlines patients' rights related to consent, which must be fully informed and given freely.

Although it is not usually the role of perioperative nurses to obtain the patient's consent for a surgical intervention as they are generally not conducting the procedure, nurses do have a responsibility to check that patients have given **consent to treatment** and that this consent is informed. This is usually substantiated by the presence of a signed consent form. For patient consent to treatment to be valid:

- it must be freely and voluntarily given
- the patient must be of the correct age, which varies from state to state/territory and in New Zealand
- the patient must have the mental capacity to understand the intended procedure
- the consent given and the information documented in the consent form must relate to the procedure to be performed
- the patient must be provided with adequate information to understand the nature and consequences of the proposed treatment, the material risks associated with the procedure, any complications and alternative treatments, and must have their questions answered (Staunton & Chiarella, 2020).

The final point was significant in the case of *Rogers v Whitaker* (1992) 175 CLR 479, which is outlined in Feature box 3.4. In Australia, this case established the standard of care required when doctors give information to patients about risks of proposed procedures.

It must be understood that the responsibility for providing information about proposed surgery and for obtaining the patient's consent remains with the surgeon or proceduralist performing the procedure or a delegated (generally medical) deputy. However, as part of the checking procedure that the patient undergoes during their perioperative experience, the perioperative nurse reviews the consent form and asks the patient to verify the surgery they are about to undergo and their understanding of this. The perioperative nurse should be alert to any signs of the patient lacking adequate understanding of the procedure. In such a situation, the perioperative nurse has an obligation to discuss this with the surgeon or another medical practitioner in charge of the patient's care, so the latter can follow up with the patient prior to surgery commencing. This

FEATURE BOX 3.4
Rogers v Whitaker (1992) 175 CLR 479

Mrs Whitaker, a woman in her 60s, was blind in her right eye following a penetrating eye injury when she was 9 years old. Despite this, she had led a normal life, was married and had raised four children. In 1983, she decided to rejoin the workforce and went for a pre-employment health check. Her general practitioner suggested that she consider investigating the possibility of a corneal graft to her damaged right eye and referred her to Dr Rogers, an expert in this area. Over the next few months, Mrs Whitaker and Dr Rogers had several consultations, and treatment options were discussed. Dr Rogers felt that surgery could significantly improve her sight and, after incessant questioning about the risk of complications, Mrs Whitaker agreed to undergo surgery. She was not, however, warned of the possibility of damage to her 'good' eye.

Surgery proceeded uneventfully, but complications developed in the postoperative period. Significantly, the left eye (the eye that had vision) developed 'sympathetic ophthalmia', a serious, although rare, inflammatory condition. Despite intensive treatment, Mrs Whitaker lost the sight in her left eye and, unfortunately, had little improvement in her right eye. She was effectively left blind. Mrs Whitaker sued Dr Rogers for negligence on the grounds that he had failed in his duty of care by not warning her of the possibility of sympathetic ophthalmia. She won her case and was awarded compensation. Dr Rogers appealed the decision against him in a case that went all the way to the High Court of Australia. In a majority judgment, the High Court upheld the decision of the lower court and, in doing so, made several significant statements that have subsequently influenced policy development in the area of informed consent (Staunton & Chiarella, 2020).

action should be documented in the patient's notes, together with the response from the surgeon/medical practitioner. While this situation clearly imposes a duty of care on the perioperative nurse to take action, it is also an example of the perioperative nurse acting as an advocate for the patient. Finally, it is important to note that patients may withdraw their consent to treatment at any time without prejudice.

Patients unable to give consent
Under common law, there is a presumption that adults are competent to make decisions about their medical treatment, including surgery. Some patients may lack the intellectual capacity to give consent to treatment because they:
- are suffering from dementia
- have an acquired brain injury
- are intellectually disabled.

However, these conditions may not automatically preclude a person giving consent, as their disability may not be serious enough to preclude them having the necessary capacity.

Other patients may be unconscious or in a physical state that prevents them from being informed and making decisions about the treatment and care options available to them. It is important to distinguish these situations.

Guardianship
To assist patients and to help staff manage patients who lack the intellectual capacity to consent, there are guardianship statutes. Guardianship legislation contains mechanisms designed to ensure that patients' rights to make decisions about their treatment are supported and the best decisions about their care are made. This is known as *substitute consent*, whereby consent to treatment is made by a designated 'person responsible'. Each jurisdiction in Australia and New Zealand has legislation setting out provisions for appointing a formal guardian and the scope of their decision-making powers. Examples of legislation include the Guardianship and Administration Act 2000 (Qld) and the Protection of Personal and Property Rights Act 1988 (NZ) (Kerridge et al., 2013; Staunton & Chiarella, 2020). There is a hierarchy of people able to give consent, ranging from a formally appointed guardian to a spouse, close friend(s) or relative(s). If a patient has no family member or other suitable person to provide substitute consent then, under the guardianship jurisdictions, a *public guardian* is appointed to make decisions on behalf of the patient (Staunton & Chiarella, 2020).

From a practical perspective, the issue of the patient's competence may not be clear. For example, on arrival in the perioperative environment, a patient may be able to communicate personal information accurately, but otherwise demonstrate a lack of capacity or understanding about the proposed surgery. Part of the handover procedure is for the perioperative nurse to check the relevant consent documentation and, if necessary, seek advice from a senior colleague about any issues relating to substitute consent. This should ensure that the patient's rights to appropriate decision-making processes are being upheld.

Advance health directive and perioperative considerations
Patients may also make their wishes for their care and treatment known through an **advance health directive** (AHD) or advance care plan (ACP), which becomes effective only when a person loses the capacity to make

or communicate those decisions for themself. Making one's own healthcare choices is a right in Australia and New Zealand, but legal requirements differ between states and territories (Advance Care Planning Australia, 2019; New Zealand Health and Disability Commissioner, 2019; New Zealand Ministry of Health, 2011). It should also be noted that there may be variation in the terms used in legislation and policy in each jurisdiction (Feature box 3.5).

AHDs can pose a dilemma for healthcare personnel when patients who have elected not to be resuscitated in the event of a cardiac arrest are scheduled for a surgical procedure. For example, terminally ill patients may

require a palliative procedure such as insertion of an access device for pain relief. An AHD stating 'not for resuscitation' should not automatically remain active in this instance; instead, the surgical team should discuss with the patient whether they wish to suspend the AHD during the perioperative period so that, if need be, active resuscitation can be instigated. The result of this discussion should be clearly documented in the patient's notes. Additionally, the surgical team must ensure that all perioperative staff members involved in the patient's care are informed of the patient's wishes prior to the latter's admission into the operating suite (Murphy, 2019). This could be noted as part of the 'Sign In' procedure on the Surgical Safety Checklist.

Consent and minors

In Australia, a person is deemed an adult at the age of 18 years and is thereafter legally empowered to give (or withhold) consent to treatment. In the case of children (minors), the age that they can give consent to health treatment varies by jurisdiction. For example, in South Australia and New Zealand a person over the age of 16 years can consent to their own treatment under the Consent to Medical Treatment and Palliative Care Act 1995 (SA) and the Care of Children Act 2004 (NZ), respectively. In New South Wales, a person over the age of 14 years can consent to medical or dental procedures, as described under the Minors (Property and Contracts) Act 1970 (NSW). In certain situations, conflict may arise between children and their parents in relation to giving consent to a medical procedure. Ideally, there should be discussion and agreement on treatment options between the child, the parents and the treating medical practitioner. The NSW Law Reform Commission has stated, 'a prudent doctor would be unlikely to continue to treat a child or young person when he or she became aware that the medical treatment was against the wishes of one of the parents' (2008, p. 142). In these circumstances, relevant courts or authorities such as the NSW Family Court or government departments can be called upon for assistance to resolve conflict over treatment or to make a determination (Staunton & Chiarella, 2020). In emergency situations requiring lifesaving intervention, doctors can override any parental objections and carry out treatment.

Emergency situations

No consent is required for a patient who arrives unconscious at the emergency department following, for example, a road accident or other type of trauma and is transferred to the operating theatre for surgery. The overriding duty is for immediate intervention to save

---

FEATURE BOX 3.5
Advance Health Directives and Perioperative Considerations

An advance health directive (AHD) is a written or oral directive by which a person sets out their choices regarding possible future healthcare services. An AHD is intended to be used in situations where the person is not competent to give informed consent.

Making one's own healthcare choices is a right in Australia and New Zealand, but legal requirements differ between states and territories. Advance care planning respects the right of an individual to decide how decisions are made about their care. There is no single way that people choose to approach how decisions should be made if they become unable to make their own healthcare decisions. Each person has their own preferences on decision making and these preferences should not be assumed. There will be variation between and within cultures.

These preferences influence how a person makes a decision and their motivations in choosing to do advance care planning (Advance Care Planning Australia, 2019).

A person who is not competent at the time of treatment to make an informed choice or give informed consent may have set out their views regarding particular services in an AHD prior to receiving treatment.

In an AHD, persons may indicate in advance their objection to, or prohibition of, treatments that would otherwise be provided. They may also specify the type of treatment they would wish to undergo should they become incompetent. A 'Do Not Resuscitate' (DNR) order is a type of AHD.

An AHD can be made only by a person who is competent at the time it is signed – it cannot be made by a person's guardian, lawyer, parent, family member or clinician on behalf of the person (New Zealand Health and Disability Commissioner – Te Toihau, Hauatanga (NZ), 2019).

their life. This action is termed 'the doctrine of emergency or necessity'. The treatment must, however, be urgent: to save life or to prevent severe or long-lasting deterioration to the patient (Staunton & Chiarella, 2020).

Consent and mental illness

Consent for treatment from patients who are deemed mentally ill is managed under relevant mental health legislation – for example, the Mental Health Act 1996 (WA), the Mental Health (Compulsory Assessment and Treatment) Act 1992 (NZ) and the Mental Health Act 2014 (Vic). Patients can voluntarily present themselves for treatment and they retain the same rights as others. In contrast, patients who threaten suicide or present as a serious threat to themselves or others may be involuntarily admitted for care and treatment. In this instance, they have no legal capacity to give or withhold consent (Staunton & Chiarella, 2020). This may include, for example, the administration of medication, surgery or electroconvulsive therapy (ECT). However, such treatments must be undertaken in accordance with the requirements of the relevant mental health legislation, because to apprehend, detain and treat a person otherwise is not legitimate (Kerridge et al., 2013). ECT is carefully regulated and requires the voluntary patient to give informed consent. For patients admitted involuntarily, the treatment must be approved by a mental health tribunal, which also determines the number of ECT treatments to be given. When the prescribed number has been given, a further review is required before any additional course of ECT can be administered (Kerridge et al., 2013).

Patients with mental illness can prove challenging when admitted into the perioperative environment. Some patients may be accompanied by specialist mental health nurses and possibly security personnel to ensure the safety of the patient and perioperative staff. They require careful management, with attention paid to ensuring that a legitimate consent process has occurred and that the consent forms and other administrative documentation related to mental health protocols are complete.

Consent and blood transfusions

Situations may arise when an adult patient refuses a blood transfusion on religious grounds (e.g. a Jehovah's Witness) or for other reasons. Adult patients have the right to refuse any treatment, including blood transfusions; however, they must be given a full explanation about the risks and alternatives should they do so. In the perioperative environment, refusal of blood products can sometimes lead to confusion and conflict among staff who do not share the same beliefs as the patient. Health professionals cannot override an adult patient's wishes to refuse blood transfusion, except by seeking legal intervention, because to do so without court sanction could expose them to actions in assault and battery (Kerridge et al., 2013). From a practical perspective, people who are Jehovah's Witnesses admitted for elective surgery have usually made their wishes clear preoperatively and have had the opportunity to discuss options for substitute intravenous products with medical staff. Advances in surgical techniques and in the development of alternative blood products have resulted in the availability of a range of alternative measures for patients who do not want to receive blood products.

When patients are admitted to hospital unconscious, their wishes may not be known unless they are carrying a 'medical directive' card indicating that they are a Jehovah's Witness. Such cards should indicate which alternative blood products they will accept, and their wishes are sacrosanct. If no notification exists, medical staff members are entitled to proceed as they would with any other patient and provide appropriate life-saving treatment, including blood transfusion (Kerridge et al., 2013).

The care of children of Jehovah's Witnesses who require blood transfusion is managed via statutory provisions, which permit blood to be administered without parental consent if necessary. These provisions also allow parental non-consent to blood transfusion to be overridden – for example, section 37 of the Care of Children Act 2004 (NZ). Parents can challenge these decisions through the courts and the outcomes are based on what is deemed to be best for the child (Staunton & Chiarella, 2020).

The South Australian cases, *Children, Youth & Women's Health Services Inc v YJL, MHL and TL (by his next friend)* [2010] SASC 175; *X & Ors v Sydney Children's Hospitals Network (Randwick and Westmead) (incorporating The Royal Alexandra Hospital for Children)* [2014] HCASL 97 (13 May 2014) and a New Zealand case with similar facts are outlined in Feature box 3.6 and illustrate this final point.

The management of patients who are Jehovah's Witnesses and the education of staff who care for them has been assisted by the Jehovah's Witness governing body publishing practical guides and setting up liaison committees within many healthcare facilities (Kerridge et al., 2013).

Culture, Religion and Surgery

Australia and New Zealand are home to millions of residents who have arrived from other countries. Respect for and sensitivity to varying religious and cultural

---

FEATURE BOX 3.6
Religion vs Science

A 10-month-old baby diagnosed with stage 4 cancer was placed under the care of the New Zealand High Court after her parents refused to consent for her to have blood transfusions to treat her cancer. In August, doctors found a large tumour in the right side of the baby's chest. They indicated that the tumour was cancer and told the parents the cancer was in her bones, but if she was treated with blood transfusions it was likely she would have a 90% chance of survival. However, if the baby did not receive the blood transfusion, life-threatening complications could occur.

Her parents would not agree to their child having a blood transfusion because they are Jehovah's Witnesses, but they did agree to the administration of chemotherapy and surgery for removal of the tumour. Consequently, the New Zealand High Court granted the application of the Auckland District Board to place the baby under its guardianship for 9 months, allowing the baby to receive the blood transfusions she needed. The baby was given an urgent blood transfusion when doctors performed a biopsy on her tumour.

Justice Helen Winkelman of the New Zealand High Court appointed the baby's parents as general agents of the court. This meant that they were still to care for the child except when it came to the administration of blood. Justice Winkelman said it was important for the parents to continue supporting their child. She hoped the court order would relieve them of their religious dilemma. Doctors were appointed as the agents for the administration of blood.

(Source: Reissa, S. (2013). Religion v science: parents denied New Zealand baby to get cancer treatment, lost court battle. *International Business Times* (Australian ed.), 10 September.)

---

beliefs during hospitalisation must be demonstrated by healthcare staff and, if necessary, guidance sought from relevant hospital departments. For example, both male and female patients of the Jewish, Muslim and Hindu faiths generally prefer to be examined by healthcare providers of the same gender where possible. Female patients in particular require sensitivity in relation to modesty concerns. Patients may also wear religious artefacts that need to be removed if they interfere with access to the operative site; for example, Hindu women may wear a sacred thread, a ring or a gold chain around their neck; while men may wear a sacred thread across their chest. However, before these items can be removed, permission must be sought from either the patient or a relative (Queensland Health, 2011).

In Māori culture, all body parts are highly revered and are either disposed of according to *tikanga* (traditional customs and beliefs) or are returned to the patient and/or the *whanau* (extended family). The Code of Health and Disability Services Consumer Rights together with individual district health boards set out specific rights in respect to the removal and use of an individual's body parts and bodily substances. Perioperative nurses should observe these cultural beliefs when disposing of resected organs or tissues (Capital & Coast District Health Board [CCDHB], NZ, 2017; New Zealand Health and Disability Commissioner, 1996). (See Chapters 1 and 7 for further information on this topic.)

Coroners' Courts

Although the outcome of the vast majority of surgical cases is positive, occasionally patients do die on the operating table or immediately postoperatively. This is a devastating event for all concerned. As well as the emotional aftermath, there are specific legal requirements to be adhered to and these fall within the jurisdiction of the coroner. The role of the coroner and the **coroners' courts** in Australia and New Zealand has been inherited from English common law, where they have existed for hundreds of years. The main role of the coroner is to detect unlawful homicides and to investigate deaths that have occurred in unusual, unexpected, violent or unnatural circumstances to ensure that there was no foul play (Staunton & Chiarella, 2020). Each Australian state/territory has a Coroners' Act, and in New Zealand there is the Coroners Act 2006.

Under these Acts, the coroner must hold inquests into deaths that occur under certain circumstances as stated in the Act. It is beyond the scope of this text to discuss these in detail; however, one circumstance that has direct implications for perioperative nurses is the death of a patient who has 'died during the process or as a result of being administered anaesthetic' and where the person's death 'was not the reasonably expected outcome of a health-related procedure carried out in relation to a person'. A 'health-related procedure' means a medical, surgical, dental or other health-related procedure (including the administration of an anaesthetic, sedative or other drug), but does not include any procedure of a kind prescribed by the regulations as being excluded (Section 6(3) Coroners' Act 2009 [NSW]).

In New South Wales, when a patient dies while under, as a result of, or within 24 hours after the administration of an anaesthetic or sedative drug for a medical, surgical or dental operation or procedure, the

NSW Public Health Act 2010 requires the health practitioner responsible for administering the anaesthetic or sedative drug to attend the Special Committee Investigating Deaths Under Anaesthesia (SCIDUA). This is an expert committee established under Section 20 of the NSW Health Administration Act 1982. It has a national focus and is represented by anaesthetists from a broad range of clinical specialties and professional organisations (Clinical Excellence Commission [CEC], 2017).

Although responsibility for the documentation related to the death of a patient in the perioperative period rests with the surgeon and the anaesthetist, perioperative nurses must be aware of the requirements related to the care of the patient after death. Essentially, these are that the patient's body should be undisturbed until a post-mortem examination has been completed (i.e. it should not be washed, and all drains, cannulae, airways, catheters and other such items should be left in place). Accessories such as drip bags, bottles, feed lines and catheter bags should accompany the patient's body to the morgue. The patient's clothing or belongings may also be required for forensic examination (and must not be returned to the family). Local policies provide guidance on the correct handling of these items, as well as the patient's body (e.g. NSW Health, 2010).

Nurses may be called as witnesses in the coroner's court if they were present at the time of the patient's death and can provide information that may assist the coroner. It is important for nurses to be fully aware of their rights and obligations to the court and they should be provided with legal advice by their hospital or professional organisation to support them in these matters.

As well as handing down findings as to the manner and cause of death, the coroner may make comments critical of the treatment and care the patient received and make recommendations for improvements. The coroner can also make comments critical of the actions of the personnel involved in the patient's care. This may give rise to disciplinary action being brought against a nurse by the appropriate regulatory agency. Should there be any doubt about the circumstances surrounding the manner of a patient's death and/or nurses' actions, it is important that the latter are aware of their rights. Until legal advice has been obtained, nurses can refuse to answer questions or give a statement if approached by a police officer assisting the coroner. While this may appear overcautious, it is prudent for the nurse to obtain legal advice when writing statements and preparing to appear in court (Staunton & Chiarella, 2020).

Documentation

Accurate records contribute to optimal patient care and provide evidence of the standard of nursing care provided. When care is delivered but not documented, it may be inferred that it was not provided to the patient (Staunton & Chiarella, 2020). **Documentation** is therefore an integral part of the role of the perioperative nurse, whether it is completing patients' records about care and treatment provided, documenting the facts of an incident in the workplace or providing a statement for a coronial inquiry or **disciplinary hearing**. The same principles of good documentation apply regardless of the context. These principles are that documentation should be:
- accurate and factual
- contemporaneous
- based on evidence and observation
- descriptive of care provided and actions taken (Staunton & Chiarella, 2020).

Within the perioperative environment, documentation includes, for example, anaesthetic records, fluid balance charts, the 'count sheet', the WHO Surgical Safety Checklist, the perioperative nursing care record, the patient observation/assessment charts used in the postanaesthesia care unit, surgeons' notes, and radiology and pathology requests and associated reports. The majority of perioperative nursing documentation is electronic, with real-time data entry completed customarily by the circulating nurse. Examples of information captured electronically include:
- patient positioning and positional aids used
- placement of electrosurgery dispersive electrode (diathermy plate or mat)
- solutions used for skin preparation (e.g. chlorhexidine solution or povidone iodine solution)
- specimens taken
- placement of drains and/or catheters
- patient's skin condition (before and after surgery)
- pressure injury prevention measures utilised.

Even though most perioperative records are electronic, the 'count sheet' and the perioperative nursing care record are likely to remain paper based for practical reasons (see the sample perioperative nursing care record in Chapter 9). The documented information gives a clear picture of the intraoperative nursing care the patient received, ensures continuity of care and provides handover information.

Electronic health record

An electronic health record (EHR) has the potential to provide all nurses with a more comprehensive and accessible means for outlining the treatment and care they deliver (Staunton & Chiarella, 2020). Many countries, including Australia and New Zealand, have adopted the EHR as a means of facilitating an efficient flow of information related to patient care across hospital departments, at a local level, and across state and national boundaries (Staunton & Chiarella, 2020). This has the potential to benefit the continuity of patient care, particularly in populations where people travel or move around for work or family reasons.

There are many advantages to maintaining an electronic record. For example, they do not require the reader to decipher handwriting, thus reducing the risk of medication-prescribing errors, misunderstandings and thereby providing a safer method of communication. However, the EHR requires computer literacy and security to enable data entry and access to the information. A number of hospitals have introduced customised software that enables the capture of specific patient information by those involved in the patient's care. Electronic record keeping can be a fast and efficient method of documenting care, as well as allowing hospitals to generate data that can assist with allocating resources, monitoring patient care and demonstrating the attainment of key performance indicators. However, staff members do need to prioritise their workloads to ensure that patient care is not compromised by data entry occurring at times when patient care activities are required. Despite the technical advances now seen in most operating rooms, issues related to privacy and patient confidentiality, as well as to the secure transmission of data, remain.

Health professionals are accountable for all documentation that is completed, whether it is electronic or paper based (Staunton & Chiarella, 2020). Staff members are assigned unique log-in details to access the computer system and it is important that care providers use their own username and password when completing data entry. Electronic records can be erroneous if staff members are not vigilant in logging out on completion of data entry (e.g. when stepping away for the computer, leaving the operating room for breaks or going off duty). Without logging off from the computer, data can be entered by other staff members and therefore wrongly attributed, with possible repercussions if such records are used in legal or professional hearings. In addition, it is important to check that the correct medical record has been opened to avoid data being entered for the wrong patient (South Eastern Sydney Local Health District, 2018).

The case in Feature box 3.7 illustrates the tragic consequences of entering information into the wrong patient's record.

FEATURE BOX 3.7
The Death of Paul Lau

A tragic example of entering data for the wrong patient led to a patient's death following routine knee surgery. While the patient, Paul Lau, was undergoing an anterior cruciate ligament (ACL) repair, the anaesthetist, using an electronic medication ordering system, ordered postoperative pain medication for the next patient on the list who was to undergo a total hip replacement. Tragically, the anaesthetist failed to properly check the EHR, and the narcotic pain protocol order was erroneously made into Paul Lau's record. Unfortunately, the error was not detected in the postoperative period and a series of subsequent systems failures contributed to Mr Lau's death from fentanyl toxicity beginning with respiratory depression, aspiration and death. The Coroner's recommendations included greater vigilance in checking the identity of patients when using EHR, as well as reviewing the software used to alert the user to an incorrect entry (Coroners Court of NSW, 2018).

In addition, vigilance is required by all perioperative staff to ensure that documentation is completed, closed and/or removed from the operating room on completion of a procedure and prior to the next patient entering. For example, patient address labels from a previous patient have the potential to be used on a subsequent patient's records or specimens, with the possibility of serious consequences. (The correct handling and labelling of specimens is addressed in Chapter 9.)

REGULATORY ACTION AND DISCIPLINARY HEARINGS
Assessment of Complaints and Notifications

As identified in Chapter 1, the nursing and midwifery councils in each state and territory of Australia, the Nursing Council of New Zealand (NCNZ) and the Health and Disability Commissioner have specific pathways to manage complaints about performance, conduct and health matters concerning practising nurses (and midwives – while acknowledging that the information in this chapter also refers to midwives, only nurses are referenced to simplify the text).

Both AHPRA and the NCNZ publish detailed data in relation to the conduct, health and competence of nurses and this is available in annual reports on the respective websites (https://www.ahpra.gov.au; https://www.nursingcouncil.org.nz).

Notifications and Complaints

All registered health practitioners have a professional and ethical obligation to protect and promote public health and safe healthcare. Protection of the community means that people (including other health professionals) have a right (and in some instances a duty) to notify the relevant health professional registration authority if they have concerns about:

- a health practitioner's conduct if it appears in some way to be putting members of the community at risk
- the health of a health practitioner if it affects their ability to practise safely
- the clinical competence or performance of a health practitioner (AHPRA, 2019a).

Notifications and complaints are managed by the NMBA in each state/territory, apart from New South Wales and Queensland, where state legislation works alongside the National Law in a co-regulatory way. In New South Wales, the Nursing and Midwifery Council (NMC) carries out its regulatory functions in conjunction with the Health Care Complaints Commission (HCCC), established under the Health Care Complaints Act (NSW) 1993. In Queensland, complaints against health professionals, including nurses and midwives, are made to the Office of the Health Ombudsman, established under the Health Ombudsman Act (Qld) 2013, which decides on subsequent action.

Fig. 3.1 shows the categories of notifications received by NMBA in 2019/20, with Fig. 3.2 identifying the outcomes of notifications received following investigation.

In New Zealand, all complaints received by the Nursing Council alleging that the practice or conduct of a nurse has affected a health consumer must be referred to the Health and Disability Commissioner (the Commissioner). The Commissioner determines jurisdiction in respect of the matter and/or whether the Commission will investigate the complaint. The Health Practitioners Competence Assurance Act 2003 requires court registrars to send a notice of conviction to the Nursing Council for a nurse convicted of an offence as stated in the Act.

Mandatory Notifications

In Australia, under the National Law (2009), health practitioners, employers and education providers also have some mandatory reporting responsibilities. These are defined in Section 140 of the National Law as:

- practising while intoxicated by alcohol or drugs
- sexual misconduct in the practice of the profession
- placing the public at risk of harm due to health impairment

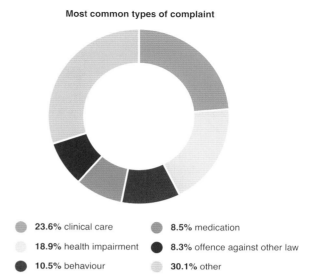

Most common types of complaint

- 23.6% clinical care
- 18.9% health impairment
- 10.5% behaviour
- 8.5% medication
- 8.3% offence against other law
- 30.1% other

FIG. 3.1 Categories of notifications. (Source: Nursing and Midwifery Board of Australia. (2020). *Annual report summary 2019/20*. Melbourne: AHPRA.)

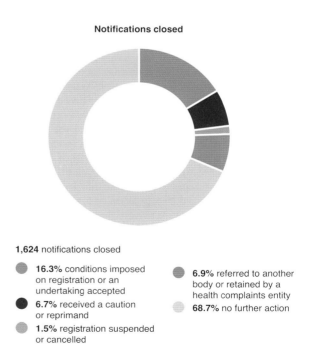

Notifications closed

1,624 notifications closed

- 16.3% conditions imposed on registration or an undertaking accepted
- 6.7% received a caution or reprimand
- 1.5% registration suspended or cancelled
- 6.9% referred to another body or retained by a health complaints entity
- 68.7% no further action

FIG. 3.2 Actions taken on notifications. (Source: Nursing and Midwifery Board of Australia. (2020). *Annual report summary 2019/20*. Melbourne: AHPRA.)

- placing the public at risk as a result of significant departure from accepted professional standards (AHPRA, 2016).

Performance

A common category of complaint received in all jurisdictions relates to nurses' performance of clinical care, as can be seen in Fig. 3.1. A non-disciplinary pathway is used to manage issues that relate to the standard of nurses' clinical performance and whether their performance has fallen significantly below the standard reasonably expected, given the individual nurse's level of training or experience. In managing performance issues, the nurse may be required to undertake a performance assessment (AHPRA, 2019b). The assessment may take place in the nurse's own workplace or in a simulated environment and is undertaken by appropriately trained assessors . If the assessment is unsatisfactory, the nurse may be referred for remediation, which may include attending relevant courses, undertaking supervision or engaging in additional continuing professional development. Conditions may also be placed on the nurse to protect the public while remediation is taking place (NMC NSW, 2017).

Conduct

Complaints related to conduct fall into two categories:
- **Unprofessional conduct** of a registered health practitioner means **professional conduct** that is of a lesser standard than that which might reasonably be expected of the health practitioner by the public or the practitioner's professional peers (AHPRA, 2010).
- **Professional misconduct** of a registered health practitioner is the more serious of the two categories and relates to unprofessional conduct by the practitioner that amounts to conduct that is *substantially* below the standard reasonably expected of a registered health practitioner of an equivalent level of training or experience. Complaints that are substantiated can result in the suspension or cancellation of the practitioner's licence to practise (AHPRA, 2010).

Conduct issues are generally related to behavioural acts or omissions. Following investigation of a complaint,

> **FEATURE BOX 3.8**
> **NZHPDT Falsifying Patient Records**
>
> The NZHPDT charged a nurse with falsification of records following the death of a patient. It was alleged that the nurse led a group of her colleagues in writing patient records that had not previously existed and rewriting existing records that were false as to dates and content. The nurse also gave instructions to destroy original patient documentation, participated in the preparation of a new Standing Order, initialling it knowing it was to be backdated and therefore false and did not exist prior to the patient's death. The nurse also failed to report to the employer the falsification of records by other staff members. The Tribunal found the charges established. The nurse was censured and her registration cancelled.

(Source: New Zealand Health Practitioners Disciplinary Tribunal. (2017). File no.: Nur17/399P.)

action may be taken by a **professional standards** committee or tribunal, depending on the seriousness of the complaint (AHPRA, 2010). Feature box 3.8 presents the outcomes of the New Zealand Health Practitioners Disciplinary Tribunal (NZHPDT) in relation to a case of falsifying patient records.

Health matters

Notifications about health matters concerning nurses can be made by a colleague, an employer or a member of the public. The notification must be related to 'a physical or mental impairment, disability, condition or disorder (including substance abuse) that detrimentally affects or is likely to detrimentally affect their capacity to practise' (AHPRA, 2019c). An independent health assessment will be carried out to establish the physical or mental impairment of the nurse and to determine a course of action. This may result in assisting nurses to manage their illness/impairment while they remain employed, place conditions on their practice, or refer the nurse to a tribunal. The aim of action is non-punitive and is taken to protect the public against the risk of harm, while supporting the nurse to manage their illness/impairment (AHPRA, 2019c).

PATIENT SCENARIOS

SCENARIO 3.3: MANDATORY NOTIFICATIONS

RN Ben Lumby walks into the sterile stock room to find EN Sammy Ravisi asleep in a chair. When woken, EN Ravisi explains that he has recently been diagnosed with narcolepsy and begs RN Lumby not to tell anyone.

> **Critical Thinking Questions**
>
> - What are the risks to patients in this situation? Provide explanations for your response.
> - What action should RN Lumby take, and why?

Immediate Action

The NMBA and the NCNZ have the power to take immediate action to suspend or place conditions upon the practice of a nurse if they are provided with information that the conduct, health or performance of the nurse is likely to pose a serious risk to the community (AHPRA, 2019d). (The NMBA can also accept an undertaking from a nurse and the surrender of their registration.) This is only an interim step while a complete investigation takes place and other action may occur after a formal hearing by a committee, panel or tribunal.

Table 3.2 lists situations where the NMBA may take immediate action. This is a serious step and is not taken lightly – the threshold is necessarily high. To take immediate action, the NMBA must reasonably believe that:

- because of their conduct, performance or health, the nurse poses a 'serious risk to persons' and that it is necessary to take immediate action to protect public health or safety, or
- the nurse's registration was improperly obtained, or
- the nurse's registration was cancelled or suspended in another jurisdiction (AHPRA, 2019d).

TABLE 3.2
Matters the NMBA May Consider Require Immediate Action

Category	Example
Police charges	Offences relating to a health practitioner's work or professional practice (e.g. assaulting a patient)
Patient outcome	A patient dies unexpectedly or a routine operation has severe adverse outcomes
Drugs	Notified by a practitioner or an independent body; includes accusations of self-administering and inappropriate prescribing of illicit or prescription drugs
Alcohol	Allegations of presenting to work under the influence of alcohol
Sexual behaviour	Inappropriate touching or professional/sexual boundary violation
Theft	Stealing drugs from the workplace
Health	Impairments (e.g. involuntary admission to hospital under the Mental Health Act) or concerns about memory/behaviour
Breach of conditions	A practitioner has conditions on their registration and the conduct/incident described may breach registration conditions

(Source: Australian Health Practitioner Regulation Agency. (2013). *A guide for practitioners: notifications in the national scheme*.)

FEATURE BOX 3.9
Immediate Action in a Professional Misconduct Case

In May 2014, the Nursing and Midwifery Board of Australia (NMBA) received a notification about an RN following the disappearance of drugs from her workplace and inadequate clinical performance. During a subsequent search of the RN's home, police seized the missing drugs and found hospital prescriptions for other drugs suspected to be forgeries. The NMBA took immediate action to ensure that the RN did not return to practise without the NMBA's approval.

A police investigation took place, which led to the RN being charged with stealing offences, for which she pleaded guilty. She was placed on a good behaviour bond and no conviction was recorded.

The Tribunal reprimanded the RN and disqualified her from applying for registration for 6 months after she admitted to professional misconduct concerning the misappropriated drugs.

(Source: *Nursing and Midwifery Board of Australia v Morey* [2017] QCAT 249.)

An example of a matter relating to a registered nurse where the NMBA took immediate action and placed conditions on the nurse's practice while a full assessment and investigation were conducted is outlined in Feature box 3.9.

Investigation

In jurisdictions in Australia, if the investigation of complaints is not conducted by an independent agency with co-regulatory responsibilities under the National Law (the HCCC in New South Wales and the Office of Health Ombudsman in Queensland), the NMBA may decide to investigate a nurse if it believes that:

- the nurse has, or may have, an impairment, and/or
- the way the nurse practises is, or may be, unsatisfactory, and/or
- the nurse's conduct is, or may be, unsatisfactory (AHPRA, 2018).

An investigator appointed by the NMBA conducts the investigation and the process depends on the facts of the case. However, the investigation must comply with nationally consistent policies and procedures. It usually involves the investigator seeking extra information to inform the NMBA's decision. An investigation will also consider whether a nurse has complied with the NMBA's registration standards, codes and guidelines (AHPRA, 2018).

It is usual for nurses being investigated to be given notice of the investigation as well as information about what is being investigated. It is also usual for nurses under investigation to be provided with regular updates on the progress of the investigation. The only exceptions to this are when there is a reasonable belief that informing the nurse may:

- seriously prejudice the investigation
- place someone's health or safety at risk, or
- place someone at risk of harassment or intimidation (AHPRA, 2013).

These processes are very similar to the requirements under the New Zealand legislation (Health Practitioners Competence Assurance Act (NZ) 2003 and Health and Disability Commissioner Act (NZ) 1994).

Panel and Committee Hearings

Under the National Law, the NMBA has the power to establish two types of panel:

- health panels for health matters if it believes that a nurse has a physical or mental impairment
- performance and professional standards panels for conduct and performance matters (AHPRA, 2019e).

Similar legislative provisions exist in New Zealand, and various policies and procedures have been established by the Nursing Council of New Zealand (NCNZ, 2012).

Tribunal Hearings

The NMBA can refer a matter to a tribunal for hearing. This happens only when the allegations involve professional misconduct and when the NMBA believes that suspension or cancellation of the nurse's registration may be warranted. Under the National Law, the NMBA must refer a matter about a nurse to a tribunal if it reasonably believes that the nurse has behaved in a way that constitutes professional misconduct. Nurses referred to a tribunal are urged to seek legal advice and representation as the tribunal procedures are formal and the consequences may have long-term impacts on a nurse's career, life and livelihood (AHPRA, 2019f). The NMBA is responsible for implementing the decisions of tribunals, such as removing a nurse's name from the Register when their registration has been cancelled. By law, tribunal proceedings are open to the public. Any decision made to suppress identifying information about the nurse is made by the tribunal (AHPRA, 2019f). The tribunal may also have a role in establishing a nurse's fitness to practise after a period of cancellation or suspension.

Serious criminal matters involving the conduct of a nurse are often dealt with in two legal jurisdictions: the criminal justice system and the health professional regulatory system.

Appeals

Nurses can appeal a decision made against them to the relevant tribunal – for example, in relation to reprimand, suspension or cancellation of registration, or conditions placed upon practice (AHPRA, 2019g).

Monitoring and compliance

In Australia, AHPRA monitors those nurses who have restrictions placed on their registration, to make sure that they are complying with them (AHPRA, 2019h). In New Zealand, this monitoring and compliance role is undertaken by the NCNZ (2012).

PRIVACY AND CONFIDENTIALITY

The legal obligations of **privacy and confidentiality** necessarily arise when creating, managing or using healthcare records. However, these two areas deal with matters that are broader than healthcare records as they extend to include relationships, trust and having adequate information to provide safe, competent care to patients while ensuring that their dignity and integrity is maintained. Furthermore, personal information is available only to those who have a legitimate right to access it.

The terms *privacy* and *confidentiality* are often used interchangeably and, while related, each has a distinct and distinguishable meaning. 'Privacy refers to one's ownership of one's body or information about one's self', whereas 'confidentiality refers specifically to restrictions upon private information revealed in confidence where there is an explicit or implicit assumption that the information shared will not be disclosed to others' (Kerridge et al., 2013, p. 298).

In relation to privacy, the Privacy Act 1988 (Cth) regulates the handling of personal information by Australian government agencies and some private sector organisations. State and territory legislation also places similar obligations on agencies and organisations, including private hospitals and health services. This applies to any sensitive information and certainly applies to patient healthcare records and health information. In New Zealand, the Privacy Act 1993 controls how agencies collect, use, disclose, store and give access to personal information. The privacy codes of practice do the same, but they apply to specific areas; namely, health, telecommunications and credit reporting (New Zealand Privacy Commissioner, 2020).

Privacy also relates to people's expectations and right to be treated with dignity and respect. Effective nurse–patient relationships are built on respect and trust (NCNZ, 2012) and the provision of treatment and care always involves some invasion of privacy (Kerridge et al., 2013). In operating rooms, the clinical team transfer patients who are clad only in a gown from trolley to operating table, place them in undignified positions and perform intimate procedures such as urinary catheterisation. These patients may be conscious, but often they are sedated or unconscious; either way, the potential for loss of dignity is great. It is important for perioperative nurses to remember that they have legal and ethical obligations and maintaining the dignity of the patients they care for is an important aspect of those obligations.

Providing perioperative nursing care necessarily means that patients are subject to breaches of their privacy and confidentiality. Taking health and social histories from patients to enable the provision of informed care often means that health professionals are in possession of information that they may share with other health professionals; this could be information that patients may not even share with their own family. Information that must remain confidential not only includes information the patient shares with health professionals, it also covers information arising from clinical assessment of the patient's physical and mental health; imaging and other investigations; and procedures. Even the fact that the person has been a patient of a health service is information that nurses must not divulge unless the patient has consented to share it.

It is recognised that it is 'difficult to maintain confidentiality in a health-care system that is increasingly team-oriented, fragmented and complex' (Kerridge et al., 2013, p. 299) and where information is stored both electronically and paper-based in multiple sites, often distant from the health professionals accessing it. However, there continues to be an obligation that this information is not accessed or shared outside the clinical team, who have a 'need-to-know' for the purposes of providing safe, effective care. Patients would not tell healthcare professionals their most intimate and private details or consent to them having access to it if they did not expect that information to be treated in the strictest confidence. When nurses need to share personal information that patients have disclosed to them in confidence – for example, with other healthcare professionals – they are obliged to seek the patient's permission to do so first. Similarly, when another healthcare professional reveals information about a patient to the nurse, the nurse must always treat the information as confidential unless advised otherwise.

These principles are distilled in the codes of professional conduct for nurses in Australia and New Zealand. For example, the code of professional conduct for nurses in Australia notes that nurses have ethical and legal obligations to protect the privacy of patients receiving treatment and care. Information obtained in the course of the relationship between nurses and patients must be kept confidential and restricted to use for professional purposes only (NMBA, 2018). In New Zealand, the code of conduct exhorts nurses to use their professional judgement to ensure that concerns about privacy do not compromise the information they give to health consumers or their involvement in care planning (NCNZ, 2012).

Breaches of Privacy and Confidentiality

There are some exceptions when healthcare professionals are required to disclose what otherwise might be confidential, highly sensitive information. For example, in cases of child abuse, notifiable diseases or professional misconduct by health professionals, legislation requires mandatory reporting by health professionals to authorities to protect individuals or populations from harm. The protection of authorised persons who make disclosures under such legislation is usually dealt with as protection from prosecution under the general common law and legislation; for example, under the Public Health and Wellbeing Act 2008 (Vic).

Except in legitimate circumstances such as those outlined above, nurses need to remain vigilant about the potential for breaching the confidentiality of people in their care. Gossiping in the operating suite tearoom about 'interesting patients' or 'amusing moments', or sharing these on social media, may seem harmless, but they are explicit breaches of privacy. They could lead to nurses having a complaint made about their conduct under the National Law or being dealt with in the court system for a breach of confidentiality or privacy. This is highlighted in the 2018 NSW Tribunal hearing outlined in Feature box 3.10.

SOCIAL MEDIA

Social media is defined as follows:

> *Social media is a term that is constantly evolving but generally refers to internet-based tools that allow individuals and groups to communicate, to advertise or share opinions, information, ideas, messages, experiences, images, and video or audio clips. They may include blogs, social networks, video and photo-sharing sites, wikis, or a myriad of other media . . . .*

(AHPRA, 2019i)

FEATURE BOX 3.10
Breach of Privacy and Confidentiality

In the case of *Health Care Complaints Commission (HCCC) v Aref* [2018] NSWCATOD 133 heard before the Tribunal in NSW, a notification was made that the RN had accessed a computer left unattended by another employee and inappropriately accessed records of himself and six other individuals. The RN did not have the credentials to log into the computer, nor did he have a legitimate reason for accessing the record. The reason for doing so concerned a long-running and acrimonious dispute in which the RN was engaged with the six patients and he was accessing the records to gain information to assist him in the dispute. One of the patients concerned became aware of the access to his records and suspected the RN of using his professional position to gain access to information for which he was not entitled.

The Tribunal found the RN in breach of privacy and confidentiality. The RN had 'unprofessionally and improperly accessed multiple health records . . . a most serious abuse of his professional position'.

The RN was reprimanded and suspended for 6 months.

(Source: *Health Care Complaints Commission (HCCC) v Aref* [2018] NSWCATOD 133.)

The use of social media has provided global opportunities to share information, form friendships, locate school friends and myriad other positive social interactions. However, with such a form of communication comes the responsibility to act appropriately while using it, particularly as a member of the nursing profession. Whether an online activity can be viewed by the general public or is limited to a specific group, health professionals need to be aware of the implications of using social media. This is because information circulated on social media may end up in the public domain and remain there, irrespective of the intent at the time of posting (AHPRA, 2019i; New Zealand Nurses Organisation [NZNO], 2019).

When using social media, nurses can meet their obligations by:
- complying with confidentiality and privacy obligations
- complying with professional obligations as defined in state/territory boards' codes of conduct
- maintaining professional boundaries
- communicating professionally and respectfully with or about patients, colleagues and employers
- not presenting information that is false, misleading or deceptive, including advertising only claims that are supported by acceptable evidence (AHPRA, 2019i).

Misuse of Social Media

Examples of how social media can be misused with possible breaches of patient confidentiality and privacy include:
- pursuing relationships with patients via social networks (e.g. befriending patients on Facebook)
- discussing patients and their families
- posting photographs of procedures, specimens, case studies, patients or other sensitive material that may enable people to be identified, without first having obtained consent (AHPRA, 2019i).

Health professionals must be aware that such actions are all possible breaches of the obligations imposed on them through specific regulatory policies or common law (AHPRA, 2019i). In addition, nurses who disseminate images or comments on social media that portray them acting in an unprofessional manner may face disciplinary action under the code of conduct. In an example from the UK, two nurses were sacked for tweeting expletive-ridden comments about patients and posting embarrassing images of themselves while at work (Davies, 2013). Such behaviour was deemed unprofessional, leading to loss of employment and possible future career advancement. Publishing complaints against colleagues about working conditions, whistleblowing or using social media also constitute inappropriate use of social media.

An Australian example of the misuse of social media is illustrated in Feature box 3.11.

Employers may access the social media history of prospective employees during the recruitment process to gain an insight into their personality and attitudes, which may influence the decision to employ or not. This scrutiny may raise issues of privacy and discrimination as the prospective employee is unaware of the screening occurring. Australian Privacy Principles (APP) published by the Australian Government Office of the Australian Information Commissioner (OAIC) (2014) include a statement requiring an organisation

FEATURE BOX 3.11
Unprofessional Conduct and Facebook

In a 2013 decision by the NMBA, a Northern Territory nurse was found guilty of unprofessional conduct and reprimanded. The nurse was found to have acted aggressively towards a patient with disabilities and subsequently published details of the incident on her Facebook page. In addition to a reprimand, conditions were placed on her practice for a period of 1 year, including counselling by a psychologist and attendance at an NMBA-approved program on legal and ethical nursing practice (NMBA, 2013).

to obtain consent from an individual prior to accessing personal information by any means. Similar provisions are in place in New Zealand through the Health Information Privacy Code 2020 (New Zealand Privacy Commissioner, 2020).

Use of Cameras Within Hospitals

Capturing photographs of the progress of a disease, a traumatic injury, an operative procedure or before-and-after results of plastic surgery has been a well-recognised practice by clinicians for many years. Clinical photography using a personal mobile device (PMD) has rapidly become commonplace in many healthcare facilities, overcoming the delays once seen with the use of professional photography units (Allen, Eleftherlou, & Ferguson, 2016). An image of a surgical wound or part of a procedure either for inclusion in the patient's medical record (primary purpose) or for teaching/research (secondary purpose) using a PMD commonly occurs in the perioperative environment, often with perioperative nurses in the role of photographer (Palacios-González, 2015). However, such practices may give rise to legal and ethical issues (i.e. breach of patient privacy and confidentiality), unless steps are taken to ensure a patient's informed consent has been obtained (OAIC, 2014).

In New Zealand, professional guidelines and legal mechanisms have been established to guide health professionals in managing patient information, including the taking and dissemination of patient images within the Code of Health and Disability Services Consumers' Rights (New Zealand Health and Disability Commissioner, 1996) and the Health Information Privacy Code 2020 (New Zealand Privacy Commissioner, 2020).

Images of patients showing medical conditions are likely to be highly sensitive and careful management of the images is necessary to avoid accidental or deliberate misuse beyond their original clinical purpose – that is, uploading onto the internet, with the resultant breaches of a patient's confidentiality and privacy. In all instances, consent to take photographs should be sought from the patient, even if the patient cannot be identified in the images (Palacios-González, 2015). Perioperative nurses acting as patient advocates should ensure that consent has been obtained for images to be taken and, if doubt exists as to consent processes, voice their concerns to their manager.

Similarly, the partners of patients undergoing a caesarean section may be eager to capture the moment of the baby's birth, believing this to be a reasonable and accepted practice. However, if the photograph includes nursing or medical staff, their permission should be sought *prior* to the photograph being taken.

FEATURE BOX 3.12
Patient Photographed in Operating Theatre

In 2015, a woman entered a Sydney private hospital to undergo a minor gynaecological procedure requiring her to be placed in the lithotomy position. During a postoperative discussion with her surgeon, it was revealed that one of the nurses in the operating theatre had taken an unauthorised photograph of the patient while in lithotomy position and shared the image with colleagues. The patient was understandably horrified and upset. When she demanded that legal action be taken against the nurse for the invasion of privacy she had suffered and deletion of the photograph, it became clear that there were limited legal options under NSW law. Other nurses present in the operating theatre had reported the actions of the nurse to hospital management, which resulted in the nurse being sacked and her actions reported to the Nursing and Midwifery Council (NMC), NSW. Following an investigation by the NMC and declaration of remorse and an apology by the nurse, no disciplinary action was taken and the nurse resumed work in another hospital.

(Source: *ABC News*, 2015, https://www.abc.net.au/news/2015-11-06/sydney-nurse-takes-explicit-photo-of-patient/6916174.)

ACORN recommends that health service organisations establish a system of governance, including policies and standardised procedures in relation to the capturing of clinical images. These should include:
- the process for obtaining and documenting informed patient consent
- security and storage of images
- correct identifying and procedure matching
- dissemination of clinical images (ACORN, 2020).

The media report in Feature box 3.12 highlights an invasion of privacy suffered by a patient when an unauthorised photograph was taken of her during surgery. The report highlights the limited legal action that the patient was able to take at the time, particularly in NSW, when they believed their privacy had been compromised. In Victoria (Privacy and Data Protection Act 2014) and Queensland (Information Privacy Act 2009), legislation does exist to protect patients from unauthorised photography in situations where it can reasonably be expected they would be afforded privacy.

Patient Care and Social Media

In contrast to previous discussion on the misuse of social media, considerable evidence exists about its positive applications. The use of social media has been embraced by a number of healthcare facilities to enhance patient care in a variety of areas (e.g. reminding patients about medical appointments or sharing general health information). Similarly, health professionals are connecting with colleagues, sharing research and seeking answers to clinical questions. Patients use social media to connect with others suffering similar medical complaints, sharing tips on management and using social media as a support mechanism (Moorhead, 2017). Several healthcare facilities have Facebook pages where events and staff achievements are announced and patient testimonials published. See, for example, The Royal Hospital for Women, Melbourne (https://www.facebook.com/theroyalwomenshospital?fref=ts) and Auckland City Hospital, New Zealand (https://www.facebook.com/akldhb).

PATIENT SCENARIOS

SCENARIO 3.4: PRIVACY AND CONFIDENTIALITY

While Mr Collins is on the operating table, the surgeon, Dr Patrick Slattery, asks RN Cohen to take a photo of the operative site using his mobile phone.

Critical Thinking Question

- How should RN Cohen respond to this request? Provide rationale(s) for your answer.

CONCLUSION

Perioperative nurses' practice is informed by and regulated within statutory and regulatory frameworks with the primary intent to protect the public. Patients entering the perioperative setting, like other healthcare settings, have the right be treated with respect and dignity, to have their information kept private and confidential, and to be cared for by safe, competent healthcare professionals. Thus, it is imperative that perioperative nurses maintain an up-to-date working knowledge of the relevant Acts, Regulations, codes and professional standards to ensure that their practice conforms to the high standards expected by the public.

RESOURCES

Australasian Legal Information Institute
https://www.austlii.edu.au
Australian College of Nursing
https://www.acn.edu.au
Australian College of Operating Room Nurses
https://www.acorn.org.au
Australian Commission on Safety and Quality in Health Care
https://www.safetyandquality.gov.au
Australian Government Department of Health
https://www.health.gov.au
Australian Health Practitioner Law Library
https://www.austlii.edu.au/au/special/healthprac
Australian Health Practitioners Regulation Agency (provides links to all state/territory nursing boards/councils)
https://www.ahpra.gov.au
Australian Institute of Health and Welfare
https://www.aihw.gov.au
Australian Nursing and Midwifery Accreditation Council
https://www.anmac.org.au

College of Nurses Aotearoa NZ
https://www.nurse.org.nz
Government of South Australia, SA Health
https://www.sahealth.sa.gov.au
Health Care Complaints Commission (NSW)
https://www.hccc.nsw.gov.au
Health Workforce New Zealand
https://www.health.govt.nz/our-work/health-workforce
International Council of Nurses
https://www.icn.ch
Jehovah's Witnesses
https://www.jw.org
National Health and Medical Research Council
https://www.nhmrc.gov.au
New Zealand Health and Disability Commissioner
https://www.hdc.org.nz
New Zealand Health Practitioners Disciplinary Tribunal
https://www.hpdt.org.nz
New Zealand Ministry of Health
https://www.health.govt.nz
New Zealand Nurses Organisation
https://www.nzno.org.nz
NSW Health
https://www.health.nsw.gov.au
Nursing Council of New Zealand
https://www.nursingcouncil.org.nz
Perioperative Nurses College of New Zealand Nurses Organisation
https://www.nzno.org.nz/groups/colleges_sections/colleges/perioperative_nurses_college

Cases

Children, Youth & Women's Health Services Inc v YJL, MHL and TL (by his next friend) [2010] SASC 175 (4 June 2010). Retrieved from <http://classic.austlii.edu.au/cgi-bin/sign.cgi/au/cases/sa/SASC/2010/175>.
Elliot v Bickerstaff [1999] 48 NSWLR 214.

Health Care Complaints Commission (HCCC) v Aref [2018] NSWCATOD 133. Retrieved from <https://www.caselaw.nsw.gov.au/decision/5b721f5be4b09e9963071b22>.

Langley & Another v Glandore Pty Ltd (in Liq) & Another (1997). Retrieved from <https://archive.sclqld.org.au/qjudgment/1997/QCA97-342.pdf>.

Nursing and Midwifery Board of Australia v George (Review and Regulation) [2015] VCAT 1878 (25 November 2015). Retrieved from <http://www8.austlii.edu.au/cgi-bin/viewdoc/au/cases/vic/VCAT/2015/1878.html?stem=0&synonyms=0&query=catherine%20george>.

Nursing and Midwifery Board of Australia v Morey [2017] QCAT 249. Retrieved from <http://archive.sclqld.org.au/qjudgment/2017/QCAT17-249.pdf>.

Rogers v Whitaker (1992) 175 CLR 479.

X & Ors v Sydney Children's Hospitals Network (Randwick and Westmead) (incorporating The Royal Alexandra Hospital for Children) [2014] HCASL 97 (13 May 2014). Retrieved from <http://classic.austlii.edu.au/cgi-bin/sign.cgi/au/cases/cth/HCASL/2014/97>.

Legislation

Care of Children Act 2004 (NZ)
Civil Law Act 2002 (NSW)
Coroners Act 2006 (NZ)
Coroners Act 2009 (NSW)
Guardianship and Administration Act 2000 (Qld)
Health and Disability Commissioner Act 1994 (NZ)
Health and Disability Commissioner (Code of Health and Disability Services Consumers' Rights) Regulations 1996 (NZ)
Health and Disability Commissioner Amendment Act 2003 (NZ)
Health (Drugs and Poisons) Regulation 1996 (Qld)
Health Practitioner Regulation National Law Act 2009 (the National Law) as in force in each state and territory
Health Practitioners Competence Assurance Act 2003 (NZ)
Health Records Act 2001 (Vic)
Health Records and Information Privacy Act 2002 (NSW)
Injury Prevention, Rehabilitation and Compensation Amendment Act (No 2) 2005 (NZ)
Information Act 2003 (NT)
Medical Treatment and Palliative Care Act 1995 (SA)
Medical Treatment Planning and Decisions Act 2018 (Vic)
Medicines, Poisons and Therapeutic Goods Act 2008 (ACT)
Mental Health Act 1996 (WA)
Mental Health Act 2014 (Vic)
Mental Health (Compulsory Assessment and Treatment) Act 1992 (NZ)
Minors (Property and Contracts) Act 1970 (NSW)
Misuse of Drugs Act 1975 (NZ)
Privacy Act 1988 (Cth)
Privacy Act 1993 (NZ)
Protection of Personal and Property Rights Act 1988 (NZ)
Public Health Act 2010 (NSW)
Public Health and Wellbeing Act 2008 (Vic)
Therapeutic Goods Act 1989 (Cth)

REFERENCES

ABC News. (2015). Sydney nurse who took explicit photo of patient under anaesthetic still practising in NSW. Retrieved from <https://www.abc.net.au/news/2015-11-06/sydney-nurse-takes-explicit-photo-of-patient/6916174>.

Advance Care Planning Australia. (2019). *Advance care planning and the law*. Melbourne: Austin Health. Retrieved from <https://www.advancecareplanning.org.au/for-health-and-care-workers/legal-requirements>.

Allen, K., Eleftherlou, P., & Ferguson, J. (2016). A thousand words in the palm of your hand: management of clinical photography on personal mobile devices. *Medical Journal of Australia, 205*(11), 499–500. Retrieved from <https://www.mja.com.au/journal/2016/205/11/thousand-words-palm-your-hand-management-clinical-photography-personal-mobile>.

Australian College of Operating Room Nurses (ACORN). (1996). *Standards, guidelines and policy statements: Standard A6: Managing accountable items*. Adelaide: Author.

Australian College of Operating Room Nurses (ACORN). (2012–13). *ACORN standards, guidelines, policy statements and competency standards*. Adelaide: Author.

Australian College of Perioperative Nurses (ACORN). (2020). *ACORN standards for perioperative nursing in Australia*. (16th ed., Vol. 1). Clinical images. Adelaide: Author.

Australian Commission on Safety and Quality in Health Care (ACSQHC/the Commission). (2008). *Australian charter of healthcare rights*. Sydney: Author.

Australian Commission on Safety and Quality in Health Care (ACSQHC/the Commission). (2017a). *National safety and quality health service standards*. Sydney: Author.

Australian Commission on Safety and Quality in Health Care (ACSQHC/the Commission). (2017b). *Australian open disclosure framework*. Sydney: Author.

Australian Government, Office of Australian Information Commissioner (OAIC) (2014). *Australian privacy principles – Privacy fact sheet 17*. Canberra: Author.

Australian Health Practitioner Regulation Agency (AHPRA). (2010). Health Practitioner Regulation National Law Act (2009). Retrieved from <https://www.ahpra.gov.au/About-AHPRA/What-We-Do/Legislation.aspx>.

Australian Health Practitioner Regulation Agency (AHPRA) (2013). A guide for practitioners: notifications in the national scheme. Retrieved from <https://www.ahpra.gov.au/Search.aspx?q=A+guide+for+practitioners%3a+Notifications+in+the+national+scheme>.

Australian Health Practitioner Regulation Agency (AHPRA). (2016). Guidelines for mandatory notification. Retrieved from <https://www.nursingmidwiferyboard.gov.au/Codes-Guidelines-Statements/Codes-Guidelines/Guidelines-for-mandatory-notifications.aspx>.

Australian Health Practitioner Regulation Agency (AHPRA). (2018). Investigation process. Retrieved from <https://www.ahpra.gov.au/Notifications/Find-out-about-the-complaints-process/Investigation.aspx>.

Australian Health Practitioner Regulation Agency (AHPRA). (2019a). How notifications are managed. Retrieved from

<https://www.ahpra.gov.au/Notifications/How-we-manage-concerns.aspx>.

Australian Health Practitioner Regulation Agency (AHPRA). (2019b). Information sheet: performance assessments. Retrieved from <https://www.ahpra.gov.au/Notifications/Further-information/Guides-and-fact-sheets/Performance-assessments.aspx>.

Australian Health Practitioner Regulation Agency (AHPRA). (2019c). Information sheet: health assessments. Retrieved from <https://www.ahpra.gov.au/Notifications/Further-information/Guides-and-fact-sheets/Health-assessments.aspx>.

Australian Health Practitioner Regulation Agency (AHPRA). (2019d). Information sheet: immediate action. Retrieved from <https://www.ahpra.gov.au/Notifications/Further-information/Guides-and-fact-sheets/Immediate-action.aspx>.

Australian Health Practitioner Regulation Agency (AHPRA). (2019e). Panel hearing. Retrieved from <https://www.ahpra.gov.au/Notifications/Further-information/Guides-and-fact-sheets/Panel-hearings.aspx>.

Australian Health Practitioner Regulation Agency (AHPRA). (2019f). Tribunal hearings. Retrieved from <https://www.ahpra.gov.au/Notifications/Further-information/Guides-and-fact-sheets/Tribunal-hearings.aspx>.

Australian Health Practitioner Regulation Agency (AHPRA). (2019g). Information sheet: appeals. Retrieved from <https://www.ahpra.gov.au/Notifications/Further-information/Guides-and-fact-sheets/Appeals.aspx>.

Australian Health Practitioner Regulation Agency (AHPRA). (2019h). Information sheet: monitoring and compliance. Retrieved from <https://www.ahpra.gov.au/Notifications/Further-information/Guides-and-fact-sheets/Monitoring-and-compliance.aspx>.

Australian Health Practitioner Regulation Agency (AHPRA). (2019i). Social media policy. Retrieved from <https://www.medicalboard.gov.au/Codes-Guidelines-Policies.aspx>.

Barnett-Davidson, M. (2013). Legal framework for nursing practice in New Zealand. In R. Beran (Ed.), *Legal and forensic medicine*. Heidelberg: Springer.

Capital & Coast District Health Board (CCDHB), NZ. (2017). *Tikanga Māori: a guide for health care workers (Kaimahi Hauora)*. Wellington: Author. Retrieved from <https://www.ccdhb.org.nz/our-services/a-to-z-of-our-services/maori-health/43875-tikanga-maori-web.pdf>.

Clinical Excellence Commission (CEC). (2017). *Activities of the special committee investigating deaths under anaesthesia. 2016 Special Report*. Retrieved from <http://www.cec.health.nsw.gov.au/__data/assets/pdf_file/0013/401341/SCIDUA-Annual-Report-2016.pdf>.

Coroners Court of NSW. (2018). Inquest into the death of Paul Lau. Retrieved from <http://www.coroners.justice.nsw.gov.au/Documents/Findings%20Paul%20Lau%20Final.pdf>.

Davies, E. (2013). Nurses sacked after posting pictures of themselves online wearing incontinence pads and tweet patients' personal details. Retrieved from <https://www.dailymail.co.uk/news/article-2433011/Nurses-sacked-posting-pictures-online-wearing-incontinence-pads-tweet-patients-personal-details.html>.

Government of South Australia, SA Health. (2016). Patient incident management and open disclosure. Policy directive. Retrieved from <https://www.sahealth.sa.gov.au/wps/wcm/connect/public+content/sa+health+internet/clinical+resources/safety+and+quality/governance+for+safety+and+quality/patient+incident+management+and+open+disclosure/patient+incident+management+and+open+disclosure>.

Government of Western Australia, Department of Health. (2016). *WA Health consent to treatment*. Perth: Author. Retrieved from <https://ww2.health.wa.gov.au/~/media/Files/Corporate/Policy%20Frameworks/Clinical%20Governance%20Safety%20and%20Quality/Policy/WA%20Health%20Consent%20to%20Treatment%20Poicy/Supporting/WA-Health-Consent-to-Treatment-Policy.pdf>.

Health Care Complaints Commission (HCCC) v Aref [2018] NSWCATOD 133. Retrieved from <https://www.caselaw.nsw.gov.au/decision/5b721f5be4b09e9963071b22>.

Henderson, V. (1964). The nature of nursing. *American Journal of Nursing, 64*(8), 62–68.

International Council of Nurses (ICN). (2012). *The ICN code of ethics for nurses*. Geneva: Author. Retrieved from <http://ethics.iit.edu/ecodes/sites/default/files/International%20Council%20of%20Nurses%20Code%20of%20Ethics%20for%20Nurses.pdf>.

Kerridge, I., Lowe, M., & Stewart, C. (2013). *Ethics and law for the health professions* (4th ed.). Sydney: Federation Press.

Medical Council of New Zealand (MCNZ). (2019). *Informed consent: helping patients make informed decisions about their care*. Retrieved from <https://www.mcnz.org.nz/assets/standards/79e1482703/Statement-on-informed-consent.pdf>.

Moorhead, A. (2017). Social media for healthcare communication. Communication. *Oxford Research Encyclopedias*. Oxford, UK: Oxford University Press. Retrieved from <https://oxfordre.com/communication/view/10.1093/acrefore/9780190228613.001.0001/acrefore-9780190228613-e-335>.

Murphy, E. (2019). Patient safety and risk management. In J. Rothrock & D. McEwen (Eds.), *Alexander's care of the patient in surgery* (16th ed., pp. 15–36). St Louis, MO: Elsevier Mosby.

National Health and Medical Research Council (NHMRC). (2019). Australian guidelines for the prevention and control of infection in healthcare. Retrieved from <https://www.nhmrc.gov.au/about-us/publications/australian-guidelines-prevention-and-control-infection-healthcare-2019>.

New Zealand Health and Disability Commissioner – Te Toihau, Hauatanga. (1996). Code of Health and Disability Services Consumers' Rights Regulations. Retrieved from <https://www.hdc.org.nz/your-rights/about-the-code/code-of-health-and-disability-services-consumers-rights/>.

New Zealand Health and Disability Commissioner – Te Toihau, Hauatanga. (2019). Consent for consumers who are not competent (fact sheet 1). Retrieved from <https://www.hdc.org.nz/media/4796/factsheet1-informedconsentforconsumersnotcompetent.pdf>.

New Zealand Health Practitioners Disciplinary Tribunal (NZHPDT). (2017). File no.: Nur17/399P. Retrieved from <https://www.hpdt.org.nz/portals/0/943Nur17399P.pdf>.

New Zealand Health Quality and Safety Commission. (2018). Surgical site infection improvement programme [webpage]. Retrieved from <https://www.hqsc.govt.nz/our-programmes/infection-prevention-and-control/projects/surgical-site-infection-improvement>.

New Zealand Ministry of Health. (2011). *Advance care planning: a guide for the New Zealand health care workforce*. Wellington: Author. Retrieved from <https://www.health.govt.nz/system/files/documents/publications/advance-care-planning-aug11.pdf>.

New Zealand Nurses Organisation (NZNO). (2019). *Guideline: social media and the nursing profession: a guide to maintain professionalism online for nurses and nursing students – 2019*. Retrieved from <https://www.nzno.org.nz/LinkClick.aspx?fileticket=mi3K2GhXMk0%3D&portalid=0>.

New Zealand Privacy Commissioner. (2020). Health Information Privacy Code 2020. Retrieved from <https://privacy.org.nz/privacy-act-2020/codes-of-practice/hipc2020/>.

NSW Health. (2010). *Coroners cases and Coroners Act 2009*. PD 2010_054. Sydney: Author.

NSW Health. (2013). *Management of instruments, accountable items and other items used for surgery or procedures*. PD2013_054. Sydney: Author.

NSW Law Reform Commission (NSWLRC). (2008). Report 119: Young people and consent to health care. Retrieved from <https://www.parliament.nsw.gov.au/tp/files/15864/r119.pdf>.

Nursing and Midwifery Board of Australia (NMBA). (2013). Panel hearing summary 2013.0173. Retrieved from <https://www.ahpra.gov.au/Publications/Panel-Decisions/Panel-hearing-summary-2013-0173.aspx>.)

Nursing and Midwifery Board of Australia (NMBA). (2016). *Registered nurse standards for practice*. Melbourne: Author.

Nursing and Midwifery Board of Australia (NMBA). (2020). *Annual report summary 2019/20*. Melbourne: Author.

Nursing and Midwifery Board of Australia (NMBA). (2018). *Code of professional conduct for nurses in Australia*. Melbourne: Author.

Nursing and Midwifery Board of Australia v George (Review and Regulation) [2015] VCAT 1878 (25 November 2015). Retrieved from <http://www8.austlii.edu.au/cgi-bin/viewdoc/au/cases/vic/VCAT/2015/1878.html?stem=0&synonyms=0&query=catherine%20george>.

Nursing and Midwifery Board of Australia v Morey [2017] QCAT 249. Retrieved from <http://archive.sclqld.org.au/qjudgment/2017/QCAT17-249.pdf>.

Nursing and Midwifery Council of NSW (NMC NSW). (2017). *Fact sheet: performance review panel*. Sydney: Author.

Nursing Council of New Zealand (NCNZ)/Te Kaunihera Tapuhi o Aotearoa. (2012). Code of conduct. Retrieved from <https://www.nursingcouncil.org.nz/Public/Nursing/Code_of_Conduct/NCNZ/nursing-section/Code_of_Conduct.aspx?hkey=7fe9d496-9c08-4004-8397-d98b-d774ef1b>.

Palacios-González, C. (2015). The ethics of clinical photography and social media. *Medicine, health care, and philosophy*, 18(1), 63–70. https://doi.org/10.1007/s11019-014-9580-y

Perioperative Nurses College of the New Zealand Nurses Organisation (PNC NZNO). (2016). Standards. Retrieved from <https://www.nzno.org.nz/groups/colleges_sections/colleges/perioperative_nurses_college/resources/standards_and_documents>.

Queensland Health. (2011). *Health care providers' handbook on Hindu patients*. Brisbane: Author.

Queensland Health. (2017). *Guide to informed decision-making in health care* (2nd ed). Brisbane: Author.

Reissa, S. (2013). Religion v science: parents denied New Zealand baby to get cancer treatment, lost court battle. *International Business Times* (Australian ed.), 10 September. Retrieved from <www.ibtimes.com.au/religion-vs-science-parents-denied-new-zealand-baby-get-cancer-treatment-lost-court-battle-1316900>.

South Eastern Sydney Local Health District. (2018). *Electronic intraoperative health care record: responsibility and accountability*. Sydney: Author.

Staunton, P., & Chiarella, M. (2020). *Law for nurses and midwives* (9th ed.). Sydney: Churchill Livingstone Elsevier.

FURTHER READING

Adrian, A., & Chiarella, M. (2010). *Professional conduct: a casebook of disciplinary decisions relating to professional conduct matters* (2nd ed.). Sydney: Nurses and Midwives Board of New South Wales.

Association of Anaesthetists of Great Britain & Ireland. (2009). Do not attempt resuscitation (DNAR) in the perioperative period. Retrieved from <https://anaesthetists.org/Portals/0/PDFs/Guidelines%20PDFs/Guidelines_DNAR_decisions_perioperative_period_2009_final.pdf?ver=2018-07-11-163758-177&ver=2018-07-11-163758-177>.

Bickhoff, L. (2014). Smart nurses' thoughtless posts on social media. *Australian Nursing and Midwifery Journal, 22*(4), 31.

Burns, K., & Belton, S. (2012). Click first, care second photography. *Medical Journal of Australia, 197*, 265.

Chiarella, M., & Vernon, R. (2019). Insights into insight: analysis of case files of nurse and midwife registrant performance complaints. *Collegian, 26*, 341–347. https://dx.doi.org/10.1016/j.colegn.2018.10.001

Finlay, A., Stewart, C., & Parker, M. (2013). Open disclosure: ethical, professional and legal obligations, and the way forward for regulation. *Medical Journal of Australia, 198*(8), 445–448.

Forrester, K., & Griffiths, D. (2015). *Essentials of law for health professionals* (4th ed.). Sydney: Elsevier Australia.

Health Care Chaplaincy. (2014). *Handbook: patients' spiritual and cultural values for health care professionals*. New York: Author. Retrieved from <http://www.healthcarechaplaincy.org/docs/publications/landing_page/cultural_sensitivity_handbook_from_healthcare_chaplaincy_network.pdf>.

Johnstone, M. J. (2019). *Bioethics: a nursing perspective* (7th ed.). Sydney: Churchill Livingstone Elsevier.

Nursing Council of New Zealand (NCNZ)/Te Kaunihera Tapuhi o Aotearoa. (2019). Keeping the public safe. Retrieved from <https://www.nursingcouncil.org.nz/Public/concerns/Keeping_the_public_safe/NCNZ/concernssection/Keeping_the_public_safe.aspx?hkey589fd89dd-681a-4d3a-a0b6-91efe858c809>.

Ramachenderan, J., & Auret, K. (2019). The challenge of perioperative advance care planning. *Journal of Pain and Symptom Management, 58(3)*, 538–542.

Ramachenderan, J., Auret, K., Smailhodzic, E., Hooijsma, W., Boonstra, A., & Langley, D. (2016). Social media use in healthcare: a systematic review of effects on patients and on their relationship with healthcare professionals. *BMC Health Services Research, 16,* 442.

Royal Australian and New Zealand College of Obstetrics and Gynaecology. (2020). Consent and provision of information to patients in Australia regarding proposed treatment. Retrieved from <https://ranzcog.edu.au/RANZCOG_SITE/media/RANZCOG-MEDIA/Women%27s%20Health/Statement%20and%20guidelines/Clinical%20-%20General/Consent-and-provision-of-information-to-patients-in-Australia-(C-Gen-2a).pdf?ext=.pdf>.

White, B., McDonald, F., & Wilmott, L., (2018). *Health law in Australia* (3rd ed.). Sydney: Thomson Reuters.

CHAPTER 4

Perioperative Patient Quality and Safety

BEN LOCKWOOD • MEREDITH GIMBLETT
EDITOR: BEN LOCKWOOD

LEARNING OUTCOMES

- Identify key clinical governance structures applicable to the perioperative environment
- Identify the nature and incidence of surgical adverse events
- Examine patient safety, risk management and quality activities as they relate to the perioperative environment
- Explore a systems approach to managing risk and patient safety
- Examine core nursing interventions aimed at ensuring patient safety

---

KEY TERMS

adverse event	patient safety
checklists	Plan Do Study Act (PDSA) cycle
clinical audit	Practice Audit Tools (PATs)
Clinical Care Standards	professional practice standards
clinical governance	quality
incident management systems	risk management
medication management	sentinel event
National Standards	surgical count
never event	WHO Surgical Safety Checklist
open disclosure	

INTRODUCTION

Every patient has the right to experience healthcare free from harm and adverse events. **Patient safety** is a paramount consideration within healthcare services, and this is particularly so in the perioperative environment owing to the vulnerability of the surgical patient and the risks associated with anaesthesia and surgery. The World Health Organization (WHO) recognises that around the world more than one million patients die every year from surgical complications, and adverse events leading to patient harm are a significant cause of the global health burden (WHO, 2019). Providing patients with safe care throughout their perioperative journey requires collaboration between nurses and other members of the multidisciplinary team. In addition to safe care, patients have a right to receive high-quality, evidence-based, effective treatment, leading to optimal outcomes and a timely return to a state of health.

This chapter explores national policy frameworks, regulatory systems, clinical governance mechanisms and professional practice standards that are used to deliver safe, high-quality patient care; it also describes how nurses work to achieve this within the perioperative setting. Described in detail are mechanisms such as the use of **checklists** to ensure safety, clinical audits to identify and measure care activities or compliance with procedures, and various approaches to managing situations when things go wrong, such as reporting systems and incident investigation.

CLINICAL GOVERNANCE

Clinical governance provides a framework through which healthcare services demonstrate accountability for the delivery of safe, high-quality patient care to ensure good clinical outcomes. It is underpinned by the concepts of clinical excellence and continuous quality and safety improvements, both of which assist healthcare services to comply with the regulatory systems and professional standards of practice (Australian Commission on Safety and Quality in Health Care [ACSQHC/the Commission], 2017a).

A national framework of clinical governance arises from bodies such as the Australian Council on Healthcare Standards (ACHS), government agencies including the Australian Commission on Safety and Quality in Health Care (ACSQHC/the Commission) and the Health Quality and Safety Commission New Zealand (HQSCNZ), and national expert bodies in health and medical research such as the National Health and Medical Research Council (NHMRC). Furthermore, quality and safety policies are driven by industry standards developed by professional bodies – for example, the International Organization

for Standardization (ISO) and Standards Australia and Standards New Zealand (AS/NZS). The ACSQHC *National model clinical governance framework* (2017b) acknowledges five essential components of the clinical governance framework:

- partnering with consumers
- governance, leadership and culture
- patient safety and quality improvement systems
- clinical performance
- a safe environment for delivery of care.

While the definition of clinical governance continues to evolve over time, the essential components remain stable, with the patient firmly placed at the core, surrounded by regulatory bodies, services and systems to ensure patient safety and high-quality healthcare (HQSCNZ, 2017a). **Quality** mechanisms, such as risk management, clinical auditing, incident reporting, open disclosure and quality improvement projects, enable perioperative nurses to identify areas of service excellence as well target areas for improvement. Staff education and training facilitate clinical effectiveness and are used to rectify gaps in practice. Clinical governance is also underpinned by the concept of **risk management**, which ensures that potential risks (preventable harm) to patients, visitors and healthcare workers can be identified, controlled or removed. Fig. 4.1 shows the essential components of clinical governance.

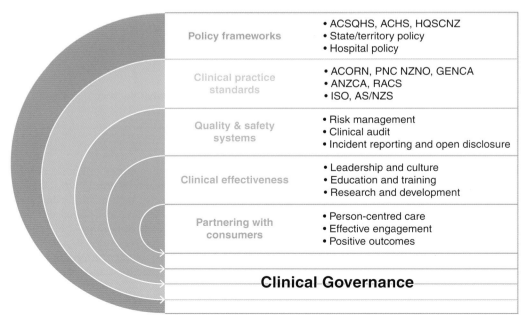

FIG. 4.1 Components of clinical governance. (Adapted from Australian Commission on Safety and Quality in Health Care. (2017b). National Model Clinical Governance Framework (p. 22). Sydney: Author.)

Professional Practice Standards and Clinical Governance

In clinical practice environments including day surgery and perioperative units, clinical governance is achieved by embedding policies, **professional practice standards** and guidelines produced by organisations including the Australian College of Perioperative Nurses (ACORN), the Perioperative Nurses College of the New Zealand Nurses Organisation (PNC NZNO), the Australian Day Surgery Nurses Association (ADSNA), the Gastroenterological Nurses College of Australia (GENCA), the Australian and New Zealand College of Anaesthetists (ANZCA) and the Royal Australasian College of Surgeons (RACS).

The development of practice standards is the core activity of many professional associations. Chapter 1 introduced the concept that standards provide the minimum requirements for practice and outlined the key professional associations established for perioperative nurses including ACORN, the PNC NZNO, the Association of periOperative Registered Nurses (AORN) and the International Federation of Perioperative Nurses (IFPN).

There are other multidisciplinary associations whose professional standards are also relevant to perioperative settings and patient safety. These include, but are not limited to, the following professional associations:

- Australian and New Zealand College of Anaesthetists (ANZCA), which produces position statements and practice guidelines such as:
  - 'Statement on roles in anaesthesia and perioperative care', which proposes that the composition of the anaesthetic and perioperative teams must support safe, high-quality patient care (ANZCA, 2015)
  - 'Guidelines on quality assurance and quality improvement in anaesthesia', which recommends evaluation of clinical care by quality assurance programs to ensure practice consistently reflects the standards and other professional documents of the College (ANZCA, 2012, 2019)
- Australasian College for Infection Prevention and Control (ACIPC), which is the peak Australasian body for infection prevention and control professionals, consulting with key stakeholders such as the ACSQHC, the ACHS and the Australian Society for Infectious Diseases (ASID). ACIPC's website provides open access to position statements such as 'Single-use devices' (ACIPC, 2016), 'Role of the infection control practitioner in antimicrobial stewardship' (ACIPC, 2017) and other resources relevant to perioperative settings

- Australian Day Surgery Nurses Association (ADSNA), which consults with government and other relevant bodies and develops the 'Day surgery best practice guidelines'
- Gastroenterological Nurses College of Australia (GENCA), which promotes excellence in gastroenterology nursing practice through the development of national standards and guidelines, and by dissemination of education and credentialling programs; GENCA members have access to discussion forums via its website and there is open access to GENCA position statements including:
  - 'Educational requirements for personnel reprocessing flexible endoscopic equipment', which recommends annual education for all personnel responsible for reprocessing flexible endoscopes (GENCA, 2012)
- Royal Australasian College of Surgeons (RACS), which supports and informs the practice of surgical trainees, members and College Fellows with a range of guidelines and position papers including:
  - 'Bullying and harassment: recognition, avoidance and management', which identifies the negative impact of workplace bullying on the quality of patient care (RACS, 2014)
  - 'Indigenous health', in which RACS identifies the disadvantage of many Aboriginal, Torres Strait Islander and Māori populations and expresses its commitment to addressing the health discrepancies of first nations communities (RACS, 2013)
  - 'Outreach surgery in regional, rural and remote areas of Australia and New Zealand', which outlines RACS' minimum requirements for the delivery of outreach surgical care to ensure that it is safe, effective and appropriate for the needs of those remote communities (RACS, 2015).

Fig. 4.2 displays the different clinical governance bodies, associations and standards in the perioperative environment.

Perioperative nursing practice in Australasia is well supported by a diverse range of professional practice standards and resources. These resources complement the standards and resources developed for perioperative nurses by ACORN and the PNC NZNO and provide guidance more broadly on the safe delivery of patient care by healthcare teams in a range of perioperative settings. Embedding quality and safety into everyday activity and ensuring that contemporary practice underpins all clinical activity ensures that perioperative nurses demonstrate the concept of clinical governance.

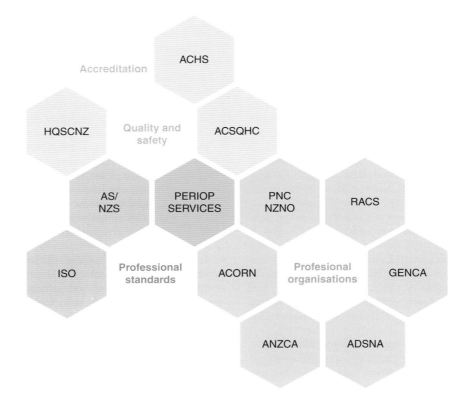

FIG. 4.2 National framework of clinical governance affecting perioperative services.

PATIENT SCENARIOS

Mr James Collins is a 78-year-old man who has been admitted for an elective right total knee replacement (TKR). Mr Collins' full history and a brief description of the healthcare setting is provided in the Introduction at the front of the book for readers to review when answering the questions in these unfolding scenarios.

SCENARIO 4.1: CLINICAL GOVERNANCE IN PRACTICE

An interdisciplinary team of three nurses, two surgeons and two anaesthetists are allocated to an all-day orthopaedic list. Surgical team members include:
- RN Ben Lumby, RN Rob Cohen and EN Pauline Noakes
- Dr Patrick Slattery and Dr Ivy West (orthopaedic surgeon and registrar)
- Dr Marion Thomas and Dr Vince De Silva (anaesthetic consultant and registrar)

- RN Margaret McCormack, anaesthetic nurse
- Theatre orderly Jimmy Montano.

Situation

Members of the team have not worked together before now. The team hold a morning briefing before the busy list commences to establish each team member's role and decide on work flows considerate of everyone's scope of practice.

Critical Thinking Questions

- As the senior RN, who will Ben Lumby be required to have clinical oversight of?
- Which professional associations will the different team members link with?

- Consider how the graduate nurse, RN Cohen, could learn more about the practice standards that underpin his role.

SCENARIO 4.2: CLINICAL GOVERNANCE – VISITORS IN THE OPERATING THEATRES

The first patient is Mr James Collins, who has been admitted for an elective right TKR (see above). Silvana Perez, a medical company representative (MCR), is due in the operating room prior to the commencement of Mr Collins' surgery to provide support for the team in the use of loan instrumentation and a new system of

hardware/prostheses that will be used to perform the procedure. While RN Ben Lumby is taking a morning tea break, RN Rob Cohen, the circulating nurse, steps out of theatre to retrieve an item from the sterile stock area. During this time, Dr Slattery asks for an instrument which is not yet opened but is in the room.

Critical Thinking Question

- Is it appropriate for EN Noakes, the instrument nurse, to ask Silvana Perez, the MCR, to open this instrument? Provide a rationale for your response.

PATIENT SAFETY AND RISK MANAGEMENT IN THE PERIOPERATIVE ENVIRONMENT

Of the 421 million episodes of hospital admissions occurring annually across the globe, approximately 42.7 million adverse events take place (WHO, 2017). Through international collaboration and engagement, the WHO is an influential global leader and advocate of equitable and safe patient care (WHO, 2017). In Australia, the Commission is committed to increasing patient safety by the provision of quality assurance mechanisms (e.g. the *National safety and quality health service standards* [NSQHS Standards]), which aim to minimise risk to the public (ACSQHC/the Commission, 2017). Similarly, New Zealand's Health Quality and Safety Commission was established in 2011 with the prime purpose of supporting and guiding healthcare facilities in continuously improving practice and minimising risk of harm to patients (Shuker et al., 2015). Globally, nationally and locally, implementation of the **WHO Surgical Safety Checklist** (SSC) (WHO, 2008) remains an important tool in mitigating risk for surgical patients (see Fig. 9.1, Chapter 9). However, despite this focus on patient safety and the availability of practice standards for the perioperative environment, clinical incidents and adverse events continue to occur (Australian Institute of Health and Welfare [AIHW], 2019) (Box. 4.1).

Adverse Events and Sentinel Events

The Australian Institute of Health and Welfare (AIHW) defines an **adverse event** as an incident that results in harm to a person receiving care and includes injury and conditions that occur during and after care (AIHW, 2018). In New Zealand, an adverse event includes any event where the outcome is unintended or unexpected and results in actual or potential harm (HQSCNZ, 2017b). The term **sentinel event** refers to 'adverse patient

safety events that are wholly preventable and result in serious harm to, or death of, a patient' (ACSQHC/the Commission, 2018a, p. 3). The Victorian State Government reports that 'retained surgical instruments or other items used during surgery requiring re-operation' is one of the most commonly reported sentinel events in the state (Safer Care Victoria, 2017, p. 4). Rather than the term sentinel event, it should be noted here that the term **never event** (i.e. an event that is 100% preventable) is used in the US and the UK when referring to these rare events.

Weiser and colleagues (2016) estimate that a total of 266–360 million surgical procedures were performed globally in 2012. Despite surgical procedures intending to improve and quality of life as well as be life preserving, the WHO (2018) noted the continuous global burden of surgical complications and mortality. Unsurprisingly, the global healthcare sector continues its focus on patient safety and further developing systems to improve outcomes for surgical patients.

Reporting on adverse events in Australasia

The AIHW publishes national data on adverse events from public and private hospitals (AIHW, 2019). These data are based on the International Classification of Diseases (ICD) version 10 Australian Modification (ICD-10-AM) discharge codes, which indicate when an adverse event has occurred during a patient's hospital stay. Many of these adverse events are thought to be preventable, including incidents such as patient falls, medication errors, pressure injuries (PI), venous thromboembolism (VTE) and healthcare-associated infections (HAIs). International data indicate that the majority of HAIs are caused by antimicrobial-resistant bacteria such as methicillin-resistant *Staphylococcus aureus* (MRSA) or multidrug-resistant Gram-negative bacteria

BOX 4.1
Australian Hospital Performance
Adverse Events, 2017–18

Adverse events are defined as incidents in which harm results to a person receiving health care. They include infections, falls resulting in injuries, and probelms with medication and medical devices. Some of these adverse events may be preventable. Similarly, the term hospital-acquired complications (HACs) refers to complications where risk mitigation strategies may reduce (not necessarily eliminate) the risk of complications occurring.

In Australia, in 2017–18:

- There was a total of 11.3 million events across the public and private sectors with 60% occurring in public hospitals.

- The most common hospital-acquired complication was healthcare-associated infections.
- 96,000 of the 11.3 events involved healthcare-associated infections.

The ACSQHC identifies 38 *complications diagnoses*. The table below outlines the 20 most common, which accounted for 89% of all hospital-acquired complications in 2017–18.

Complications	Public hospital	Private hospital	Total
Delirium	24 937	7 927	32 864
Arrhythmia	19 594	9 466	29 060
Urinary tract infection	20 208	8 160	28 368
Pneumonia	19 737	3 728	23 465
Blood stream infection	16 462	2 948	19 410
Hypoglycaemia	10 090	1 273	11 363
Aspiration pneumonia	7 503	1 213	8 716
Gastrointestinal bleeding	6 509	1 966	8 475
Heart failure and pulmonary oedema	5 352	1 814	7 166
Surgical site infection	4 989	1 928	6 917
Acute coronary syndrome	5 065	1 046	6 111
3rd/4th degree perineal laceration during deliver	5 491	534	6 025
Respiratory failure	4 767	867	5 634
Malnutrition	4 171	1 286	5 457
Surgical wound dehiscence	4 137	1 217	5 354
Multiresistant organism	4 206	1 056	5 262
Postoperative haemorrhage/haematoma requiring return to OR or transfusion	3 496	1 761	5 257
Central- and peripheral-line-associated bloodstream infection	3 698	746	4 444
Infection associated with prosthetic/implantable device	3 386	827	4 213
Deep vein thrombosis	2 473	1 610	4 083
TOTAL COMPLICATIONS	**198 696**	**58 066**	**256 762**

(Source: Adapted from Australian Institute of Health and Welfare. (2019). *Admitted patient care 2017–18: Australian hospital statistics*. Health services series no. 90. Cat. no. HSE 225. Canberra: Australia.)

(WHO, 2018). It is important to note that antibiotic resistance is not discriminatory; it can affect anyone, at any age (WHO, 2018). Australian hospitals are required to report on rates of HAIs including MRSA and *S. aureus* bacteraemia (SAB). Most people carry *S. aureus* with only minor ill effect; however, when the microorganism enters the bloodstream it causes serious infections (SAB), with mortality rates reported to be 15%–35% (ACSQHC/the Commission, 2014a). Between 2012–13 and 2016–17, the national rate of SAB declined from 0.9 cases to 0.8 cases per 10,000 days of patient care (AIHW, 2018). While the decline in SAB incidence is encouraging, healthcare-acquired complications constitute a disproportionate number of overall complications, many of which are preventable (see Box 4.1).

Reporting on sentinel events in Australia and New Zealand

Reporting on sentinel events was first proposed in 2002 by the Australian health ministers, following a historic agreement by the states and territories to standardise terminology and report their incidence annually. It has been mandatory since 2007 (ACSQHC/the Commission, 2018a). Sentinel events are reported and investigated to ensure public accountability, share knowledge, provide transparency of practice and drive continuous improvements in patient safety (ACSQHC/the Commission, 2018a, 2018b). The original eight sentinel events that were required to be reported have undergone revision and now comprise ten sentinel reportable events (ACSQHC/the Commission, 2018a). The current reportable sentinel events, as defined by the Commission, are:

1. Surgery or other invasive procedure performed on the wrong site – resulting in serious harm or death.
2. Surgery or other invasive procedure performed on the wrong patient – resulting in serious harm or death
3. Wrong surgical or other invasive procedure performed on a patient – resulting in serious harm or death
4. Unintended retention of foreign object in a patient after surgery or other invasive procedure – resulting in serious harm or death
5. Haemolytic blood transfusion reaction resulting from ABO incompatibility – resulting in serious harm or death
6. Suspected suicide of a patient in an acute psychiatric unit or acute psychiatric ward

7. Medication error – resulting in serious harm or death
8. Use of physical or mechanical restraint – resulting in serious harm or death
9. Discharge or release of an infant or child to an unauthorised person
10. Use of an incorrectly positioned oro- or naso-gastric tube resulting in serious harm or death (ACSQHC/the Commission, 2018a, p. 7).

In 2014–15, the AIHW reported 99 sentinel events in Australian public hospitals, with the most commonly reported sentinel event being a *retained instrument or other material after surgery requiring re-operation or further surgical procedure* (NB: this terminology predates the current reportable sentinel events list) (AIHW, 2018). (See Chapter 9 for further details of retained surgical items.) More recent data show that sentinel events are becoming less frequent in Australia, with the Commission indicating an overall drop in reported sentinel events across 2012–17 (ACSQHC/the Commission, 2019a) (Fig. 4.3). Safer Care Victoria (2018) notes that sentinel events spiked in conjunction with

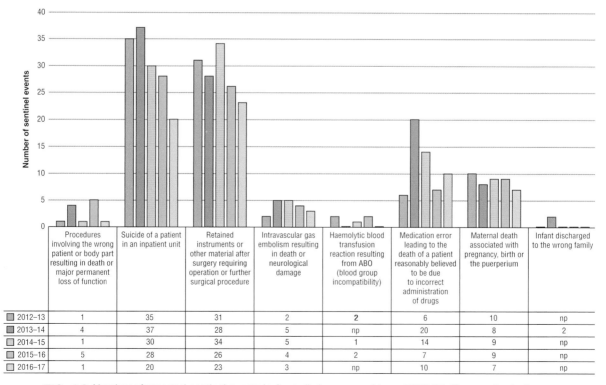

	Procedures involving the wrong patient or body part resulting in death or major permanent loss of function	Suicide of a patient in an inpatient unit	Retained instruments or other material after surgery requiring operation or further surgical procedure	Intravascular gas embolism resulting in death or neurological damage	Haemolytic blood transfusion reaction resulting from ABO (blood group incompatibility)	Medication error leading to the death of a patient reasonably believed to be due to incorrect administration of drugs	Maternal death associated with pregnancy, birth or the puerperium	Infant discharged to the wrong family
2012–13	1	35	31	2	2	6	10	np
2013–14	4	37	28	5	np	20	8	2
2014–15	1	30	34	5	1	14	9	np
2015–16	5	28	26	4	2	7	9	np
2016–17	1	20	23	3	np	10	7	np

FIG. 4.3 Number of reported sentinel events in Australia by year and type, 2012–17. (Source: Australian Commission on Safety and Quality in Health Care (2019a). *The state of patient safety and quality in Australian hospitals 2019* (p. 22) Sydney: Author.)

TABLE 4.1
Surgical Adverse Events From the NZ National Minimum Dataset, 2007–8 to 2015–16

External cause of injury code and label	07–08	08–09	09–10	10–11	11–12	12–13	13–14	14–15	15–16	16–17
Y61.0 – Foreign object accidentally left in body during surgical operation	40	17	40	50	57	57	42	46	59	24*
Y65.5 – Performance of inappropriate operation	4	6	1	0	6	7	7	10	8	2*
Total	44	23	41	50	63	64	49	56	67	26*

*Note: the results for 2016/17 are for July to December 2016 only and so represent half a year
Source: The National Minimum Dataset; extracted by the Health Quality and Safety Commission, September 2016 and April 2017

improvements in reporting systems; however, this is likely evidence of the increasing understanding and appreciation of reporting systems, rather than healthcare becoming less safe. Nonetheless, perioperative staff must remain vigilant, as retained surgical items and medication errors remain the second and third highest occurring sentinel events respectively across Australia (ACSQHC/the Commission, 2019a).

New Zealand health services report on serious adverse events in the HQSCNZ annual reports. Table 4.1 depicts New Zealand data from 2007–08 to 2015–16, during which time 483 serious adverse events were reported. Of these events, 432 were retained surgical items and 51 were performance of an inappropriate operation (wrong site surgeries or wrong patients/wrong procedures). While these data show an upward trend in events from previous reporting periods, this trend most likely reflects improvements in adverse event reporting rather than increases in actual events (HQSCNZ, 2018a). As at 2017, New Zealand district health boards (DHBs) are required to disclose *always report and review events*, which are events that must be reported whether or not harm has resulted (HQSCNZ, 2018a). Of the 84 reported events in 2017, there were 54 reports of *wrong site, wrong implant, wrong prosthesis, wrong consumer/procedure* and 27 reports of *retained foreign object post-procedure* (HQSCNZ, 2018a).

Although healthcare facilities across Australasia are required to report and investigate sentinel events when they occur, comparisons between reports are not always helpful owing to variations in the reporting practices between the two national jurisdictions. Despite this lack of a standardised reporting process, there *are* consistencies in approach across jurisdictions. For example, healthcare workers in Australia and New Zealand are required to:

- report patient safety incidents
- classify the severity of the incident using standardised Severity Assessment Code (SAC) tools
- collect incident data and report on incident management using electronic reporting systems
- investigate high-severity patient safety incidents using root cause analysis (RCA) processes (ACSQHC/the Commission, 2009a).

It is beyond the scope of this text to further explore the use of SAC tools and RCA processes generally. More information from state and territory health departments and safety and quality entities can be found in the Resources section at the end of this chapter.

In acknowledging the rise of metadata in driving healthcare improvements, several Australian hospitals have recently joined the National Surgical Quality Improvement Program (NSQIP), which is administered by the American College of Surgeons (ACS, 2019). The NSQIP is an international, risk-adjusted, program built to measure and improve the quality of surgical outcomes around the globe. Not only acting as a database registry, the NSQIP also provides participating hospitals with comprehensive data analysis reports and quality improvement implementation guidelines and tools. It allows hospitals to identify preventable surgical complications by using validated, risk-adjusted clinical data. Since its inception in the late 1990s, the program has shown that participating hospitals can prevent 250–500 complications annually, save 12–36 lives annually and reduce by millions the costs associated with health-acquired complications (ACS, 2019; Agency for Clinical Innovation [ACI], 2019).

PATIENT SCENARIOS

SCENARIO 4.3: REVIEW OF A SENTINEL EVENT

The operating team described in Scenario 4.1 have been asked to participate in an investigation of a recent sentinel event in which a wrong site surgery occurred at another facility in their region. The investigation reveals that team communication and distractions contributed to this event. In particular, it was noted that the surgeon was called to the telephone during the team 'Time Out'.

Critical Thinking Questions

- What actions would the team take if a disruption occurred during team 'Time Out'? Provide rationales to explain why you believe these actions are important.
- List two other factors that may contribute to wrong site surgeries.

SAFETY AND QUALITY FRAMEWORKS

The evolution of safety and quality in healthcare is a process of reform, with the imperative to reduce harm to patients and improve clinical outcomes (ACSQHC/the Commission, the Commission, 2009a). Over the past two decades, there has been significant research demonstrating how errors and serious mishaps occur in healthcare settings, with research noting that such errors frequently have their roots in system failures (including equipment failures) and are attributed to human factors, most notably communication failures (Berger, Greenberg, & Bilimoria, 2015; Gawande, 2010; Gjeraa, Spanager, Konge, Petersen, & Ostergaard, 2016; Kumar & Raina, 2017; Reason, 2000). (Refer to Chapter 2 for information on human factors in the perioperative environment.) Continued investigation into safety and quality has increased knowledge and understanding of the nature of error, as well as highlighted the importance of improvement systems to address issues and change management processes to embed and sustain improvements (ACSQHC/the Commission, 2009b; Griffin et al., 2016; Reason 2000). By using techniques from other high-risk industries where safety is paramount, such as the nuclear and aviation industries (Kapur, Parand, Soukup, Reader, & Sevdalis, 2015; Powell-Dunford et al., 2017), the healthcare sector has developed techniques to identify risk, investigate and analyse incidents, and use the knowledge gained to improve clinical practice and patient outcomes.

Significant quality and safety changes began in 2010, when Australian health ministers endorsed a safety and quality framework articulating the actions that clinicians should take to improve the quality of healthcare for all Australians (ACSQHC/the Commission, 2010). The framework indicated that safe, high-quality healthcare must always be consumer-centred, driven by information and organised for safety (ACSQHC/the Commission, 2010). Similarly, in 2010 New Zealand established the HQSCNZ, which was designed to ensure healthcare consumers receive high-quality, best-value and equitable care (HQSCNZ, 2015). The HSQCNZ considered measures of equity, safety, patient experience and effectiveness, while addressing the social determinants of health (HQSCNZ, 2018b).

In 2010 in Australia, the Commission produced the first edition of the *National safety and quality health service standards* (the **National Standards**), which provide statements about the level of healthcare that patients can expect and how hospitals are to deliver safe and quality care for their consumers (ACSQHC/the Commission, 2011a, 2011b). Hospitals are assessed and accredited against these National Standards to ensure quality and safety practices meet the requirements. In conjunction with the formation of the National Standards, the Commission created the Australian Health Service Safety and Quality Accreditation Scheme (the AHSSQA Scheme), which was tasked to coordinate accreditation processes nationally, and collect and analyse feedback on the lessons learnt through accreditation cycles (ACSQHC/the Commission, 2019b). Healthcare services across Australia were first assessed against the National Standards in 2013.

The National Standards were first developed as a set of 10 mandatory standards. In 2014, they were reviewed by the Commission over six stages, with drafting and national consultation undertaken during the second half of 2015. Together with collaboration from the Australian Government, the private sector, clinical experts, patients and consumers, the second edition of the National Standards was published by the Commission in 2017 and updated in 2021 in response to the SARS-CoV2 (COVID-19) global pandemic (ACSQHC/the Commission, 2017a, 2021). The second edition of the National Standards is a set of eight mandatory standards that aim to protect patients from adverse events

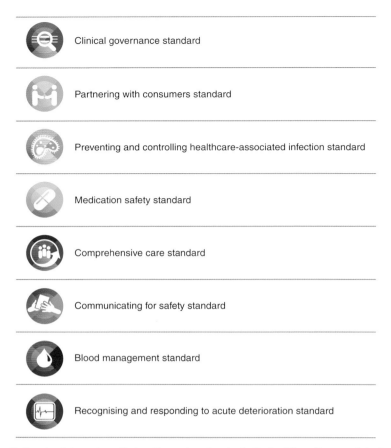

Clinical governance standard

Partnering with consumers standard

Preventing and controlling healthcare-associated infection standard

Medication safety standard

Comprehensive care standard

Communicating for safety standard

Blood management standard

Recognising and responding to acute deterioration standard

FIG. 4.4 The *National safety and quality health service standards*, 2nd edition. (Source: Adapted from Australian Commission on Safety and Quality in Health Care. (2017a). *National safety and quality health service standards*, 2nd ed. Sydney: Author.)

by establishing a nationally consistent framework for the delivery of safe, quality care and best practice (ACSQHC/the Commission, 2017a). Fig. 4.4 outlines the second edition of the National Standards.

The key objective of the National Standards is to ensure that health service organisations have safety and quality systems to manage risk (ACSQHC/the Commission, 2017a). Furthermore, by establishing systems to acknowledge, report and analyse adverse events in a transparent fashion, opportunity is created to change systems (and cultures) and subsequently to develop and implement policies to reduce or prevent adverse events.

A 2018 report on the impact of the implementation of the National Standards in Australia marked a milestone in the history of safety and quality efforts, noting that the creation of the first edition of the National Standards was a groundbreaking initiative with demonstrated improvements to the safety and quality of healthcare provision across Australia, including drops in the rates of drug-resistant bacteraemia and in-hospital cardiac arrest (ACSQHC/the Commission, 2017a, 2018c). The report, however, provided evidence that more work was still needed to continue to see improvement in healthcare outcomes, especially for high-risk patients and marginalised populations (ACSQHC/the Commission, 2018a). In collaboration with the AIHW, the Commission produced the first Australian *Atlas of healthcare variation* in 2015, and subsequently released the third Atlas in 2018 (ACSQHC/the Commission & AIHW, 2018). The Atlas explores the extent to which healthcare usage in Australia varies depending on where people live, with an aim to encourage further investigation into healthcare disparities and to promote equity to healthcare resources (ACSQHC/the Commission & AIHW, 2018). Notably, the Atlas highlights that the health of Aboriginal and Torres Strait Islander people has improved overall; however, on every indicator they experience poorer health outcomes than other Australians owing to complex and interrelated risk factors, social determinants of health and access to culturally appropriate services (ACSQHC/the Commission, 2017c). The revision of the National Standards into the second edition sought to addresses gaps identified in the first edition, including the areas of mental health and cognitive impairment, health literacy, end-of-life care and Aboriginal and Torres Strait Islander health. Healthcare organisations began to be assessed against the second edition of the National Standards from 2019. The National Standards are broad and designed to cover all aspects of healthcare. That said, each Standard has relevance for perioperative practice, though this is more overt in some compared with others.

Clinical Governance Standard

This Standard describes how organisations are required to implement and govern quality and safety systems. This Standard, together with the Partnering with Consumers Standard, applies to the implementation of all the other Standards. In the perioperative setting, the Clinical Governance Standard is demonstrated by a range of systems and practices, including:

- systems to ensure the workforce has the right qualification, skills and supervision to provide safe, high-quality healthcare
- development, review and compliance with policies, procedures and protocols that guide appropriate care, such as ACORN Standards, ANZCA guidelines and the Sterilisation Standard AS/NZS 4187 (Standards Australia, 2014)
- clinical audit cycles to observe, measure, evaluate and report on clinical care activities and performance indicators (such as hand hygiene compliance)
- implementation of an effective incident management system to ensure that adverse events are reported, analysed and used to improve patient safety
- monitoring the prescription and administration of antibiotics in accordance with surgical prophylactic antibiotics guidelines (see Feature box 4.3 later in the chapter).

Essentially, the Clinical Governance Standard ensures that everyone has a responsibility to work together to keep themselves and their patients safe. The Commission reports that since implementation of the National Standards many hospital boards agree that they have improved patient safety by better integration of governance and quality systems, clarified roles and responsibilities, and increased engagement with clinicians and consumers (ACSQHC/the Commission, 2018a).

Partnering with Consumers Standard

This Standard describes how organisations and healthcare professionals engage with their patients, by providing frameworks to raise the profile of consumer participation in healthcare and empowering staff to act as strong patient advocates. In the perioperative field, this engagement may include:

- patient representation on operating theatre governance committees where decisions are made about service delivery
- patient input and review of perioperative patient information resources
- consultation with patients in the design and redevelopment of operating theatre suites.

An example of partnering with patients is via patient satisfaction surveys. These can be paper based, online questionnaires or, in the case of day surgery patients, may involve perioperative nurses making follow-up phone calls to check on patients' progress, when there is also an opportunity to determine their level of satisfaction with the care they received by using a predetermined set of questions. Measuring patient satisfaction provides valuable information about the quality of healthcare services; however, the information given is often subjective and requires structured and validated tools to provide meaningful and useful information (Burt et al., 2017).

Preventing and Controlling Infections Standard

This Standard focuses on infection control, which is at the core of many activities in perioperative nursing. The Standard recognises that patients and staff in healthcare services have infection control risks, which provide infectious agents with the opportunity to spread and adapt (ACSQHC/the Commission, 2021). These risk factors include:

- treatment in close proximity to another patient
- invasive devices and surgical procedures
- prescription of broad-spectrum antibiotics and immunosuppressive drugs
- mechanisms for transmission of infectious agents
- reservoirs of pathogens.

The Standard is understandably large in scope, covering the concepts of aseptic technique, standard and transmission-based precautions, hand hygiene, antimicrobial stewardship, surveillance, workforce immunisation, responding to infections that cause outbreaks, epidemics or pandemics, environmental cleaning, and the reprocessing and sterilisation of surgical instruments, which is also directed by AS/NZS 4187: *Reprocessing of reusable medical devices in health service organisations* (Standards Australia, 2014). The infection prevention concepts and practices at the core of this AS/NZS Standard are explored in more detail in Chapter 6. Other examples of how the Standard relates to the perioperative setting include:

- using the WHO (2008) SSC to determine the need for antibiotic prophylaxis and to ascertain whether antibiotics have been administered appropriately (timing and duration of administration) (see Feature box 4.3 later in chapter)
- ensuring perioperative nurses maintain vigilance when using aseptic techniques during invasive procedures such as the insertion of an arterial line for blood pressure monitoring, or the set-up of an aseptic field for a surgical procedure, in order to reduce the likelihood of contamination leading to surgical site infection (SSI)
- auditing and reporting of perioperative staff hand hygiene compliance in accordance with Hand Hygiene Australia's 5 Moments for Hand Hygiene (see Chapter 6 for further information), as well as the concept of being 'bare below the elbows'
- assessing perioperative nurses' compliance with correct practices for validating, opening and dispensing sterile items to prevent contamination of aseptic field
- the storage of sterile equipment and consumable items in appropriate spaces and environmental conditions
- workforce immunisation processes and outbreak prevention strategies
- the identification and appropriate management of patients known to harbour multiresistant organisms, such as MRSA, in order to minimise the risk for SSI and environmental contamination.

Medication Safety Standard

This Standard is about implementing systems to promote medication safety and to reduce the incidence of medication errors and harm from medicines. In the perioperative setting, it directs the handling and administration of medications, as well as the secure management of opioids, narcotics, sedatives and other restricted medications, to prevent misuse. Of note for perioperative nurses is the labelling of medications (including those on the aseptic field) and lines to reduce the likelihood of errors. This Standard is explored in detail in the section on medication management later in this chapter.

Comprehensive Care Standard

This second edition Standard is a combination of Standards 8 and 10 from the first edition of the National Standards, as well as inclusion of important new information. It requires healthcare services to address the issues underlying many adverse events, such as failures to provide continuous and collaborative care, work in partnership with patients, or to communicate and work as a team (ACSQHC/the Commission, 2017a). The Comprehensive Care Standard seeks to minimise harm to patients, by highlighting actions to safely care for patients at risk of a variety of situations or factors, specifically:

- pressure injuries
- falls
- poor nutrition and malnutrition
- cognitive impairment
- unpredictable behaviours and preventing aggression from violence
- restrictive practices.

The Standard seeks to engage consumers in the decision-making processes regarding their healthcare needs to coordinate a customised and patient-focused approach that is appropriate and cognisant of the impact to the patient's life and well-being. Importantly for perioperative services, staff should have regard to international guidelines for the prevention of pressure injuries, which make specific recommendations for patients having surgery. The National Pressure Ulcer Advisory Panel, in association with the European Pressure Ulcer Advisory Panel and Pan Pacific Pressure Injury Alliance, recognises perioperative patients as a special needs population (National Pressure Ulcer Advisory Panel, European Pressure Ulcer Advisory Panel and Pan Pacific Pressure Injury Alliance [NPUAP-EPUAP-PPPIA], 2019). Indeed, all surgical patients face increased risk of sustaining tissue damage caused by pressure, friction or shearing forces. This is due to a combination of intrinsic patient-related risk factors and extrinsic environment or practice-related risk factors. Thus, perioperative clinicians must be able to assess a patient's potential risk of sustaining tissue damage or a pressure injury and put in place strategies to mitigate these risks (see Chapter 9 for further information). If a pressure injury does occur, clinicians must report this as an adverse event and take measures to support restoration of tissue integrity.

In the perioperative environment, falls can occur when patients are ambulatory, often during transfer and admission to the service. Moreover, if intraoperative patient positioning is not well planned and closely monitored, the patient's limbs may fall over the edge of the OR table, with potential to cause tissue, nerve or musculoskeletal injury (see Chapter 9 for further information). Healthcare workers are also at risk of falls. For example, the perioperative environment presents potentially dangerous clinical situations such as:

- when staff rush to prepare the OR between patients, particularly if the OR floor has not dried completely after cleaning
- the potential for slipping on wet floors around scrub bays
- the impact of large fluid spills during procedures such as those undertaken during closed urology surgery or orthopaedic arthroscopy
- the presence of trip hazards from power cords or leads in cramped physical spaces such as the anaesthetic bay.

Perioperative nurses should comply with workplace policies to assess individual patient risks for falls (as well as for pressure injuries) and should be familiar with the use of **incident management systems**. There are a variety of systems in use, including:

- Risk Manager used by QLD Health
- the Clinical Incident Management System (Datix CIMS) used by WA Health (Western Australia Department of Health, 2019)

- the Incident Information Management System (IIMS) used by NSW Health
- Safety Learning System (SLS) used by SA Health
- the RL6 reporting system used by all five district health boards in New Zealand.

Communicating for Safety Standard

This second edition Standard is a combination of Standards 5 and 6 from the first edition of the National Standards. The Standard focuses on correct patient identification and procedure matching processes, as well as clinical handover and organisational processes to support effective communication. In the perioperative setting, patient identification and procedure matching is crucial in order to avoid performing the wrong procedure on the wrong site or the wrong patient (see Feature box 4.1). Patient identification in medical records and on patient wristbands requires at least three nationally recognised identifiers: the patient's full name, date of birth and hospital/medical record number. Furthermore, this Standard describes how healthcare services must ensure that structured approaches are used for information exchange and clinical handover. Unstructured clinical communications and handovers can pose significant risk to patients because critical information may be omitted, responsibility

---

FEATURE BOX 4.1
A Case of Mistaken Identity

A report from the Health Quality and Safety Commission New Zealand in 2014 describes an incident where the wrong patient was taken for a chest X-ray. Two patients with the same first name (Bill Adams and Bill Smith) were sharing a hospital room. An orderly arrived to pick up Bill Adams for his chest X-ray, but when the orderly asked simply for 'Bill', Bill Smith replied, as Bill Adams was out of the room. Thus, the wrong Bill accompanied the orderly to the radiology department where the radiographer also identified the patient by his first name only. The X-ray was taken and the error was picked up 3 days later when a subsequent CT scan was ordered for Bill Adams. The report noted that errors in correct patient identification procedures led to the incident and, as a result, formal patient identification systems were put in place at the facility.

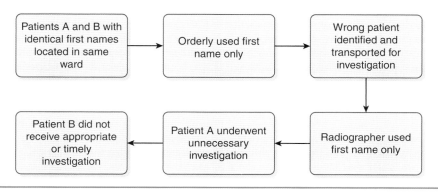

(Source: Health Quality and Safety Commission New Zealand. (2014). *Open book: accurate patient identification, December 2014*. Wellington: Author.)

and accountability may not be recognised and adverse patient events can ensue. Often in the perioperative setting, patient information is communicated via a variety of methods. These include the use of checklists in perioperative documentation, as well as face-to-face clinical handovers using frameworks such as Identification, Situation, Background, Assessment, Recommendation (ISBAR) or Identification, Situation, Observation, Background, Assessment, Recommendation (ISOBAR) (with the latter being recommended by ANZCA (2013, 2019)). Clinical handover in the perioperative setting occurs when patients are admitted to the operating suite and when they are transferred from the operating room (OR) to the postanaesthesia care unit (PACU) (ANZCA, 2020). Nurses should conduct a structured clinical handover when acting in relief roles because the incoming nurse may not have participated in a patient identification process such as 'Time Out'. When information is provided in a structured manner, there is less likelihood of miscommunication or omissions. (Clinical handover is further discussed in Chapters 7 and 12, and patient identification and procedure matching is explored in more detail in the section on the use of checklists in this chapter; or see Chapter 9 for further information.)

Blood Management Standard

This Standard is concerned with the safe administration, patient monitoring, documentation and disposal of blood products. Transfusion-related adverse events and acute haemolytic reactions can occur if stringent cross-matching and positive patient identification processes are not observed (Australian Red Cross Life Blood, 2019). Blood products require additional processes for correct handling and storage to reduce contamination, staff exposure and wastage. In Australia, blood supply services are coordinated and managed by the National Blood Authority (NBA), a statutory agency established under the National Blood Authority Act 2003 (NBA, n.d.a). The NBA has developed six patient blood management guidelines (NBA, 2019) and a national education program. The latter includes the BloodSafe program, comprising several e-learning modules, which all Australian healthcare workers involved in blood transfusions must complete (NBA, n.d.b). For example, this mandatory program is applicable to:

- orderlies and patient care assistants who are required to correctly identify and transport blood products within the healthcare facility
- doctors and nurses who are required to check and administer blood products or manage the storage of blood products in the perioperative setting.

A common occurrence in many perioperative settings is the administration of large volumes of blood via a mass transfusion pack for critical bleeding. In these instances, perioperative nurses must apply stringent processes for accurate cross-checking and documentation, and ensure that blood products are stored appropriately to reduce wastage caused by temperature variations or packaging contamination. ANZCA has endorsed six of the NBA's evidence-based patient blood management guidelines, including Module 1: Critical bleeding/massive transfusion and Module 2: Perioperative (ANZCA, 2019).

Recognising and Responding to Acute Deterioration Standard

The second edition revision of this Standard seeks to ensure that acute deterioration is recognised in a patient's physical condition as well as in their mental or cognitive condition, and that prompt and appropriate action is taken. This Standard is paramount to safe and high-quality patient care in the perioperative setting. Systems such as criterion-based patient monitoring tools and observation charts can help nurses (and other healthcare workers) to identify and respond to a deteriorating patient in a structured, consistent and timely manner. Recognition of deterioration is especially relevant for nurses caring for patients in the postoperative phase, where adverse events are more likely to occur and where clinical deterioration can occur rapidly. Furthermore, perioperative nurses need educating to recognise and respond appropriately to situations that are unique to acute care settings, including airway emergencies such as 'can't intubate, can't oxygenate' (CICO) and crises such as malignant hyperthermia (Feature box 4.2). See Chapter 8 for further information.

Australian Council on Healthcare Standards

The Australian Council on Healthcare Standards (ACHS) is an independent council and accreditation agency representing governments, peak health bodies and healthcare consumers in Australia. In tandem with the Commission and the National Standards, the ACHS is tasked with the process of accrediting healthcare organisations using the Evaluation and Quality Improvement Program (EQuIP) which has been recently updated to the latest edition EQuIP6 (ACHS, 2018). In New Zealand, the certification of healthcare services is provided by HealthCERT, under the Health and Disability Service (Safety) Act 2001 (Ministry of Health, New Zealand, 2019). Healthcare facility accreditation occurs in either a fixed-term or ad hoc cycle by means of organisation-wide surveys involving

FEATURE BOX 4.2
The Hidden Dangers of Malignant Hyperthermia

A 35-year-old woman with no significant medical history was admitted to hospital for a routine hernia repair. Her only previous surgery was a caesarean section under spinal anaesthesia. Upon induction, the anaesthetist noticed some unusual cardiac arrhythmias followed by a dramatic rise in expired CO_2 levels. The symptoms continued to escalate, with muscle rigidity and an increase in body temperature occurring. Recognising the symptoms, the anaesthetist declared a malignant hyperthermia (MH) emergency.

Due to the rarity of such a crisis, the perioperative team was unprepared. There was delay in obtaining the supply of dantrolene (the muscle relaxant required to treat the symptoms) and staff members were inexperienced in the correct process for its reconstitution and administration. Lack of clinical leadership on the part of the anaesthetist contributed to poor team cohesiveness; consequently, the team did not commence cooling strategies in a timely fashion and the patient's temperature continued to rise. The patient's condition deteriorated further, until this metabolic crisis precipitated a cardiac arrest. Fortuitously, the patient was successfully resuscitated, her condition stabilised and she was admitted to the intensive care unit where she spent a further 7 days recovering.

Although rare, MH represents a significant risk to surgical patients (Malignant Hyperthermia Australia and New Zealand [MHANZ], 2019). This example demonstrates the importance of early recognition and appropriate response to clinical deterioration in the perioperative setting. It further highlights that perioperative staff require periodic training to deal with unexpected crises and need clear action plans for managing them. A guide to the appropriate management of malignant hyperthermia can be found at http://malignanthyperthermia.org.au/.

(Source: B. Lockwood, personal communication, 23 July 2015.)

processes of audit, evaluation and assessment (ACHS, 2015, 2018; Ministry of Health, New Zealand, 2019). This cyclical accreditation process ensures that healthcare services can demonstrate adherence to relevant regulatory frameworks. As part of the accreditation cycle, perioperative services are expected to implement, audit and improve patient safety and quality systems continuously, culminating in the accreditation survey, when all evidence of the service's compliance is assessed.

Open Disclosure

Within the National Standards framework, **quality** comes from the ability to identify risks to patient safety and act upon them to reduce the likelihood that they will occur. Moreover, if adverse events do occur, a quality system allows for **open disclosure** so patients are fully informed and an examination of the event can take place, thus mitigating against future occurrences.

The Australian Open Disclosure Framework, endorsed in 2013, assists health services to communicate openly with consumers when their care results in harm or does not go according to plan (ACSQHC/the Commission, 2013a). The framework provides steps and processes for healthcare workers to maintain their ethical responsibility to provide honest and open communication with patients and their families. Importantly, open disclosure is a means to acknowledge accountability and provide pathways to remediation and quality improvement. Open disclosure is a discussion and an exchange of information that may take place over several meetings (ACSQHC/the Commission, 2013b).

The elements of open disclosure are:
- an apology or expression of regret (including the word 'sorry')
- a factual explanation of what happened
- an opportunity for the patient to relate their experience
- an explanation of the steps being taken to manage the event and prevent recurrence.

Clinical Care Standards

In 2013, the Commission established the **Clinical Care Standards** program outlining quality statements that support clinical experts and consumers in managing conditions that would benefit from a nationally coordinated approach (ACSQHC/the Commission, 2013b). The Clinical Care Standards of Antimicrobial Stewardship, Acute Coronary Syndromes, Hip Fracture Care, Venous Thromboembolism Prevention, Colonoscopy, and Third and Fourth Degree Perineal Tears have key relevance to the perioperative setting and provide perioperative health workers nationwide with best-practice guidelines to achieve safe, high-quality patient care (Feature box 4.3).

USE OF CHECKLISTS

Checklists provide a mechanism to safeguard against human failure and have been used successfully in many industries including healthcare to reduce adverse events, complications and mortality (Gawande, 2010). As in other high-risk industries, checklists used in healthcare are designed to ensure that essential task components are undertaken in a specific order, before the next activity can occur, thus reducing the likelihood of error occurring due to omission of process or activity. The

---

FEATURE BOX 4.3
Clinical Care Standards Relevant to Perioperative Services

Clinical Care Standards aim to standardise the delivery of care for specific clinical conditions in line with current best evidence so as to avoid unwarranted variation (ACSQHC, 2019c). The Clinical Care Standards are continuously being improved with additions and updates. The following list is an overview of some of the Clinical Care Standards relevant to perioperative services.

- **Acute Coronary Care Syndromes Clinical Care Standard** – provides statements about the requirement for patients with an acute ST-segment myocardial infarction (STEMI) to have access to timely percutaneous coronary intervention, usually in less than 90 minutes
- **Antimicrobial Stewardship Clinical Care Standard** – provides instructions for the use of antimicrobials for surgical prophylaxis, including statements for prescribing in accordance with current therapeutic

guidelines cognisant of the patient's clinical condition, and the timing and duration of doses
- **Colonoscopy Clinical Care Standard** – provides statements about the use of procedural sedation and the associated clinical risk assessments required beforehand, as well as requirements for the post-procedure recovery care and discharge
- **Hip Fracture Care Clinical Care Standard** – provides quality statements associated with pain assessment and treatment, and recommendations for the timing of surgery to be within 48 hours
- **Venous Thromboembolism Prevention Clinical Care Standard** – provides statements regarding venous thromboembolism (VTE) risk assessment, documentation and communication, as well as key considerations for the use of VTE prevention strategies such as mechanical and pharmacological prophylaxis.

(Sources: Australian Commission on Safety and Quality in Health Care. (2014b). *Acute Coronary Syndromes Clinical Care Standard*; (2016). *Hip Fracture Care Clinical Care Standard*; (2018d). *Venous Thromboembolism Prevention Clinical Care Standard*; (2018e). *Colonoscopy Clinical Care Standard*; (2019c). *Overview of the Clinical Care Standards*; (2020). *Antimicrobial Stewardship Clinical Care Standard*. Sydney: Author.)

---

checklist approach has several advantages. Checklists aid memory recall, particularly for mundane matters that can easily or routinely be overlooked (WHO, 2019). Checklists clarify the minimum expected steps in a complex process and help teams to work together to establish a high standard of baseline performance (WHO, 2019). Preoperative checklists guide healthcare workers in the preparation of patients for surgery. They can be as simple as tools that confirm a patient's readiness for surgery (e.g. the pre-op checklist), through to more comprehensive documents that follow the entire surgical patient journey from pre-admission clinic through the operating suite and onto the discharge ward. Checklists also include tools used intraoperatively and during the patient's stay in the PACU. (See Chapters 8, 9 and 12 for further information.)

PATIENT SCENARIOS

SCENARIO 4.4: TRAY LISTS AS CHECKLISTS

Consider again the scenario with Mr James Collins, admitted for elective TKR. There will be several instrument trays as well as loan instrument sets for EN Noakes, the instrument nurse, and RN Lumby and RN Cohen, the circulating nurses, to manage through this procedure. EN Noakes and RN Cohen are checking the loan instruments prior to the beginning of the case. Silvana Perez, the MCR who is here to support staff in the use of new instrumentation/prostheses, tells EN Noakes and RN Cohen that they do not need to check the loan trays because she knows the trays are correct and Dr Slattery wants to get started as soon as possible. It will take time to check the trays thoroughly.

> **Critical Thinking Question**
>
> - Should EN Noakes and RN Cohen continue to check the loan trays, or simply mark on the checklist that all items are present? Provide justification for your response.

Mr Collins' surgery has been successfully completed, and RN Ben Lumby says that he will take his lunch break now so that he can scrub for the next case, leaving the circulating nurse, RN Cohen, and instrument nurse, EN Noakes, to check the instrument tray lists. During the tray list checks, RN Cohen has been asked by Dr De Silva, the anaesthetic registrar, to help move the bed back into the room; however, the tray lists are incomplete and some of the loan trays still need to be checked.

Critical Thinking Questions
• How would RN Cohen, as the circulating nurse, manage these competing priorities? • What are the risks for Mr Collins if the tray lists are not completed accurately?

WHO Surgical Safety Checklist

WHO introduced the Safe Surgery Saves Lives initiative in 2008, promoting the use of the Surgical Safety Checklist (SCC) (WHO, 2008). Auckland City Hospital was one of the eight pilot sites involved in the initial participation of this WHO initiative (Weiser & Haynes, 2018). Improving patient safety in the perioperative environment by the use of checklists has the added benefits of improving teamwork and communication (WHO, 2019). Once a patient has entered the OR, the SSC identifies three occasions when clinicians are required to pause and check that specific activities have occurred. These are:

- the period before induction of anaesthesia ('Sign In')
- the period after induction and before surgical incision ('Time Out')
- the period during or immediately after wound closure, before the patient leaves the OR ('Sign Out') (WHO, 2008, p. 6).

The RACS adopted the SSC in early 2009, following consultation with the ANZCA, the Royal Australian and New Zealand College of Obstetricians and Gynaecologists (RANZCOG), ACORN and the Commission (Gough, 2010). The Australian and New Zealand edition of the SSC was developed and endorsed in late 2009 by health ministers in both countries, and its use is now standard perioperative practice (Gough, 2010) (see Chapter 9, Fig 9.1 for an image of the WHO Surgical Safety Checklist). An international systematic review and meta-analysis into the use of the SSC found that patients in hospitals where the SSC is implemented have overall better postoperative outcomes than those in hospitals that do not (Abbott et al., 2018). Complementing these findings, an Australian prospective longitudinal study by Gillespie and colleagues (2018) highlighted that team communication and overall team culture, which both have an impact on patient safety, improved following the implementation of a structured program to increase compliance with conducting the SSC.

Checklists are used in the PACU to assess a patient's readiness for discharge back to the ward, or in day-surgery cases to a stage two (step-down) recovery unit prior to discharge home (ACORN, 2020a; ANZCA, 2020). The concept of a postanaesthesia discharge scoring system was first introduced as the Aldrete Score by Aldrete and Kroulik in 1970. Such checklists enable the PACU nurse to use clinical judgement in combination with the objective scoring of physiological parameters to determine patient readiness for discharge (Street, Phillips, Mohebbi, & Kent, 2017). The use of criterion-based discharge tools helps avoid the potentially dangerous case of discharging postoperative patients prematurely (Street et al., 2017).

Management of Accountable Items

Another paramount checklist in the perioperative environment is the document used to ensure that all surgical items are accounted for on completion of a surgical intervention. The instruments, sponges, swabs and consumable items used during surgery are at risk of being retained in patients' body cavities and/or wounds. Therefore, an integral aspect of patient safety in the perioperative settings is the performance of the **surgical count**. The presence of all items on the surgical field and their use within the patient require the careful attention of all team members and the use of a risk management tool. Conducting a count of all surgical items before the commencement of surgery, on closure of a body cavity, on commencement of skin closure and on surgery completion, and then documenting the outcomes, enables the perioperative nurse to account for and manage this risk (ACORN, 2020b; Association of periOperative Registered Nurses [AORN], 2016). Despite this activity, the inadvertent retention of surgical items still occurs. (See Chapter 9 for further information on the conduct of the surgical count.)

As discussed in the previous Scenario, standardised checklists for the inventory of surgical instrument trays facilitate perioperative nurses in counting, checking and documenting instruments used in surgical procedures (ACORN, 2020b; AORN, 2016). Instruments, and in some cases their components (e.g. screws, pins, bolts), must be accounted for before a procedure commences and at the completion of the surgery. Feature box 4.4 describes the case of an item retained in a patient having surgery in an Australian Hospital. Sterilisation staff also account for

FEATURE BOX 4.4
Retained Surgical Item

A patient was admitted for an elective cardiothoracic procedure. At the end of the procedure, the surgical count was noted to be correct. However, a routine post-operative X-ray detected a nut from the valve replacement deployment device in the patient's pericardium. These items are not routinely counted as individual components. The patient returned to theatre to have the nut removed.

An investigation cited contributing factors to be that the device was disassembled during the procedure, but was counted as one whole item on the count sheet (as opposed to the number of its parts). The Victorian Surgical Consultative Council (VSCC) recommends that all detachable components of a device/instrument/retractor should be included in the surgical count.

(Source: Victorian Surgical Consultative Council. Retained materials in surgery. Information bulletin, January 2019.)

instruments when they are received into the sterilising department. This multi-tier checking system mitigates the risk of instruments or parts thereof being inadvertently retained in a patient, or discarded accidentally.

MEDICATION MANAGEMENT

Medications pose a risk to patients, and **medication management** (the safe handling and administration of pharmacological preparations) is both regulated and widely researched in healthcare (ACSQHC/the Commission, 2017a; ANZCA, 2019; Johnson et al., 2017). Table 4.2 identifies relevant regulations in Australia and New Zealand.

Complications from medication errors are reportable incidents. In 2017–18, *medication complications* accounted for 0.2% of all reported hospital-acquired complications in Australian hospitals (AIHW, 2019). Errors in medication administration can occur at any point in the process, from ordering to transcribing, dispensing, administering and monitoring, and they

TABLE 4.2
Relevant Legislation and Regulations in Relation to Perioperative Medication Safety

Area	Relevant Legislation and Regulations in Relation to Perioperative Medication Safety
NZ	Medicines Act 1981 https://www.legislation.govt.nz/act/public/1981/0118/69.0/DLM53790.html
ACT	Medicines, Poisons and Therapeutic Goods Act 2008
NSW	Poisons and Therapeutic Drugs Act 1966 and Poisons and Therapeutic Goods Regulations 2008
NT	Medicines, Poisons and Therapeutic Goods Act 2012 (Mo. 13 of 2012) https://www.austlii.edu.au/au/legis/nt/num_act/mpatga201213o2012425
Qld	Queensland Health Act 1937 https://www.austlii.edu.au/au/legis/qld/consol_act/ha193769 and Health (Drugs and Poisons) Regulation 1996
SA	Controlled Substances Act 1984 https://www.austlii.edu.au/au/legis/sa/consol_act/csa1984242 Controlled Substances (Poisons) Regulation 2011 https://www.corrigan.austlii.edu/au/au/legis/sa/num_reg/csr2011140o2011497/index.html#s4
Tas	Poisons Act 1971 https://www.legislation.tas.gov.au/view/html/inforce/current/act-1971-081
Vic	Drugs, Poisons and Controlled Substances Act 2006 https://www.austlii.edu.au/au/legis/vic/consol_act/dpacsa1981422/
WA	Poisons Act 2014 https://www.legislation.wa.gov.au/legislation/statutes.nsf/main_mrtitle_13172_homepage.html Poisons Regulations 1965 https://www.legislation.wa.gov.au/legislation/statutes.nsf/main_mrtitle_1920_homepage.html

(Sources: Adapted from Australian College of Perioperative Nurses. (2020c). *ACORN Standards for perioperative nursing in Australia.* (16th ed., Vol. 1). Clinical standards. Adelaide: Author; Ministry of Health, New Zealand. (1981). New Zealand Medicines Act, 1981. http://www.legislation.govt.nz/act/public/1981/0118/69.0/whole.html#DLM53790.)

are largely preventable (Li, 2018; Wahr et al., 2017). This is particularly evident in the perioperative setting where medications are uniquely managed (Burlingame, 2018). Understanding the specific risks to surgical patients will help perioperative nurses to recognise threats to patient safety and employ strategies to mitigate such adverse medication events (Le, 2017).

Medication errors can occur at any point in a patient's perioperative journey. Preoperatively, oral medications may be inadvertently withheld by a fasting patient. Alternatively, medications that should have been withheld, such as anticoagulants, may instead be administered to the preoperative patient, resulting in an increased risk of intraoperative bleeding (Queensland Department of Health, 2016). Drugs of dependence including opioids, narcotics and sedatives are routinely administered to patients in the perioperative setting. State and national legislation describes the controlled access to these medications, and perioperative nurses should always ensure that medication dispensing and administration practices are within relevant medication legislation (ACORN, 2020c) (see Table 4.2). Due to the flow of activities in the perioperative environment, particularly during anaesthetic and surgical procedures, the circulating, instrument or anaesthetic nurse may be required to prepare medications for subsequent administration by a medical officer. NSW Health (2018) notes that this practice poses considerable risk – for example:

- The anaesthetic nurse may be required to obtain a medication from a locked drug cupboard, per anaesthetist preference, prior to the patient arriving in the anaesthetic bay or OR, resulting in documentation errors or potential loss.
- The circulating nurse may supply an incorrect medication onto the aseptic field.
- The instrument nurse may prepare an incorrect dose/concentration for the surgeon.
- The instrument nurse may fail to label the medication correctly, resulting in an error.

The perioperative environment and other procedural areas (e.g. endoscopy suites) are considered closed-practice environments, where patients are treated in isolated areas. As such, each patient's identity is definitively established when entering the area (ACSQHC/the Commission, 2015). From this closed environment, patients eventually transition into open-practice environments (e.g. the PACU). Differences in clinical care areas and their patient flows dictate specific medication/fluid labelling and patient identification requirements. Fig. 4.5 shows the different labelling requirements for open- and closed-practice environments.

While recommendations exist within Australia and New Zealand, there are no national policies for the preparation of medications in the perioperative setting. However, new procedures in some states such as New South Wales provide a safety framework for the perioperative setting (NSW Health, 2018). Professional organisations such as ACORN (2020c) and AORN (Burlingame, 2018) have developed best-practice standards that also guide perioperative nurses in this regard.

Labelling of Injectable Medicines, Fluids and Lines

In 2010, the Commission produced the *National recommendations for user-applied labelling of injectable medicines, fluids and lines*. The document, revised in 2012 and further reviewed and updated in 2015, outlines the minimum requirements for the safe handling, identification and administration of injectable medicines both on and around the aseptic field (ACSQHC/the Commission, 2015). Most recent updates include specific guidance for labelling of locked catheters, liquid medicines for oral, enteral and inhalational routes, labelling of non-injectable medicines and fluids that are prepared in the same area as injectable medicines (e.g. surgical preparation solutions) (Government of South Australia, SA Health, 2019).

The Commission's national labelling recommendations also reflect AORN's *Recommended practices for medication safety* (Burlingame, 2018) and continue to provide guidance to perioperative nurses in New Zealand. On the aseptic field, perioperative nurses must be able to identify medicines and fluids within containers and syringes, as medication mix-ups resulting in the administration of the wrong drugs have been reported, resulting in critical outcomes (ANZCA, 2020). A short film by Doncaster and Bassetlaw Hospitals NHS Foundation Trust (2014), 'The human factor: learning from Gina's story', discusses the tragic story of a how a simple human and procedural mistake involving medication errors caused a terrible incident in February 2013 (see Resources at the end of this chapter).

Preprinted sterile medication labels provide a standardised methodology for identifying medications on the aseptic field. The Commission notes several requirements for the safe usage of sterile medication labels:

- Labels should be pre-printed with the name of the medicine or fluid.
- Sheets of pre-printed routinely used medication and fluid labels are preferred over blank labels that require notation by the instrument nurse.
- On the pre-printed sheet, labels for injectable medications and non-injectable fluids (such as hydrogen peroxide) should be kept separate, and the non-injectables' labels should have a red watermark of the St Andrew's Cross.

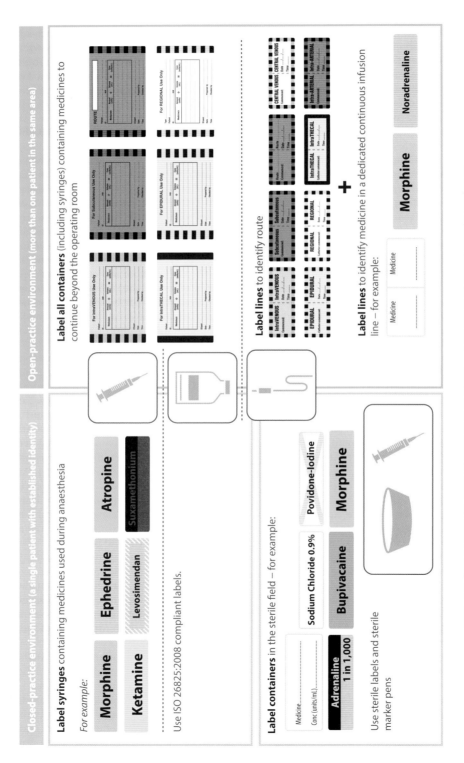

FIG. 4.5 Perioperative labelling of medicines and fluids – comparison of closed-practice and open-practice labels. (Source: Australian Commission on Safety and Quality in Health Care. (2015). *National standard for user-applied labelling of injectable medicines, fluids and lines* (p. 26, Figure 2). Sydney: Author.)

- Sterile blank labels and a sterile marking pen should be included in all pre-printed label packs, or available separately, to allow the instrument nurse to write on abbreviated container labels (when pre-printed labels are not available).
- Labels should be able to be removed from reusable containers without leaving a residue.

- Labels must be durable when wet so they do not peel off throughout the surgical procedure.
- Colour coding must comply with ISO 26825: 2008 User-applied labels for syringes containing drugs used during anaesthesia (ACSQHC/the Commission, 2015).

Fig. 4.6 provides an example of pre-printed sterile medication labels and sterile abbreviated container

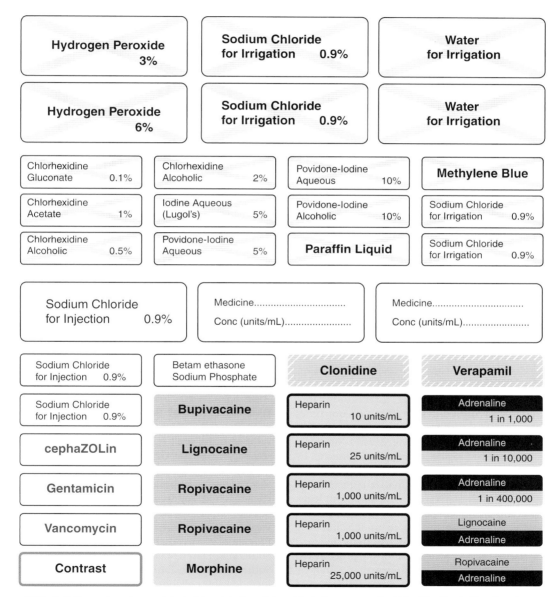

FIG. 4.6 Examples of pre-printed abbreviated container labels for user-applied identification in the closed-practice environment. (Source: Australian Commission on Safety and Quality in Health Care. (2015). *National standard for user-applied labelling of injectable medicines, fluids and lines* (p. 27). Sydney: Author.)

labels that may be used on the aseptic field (ACSQHC/the Commission, 2015). Despite systems such as medication labelling and double-checking protocols, medication errors still occur (Wahr et al., 2017). Precautions should be taken to decrease the risk of errors, particularly during transitions in patient care. Perioperative nurses must be cognisant of this fact, whether they are caring for patients in closed-practice environments such as the OR, procedure room, catheter laboratory or endoscopy suite, or in open-practice environments such as the PACU or postoperative ward (ACSQHC/the Commission, 2015).

PATIENT SCENARIOS

SCENARIO 4.5: MEDICATION MANAGEMENT

RN Rob Cohen has 'scrubbed-in' to take over the instrument nurse role for a patient undergoing a complex lower limb reconstruction involving a free flap. RN Cohen is relieving EN Noakes while she has a lunch break. The procedure is at the mid-way point when RN Cohen 'scrubs-in'. The instrumentation set-up has multiple receivers (i.e. gallipots) and syringes containing a variety of fluids, which EN Noakes has verbally handed over to RN Cohen as local anaesthetic, heparinised saline and adrenaline solutions. None of the containers or syringes is labelled.

Critical Thinking Questions

- Describe the potential adverse events that might occur in this circumstance.
- How could RN Cohen safely identify the medications on the set-up? Provide rationales to explain why you believe these actions are important.

CLINICAL AUDIT

Clinical audits have a long-established history in healthcare, with early clinicians such as Nightingale and Codman monitoring mortality and morbidity by means of epidemiological or patient record review (Travaglia & Debono, 2009). Today, clinical auditing is a component of a quality and safety framework and is vital to ensure health systems and practices are safe. Fig. 4.1 illustrates how clinical auditing is a central component of clinical governance. Audits are cyclical processes that involve a systematic gathering of information by observation or data analysis. The information is used to review performance, assess compliance with standards or procedures, or compare outcomes against previous results or benchmarked standards (Pozo-Rodríguez, Castro-Acosta, & Álvarez-Martínez, 2015). Perioperative nursing is shaped and directed by many standards, policies and clinical procedures and it is important to understand whether clinicians are complying with these standards, procedures and legislative requirements. It is equally important for patient safety and practice improvement to understand why clinicians fail to comply with these requirements.

Perioperative nurses engage in auditing processes in a wide variety of ways. These auditing activities may be part of a clinical portfolio that a nurse holds (e.g. a perioperative infection control portfolio), or they may be completed as part of the regular practice audits required of hospital departments, such as hand hygiene compliance or review of medication documentation.

Research box 4.1 describes a series of clinical audits to assess staff compliance with best practice.

For audits to be meaningful, they must be relevant to clinical practice, patient and staff safety, or guide the improvement of patient outcomes (ACSQHC/the Commission, 2017b). Audits should seek to ensure that practice is in line with relevant standards, policies, procedures, guidelines or recommendations. To this end, clinical audit tools can be developed by clinicians within perioperative services based on these resources; alternatively, clinical audit tools can be adopted from those already created and validated by external organisations.

ACORN Practice Audit Tools (PATs)

ACORN's suite of **Practice Audit Tools (PATs)** was developed to be used by perioperative services, enabling standardisation and benchmarking across organisations. The ACORN Audit Project had its foundations in a practice improvement project that began in 2015 across 14 Pacific Island countries (PICs) and was facilitated by Strengthening of Specialised Clinical Services in the Pacific (SSCSiP), one of the Regional Clinical Services Programs of the Pacific Community in Fiji (Davies, Sutherland-Fraser, Mamea, Raddie, & Taoi, 2017; Davies, Sutherland-Fraser, Taoi, & Williams, 2016). The project included the collaboration of Australian perioperative nurse consultants. The project successfully developed and implemented a small bundle of standards on infection prevention practices for Pacific perioperative settings, along with a small set of observational tools

---

RESEARCH BOX 4.1
Auditing Clinical Practice
Ensuring High Reliability at an Australian Hospital

This article outlines the development of a series of clinical audits in the perioperative setting of a tertiary hospital in Brisbane. The audits, which aligned to the National Standards, collected evidence of staff compliance with best practice and gave insights into strategies used to minimise risks to patient safety. The audits were aimed at four key areas of perioperative practice:

- *Surgical Safety Checklist:* the observational audit tool captured information that previous audits had missed, including the name of the person initiating the 'Time Out', which helped to identify occasions when key staff did not participate in the conduct of the checklist.
- *Intraoperative medication labelling:* real-time observational audits were conducted of staff compliance with pre-populated sterile labels.
- *Surgical aseptic technique:* nurses' practice and techniques were observed for compliance with standards

on gowning, gloving, and establishing and maintaining surgical aseptic practices. Facilitators suspended the audit to address breaches in practice when required.

- *Clinical handover from the OR to the PACU:* each month, facilitators conduct 20 audits of the information and efficacy of clinical handover between OR and PACU nurses.

The article describes the aims of each clinical audit as well as the methodology for data collection. The article discusses the insights gained from each audit and describes how the results were used to improve clinical practice. Of importance, the article notes that the audits were used as tools to create positive change in the perioperative setting, rather than as a punitive measure, thus empowering staff to engage in quality improvement activities.

(Source: Steel, C. (2015). Auditing clinical practice: ensuring high reliability at an Australian hospital. *AORN Journal, 102*, 81–84.)

for the PICs to audit perioperative nurses' practice and measure baseline compliance with the new standards. Following the success of the project in the Pacific, and in recognition of the potential benefits for the Australian perioperative nursing community, ACORN embarked on a similar project with Australian perioperative nurse consultants to develop practice audit tools for use within Australian practice settings (Sutherland-Fraser & Davies, 2018). The ACORN PATs are customised spreadsheets to record evidence of clinical practice during real-time observational audits of perioperative nurses. The PATs are divided into two bundles covering asepsis and clinical care, and staff and patient safety.

Table 4.3 outlines the ACORN Practice Audit Tools, and Feature box 4.5 describes one user's experience of the ACORN Practice Audit Tools in a large tertiary hospital.

An important component of audit programs is the audit reports, which detail their purpose and scope, and discuss the outcomes and findings. Audit reports also contain action plans that detail specific tasks to be completed based on audit findings. Perioperative nurses are often engaged in the implementation phase of the clinical audit cycle, by enacting recommendations, strategies or activities to improve practice.

Plan-Do-Study-Act (PDSA) Cycle

A commonly used tool in clinical auditing and the implementation of the resultant actions is the **Plan-Do-Study-Act (PDSA) cycle** (Christoff, 2018). This four-step cyclical

TABLE 4.3 ACORN Practice Audit Tools

Practice Audit Tools 1: Asepsis and Clinical Care	Practice Audit Tools 2: Staff and Patient Safety
Perioperative attire Asepsis and infection prevention Surgical hand antisepsis, gowning and gloving Preoperative patient skin antisepsis Specimen identification, collection and handling	Documentation Surgical safety Medication safety Management of sharps in the preoperative environment Safe patient positioning in the perioperative environment and safe manual handling Management of accountable items used during surgery and procedures Surgical plume and electrosurgical equipment

(Source: Australian College of Perioperative Nurses (ACORN) (2018d) PATS.)

model facilitates breaking an improvement plan down into its component steps, each worked through in turn. The first step is the development of the 'plan', where the need for change is identified, goals are stated and tasks are outlined and delegated (Christoff, 2018). In the next 'do' phase, the plan, or a component of the plan, is implemented; it is directly followed by the collection and analysis of data in

---

FEATURE BOX 4.5
ACORN PATs User Experience

Using the ACORN PATs has significantly enhanced our processes for quality improvement. Prior to the ACORN PATs we wrote our own audits, which was time consuming and, depending on the writer, had the potential to provide flawed data, as not all staff have the skills to write clear, unambiguous and jargon-free questions that provide a measurable answer.

Having staff pre-read the ACORN Standard prior to undertaking the audit ensures that the audit means one thing to everyone; namely, auditors are all on the same page. Ensuring that Standards are read prior to auditing also improves the knowledge of staff. Surprisingly, most staff comment that they know the Standards; however, after they undertake the pre-reading, many staff make comments about something they didn't know.

The ACORN PATs have expanded our thinking into the responsibilities of the organisation in regard to quality improvement. Prior to the PATs we only looked at what happened inside the theatre; now we are more critical and aware of organisational responsibilities and processes that impact on patient outcomes from outside the service too. Results are presented to staff with an action plan to manage compliance and improvement. Each audit cycle sets the bar higher for improvement, with regional benchmarking between other local health networks to commence soon.

Our service is now always 'accreditation ready' as we can easily demonstrate that we are complying with recognised practice standards and are continuously improving patient care and outcomes within a clear framework. The ACORN PATs are the cornerstone of our clinical governance program and are recognised by our clinicians and management as a systematic, critical and objective examination of our practice.

(Source: J. Booth, Personal Communication, 23 May 2019.)

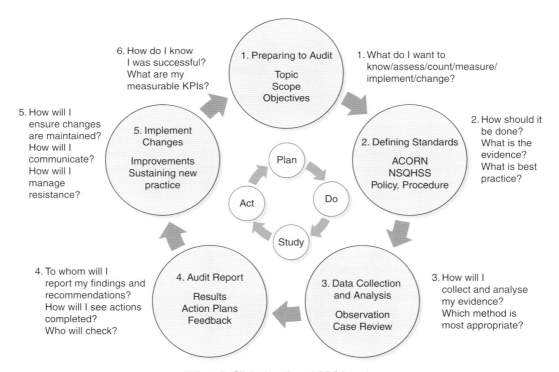

FIG. 4.7 Clinical audit and PDSA cycle.

the 'study' phase. This step provides an opportunity to determine what has worked, and what might need to be changed. The final step is 'act', where either the plan is adopted or the changes to the plan are implemented, leading into another PDSA cycle (Christoff, 2018).

Perioperative nurses may choose to engage in informal audit processes by means of self-evaluation or practice reflection by asking questions such as: 'Did I complete that procedure correctly?', 'What went well/wrong?' or 'How can I improve?' Fig. 4.7 details the clinical audit cycle.

PATIENT SCENARIOS

SCENARIO 4.6: CLINICAL AUDITS

RN Jenny Sang has been assigned to investigate whether nurses in the operating suite are performing adequate hand hygiene before and after patient contact in the PACU in an effort to improve compliance and patient outcomes. RN Sang decides to conduct a practice audit.

Critical Thinking Questions

- Describe the objectives of an audit in relation to the 5 Moments of Hand Hygiene and identify at least two other standards that might inform this practice audit.

- Describe how you would conduct an audit on hand hygiene in your own workplace. Provide rationales to explain why you believe your collection methods are necessary.

- How would you report your findings and recommendations to your manager?

- If changes were implemented as a result of your audit, how would you know whether they were sustained into the future?

CONCLUSION

Patients admitted to hospital should feel safe and not have concerns that something may go wrong while they are receiving treatment. The evidence, however, demonstrates that patients do experience adverse events, many of which are preventable. This chapter has explored the concepts of clinical governance and national safety and quality frameworks for healthcare workers, as well as the strategies commonly used to prevent adverse events and ensure perioperative patients are provided with the safest possible care.

At a time of intense public scrutiny and professional interest in safety and quality in healthcare, ways to ensure patient safety in the high-risk setting of the operating suite remain paramount. Indeed, this chapter has shown that perioperative patient safety is of concern globally, with particular attention focused on reducing sentinel events such as wrong site surgery and retained surgical items. The ongoing implementation of the National Standards, Clinical Care Standards and ACORN Practice Audit Tools as part of a wider clinical governance framework is crucial to ensure positive patient outcomes. Patient safety is the ultimate aim of every healthcare professional and will continue to be a primary focus of perioperative practice into the future.

RESOURCES

Australasian College for Infection Prevention and Control Ltd (ACIPC)
https://www.acipc.org.au
Australian College of Perianaesthesia Nurses
https://acpan.edu.au/
Australian College of Perioperative Nurses
https://www.acorn.org.au/
Australian Commission on Safety and Quality in Health Care (ACSQHC/the Commission)
www.safetyandquality.gov.au
Australian Day Surgery Nurses Association (ADSNA)
https://adsna.info
Australian Institute of Health and Welfare (AIHW)
https://www.aihw.gov.au/search?%7B%22SearchText%22:%22online%20reports%22%7D
Gastroenterological Nurses College of Australia (GENCA)
https://www.genca.org
Health Quality and Safety Commission New Zealand (HQSCNZ)
https://www.hqsc.govt.nz
Hoyt, D. B., & Ko, C. Y. (Eds.). 2017. *Optimal resources for surgical quality and safety.* Chicago: American College of Surgeons.
Implementation toolkit for clinical handover improvement
https://www.safetyandquality.gov.au/implementation-toolkit-resource-portal
Labelling recommendations
https://www.safetyandquality.gov.au/sites/default/files/migrated/National-Standard-for-User-Applied-Labelling-Aug-2015.pdf
On the radar
https://www.safetyandquality.gov.au/publications-resources/on-the-radar
Resources for the NSQHS Standards
https://www.safetyandquality.gov.au/standards/national-safety-and-quality-health-service-nsqhs-standards/resources-nsqhs-standards

Incident Management and Reporting Systems

New Zealand
https://www.hqsc.govt.nz/our-programmes/reportable-events
NSW Health
https://www.cec.health.nsw.gov.au/Review-incidents/incident-management
WA Health
https://ww2.health.wa.gov.au/Articles/A_E/Clinical-incident-management-system
Malignant Hyperthermia Resource Kit, Malignant Hyperthermia Australia & New Zealand
https://malignanthyperthermia.org.au/resource-kit/

Patient Safety Reports and Sentinel Event Reporting

New Zealand
https://www.hqsc.govt.nz/our-programmes/adverse-events/news-and-events/news/3888/
Perioperative Nurses College – New Zealand Nurses Organisation
https://www.nzno.org.nz

South Australia
https://www.sahealth.sa.gov.au/wps/wcm/connect/72093780
    46aaedec99a4fb2e504170d4/1_Patient%2BSafety%2B
    Report%2528v4%2529LR.pdf?MOD=AJPERES&CACHE=
    NONE&CONTENTCACHE=NONE
Victoria
https://www.bettersafercare.vic.gov.au/notify-us/sentinel-
    events
Western Australia
https://ww2.health.wa.gov.au/Articles/S_T/Sentinel-events

Safe Surgery
ACSQHC/the Commission
https://www.safetyandquality.gov.au/our-work/patient-
    identification/patient-procedure-matching-protocols/
    surgical-safety-checklist
Reducing Perioperative Harm (HQSCNZ)
https://www.hqsc.govt.nz/our-programmes/reducing-
    perioperative-harm
The Human Factor: Learning from Gina's Story
https://www.youtube.com/watch?v=IJfoLvLLoFo&app=
    desktop
World Health Organization (WHO) Safe Surgery
https://www.who.int/patientsafety/safesurgery/en/

REFERENCES

Abbott, T. E. F., Ahmad, T., Phull, M. K., Fowler, A. J., Hewson, R., Biccard, B. M., . . . International Surgical Outcomes Study (ISOS) group. (2018). The surgical safety checklist and patient outcomes after surgery: a prospective observational cohort study, systematic review and meta-analysis. *British Journal of Anaesthesia, 120*(1), 146–155. https://dx.doi.org/10.1016/j.bja.2017.08.002

Agency for Clinical Innovation (ACI). (2019). National Surgical Quality Improvement Program (NSQIP). Retrieved from <https://www.aci.health.nsw.gov.au/__data/assets/pdf_file/0006/445740/NSQIP-one-pager_v1.0.pdf>.

Aldrete, J. A., & Kroulik, D. (1970). A postanesthetic recovery score. *Anesthesia and Analgesia, 49*(6), 924–934.

American College of Surgeons. (2019). ACS National Surgical Quality Improvement Program. Retrieved from <https://www.facs.org/quality-programs/acs-nsqip>.

Association of periOperative Registered Nurses (AORN). (2016). Guidance at a glance: retained surgical items. *AORN Journal, 104*(5), 474–477.

Australasian College for Infection Prevention and Control (ACIPC). (2016). *Single-use devices* [Position statement]. Brisbane: Author. Retrieved from <http://www.acipc.org.au/wp-content/uploads/2017/06/Single-Use-Items.pdf>.

Australasian College for Infection Prevention and Control (ACIPC). (2017). *The role of the infection control practitioner in antimicrobial stewardship* [Position statement]. Brisbane: Author. Retrieved from <http://www.acipc.org.au/wp-content/uploads/2017/07/20170622_ACIPC_Position_Statement-_AMS_-Final.pdf>.

Australian and New Zealand College of Anaesthetists (ANZCA). (2012). *PS58 Guidelines on quality assurance and quality improvement in anaesthesia*. Melbourne: Author. Retrieved from <https://www.anzca.edu.au/resources/professional-documents/guidelines/ps58-guidelines-on-quality-assurance-and-quality-i>.

Australian and New Zealand College of Anaesthetists (ANZCA). (2013). *PS53 Background paper: statement on the handover responsibilities of the anaesthetist*. Melbourne: Author. Retrieved from <https://www.anzca.edu.au/getattachment/74eae67f-3d96-4a81-a737-5b2cc9c1b261/PS53-Statement-on-the-handover-responsibilities-of-the-anaesthetist>.

Australian and New Zealand College of Anaesthetists (ANZCA). (2015). *PS59 Statement on roles in anaesthesia and perioperative care*. Melbourne: Author. Retrieved from <https://www.anzca.edu.au/getattachment/59e8e8b0-0c6b-4ef7-9908-fa42d5f5110a/PS59BP-Statement-on-roles-in-anaesthesia-and-perioperative-care-Background-Paper>.

Australian and New Zealand College of Anaesthetists (ANZCA). (2018). *PS58 Guidelines on quality assurance and quality improvement in anaesthesia*. Melbourne: Author. Retrieved from <https://www.anzca.edu.au/8d0de69a-661c-4b92-9deb-20b9709caa0f>.

Australian and New Zealand College of Anesthetists (ANZCA). (2019). Guidelines and standards. Retrieved from <https://www.anzca.edu.au/safety-advocacy/standards-of-practice/policies,-statements,-and-guidelines>.

Australian and New Zealand College of Anaesthetists (ANZCA). (2020). *PS04 Statement on the post-anaesthesia care unit*. Melbourne: Author. Retrieved from <https://www.anzca.edu.au/getattachment/7045495a-0f12-4464-852c-b93c0453e1ed/PS04-Statement-on-the-post-anaesthesia-care-unit>.

Australian College of Perioperative Nurses (ACORN). (2020a). *ACORN standards for perioperative nursing in Australia* (16th ed., Vol. 1). Professional standards – post anaesthesia care unit nurse. Adelaide: Author.

Australian College of Perioperative Nurses (ACORN). (2020b). *ACORN standards for perioperative nursing in Australia* (16th ed., Vol. 1). Clinical standards – accountable items. Adelaide: Author.

Australian College of Perioperative Nurses (ACORN). (2020c). *ACORN standards for perioperative nursing. nursing in Australia* (16th ed., Vol. 1). Clinical standards – medication safety. Adelaide: Author.

Australian College of Perioperative Nurses (ACORN). (2020d). PATS. Retrieved from <https://www.acorn.org.au/index.cfm?display5786019>.

Australian Commission on Safety and Quality in Health Care (ACSQHC/the Commission). (2009a). Developing a safety and quality framework for Australia. Retrieved from <https://www.safetyandquality.gov.au/wp-content/uploads/2009/01/Developing-a-Safety-and-Quality-Framework-for-Australia.pdf>.

Australian Commission on Safety and Quality in Health Care (ACSQHC/the Commission). (2009b). Windows into safety and quality in health care, 2009. Retrieved from <https://www.safetyandquality.gov.au/sites/default/files/migrated/windows-2009-web-version.pdf>.

Australian Commission on Safety and Quality in Health Care (ACSQHC/the Commission). (2010). Australian safety and quality framework for health care. Retrieved from <https://www.safetyandquality.gov.au/sites/default/files/migrated/ASQFHC-Guide-Policymakers.pdf>.

Australian Commission on Safety and Quality in Health Care (ACSQHC/the Commission). (2011a). Windows into safety and quality in health care, 2011. Retrieved from <https://www.safetyandquality.gov.au/publications/windows-into-safety-and-quality-in-health-care-2011>.

Australian Commission on Safety and Quality in Health Care (ACSQHC/the Commission). (2011b). *National safety and quality health service standards*. Sydney: Author.

Australian Commission on Safety and Quality in Health Care (ACSQHC/the Commission). (2013a). Australian Open Disclosure Framework – better communication, a better way to care. Retrieved from <https://www.safetyandquality.gov.au/publications/australian-open-disclosure-framework>.

Australian Commission on Safety and Quality in Health Care (ACSQHC/the Commission). (2013b). Clinical Care Standards. Retrieved from <https://www.safetyandquality.gov.au/our-work/clinical-care-standards>.

Australian Commission on Safety and Quality in Health Care (ACSQHC/the Commission). (2014a). Report on healthcare associated *Staphylococcus aureus* bacteraemia workshop. Retrieved from <https://www.safetyandquality.gov.au/sites/default/files/migrated/SAB-background.pdf>.

Australian Commission on Safety and Quality in Health Care (ACSQHC/the Commission) (2014b). *Acute coronary syndromes clinical care standard*. Sydney: Author.

Australian Commission on Safety and Quality in Health Care (ACSQHC/the Commission). (2015). *National standard for user-applied labelling of injectable medicines, fluids and lines*. Sydney: Author. Retrieved from <https://www.safetyandquality.gov.au/wp-content/uploads/2015/10/Perioperative-labelling-of-medicines-and-fluids-poster-December-2016.pdf>.

Australian Commission on Safety and Quality in Health Care. (ACSQHC/the Commission). (2016). *Hip fracture care clinical care standard*. Sydney: Author.

Australian Commission on Safety and Quality in Health Care (ACSQHC/the Commission). (2017a). *National safety and quality health service standards* (2nd ed.). Sydney: Author.

Australian Commission on Safety and Quality in Health Care (ACSQHC/the Commission). (2017b). *National Model Clinical Governance Framework*. Sydney: Author. Retrieved from: <https://www.safetyandquality.gov.au/sites/default/files/migrated/National-Model-Clinical-Governance-Framework.pdf>.

Australian Commission on Safety and Quality in Health Care (ACSQHC/the Commission). (2017c). *Vital signs 2017: the state of safety and quality in Australian health care*. Sydney: Author.

Australian Commission on Safety and Quality in Health Care (ACSQHC/the Commission), Australian Institute of Health and Welfare (AIHW). (2018). *The third Australian atlas of healthcare variation*. Sydney: Author.

Australia Commission on Safety and Quality in Health Care (ACSQHC/the Commission). (2018a). Australian sentinel events list (version 2). Retrieved from <https://www.safetyandquality.gov.au/our-work/indicators/australian-sentinel-events-list>.

Australian Commission on Safety and Quality in Health Care (ACSQHC/the Commission). (2018b). Hospital-acquired complications (HACs). Retrieved from <https://safetyandquality.govcms.gov.au/our-work/indicators/hospital-acquired-complications>.

Australian Commission on Safety and Quality in Health Care (ACSQHC/the Commission). (2018c). Creating safer, better health care – the impact of the national safety and quality health service standards. Sydney: Author.

Australian Commission on Safety and Quality in Health Care (ACSQHC/the Commission). (2018d). *Venous thromboembolism prevention clinical care standard*. Sydney: Author.

Australian Commission on Safety and Quality in Health Care (ACSQHC/the Commission). (2018e). *Colonoscopy clinical care standard*. Sydney: Author.

Australian Commission on Safety and Quality in Health Care (ACSQHC/the Commission). (2019a). *The state of patient safety and quality in Australian hospitals 2019*. Sydney: Author.

Australia Commission on Safety and Quality in Health Care (ACSQHC/the Commission). (2019b). Australian Health Service Safety and Quality Accreditation Scheme. Retrieved from <https://www.safetyandquality.gov.au/standards/nsqhs-standards/assessment-nsqhs-standards/australian-health-service-safety-and-quality-accreditation-scheme>.

Australian Commission on Safety and Quality in Health Care (ACSQHC/the Commission). (2019c). Overview of the Clinical Care Standards. Retrieved from <https://www.safetyandquality.gov.au/standards/clinical-care-standards/overview-clinical-care-standards>.

Australian Commission on Safety and Quality in Health Care (ACSQHC/the Commission). (2020). Antimicrobial Stewardship Clinical Care Standard. Retrieved from <https://www.safetyandquality.gov.au/our-work/clinical-care-standards/antimicrobial-stewardship-clinical-care-standard>.

Australian Commission on Safety and Quality in Health Care (ACSQHC/the Commission). (2021). *National safety and quality health service standards*. (2nd ed.). Sydney: Author.

Australian Council on Healthcare Standards (ACHS). (2015). Overview of accreditation programs and services. Retrieved from <https://www.achs.org.au/programs-services/overview>.

Australian Council on Healthcare Standards (ACHS). (2018). EQuIP6 information pack. Retrieved from <https://www.achs.org.au/media/114456/equip6_information_pack_final.pdf>.

Australian Institute of Health and Welfare (AIHW). (2018). *Australia's health 2018*. Australia's health series no. 16. Canberra: Author.

Australian Institute of Health and Welfare (AIHW). (2019). *Admitted patient care 2017–18: Australian hospital statistics*. Health services series no. 90. Cat. no. HSE 225. Canberra: Author.

Australian Red Cross Life Blood. (2019). Factors contributing to transfusion-related adverse events [webpage]. Retrieved from <https://transfusion.com.au/adverse_events/risks>.

Berger, E. R., Greenberg, C. C, & Bilimoria, K. Y. (2015). Challenges in reducing surgical 'never events'. *Journal of the American Medical Association*, *314*(13), 1386–1387.

Burlingame, B. L. (2018). Guideline implementation: medication safety. *AORN Journal*, *107*(4), 477–484.

Burt, J., Campbell, J., Abel, G., Aboulghate, A., Ahmed, F., Asprey, A., … Roland, M. (2017). *Improving patient experience in primary care: a multimethod programme of research on the measurement and improvement of patient experience*. Southampton, UK: NIHR Journals Library. (Programme Grants for Applied Research, No. 5.9.) Retrieved from <https://aornjournal.onlinelibrary.wiley.com/doi/10.1002/aorn.12096>.

Christoff, P. (2018). Running PDSA cycles. *Current Problems in Pediatric and Adolescent Health Care*, *48*(8), 198–201. https://dx.doi.org/10.1016/j.cppeds.2018.08.006

Davies, M., Sutherland-Fraser, S., Mamea, N., Raddie, N., & Taoi, M. H. (2017). Implementing standards in Pacific Island countries: the Pacific perioperative practice bundle (Part 2). *Journal of Perioperative Nursing in Australia*, *30*(1), 41–48.

Davies, M., Sutherland-Fraser, S., Taoi, M. H., & Williams, C. (2016). Developing standards in Pacific Island countries: the Pacific perioperative practice bundle (Part 1). *ACORN Journal*, *29*(2), 42–47.

Doncaster and Bassetlaw Hospitals NHS Foundation Trust. (2014). The human factor: learning from Gina's story [video file]. Retrieved from <https://www.youtube.com/watch?feature=youtu.be&v=IJfoLvLLoFo&app=desktop>.

Gastroenterological Nurses College of Australia (GENCA). (2012). *Educational requirements for personnel reprocessing flexible endoscopic equipment* [position statement]. Beaumaris, Victoria: Author. Retrieved from <https://www.genca.org/public/5/files/PS_Educational_Requirements.pdf>.

Gawande, A. (2010). *The checklist manifesto: how to get things right*. New York: Metropolitan Books.

Gillespie, B. M., Harbeck, E. L., Lavin, J., Hamilton, K., Gardiner, T., Withers, T. K., & Marshall, A. P. (2018). Evaluation of a patient safety programme on Surgical Safety Checklist Compliance: a prospective longitudinal study. *British Medical Journal Open Quality*, *7*(3), e000362. https://dx.doi.org/10.1136/bmjoq-2018-000362

Gjeraa, K., Spanager, L., Konge, L., Petersen, R. H., & Ostergaard, D. (2016). Non-technical skills in minimally invasive surgery teams: a systematic review. *Surgical Endoscopy*, *30*, 5185–5199.

Gough, I. (2010). A surgical safety checklist for Australia and New Zealand. *Australia and New Zealand Journal of Surgery*, *80*, 1–2.

Government of South Australia, SA Health. (2019). Labelling medicines: national labelling recommendations. Retrieved from <https://www.sahealth.sa.gov.au/wps/wcm/connect/Public+Content/SA+Health+Internet/Clinical+Resources/Clinical+Programs+and+Practice+Guidelines/Medicines+and+drugs/Labelling+medicines/>.

Griffin, P., Nembhard, H., Deflitch, C., Bastian, N., Kang, H., & Munoz, D. (Eds.). (2016). Reliability and patient safety. In *Healthcare systems engineering* (pp. 217–244). Hoboken, NJ: John Wiley & Sons.

Health Quality and Safety Commission New Zealand (HQSCNZ). (2014). *Open book: accurate patient identification, December 2014*. Wellington: Author. Retrieved from <https://www.hqsc.govt.nz/assets/Reportable-Events/Publications/Open-book/OB-accurate-patient-identification-Dec-2014.pdf>.

Health Quality and Safety Commission New Zealand (HQSCNZ). (2015). Health Quality and Safety Commission New Zealand [webpage]. Retrieved from <https://www.hqsc.govt.nz>.

Health Quality and Safety Commission New Zealand (HQSCNZ). (2017a). *Clinical governance: guidance for health and disability providers*. Wellington: Author.

Health Quality and Safety Commission New Zealand (HQSCNZ). (2017b). National Adverse Events Reporting Policy 2017. Retrieved from <https://www.hqsc.govt.nz/assets/Reportable-Events/Publications/National_Adverse_Events_Policy_2017/National_Adverse_Events_Policy_2017_WEB_FINAL.pdf>.

Health Quality and Safety Commission New Zealand (HQSCNZ). (2018a). *Learning from adverse events: adverse events reported to the Health Quality & Safety Commission 1 July 2017–30 June 2018*. Wellington: Author.

Health Quality and Safety Commission New Zealand (HQSCNZ). (2018b). A window on the quality of New Zealand's health care. Retrieved from <https://www.hqsc.govt.nz/assets/Health-Quality-Evaluation/Windows_Document/Window-Jun-2018.pdf>.

Johnson, M., Sanchez, P., Langdon, R., Manias, E., Levett-Jones, T., Weidemann, G., Aguilar, V., & Everett, B. (2017). The impact of interruptions on medication errors in hospitals: an observational study of nurses. *Journal of Nursing Management*, *25*, 498–507.

Kapur, N., Parand, A., Soukup, T., Reader, T., & Sevdalis, N. (2015). Aviation and healthcare: a comparative review with implications for patient safety. *Journal of the Royal Society of Medicine Open*, *7*(1), 2054270415616548.

Kumar, J., & Raina, R. (2017). 'Never events in surgery': mere error or an avoidable disaster. *Indian Journal of Surgery*, *79*(3), 238–244. https://dx.doi.org/10.1007/s12262-017-1620-4

Le, L. K.-D. (2017). Evidence summary: medication safety in the perioperative setting. The Joanna Briggs Institute EBP Database, JBI@Ovid, JBI5466.

Li, Y. (2018). Medication errors: contributing factors. The Joanna Briggs Institute EBP Database, JBI@Ovid, JBI1665.

Malignant Hyperthermia Australia and New Zealand (MHANZ). (2019). Malignant hyperthermia resource kit. Retrieved from <http://malignanthyperthermia.org.au/wp-content/uploads/2018/09/MALIGNANT-HYPERTHERMIA-RESOURCE-KIT-2018.pdf>.

Ministry of Health, New Zealand. (1981). New Zealand Medicines Act, 1981 Retrieved from <http://www.legislation.govt.nz/act/public/1981/0118/69.0/whole.html#DLM53790>.

Ministry of Health, New Zealand. (2019). Certification of health care services [webpage]. Retrieved from <https://

www.health.govt.nz/our-work/regulation-health-and-disability-system/certification-health-care-services>.

National Blood Authority Australia (NBA). (n.d.a). Overview and role of the NBA. Retrieved from <https://www.blood.gov.au/about-nba>.

National Blood Authority Australia (NBA). (n.d.b). Education and training. Retrieved from <https://www.blood.gov.au/education-and-training>.

National Blood Authority Australia (NBA). (2019). Patient blood management guidelines. Retrieved from <https://www.blood.gov.au/pbm-guidelines>.

National Pressure Ulcer Advisory Panel, European Pressure Ulcer Advisory Panel and Pan Pacific Pressure Injury Alliance (NPUAP-EPUAP-PPPIA). (2019). In E. Haesler (Ed.), *Prevention and treatment of pressure ulcers: quick reference guide*. Perth: Cambridge Media.

NSW Health. (2018). South Eastern Sydney Local Health District (SESLHD) procedure: medicine. Managing intraoperative medications. SESLHDPR/209. Retrieved from <https://www.seslhd.health.nsw.gov.au/Policies_Procedures_Guidelines/Clinical/Medicine/documents/SESLHDPR209-MedicineManagingIntraoperativeMedications.pdf>.

Powell-Dunford, N., Brennan, P. A., Peerally, M. F., Kapur, N., Hynes, J. M., & Hodkinson, P. D. (2017). Mindful application of aviation practices in healthcare. *Aerospace Medicine and Human Performance, 88*(12), 1107–1116.

Pozo-Rodríguez, F., Castro-Acosta, A. A., & Álvarez-Martínez, C. J. (2015). Clinical audit: why, where and how? *Archivos de Bronconeumología, 51*(10), 479–480.

Queensland Department of Health. (2016). *Guideline for anticoagulation and prophylaxis using low molecular weight heparin (LMWH)*. Version 4. Document Number QH-GDL-951:2015. Retrieved from <https://www.health.qld.gov.au/__data/assets/pdf_file/0023/147533/qh-gdl-951.pdf>.

Reason, J. (2000). Human error; models and management. *British Medical Journal, 320*, 768–770.

Royal Australasian College of Surgeons (RACS). (2013). Indigenous health. Ref. no. FES-FEL-001 [position paper]. Melbourne: Author. Retrieved from <https://www.surgeons.org/policies-publications/publications/position-papers/#b>.

Royal Australasian College of Surgeons (RACS). (2014). *Bullying and harassment: Recognition, avoidance and management* [position paper]. Melbourne: Author.

Royal Australasian College of Surgeons (RACS). (2015). *Outreach surgery in regional, rural and remote areas of Australia and New Zealand, Ref. No. FES-FEL-033* [position paper]. Melbourne: Author. Retrieved from <https://www.surgeons.org/about-racs/position-papers/outreach_surgery_in_regional_rural_and_remote_australia_and_new_zealand_2015>.

Safer Care Victoria. (2017). *Supporting patient safety: sentinel event program triennial report 2013–2016*. Victoria, Australia: Victoria State Government.

Safer Care Victoria. (2018). *Sentinel events annual report, 2016–17*. Victoria, Australia: State of Victoria.

Shuker, C., Bohm, G., Bramley, D., Frost. S., Galler, D., Hamblin, R., … Merry, A. F. (2015). The Health Quality and Safety Commission: making good health care better. *New Zealand Medical Journal, 128*(1408), 98–109.

Standards Australia. (2014). *AS/NZS 4187 Reprocessing of reusable medical devices in health service organisations*. Sydney: Author.

Steel, C. (2015). Auditing clinical practice: Ensuring high reliability at an Australian hospital. *AORN Journal, 102*, 81–84. https://dx.doi.org/10.1016/j.aorn.2015.05.013

Street, M., Phillips, N. M., Mohebbi, M., & Kent, B. (2017). Effect of a newly designed observation, response and discharge chart in the Post Anaesthesia Care Unit on patient outcomes: a quasi-experimental study in Australia. *British Medical Journal Open, 7*(12), e015149.

Sutherland-Fraser, S., & Davies, M. (2018). The ACORN practice audit tools project: using standards to drive improvement in perioperative practice. *Journal of Perioperative Nursing in Australia, 31*(2), 37–45.

Travaglia, J., & Debono, D. (2009). *Clinical audit: a comprehensive review of the literature*. Sydney: University of New South Wales, Centre for Clinical Governance Research in Health, Faculty of Medicine.

Victorian Surgical Consultative Council (VSCC). (2019). Retained materials in surgery. Information bulletin, January 2019. Retrieved from <https://www.bettersafercare.vic.gov.au/sites/default/files/2019-01/INFORMATION%20BULLETIN_Retained%20materials%20in%20surgery_FINAL.pdf>.

Wahr, J. A., Abernathy III., J. H, Lazzara, E. H., Keebler, J. R., Wall, M. H., Lynch, I., … Cooper, R. L. (2017). Medication safety in the operating room: literature and expert-based recommendations. *British Journal of Anaesthesia, 118*(1), 32–43.

Weiser, T. G., & Haynes, A. B. (2018). Ten years of the Surgical Safety Checklist. *British Journal of Surgery, 105*(8), 927–929.

Weiser, T. G., Haynes, A. B., Molina, G., Lipsitz, S. R., Esquivel, M. M., Uribe-Leitz, T., … Gawande, A. A. (2016). Size and distribution of the global volume of surgery in 2012. *Bulletin of the World Health Organization, 94*, 201F–209F. https://dx.doi.org/10.2471/BLT.15.159293

Western Australia Department of Health. (2019). Clinical incident management system [online]. Perth: Author. Retrieved from <https://ww2.health.wa.gov.au/Articles/A_E/Clinical-incident-management-system>.

World Health Organization (WHO). (2008). *Implementation manual surgical safety checklist*. Geneva: Author.

World Health Organisation (WHO). (2017). *Patient safety: faking health care safer*. Geneva: Author.

World Health Organization (WHO). (2018). *Antimicrobial resistance* [Fact sheet, February]. Geneva: Author. Retrieved from <https://www.who.int/news-room/fact-sheets/detail/antimicrobial-resistance>.

World Health Organization (WHO). (2019). *10 Facts on patient safety*. Geneva: Author. Retrieved from <https://www.who.int/features/factfiles/patient_safety/patient-safety-fact-file.pdf?ua=1>.

FURTHER READING

Agency for Clinical Innovation (ACI). (2019). National Surgical Quality Improvement Program (NSQIP). About NSQIP. Retrieved from <https://www.aci.health.nsw.gov.au/resources/surgical-services/efficiency/nsqip>.

Australian Commission on Safety and Quality in Health Care (ACSQHC/the Commission). Sentinel events list. Retrieved from <https://www.safetyandquality.gov.au/our-work/indicators/australian-sentinel-events-list>.

Australian Institute of Health and Welfare (AIHW). (2020). Australian hospital statistics. Retrieved from <https://www.aihw.gov.au/reports-data/myhospitals>.

Gordon, S., Mendenhall, P., & O'Connor, B. B. (2013). *Beyond the checklist: what else health care can learn from aviation teamwork and safety*. New York: Cornell University Press.

Health Quality and Safety Commission New Zealand (HQSCNZ). (various dates). *Serious sentinel events in New Zealand hospitals (2006–2007, 2007–2008, 2008–2009); Making our hospitals safer: serious sentinel events (2009–2010, 2010–2011, 2011–2012);* and *Making health and disability services safer: serious sentinel events (2012–2013, 2013–2014).* Retrieved from <https://www.hqsc.govt.nz/search?q=serious+sentinel+events&action_search=>.

Hemingway, M. W., O'Malley, C., & Silvestri, S. (2015). Safety culture and care: a program to prevent surgical errors. Continuing education. *AORN Journal, 101*(4), 404–415.

Jensen, J., & Shipp, D. (2015). Labelling in perioperative areas: an evolving process. *ACORN Journal, 28*(4), 10–13.

National Health and Medical Research Council (NHMRC). (2019). *Australian guidelines for the prevention and control of infection in healthcare*, Canberra: Author.

Pearse, R. M., Moreno, R. P., Bauer, P., Pelosi, P., Metnitz, P., Spies, C., … European Surgical Outcomes Study (EuSOS) group for the Trials groups of the European Society of Intensive Care Medicine and the European Society of Anaesthesiology. (2012). Mortality after surgery in Europe: a 7-day cohort study. *Lancet, 380,* 1059–1065. https://dx.doi.org/10.1016/S0140-6736(12)61148-9

Safe Surgery 2020 – a collaboration of foundations, nonprofits, educational institutions and local governments who want to make surgery safe, affordable and accessible across the world. Retrieved from <https://www.safesurgery2020.org/>.

CHAPTER 5

The Perioperative Environment and Staff Safety

MICHELLE LOVE • MICHELLE SKRIVANIC • PENNY J. SMALLEY
• SALLY SUTHERLAND-FRASER
EDITOR: SALLY SUTHERLAND-FRASER

LEARNING OUTCOMES

- Outline the rationales for the design, layout and traffic patterns of perioperative environments
- Identify the parameters of environmental controls including temperature, humidity, ventilation and air-handling systems
- Describe the requirements for waste management and identify sustainable practices within the perioperative environment
- Examine workplace health and safety issues for perioperative nurses including manual handling, electrical equipment, sensitivities or allergic reactions, occupational exposures and impacts on performance and well-being
- Describe the preparation and cleaning requirements of perioperative environments

KEY TERMS

administrative controls

electrosurgical unit

engineering controls

environmentally controlled unit

hazards

hierarchy of control measures

laser

operating suite design

procedural controls

radiation safety

risk

surgical plume

sustainable practice

INTRODUCTION

The perioperative environment is a purpose-built and highly regulated environment with design features that play a significant role in staff and patient safety. These features include traffic patterns to manage the flow of patients, as well as staff and materials, and to segregate or restrict entry of external contaminants and cross-contamination; floor and wall surfaces that are easy to clean and maintain; and air-handling systems – all of which can reduce the **risk** of infection for the surgical patient. Safety features and recommended practices also protect the perioperative team from physical and manual **hazards** within this highly technical workplace, as well as those that may affect their performance and well-being.

The perioperative environment refers collectively to many individual departments, which provide diverse yet related services for patients during the perioperative journey. In addition to the operating suite, the perioperative environment may include departments where day procedures, endoscopy or interventional services are provided, as well as the sterilising services department (SSD) and interventional radiology. The operating suite, which itself may comprise many individual theatres or operating rooms (ORs), is a high-risk area that places patients at risk of surgical site infections (SSI) and exposes staff to many hazards and potential injuries.

The first half of this chapter explores the structural components present in most perioperative environments and identifies the impact that design and environmental features have on the safety of staff and patients. The second half of the chapter focuses on the operating suite, and the principles described will also be relevant for nurses working elsewhere in the perioperative environment. These principles include the workplace health and safety (WH&S) issues for perioperative nurses, including manual handling, the safe use of electrosurgery and lasers generating surgical plume, and the prevention of fires in the operating suite. The management of latex and chlorhexidine sensitivity are discussed for both staff and patients, while the management of occupational exposures focuses on the risks to staff from waste anaesthetic gases, radiation, chemicals and noise. Potential staff exposure to biohazards and standard sharps safety measures are also described. Readers will find information about waste management and potential ways to implement sustainable practices in the perioperative environment. Cleaning systems, which provide a safe working environment for staff, patients and visitors to the perioperative environment, are also detailed. The chapter concludes with a description of the perioperative nurse's role in preparation of the OR for patients undergoing surgery.

OPERATING SUITE DESIGN

The **operating suite design** and layout must accommodate the day-to-day workload and the corresponding fluctuations in staff and patient numbers while allowing for the addition of emerging technology, equipment and procedures (Australasian Health Infrastructure Alliance [AHIA], 2018a). The operating suite is a self-contained, **environmentally controlled unit** that consists of many physically distinct functional areas (AHIA, 2018a). It may be adjacent to a pre-admission area (or a perioperative unit), through which patients for day surgery and those requiring admission are admitted.

The Australian states and territories and New Zealand have their own set of building codes, infection prevention and control guidelines and capital works guidelines. Such guidelines assist with hospital design when new hospitals are being planned or refurbishments are commissioned. For example, the Western Australia Department of Health (WA DoH) guidelines provide direction not only for planning of public and private hospitals, but also for day procedure hospitals, psychiatric hospitals and nursing homes (WA DoH, 2018). The *Australasian health facility guidelines*, an initiative of the AHIA, are also available to assist Australian and New Zealand health departments undertaking health facility projects to achieve the standards for building, space, equipment, fitting out and furnishings, and these are the minimum standards for design (AHIA, 2018a).

Professional colleges also identify best practices for the physical environments where patient care is provided. For example, the Australian College of Perioperative Nurses (ACORN) recommends that perioperative nurses, surgeons and anaesthetists are involved in the planning and design of perioperative departments along with other interested parties such as engineers, infection prevention and control personnel and WH&S representatives (ACORN, 2020a; Link, 2019). Relevant position statements from medical colleges pertain to the commissioning of medical gas pipelines (Australian and New Zealand College of Anaesthetists [ANZCA], 2020), the minimum requirements for physical environments such as the post-anaesthesia care unit (PACU) and day procedure units (ANZCA, 2018a, 2018b) as well as adult cardiac surgery units (Australian and New Zealand Society of Cardiac and Thoracic Surgeons [ANZSCTS], 2014).

Planning the built environment of the operating suite should incorporate human factors and ergonomics (HFE) in the design to eliminate hazards and performance obstacles known to impact on patient safety (Xie & Carayon, 2015). Chapter 2 provides the reader with more information about human factors and patient safety. Studies have identified that OR layout and configuration of equipment resulting in unnecessary movement and obstructed pathways has a negative effect on surgical team members' performance by causing increased distractions, tension and frustrations in the team (Ahmad et al., 2016). Environmental factors such as light, temperature, movement and noise have also been found to contribute to the error rate within the OR (Zabihirad, Mojdeh, & Shahriari, 2019). Other considerations in operating suite design include the flow of the patients, staff, consumables and equipment. Such considerations can minimise delays, maintain patient privacy and allow for segregation of some patient cohorts; for example, paediatric patients, immunocompromised patients and patients with a known status of multi-resistant organism (MROs), and/or communicable diseases (National Health and Medical Research Council [NHMRC], 2019), who may require specific or individualised flow patterns.

When designing the operating suite, the decision regarding the number of ORs and PACU bed capacity is governed by many factors, including:
- number of surgical procedures, factoring in potential for cancellations and emergency surgery
- case mix and complexity of surgical procedures, which also influences recovery time
- changeover times in between surgical procedures
- planning for future trends and technology
- anticipated hours of activity per day (AHIA, 2018a).

There are several design models for the operating suite layout that achieve a balance between the environmental needs of the staff, infection prevention and control, operational flow and functional requirements. The *Australasian health facility guidelines* (AHIA, 2018a) describe three design models which have been used commonly in past decades:

- *Single corridor.* This model has a central corridor that divides the ORs and storage areas and allows the passage of all patients, staff, supplies and equipment. This model, however, may not be appropriate if the corridor is not wide enough to permit the passage of clean and contaminated supplies within a common area. There is also the risk that preoperative patients transported in the same corridor may be exposed to distressing sights and sounds. Keeping doors closed and incorporating other methods to maintain patient privacy can minimise these risks.

- *Racetrack style (dual corridor).* In this model, the ORs are usually placed around a corridor containing equipment and supply areas. An outside 'racetrack' maybe used for the passage of contaminated equipment and

supplies. The aim is to manage the use of each corridor, reducing the presence or flow of clean and contaminated items without duplicating equipment, supplies and staff.

- *Small clusters.* This model clusters between two and four ORs with a shared sterile stock room and corridors. Disadvantages include the additional costs associated with duplicating supplies in multiple sterile stock rooms.

The *Australasian health facility guidelines* (AHIA, 2018a) also describe the more common design models in contemporary projects:

- *Single-handed layout.* In this model, each OR layout is the same, with the identical placement of OR doors, equipment and fittings inside each OR. This model may enhance safety, with team members familiar with the same layout in any OR; however, the limitations include restrictions in sharing support areas, such as scrub bays and clean-up areas (Fig. 5.1).

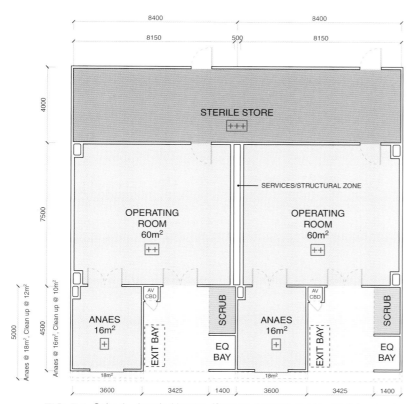

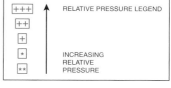

FIG. 5.1 Suite 1 – handed layout. (Source: Australasian Health Infrastructure Alliance. (2018a). *Australasian Health Facility Guidelines. Part B: Health Facility Briefing and Planning 0520 – Operating Unit*. Version 6, p. 47 5.5.1 Suite 1 – Handed layout.)

- *Mirrored layout.* This model refers to a pair of ORs designed in mirror image of each other, which allows for easy sharing of support areas. The mirrored layout may be configured in a number of different ways, depending upon the adjacent services and floor plan (Figs 5.2 and 5.3).

Design of the operating suite should also incorporate close or direct links with other units for convenience, practicality, patient safety and privacy, including:
- sterilising services department (SSD)
- emergency department (ED)
- intensive care unit (ICU)/high-dependency unit (HDU)
- surgical wards
- delivery suite
- pathology – may also include an area for frozen section testing inside the operating suite, blood bank – or a designated blood storage unit may be located inside the operating suite
- biomedical engineering (or an area for equipment testing and repair)
- medical imaging departments (AHIA, 2018a).

Traffic Patterns

Traffic patterns define the movement of personnel, equipment, supplies and instrumentation through the operating suite. Traffic patterns also aim to prevent the introduction of potential sources of contamination through the segregation of some activities as part of infection prevention and control recommendation, as well as quality and safety standards (Australian Commission on Safety and Quality in Health Care [ACSQHC/the Commission], 2020a) (Fig. 5.4). For example, waste, contaminated supplies and soiled reusable medical devices (RMDs) should not travel down the same corridor as clean and sterile supplies. If this is necessary because of the operating suite's design, measures must be taken to minimise any potential contamination between clean and contaminated supplies. Such measures include the use of a 'closed cart' system for transporting soiled and contaminated RMDs to the SSD for decontamination and reprocessing (AHIA, 2018a). Chapter 6 provides the reader with more information about the handling of RMDs.

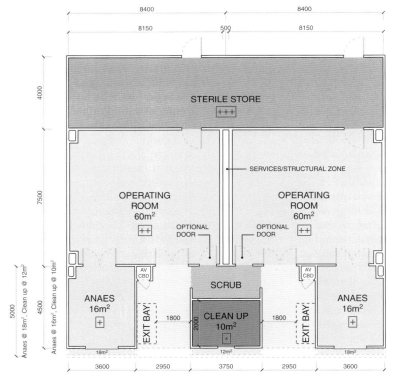

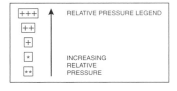

FIG. 5.2 Suite 1 – mirrored layout. (Source: Australasian Health Infrastructure Alliance. (2018a). *Australasian Health Facility Guidelines. Part B: Health Facility Briefing and Planning 0520 – Operating Unit*. Version 6, p. 48 5.5.2 Suite 1 – Mirrored layout.)

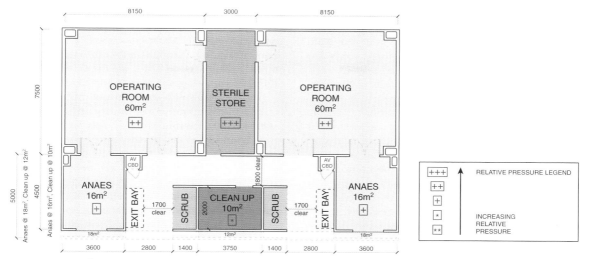

FIG. 5.3 Suite 2 – mirrored layout. (Source: Australasian Health Infrastructure Alliance. (2018a). *Australasian Health Facility Guidelines. Part B: Health Facility Briefing and Planning 0520 – Operating Unit*. Version 6, p. 49 5.5.3 Suite 2 – Mirrored layout.)

	PATIENT	STAFF	SUPPLIES
Unrestricted	Emergency/ ICU/ wards/ admissions send patients to the operating suite (OS) Theatre reception greet visitors and staff	Change rooms Tea rooms Staff education rooms (or may be in the semi restricted area)	Supplies and consumables received from stores. Decanted from boxes before transfer to inside OS Loan set delivery to SSD
Semi restricted	Patients enter holding bay Induction rooms maybe used	Staff gather necessary reusable medical devices (RMDs), consumables and equipment for surgery	Cleaning → sterilisation of RMDs undertaken in SSD Sterile consumables and RMDs enter sterile stock room Sterile supplies are gathered in preparation for operation
Restricted	Patient enters operating room (OR)	Check and prepare OR prior to list Surgical hand antisepsis, gowning and gloving Prepare and set up aseptic field Surgery performed	Setup taken into the OR for surgery (should be checked by nursing staff) OR waste segregation (e.g. recycling) practices implemented
Semi restricted	Patients enter post anaesthetia care unit after surgery Discharged to ward or home	Cleaning OR in between patients Terminal cleaning of OR at end of list Environmental cleaning	Unused consumables and RMDs returned to sterile stock room Dirty RMDs taken into OR cleanup area for transportation to SSD Dirty linen and segregated waste removed

FIG. 5.4 Correct traffic flow in and out of the operating suite. (Created by Michelle Love)

Operating Suite Zones

The **operative suite** commonly features three areas, or 'zones', which ACORN (2020a) defines as unrestricted, semi-restricted and restricted zones. These zones are determined by the activities performed therein, each requiring different environmental controls, such as air-handling, and different perioperative practices and attire. In many hospitals, signage outside the operative suite indicates to personnel that they are entering a restricted area (AHIA, 2018a). All perioperative staff should be aware that the boundaries and areas of transition between these zones may not be immediately clear within the operating suite, especially for new staff and visitors who may be unfamiliar with the perioperative environment or the functions of each zone.

Unrestricted

Entry points to the operating suite are considered unrestricted zones because they provide access for personnel and patients as well as movement of equipment, delivery of supplies and removal of waste. Public areas such as reception are also unrestricted because they provide access for external visitors (AHIA, 2018a). Staff changing rooms are also considered unrestricted zones because these rooms are the entry point and act as a transition zone for personnel, where both street clothes and perioperative attire are permitted (ACORN, 2020a).

Semi-restricted

Semi-restricted areas may include peripheral support areas, such as the medicine and pharmacy storage rooms, holding bays, the PACU and the corridors leading to restricted areas (AHIA, 2018a). Semi-restricted zones are limited to personnel usually wearing perioperative attire (ACORN, 2020a), although some hospitals may allow personnel wearing hospital uniforms to access these areas – for example, PACU staff and ward staff accessing the PACU for clinical handover and patient transfer.

Restricted

Restricted areas are limited to authorised personnel wearing perioperative attire and include sterile stock rooms, procedural rooms and OR modules and areas for the processing of sterile items (ACORN, 2020a; AHIA, 2018a). Visitors may also be permitted in restricted areas under certain circumstances. More information about visitors to the operating suite is provided at the end of this chapter.

OPERATING SUITE LAYOUT

There are many possible layouts for the operating suite; however, the specific requirements for the common components should be informed by the relevant building codes and guidelines – for example the *Australasian health facility guidelines* (AHIA, 2018a) – as well as nationally endorsed infection prevention and control guidelines, such as those produced by NHMRC, and the recommendations of professional colleges such as ACORN and ANZCA.

The following components are outlined in sequence, working from the entrance of the operating suite, where unrestricted and semi-restricted areas are likely to be located, through to the centre of the operating suite and restricted areas.

Changing Rooms

Secure designated male and female changing rooms must be provided for staff and other authorised personnel to store their belongings such as mobile phones securely in lockers. Personal communication devices and mobile technology in particular are potential sources of contamination when brought into the perioperative environment (Corrin, Lin, MacNaughton, Mahato, & Rajendiran, 2016; Qureshi et al., 2020) and, subsequently, may be an infection risk when taken back into the wider community and used without adequate cleaning (White, 2017). Similarly, larger personal items such as backpacks, handbags and briefcases may not be permitted in the anaesthetic room and the OR because of the recommended practices that apply to these restricted areas of the operating suite (ACORN, 2020b).

Changing rooms should be supplied daily with adequate volumes of freshly laundered perioperative attire in a range of sizes for the anticipated staffing of the department. Staff amenities should also include showers, which staff can use when additional infection prevention and control measures are required (AHIA, 2016a).

Reception

The reception area is the boundary between the operating suite and the rest of the hospital. It is a key information hub for personnel, where the OR schedules are created, confirmed and amended. It may also incorporate a waiting area for patients and families. The reception area is also a place to document the passage of visitors including students and medical company representatives (MCRs) (ACORN, 2020c). Staff duress alarms, which silently summon security in the event of a personal threat or physical assault, are required in reception areas (AHIA, 2018b), as well as postanaesthesia and recovery areas (Ministry of Health, New South Wales (NSW), 2017a).

Preoperative Holding Bay

The preoperative holding bay is an admission area for patients where the preoperative ward nurse and the perioperative nurse conduct patient clinical handovers.

Some patients may need the presence of an interpreter in the holding bay to assist communication, while paediatric patients may be accompanied by a parent or carer, who may be permitted to wait in the holding bay. Recommended minimum staffing for the holding bay is one nurse (ACORN, 2020d) who is responsible not only for patient admission and ongoing monitoring but also for coordination of patient flow through timely communication and liaison between each OR and the preoperative patient areas.

Storage Areas

A range of storage areas is required for the diverse equipment and supply needs of the operating suite. Storage areas located on the periphery of the operating suite are needed for the receipt of bulk supplies from the outside. These storage areas must provide adequate space to de-box and decant these supplies from any external packaging before they are distributed further. Storage areas located deeper within the restricted areas of the operating suite are needed for those supplies and equipment which may require specialised environmental controls (e.g. in sterile stock rooms or fume cabinets), or strict access and security measures (e.g. pharmacy supplies and gas cylinders). Most of the daily supplies and frequently used specialty equipment, such as lead gowns, microscopes, lasers and positioning devices, must be stored in areas that are easily accessible from the ORs and anaesthetic rooms. Such areas include equipment bays located throughout the operating suite for staff access close to point of use. Suitable areas are also required for staff to sort and manage waste (AHIA, 2018a).

Sterile Stock Room

The sterile stock room is a restricted area used primarily for the storage of supplies and equipment which have been sterilised for use during aseptic procedures. Healthcare facilities are expected to manage the risks of contamination in such storage areas (ACSQHC/the Commission, 2020a) through adherence to national and international technical standards which outline the environmental controls in these rooms, such as recommended ranges for temperature and humidity levels (Standards Australia, 2014). The ranges for environmental controls are also cited by professional colleges in recommended practices for perioperative nurses (ACORN, 2020a, 2020e). Environmental controls are also an important part of stock management in the operating suite, which is described in more detail in Box 5.1 (see also Chapter 6). The sterile stock room must be in a central location and easily accessible from all ORs. It must be cleaned regularly and kept free of dust, vermin and insects. Setups of RMDs and sterile

supplies gathered in preparation for the next day's planned surgical procedures, and may be placed on a trolley or in a closed case cart and stored in the sterile stock room or a dedicated storage area overnight (AHIA, 2018a). The sterile stock room may also be where surgical prostheses are stored and may serve an additional function as the designated prosthesis management area.

Staff Rooms

Regular rest and meal breaks can reduce the risk of workplace fatigue (Safe Work Australia, 2013). Professional colleges also recognise the risk of fatigue for the perioperative team (ACORN, 2020f) and, to this end, recommend that staff rooms are located within the operating suite. This provides a place for the perioperative team to relax and have a meal break without the need to change from perioperative attire. Another designated room is also recommended for staff meetings and in-service

---

BOX 5.1
Design Features for Storing Sterile Supplies

The sterile storage area is not to be used as a shared equipment storage space, and outer packaging boxes should not be placed on the sterile stock shelves owing to the potential of contamination from the packaging with dust, insect infestations or other contaminants.

Sterile packages and trays are ideally stored on a smooth, non-porous surface, such as open wire shelving which is at least 250 mm above the floor and 440 mm from the ceiling.

The open shelving allows dust to fall to the floor and permits cleaning to take place more effectively. Shelving must protect the integrity of the sterile stock, facilitate inventory management and stock rotation and not allow dust to collect (e.g. no solid containers).

The sterile stock room must be kept cool and dry, with a temperature of 18°C–25°C and a relative humidity of 35%–70% to prevent compromising the integrity of the sterile packages.

Sterile supplies need to be kept away from direct sunlight; therefore, windows within the sterile stock area are not considered ideal.

To maximise storage space, many operating suites use mobile compactors.

Consideration must be given to work health and safety concerns for staff regarding the height of shelving, weight of trays and the placement of heavy stock items.

(Sources: Australian Commission on Safety and Quality in Health Care. (2020a). AS18/07: *Reprocessing of reusable medical devices in health service organisations*. Sydney: Author; Australasian Health Infrastructure Alliance. (2018a). *Australasian healthcare facility guidelines – part B Health facility briefing and planning*, Version 4; Standards Australia. (2014). AS/NZS 4187 *Reprocessing of reusable medical devices in health service organizations*. Sydney: Author.)

education, and for continuing education purposes where the perioperative team can access journals and textbooks, organisational intranet and the internet (AHIA, 2018a).

The Postanaesthesia Care Unit (PACU)

The PACU is classified as a semi-restricted area which also functions as a transition zone in the operating suite. It is accessed by staff dressed in hospital uniforms or civilian clothes and staff wearing perioperative attire (ACORN, 2020a). The PACU needs to be accessible to all staff to facilitate patient transfers to postoperative areas (or discharge home in day procedure facilities) and also in the event of emergencies and medical team response.

The PACU is where nurses provide care to postanaesthetic patients. It may be separated into different areas or stages with postoperative beds, or recliner chairs in day procedure facilities, and needs to be located close to the operating/procedure rooms (AHIA, 2018a; ANZCA, 2018a). The layout and design of the PACU also need to facilitate good observation of all patients simultaneously (ANZCA, 2018a, 2018b). Curtained cubicles may allow privacy for patients while still maintaining adequate workspace. Paediatric patients should be recovered in a dedicated area within the PACU and provide enough space for a parent or carer to be present and seated (AHIA, 2018a; ANZCA, 2018a,). Patients requiring isolation and transmission-based precautions should be nursed in dedicated bays (AHIA, 2018a). The PACU requires appropriate lighting and wall colouring to facilitate accurate assessment of patients' skin colour (ANZCA, 2018a), which may indicate changes in the patient's physiological status. Chapter 12 provides the reader with more information about PACU.

Operating Room Module

Surgical procedures are performed within specialised rooms of the operating suite. An OR module is a group of areas that are configured closely together to optimise patient flow and minimise the distances that staff need to travel to perform their duties. Modules include patient care areas such as an anaesthetic bay and an OR, as well as a staff scrub bay, clean-up area and exit bay.

Anaesthetic rooms

Anaesthetic rooms are located proximal to the OR and patients are transferred here from the holding bay when the anaesthetist is ready to prepare a patient for surgery (ANZCA, 2021). Insertion of intravenous lines, invasive monitoring devices and regional anaesthesia may be performed in the anaesthetic room. In some facilities, general anaesthesia may be induced in the anaesthetic room before transferring the patient to the

OR table (Joseph, Joshi, & Allison, 2018). In other facilities, the patient may be transferred onto the operating table for induction – this may happen in smaller facilities without anaesthetic rooms, or because of anaesthetic preference and local protocol. Use of anaesthetic rooms provides patient privacy, increases throughput and reduces OR changeover time (Joseph et al., 2018). Chapter 8 provides the reader with more information about anaesthesia.

Scrub bays

Scrub bays are required for each OR and may be shared between two ORs, depending upon workload and layout. Small supplies of PPE should be available in scrub bays, as well as a mirror for staff to check their PPE application and ensure all hair is contained in headwear (AHIA, 2016b). Scrub bays provide staff with a deep sink or trough with running water, and access to a range of antiseptic solutions in an area large enough to accommodate several members of the surgical team undertaking the surgical hand antisepsis procedure simultaneously (AHIA, 2016b). The location of scrub bays directly outside the OR door facilitates staff adherence to aseptic technique (Joseph et al., 2018). This layout also facilitates staff access to sterile gown and glove trolleys located generally within the OR away from wet areas. Staff should be aware of the risks of contamination of supplies from moisture in scrub bays, soaking of perioperative attire and splashes to PPE, as well as the risk of slip and falls. To prevent slip injuries to personnel, the floor coverings in the scrub areas should be of a non-slip texture (AHIA, 2018a).

Clean-up areas

Located adjacent to the OR, this area is where sharps, fluids, waste, instrument trays and other RMDs are transferred immediately following surgery. Trays and other RMDs are checked, then placed in another trolley or closed cart system to be transported to the SSD for reprocessing (AHIA, 2018a). Sharps are emptied in an appropriate receptacle, fluids are discarded and waste, such as segregating recyclable, general, clinical and cytotoxic waste, is streamlined for disposal (AHIA, 2018a).

Exit bays

Exit bays function primarily as the exit point for the patient to be transferred from the OR to PACU. They also facilitate the unidirectional flow of used RMDs and removal of waste from the ORs, and commonly function as the temporary location of the patient trolley or bed during surgery. Where space allows, exit bays may also be used to store clean linen, patient-positioning aids and fluid-warming cabinets (AHIA, 2018a). In such layouts, the requirement to segregate clean and dirty activities must be addressed for compliance with standards (ACSQHC/the Commission, 2020a).

Standard Operating Rooms

The standard OR (sometimes called the operating 'theatre') should have a designated entry point for the patient and clean supplies, and a separate exit point for the patient and waste (AHIA, 2018a). The minimum size recommended for a general OR is 42 m^2, whereas 55 m^2 is recommended for a large OR (AHIA, 2018a) (Fig. 5.5). The configuration of the OR should facilitate safe patient care and efficient work flows, particularly around the aseptic field to reduce inadvertent contamination from movement of staff or equipment.

Dedicated Operating Rooms

Some facilities, such as large tertiary-referral hospitals, use dedicated ORs for specialty surgery such as endoscopy, closed urology, ophthalmics, orthopaedics, cardiothoracics, or robotic and/or hybrid surgery. This approach is beneficial as it allows specialised equipment, such as microscopes and non-standard operating tables, to remain within the OR. This may reduce the potential for damage due to frequent movement, although fixed equipment may limit the flexibility that is often required of operating suites in smaller hospitals. Building codes and professional colleges also provide recommendations for dedicated ORs. For example, cardiothoracic ORs should be located to facilitate access and support to specialised services such as perfusion rooms (AHIA, 2018a), while the ANZSCTS recommends using large ORs of 55 m^2 for adult cardiac surgery (ANZSCTS, 2014). Another common example of a dedicated OR is for obstetric patients. As labouring women may present with urgency for emergency care, it is common practice for such rooms to be ready for immediate use with all equipment and supplies available. These rooms should provide adequate space for the midwife and presence of a support person, as well as additional fixtures and gas outlets for the neonatology and/or paediatric team to care for the newborn baby.

Hybrid Operating Rooms

The hybrid OR is an 'operating room with a fixed imaging platform designed to perform minimally invasive surgery and enable conversion to an open procedure' (AHIA, 2018a, p. 6). Hybrid OR technology is used in neurosurgery, orthopaedics, otolaryngology, cardiovascular and thoracic surgery (Casar Berazaluce, Hanke, von Allmen, &

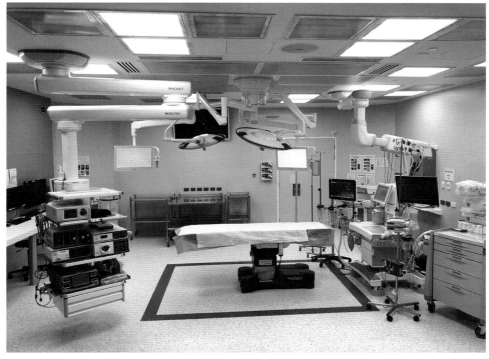

FIG. 5.5 Modern operating room. (Source: Reproduced with permission of Flinders Hospital, Adelaide.)

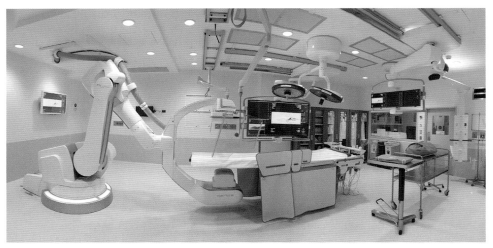

FIG. 5.6 Hybrid operating room. (Source: Reproduced with permission of Concord Repatriation General Hospital, Sydney.)

Racadio, 2019). These ORs (sometimes called interventional ORs) combine the features of the cardiac catheter unit or angioplasty suite with those of a standard OR. They provide an environment for highly advanced imaging technology and enable the surgeon to manipulate and reposition the imaging equipment during minimally invasive procedures (Schuetze et al., 2019). Hybrid ORs may also provide additional infection prevention and control measures because of the restricted entry policies and wearing of complete perioperative attire required in the perioperative environment (Kaneko & Davidson, 2014).

The size of the hybrid OR will be influenced by the procedures and equipment needs, as well as the existing infrastructure. The AHIA (2018a) recommends a space of 75 m^2 to accommodate the fixed imaging equipment in the hybrid OR, with additional space recommended for the attached control room and the equipment room. The ANZSCTS (2014) recommends that adult cardiac surgery requires 150 m^2 in total, comprising a hybrid OR measuring 70 m^2, with the control room and storage accounting for the remaining area.

A radiographer will work from the control room, which facilitates a direct view of the surgical field as well as a view of the monitors, enabling simultaneous viewing of multiple radiological images. Instead of mobile X-ray machines, most hybrid ORs have a ceiling or floor-fixed intraoperative X-ray machine (also referred to as the 'C-arm' because of its shape), which moves in a parallel plane to the OR table, capturing radiological images of the patient. The C-arm should be designed so it can be moved away from the aseptic field to improve the surgeon's access (Casar Berazaluce et al., 2019). Lead-

lined walls and doors are recommended to minimise radiation scatter (Kaneko & Davidson, 2014) and illuminating warning signs are required to alert staff when the radiological screening is in progress (Australian Radiation Protection and Nuclear Safety Agency [ARPANSA], 2020) (Fig. 5.6).

Hybrid ORs display high-quality images; however, the radiation levels should be closely monitored because the exposure is greater than in a standard OR using a mobile C-arm. Hybrid ORs should also be fitted with extra equipment such as suspended lead shields and mobile lead screens to reduce the levels of radiation exposure. Additionally, lead drapes may be fitted to the sides of the OR table to shield the legs of personnel standing close to the table during radiographic screening. Specialised protective head scarves and eye protection can also be used in hybrid ORs (Guillou et al., 2018) (see also the later section on radiation). Additional work health and safety considerations for the perioperative environment are discussed in later sections of this chapter.

Sterilising Services Department (SSD)

The operating suite is the primary user of the SSD. The efficient transport of clean and contaminated RMDs between the two departments will be facilitated by their relative location and proximity. In some facilities, the SSD is located within the operating suite. Regardless of its location, contaminated RMDs should be enclosed in carts or puncture-resistant containers with lids during transport to the SSD (AHIA, 2016c). Separate lifts and hoists should be used to transport clean and contaminated RMDs to and from the SSD when it is located on a different floor from the operating suite (AHIA, 2016c). Loan sets of RMDs and prostheses are in frequent use, and a dedicated area should be provided for receipt, inventory management and return of loan sets to medical companies (ACORN, 2020g; AHIA, 2016c).

The SSD layout must be clearly defined to distinguish the decontamination (dirty) and packaging/sterilising (clean) areas to ensure a unidirectional work flow and reduce the risk of cross-contamination (Standards Australia, 2014). Contaminated RMDs should be delivered directly into the cleaning or decontamination room for processing (AHIA, 2016c). All personnel within this area must wear personal protective equipment (PPE) while handling contaminated RMDs and chemicals (Standards Australia, 2014). Additionally, hearing protection should be included as part of PPE wherever noise levels are a WH&S hazard (Safe Work Australia, 2018a). Decontamination areas incorporate negative air pressure to contain potentially harmful substances within the area, whereas positive air pressure is used within the designated clean packaging/storage areas (Ministry of Health, NSW, 2016). After the RMDs have been processed, they enter the clean side of the SSD, where specially trained staff are required to check them for completeness and mark their inclusion on the tray checklists (ACORN, 2020e) before packaging and sterilisation. Following sterilisation processes (which may include time on cooling racks), the items must be handled, transported and stored in a manner that minimises the risk of contamination (Standards Australia, 2014). Chapter 6 provides the reader with more information about asepsis and sterilisation.

OPERATING SUITE ENVIRONMENTAL CONTROLS

The following environmental controls and design considerations are required to ensure that the operating suite complies with relevant building standards and infection prevention and control practices, and to facilitate cleaning regimens. Different areas of the operating suite will have specific recommendations for environmental controls depending upon the current standards (ACORN, 2020a), as well as the policies and guidelines for each jurisdiction AHIA (2018a). For example, the settings and ranges for temperature and humidity will vary according to the function of that area of the operating suite. Before exploring these controls, the following section will describe architectural features of the operating suite and will outline the different requirements of relevant building standards. The section also outlines the recommended cleaning principles and schedules for cleaning the perioperative environment.

Windows

Natural light from sealed windows is recommended wherever possible in the perioperative environment, including individual ORs, the PACU and staff areas (AHIA, 2018a). Building codes for perioperative environments recognise that many people work in such areas, and professional colleges also acknowledge reports that natural light can boost morale, motivation and comfort of the perioperative team (ACORN, 2020a). Furthermore, windows from corridors into the OR allows for supervision of practice and opportunities for training (AHIA, 2018a), while limiting the number of personnel inside the OR. Clear sight-lines, with a view of the OR table and the patient from adjacent spaces such as scrub bays with windows or glazed doors, can be beneficial for staff preparing to join the team (Joseph et al., 2018). The dignity and privacy of perioperative patients must also be considered with windows and sight lines, particularly when the patient is uncovered or exposed for surgery.

While there are benefits from natural lighting, most surgical techniques and approaches require specifically tailored surgical lighting (Knulst & Dankelman, 2017). For example, minimally invasive surgery is performed in low-light ORs where windows are fitted with coverings to control light and glare. These measures can improve the team's view of images displayed on digital screens and monitors (AHIA, 2018a). Protective window covers are also required in ORs where laser technologies are used, and these covers must be kept closed when lasers are in use (Standards Australia, 2018a).

Ceilings, Doors, Floors and Walls

Building codes require that ceilings should be made of seamless, non-reflective, non-porous material to facilitate cleaning and prevent accumulation of dirt. Similarly, light fittings must be flush fitting and sealed, while walls should be seamless and tightly sealed at floor level to minimise entry of insects and to facilitate effective cleaning (AHIA, 2016b, 2018a; WA DoH, 2018). Neutral-coloured ceilings and walls can assist with visual assessment of patient skin tone and body fluids indicating changes to patient oxygenation, while a semi-matt finish reduces glare for the perioperative team (AHIA, 2018a; WA DoH, 2018).

Automatic opening doors in areas where patient beds pass, such as exit bays, may reduce ergonomic injuries to staff (AHIA, 2018a), while swing-type doors allow easy access for hands-free entry to the OR. In all instances, robust door seals are required to maintain positive air pressure within the OR and protective strips are required to prevent damage to doors and walls from heavy traffic and cleaning regimens (ACORN, 2020a; AHIA, 2016c, 2018a).

The floors should be made from smooth, seamless materials, such as vinyl, which is impervious to moisture, easily cleaned, stain resistant, comfortable for long periods of standing and suitable for wheeled traffic (AHIA, 2016c, 2018a). The colour of the OR floor must allow for contrast between different materials, which will assist personnel to locate small items that have been dropped on the floor, such as suture needles. It is also recommended that light-coloured vinyl floor coverings are avoided owing to their potential for discoloration from surgical skin preparations and other fluids (AHIA, 2018a). The floors in wet areas of the perioperative environment, including scrub bays, cleaning areas and the sterilising department, should be non-slip (AHIA, 2016b, 2018a,; WA DoH, 2018).

Temperature

The ranges for ambient temperatures within the operating suite are described by Australian agencies and recommended in the specific policies and guidelines for each jurisdiction (AHIA, 2018a). ACORN recommends a general temperature range of 18°C–24°C, with a narrower range of 20°C–22°C within the OR to inhibit bacterial growth (ACORN, 2020a). Individual ORs should also be built with a capacity for temperature adjustment beyond this range to accommodate some types of surgery and/or the condition of individual patients. For example, the potential for hypothermia in burns patients means that the OR temperature may need to be increased to as high as 42°C (Queensland Health, 2017a). Similarly, neonates as well as paediatric, geriatric, obstetric and trauma patients are also highly susceptible to hypothermia and require higher ambient temperatures in the OR (Katz, 2017; Ministry of Health, NSW, 2016).

Maintaining the temperature comfort of staff working in the operating suite can also be challenging because of the different requirements for perioperative attire depending upon the staff role (Külpmann et al., 2016). For example, scrubbed team members wearing surgical gowns and working in close proximity under OR lights may be more comfortable in a cooler and dryer OR, whereas non-scrubbed team members may not have the added layers of attire or close proximity (Katz, 2017). While staff comfort may be a consideration in temperature regulation of the environment, the patient's safety and comfort should always be the priority (Collins, Budds, Raines, & Hooper, 2019). Perioperative patients may be transferred into the OR wearing as little as a hospital gown without any undergarments or other layer of clothing to provide warmth and privacy. They may have large areas of skin, tissue or open wounds exposed to low ambient temperatures. Patient temperature regulation may also be altered by anaesthetic agents (Katz, 2017) so the perioperative team needs to understand these risk factors for hypothermia and must work together to maintain patient comfort and prevent further heat loss (Collins et al., 2019). Inadvertent perioperative hypothermia (IPH) is discussed in more detail in the second half of this textbook.

Humidity

Recommendations for the range of humidity levels also differ according to the primary function of the area. Australian agencies recommend that general levels of humidity in the operating suite are maintained between 35% and 60% (Ministry of Health, NSW, 2016; Queensland Health, 2017a), while American guidelines followed in New Zealand recommend a wider range between 20% and 60% (Katz, 2017; Phillips, 2017). Standards Australia (2014) cites a range of 35%–70% humidity for storage areas in the operating suite; however, high humidity levels may produce condensation and compromise the pack integrity of the sterile stock (Phillips, 2017). High humidity can also increase fatigue among the surgical team and may encourage insect infestations (Queensland Health, 2017a). Furthermore, perioperative patients are at increased risk of surgical site infections (SSIs) in humid environments where pathogenic bacteria can thrive (Katz, 2017). ACORN (2020a) therefore recommends a narrow range of 50%–60% humidity within the OR where aseptic procedures are performed. Restricting the humidity range not only inhibits bacterial growth but also inhibits the development of condensation and mould (Phillips, 2017; Queensland Health, 2017a).

In areas where flammable agents are being used or stored, humidity should be maintained at 55% (Queensland Health, 2017b). Low humidity levels have been associated with static electricity and flammable agents in the past; however, modern anaesthetic agents and techniques have reduced the risk of fires generated from static sparks in the OR (Katz, 2017; Phillips, 2017).

Air-Handling Systems and Ventilation

Air handling refers to air-flow management, air filtration and pressure gradients (AHIA, 2018a). In conjunction with humidity levels, air-handling systems and ventilation within the operating suite are controlled to reduce the spread of airborne infectious organisms from one area to another. Within an individual OR, they are used to minimise the patient's risk of acquiring an SSI due to airborne contaminants and from bacteria as well as to provide a comfortable environment for the OR personnel (AHIA, 2018a; Khankari, 2018).

During surgery, dust particles, textile fibres, skin squames and respiratory aerosols that contain microorganisms are released from surgical team members into the air of the OR (Armellino, 2016). A positive air pressure system is recommended for the OR (AHIA, 2016b) to direct the air out from the centre of the room, hence minimising the potential for particles and micro-organisms to settle on the aseptic field or enter the operative site. The air supplied to the individual OR should pass through the aseptic zone and exit through low-lying wall grids in the OR, without recirculation (Khankari, 2018). The bottom of the wall grids must be no lower than 300 mm from the floor (Standards Australia, 2012).

Positive air pressure systems sweep the air out from the cleanest areas to the less clean areas – that is, from the OR out into the adjacent areas, including the corridors and scrub areas. Sterile stock areas have similar needs to the OR and should therefore have an equal or higher air pressure than inside the OR (Standards Australia, 2012) to prevent the contamination of supplies.

Microbial counts can be high in the air circulating outside the OR (Bashaw & Keister, 2019; Ministry of Health, NSW, 2016) – hence the recommendation that OR doors *must* be kept closed at all times (other than the *necessary* passage of staff, supplies and the patient) to reduce the risk of airborne contaminants entering the surgical field (ACORN, 2020h) (Research box 5.1). The microbial count in the OR itself is usually at its peak during skin incision, which follows a period of maximum air disturbance in the OR created during staff gloving and gowning, patient draping, the movement of staff and the frequent opening and closing of doors (Loison et al., 2017; Phillips, 2017). Staff movements and door opening can be reduced when the minimum predictable supplies are available in reach within the OR during the course of surgery (Loison et al., 2017).

A negative air pressure system is recommended for rooms where bronchoscopies and sputum collections occur (AHIA, 2016d). In this system, the pressure gradient means that air flows into the room, and this can minimise the dispersal of procedure-generated micro-organisms into adjacent areas.

ACORN (2020a) describes three types of **ventilation systems** used within the perioperative environment. Each system is differentiated by the frequency of air changes per hour, as well as the type of filter, location of air entry and exit, and the direction of air flows.

- *Conventional air-conditioning system.* This system is used in the unrestricted areas of the perioperative environment such as the reception area and offices. This system uses filtered and recirculated air, with a minimum of four fresh air changes each hour.
- *Ultra-clean air system.* This system is used in the restricted areas of the perioperative environment such as the sterile stock room, anaesthetic bay and the OR, as well as some parts of the SSD. In many instances, high-efficiency particulate-arresting (HEPA) air filters

---

RESEARCH BOX 5.1
Operating Room Doors and Air-handling Systems

Airborne contaminants in the OR have been associated with surgical site infections (SSI), and movements of staff, equipment and supplies in the OR may be associated with increased risk of contamination. Researchers have found that, as the number of people inside the OR increases, so too does the number of pathogens in the OR, which consequently increases the incidence of SSIs (Bashaw & Keister, 2019; Loison et al., 2017). The evidence suggests that air-conditioning efficacy decreases when OR doors are opened; however, more research is required to determine whether it is the number of people inside the OR that reduces the efficacy of the system, or the increased traffic through the OR doors (Bashaw & Keister, 2019; Blocker, Forsyth, Branaghan, & Hallbeck, 2017).

Numerous studies have explored the frequency and reasons that OR doors are opened during surgery. In one such study, all surgical specialties recorded a high frequency of door openings during surgery; spinal surgery (50 door openings per hour) and cardiac surgery (48 door openings per hour) were the highest, with neurosurgery (42 door openings per hour) and joint replacement surgery (40 door openings per hour) also high (Rovaldi & King, 2015). Opening of OR doors was related to equipment and supply issues (44%), staff meal breaks and/or team members entering and leaving the OR (16%) and communication (13%), while there was no detectable reason for 28% of occasions studied (Loison et al., 2017). Temporary signage over doors highlighting 'joint in progress' or 'implants in use' may serve as an alert to staff; however, the effectiveness of these signs to reduce the frequency of door openings has been found to diminish over time, especially when signs were not removed following the surgery (Rovaldi & King, 2015).

---

are used, which have a minimum filtration efficiency of 99.99%. This system must not use recirculated air and is required to deliver a minimum of 20 air changes per hour (Standards Australia, 2012). If normal efficiency particulate air filters are used for this system instead of HEPA filters, the clean air must be moved in a unidirectional flow (Research box 5.2).

- *Laminar air flow (LAF).* This system also uses HEPA filters to produce unidirectional air flows into the OR. In the LAF system, the filtered air flows in from the centre of the OR, above the operating table, then downwards and out through low wall vents. It requires as many as 400 air changes per hour (Standards Australia, 2012).

Lighting

Operating lights are ceiling mounted directly above the OR table to provide shadowless light on the surgical site.

RESEARCH BOX 5.2
Ultra-clean Air and Laminar Air-flow Systems

The ultra clean air environment was created in 1962 by Sir John Charnley and a colleague to address a rise in the rate of joint infections. Over the years, the original design has been modified, with the addition of walls to cocoon the surgical team members inside a chamber, followed by the reduction of walls to improve traffic patterns of the surgical team members (Thomas & Simmons, 2018).

Although now commonly referred to as laminar air flow (LAF), this is technically inaccurate from an engineering perspective. True laminar air flow occurs in parallel layers with no disruptions occurring between layers; however, regardless of its design, all air flow in the OR is turbulent. Hence, the system might instead be called the ultra-clean air (UCA) system (Thomas & Simmons, 2018).

While the principle of the LAF is biologically sound and supported by previous studies, recent research and meta-analysis can no longer establish the effectiveness of LAF in preventing SSIs following joint replacement surgery (Bischoff, Zeynep Kubilay, Allegranzi, Egger, & Gastmeier, 2017; Singh, Reddy & Shrivastava, 2017; Weinstein & Bonten, 2017). Having an increased number of air changes, long thought to be best for reducing SSI rates, has always had a negative impact owing to the increased turbulence, drafts and noise, unwanted low humidity and the thermal discomfort to personnel within the OR (Katz, 2017), as well as financial burden on the healthcare facility (Khankari, 2018).

Historically, incandescent lights were used; however, these radiated heat onto the surgical team. The use of light-emitting diodes (LEDs) aims to eliminate this undesired effect (Knulst & Dankelman, 2017). Furthermore, the use of blue-enriched white lights is to reduce optical strain during laparoscopic surgery, having been found to be effective in highlighting mucosal patterns and microvascular details during endoscopy (Wong, Smith, & Crowe, 2010). During minimally invasive surgery, room lights are often dimmed to allow the surgical site to be highly illuminated on the monitors. This low lighting can pose an occupational risk to staff where hazards on the floor, for example, cannot be seen. Another risk associated with reduced room lights comes from the difficulty staff may have in reading fine print on packages and ampoules, which may lead to selection and opening of incorrect items. Green light filters provide some source of light for other perioperative members by minimising the reflection off the monitors (Smith, 2019).

The position of the operating light may require manipulation during surgery, and there is a risk of contamination if unscrubbed personnel re-adjust the light, owing to their proximity to the aseptic field (Knulst & Dankelman, 2017). Sterile light handles allow the surgical team to adjust the light from within the aseptic field. In seeking to control the position of the light themselves, the surgical team's movements may also create a contamination risk or an interruption or distraction from the procedure under way. Anticipation of the required light position may be confirmed during team briefings, and attentive supervision during the surgical procedure is an effective way that perioperative nurses manage these risks. Members of the surgical team may also wear headlights to improve illumination and visibility when working in deep cavities or in confined surgical sites and incisions. Surgeons routinely don and adjust their headlight prior to scrubbing to confirm full function and ensure the required range of movement. Perioperative nurses may need to connect the light lead to the light source and/or reposition the equipment to follow the progress of surgery around changing surgical sites. Technology such as touchless OR surgical lights may alleviate these risks by using gesture recognition or hand tracking to move the light to where it is required during surgery (Knulst & Dankelman, 2017).

PATIENT SCENARIOS

A brief description of the healthcare setting is provided at the front of the book for readers to review when answering the questions in these unfolding scenarios relating to these four patients:

1. Mr James Collins is a 78-year-old man scheduled for a right total knee replacement – TKR.
2. Mrs Patricia Peterson is a 42-year-old Indigenous woman who requires an emergency laparoscopic cholecystectomy – lap chole.
3. Mrs Janine Clark is a 35-year-old woman scheduled for an elective lower segment caesarean section – LSCS.
4. Master Thanh Nguyen is a 3-year-old boy admitted as a day surgery patient for a left orchidopexy.

SCENARIO 5.1: ENVIRONMENTAL CONTROLS

Critical Thinking Question

- Which of the patients from the four scenarios might need the OR temperature to be raised higher than standard levels? Provide your rationale for this adjustment to the perioperative environment in your answer.

WASTE MANAGEMENT

Malik and colleagues (2018) estimated that 7% of Australia's entire carbon footprint stems from the healthcare sector. This figure includes carbon emissions generated by public and private healthcare facilities, as well as capital expenditure on the built environment and the production of pharmaceuticals. Healthcare waste not only affects organisations financially; it also has broader effects on the community and the environment.

The perioperative environment is responsible for a large proportion of that healthcare waste, with some authors suggesting this may be as high as 20%–30% (Hubbard, Hayanga, Quinlan, Soltez, & Hayanga, 2017). The treatment and disposal of clinical waste by incineration or autoclaving and shredding uses more energy and represents a further environmental cost. For example, in 2017–18, half of the total cost for disposal of solid waste generated in Victorian public health services was for clinical waste, which represented only 12% of the overall waste generated (State of Victoria, 2018).

Sustainable practice for perioperative nurses begins with awareness of environmentally responsible use of resources and the correct segregation of waste streams according to the relevant state and jurisdictional policies (ACORN, 2020i). In some jurisdictions, non-segregation of waste is an offence, incurring penalties to the organisation (Queensland Government, 2019). By reducing, reusing, recycling and rethinking definitions of waste, small changes can take place to reduce the amount of healthcare waste produced, which in turn can reduce the overall impact on the environment. Even small changes in clinical practices are worthwhile because of the subsequent reduction in associated costs to the facility. This can create a 'win–win' situation for the healthcare system and the community (Kagoma, Stall, Rubinstein, & Naudie, 2012; Wyssusek, Foong, Steel, & Gillespie, 2016). More practical tips for waste management and sustainable practices are discussed in Feature box 5.1.

Waste Streams

Healthcare waste can be divided into the following streams:

- general waste
- clinical waste
- recyclable/reposable waste streams
- cytotoxic waste.

Regardless of the specific waste stream, infection prevention measures, including the use of PPE, apply whenever handling waste in the perioperative environment (ACORN, 2020j).

General waste

Waste items in this category are those not heavily soiled or saturated by chemicals or radiation, or infectious substances such as blood or body fluids (Ministry of Health, NSW, 2017b). Examples of general waste generated in the perioperative environment include paper, packaging, surgical face masks, gloves and wound dressings, depending on the degree of contamination (State of Victoria, 2020). General waste is generally considered non-hazardous and may include whole unbroken glass bottles, whereas broken glass and other sharps are classified as sharps clinical waste.

Clinical waste

Items with large amounts of blood or body fluid (such as suction fluid containers), or visibly blood-stained items (such as used swabs and sponges), are considered clinical waste. Clinical waste is collected in yellow-coloured bags marked with a black biohazard symbol (Standards Australia, 2018b) and is disposed by incineration or autoclaving and shredding (Ministry of Health, NSW, 2017b). Clinical waste also includes pharmaceutical waste, sharps and anatomical waste. Perioperative nurses should be aware of exceptions for the return of excised tissue to the patient and/or family in facilities which have implemented a culturally sensitive and well-regulated process (Canterbury District Health Board [CDHB], 2016).

Recyclable/reposable waste

There are many clean and contaminated items from the perioperative environment that are suitable for recycling. However, the suitability for waste item choices may depend on the waste contracts for each facility. Reposable items include surgical instruments which are disposable and manufactured for reuse for a small number of occasions, or may be partly disposable and reusable (Mangeshikar & Mangeshikar, 2018).

Each waste stream must be separated into specific receptacles (Fig. 5.7). The prompt removal of multiple waste stream receptacles is imperative to maintain adequate space and a well-functioning perioperative environment. Labelling and colour coding are part of national standards (Standards Australia, 2018b), which ensure the waste streams are transported to the appropriate areas to avoid being sent to general waste. Many facilities have discovered that recycling waste streams can generate income and cost less than general or clinical waste removal (Global Green and Healthy Hospitals [GGHH], n.d). Bailing on site may also reduce the bulk of the waste to be transported, thereby reducing the cost.

Some recycling waste streams include, but may not be limited to:

- polypropylene materials (e.g. sterile wrap for instruments/equipment, perioperative attire hats, overboots and unsterile protective gowns)

FEATURE BOX 5.1
Environmental Sustainability in Healthcare

The world's climate has an impact on the health outcomes of all populations throughout the world, affecting food and water supplies, producing weather extremes and increasing the spread of infectious diseases (International Council of Nurses [ICN], 2018). A commitment from healthcare professionals has been recognised as one way to reduce the adverse effects of climate change (Guetter et al., 2018; Rychetnik, Sainsbury, & Stewart, 2018). The World Health Organization (WHO) identifies waste management as one of seven elements which it believes can drive environmental sustainability in healthcare. The other elements are energy efficiency practices, green building design and alternative energy generation, as well as transportation, food and water (WHO, 2019).

The healthcare sector can influence such change in several ways:

- Healthcare organisations can implement procurement processes to source more environmentally friendly products and packaging from manufacturers in the medical industry.
- Perioperative managers can work with hospital engineers to minimise energy consumption wherever possible, for example:
  - Preset the air conditioning to 22°C in unused ORs between 6 pm and 6 am.
  - Ensure that all non-essential computers, equipment and lights are turned off after hours.
  - Install scrub sinks with automatic motion sensors to limit the volume of water wasted during the surgical scrub.
- Perioperative nurses can reduce energy consumption and minimise the overall production of waste by:
  - being more considered in their usage and opening the minimum number of supplies
  - ensuring the timely rotation of stock to avoid expiring products and wastage

- turning off the tap between steps in the surgical scrub where water-less scrub solutions are not already provided as an alternative
- being thoughtful in their waste separation and disposal processes, especially with clinical waste
- leading behavioural change as positive role models, and by increasing their colleagues' awareness of waste management and sustainable practices (Weiss et al., 2016).

There are many organisations providing information and resources to support environmental sustainability in healthcare settings, including Health Care Without Harm (HCWH), an international non-government organisation, and the Climate and Heath Alliance (CAHA) based in Australia. Both groups support the Global Green and Healthy Hospitals (GGHH) group, whose members represent more than 1700 health districts, hospitals and healthcare services within Australia and New Zealand. The GGHH website publishes a range of case studies on waste management strategies as well as sustainable practices for chemicals, energy and water usage in hospitals. Another organisation providing web-based access to resources and an innovation exchange is the Agency for Clinical Innovation (ACI), which also supports a webpage for Green Operating Theatres.

Further information is available from:

Agency for Clinical Innovation (ACI) Green Operating Theatres

https://aci.health.nsw.gov.au/networks/anaesthesia-perioperative-care/green-theatres

Climate and Health Alliance (CAHA) Global Green and Healthy Hospitals (GGHH)

https://www.caha.org.au/globalgreen_healthyhospitals

Healthcare Without Harm (HWH)

https://noharm.org

- PVC (e.g. oxygen tubing and masks with metal and elastic removed and IV fluid bags with bungs removed)
- hard plastics (clean and contaminated must be separated)
- soft plastics (e.g. outer packaging material)
- paper and cardboard
- metal and plastic items (e.g. disposable trocars, diathermy pencils, endo-staplers or disposable instruments)
- batteries
- ink cartridges

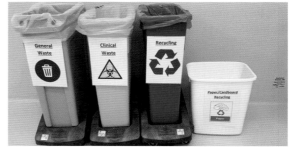

FIG. 5.7 Waste and recycling bins. (Source: Reproduced with permission of Concord Repatriation General Hospital, Sydney.)

- glass, aluminium and other materials used for food and beverages (in local facilities with co-mingling recycling programs to manage tea-room waste).

Cytotoxic waste

Items that have been contaminated by cytotoxic substances used during chemotherapy or surgical procedures are treated as cytotoxic waste and require disposal in specially marked cytotoxic bags or containers which are purple or orange in colour with a white 'telophase' symbol (Ministry of Health, NSW, 2017b). Cytotoxic waste includes the used PPE such as gloves and gowns worn by staff preparing or handling cytotoxic substances, as well as the equipment used during medication administration such as ampoules, syringes, caps and lines, and the equipment used during the clean-up and management of any spills (State of Victoria, 2020). Cytotoxic waste has the potential to cause harm to healthcare clinicians, waste management handlers and the public, so strict disposal methods are required – such as incineration at high temperatures (Queensland Government, 2019).

Perioperative nurses should complete relevant training prior to working with cytotoxic substances, covering the relevant WH&S legislation, protective measures, record keeping and waste management (State of Queensland, 2018). They should also refer to the specific substance labels, relevant safety data sheets and local policies for detailed WH&S information (Safe Work NSW, 2017). Alternative workplace allocations may also be a consideration for some female staff, owing to the potential adverse effects from exposure to cytotoxic substances during pregnancy and breastfeeding (Safe Work NSW, 2017).

The perioperative team should also consider the potential risks associated with the care of chemotherapy patients undergoing surgical procedures. This is because the excreted body fluids of chemotherapy patients may contain cytotoxic residues for up to 7 days (Government of South Australia, 2015). The following actions can reduce the risks of exposure for the perioperative team when caring for chemotherapy patients in the operating suite:

- Use cytotoxic PPE whenever handling excreted body fluids of chemotherapy patients, such as vomitus, urine and faeces, and when handling vomit bowls, urine bags, colostomy bags, bed pans or urinals.
- Decontaminate bed pans and urinals in an automated sluice machine for two cycles before releasing.
- Consider the chemotherapy patient's linen as cytotoxic waste and discard it into cytotoxic waste

containers (St George Hospital and Community Health Service, 2019).

CLEANING SYSTEMS IN THE OPERATING SUITE

Environmental cleaning systems are an important component of infection prevention and control programs, which facilitate the provision of a safe and clean environment for all patients and can reduce the risk of hospital-acquired infections (ACSQHC/the Commission, 2017a; Ministry of Health, NSW, 2020; NHMRC, 2019). The operating suite is an extreme-risk environment where vulnerable patients undergo highly invasive procedures and healthcare workers are exposed to blood and body fluids (Ministry of Health, NSW, 2020). A clean and well-maintained operating suite requires a team approach including clinical staff as well as support staff, who may be deployed from the facility's cleaning and environmental services or by external contractors. Facilities should ensure that all staff who undertake environmental cleaning have been trained and should monitor staff compliance through regular cleaning audits (Government of South Australia, 2017; Ministry of Health, NSW, 2020).

Microfibre cloths and mops have been replacing the traditional cotton string mops as one of the most frequently used methods for routine and terminal cleaning in healthcare settings (Kenters et al., 2019). However, staff should be aware that laundering of reusable microfibre products is not sufficiently standardised and the products can become degraded when in contact with sodium hypochlorite, limiting their use within specialised environments. The environmental cleaning routines for the operating suite follows those routines for healthcare facilities more generally, and include the following principles:

- assessment of risks such as manual handling, biohazards, etc.
- application of PPE according to risk
- colour coding and segregation of reusable equipment for different functional areas
- specified dilutions for cleaning products (e.g. neutral detergents and disinfectants) (ACSQHC/the Commission, 2020b)
- recommended techniques to reduce aerosolisation of dust particles (e.g. damp cleaning with lint-free materials, pour bottles instead of aerosol spray bottles)
- recommended cleaning schedules (Government of South Australia, 2017; Clinical Excellence Commission [CEC], n.d.).

Specific cleaning schedules for the operating suite may vary between jurisdictions and facilities; however, they should comply with national and state authorities (ACSQHC/the Commission, 2017a; NHMRC, 2019; CEC, n.d.) and reflect the recommendations of professional associations (ACORN, 2020k). Schedules typically include:

- minimum daily cleaning routines
  - cleaning before patient care and after patient care
  - terminal cleaning at the end of the day
- periodic cleaning routines for different functional areas, equipment and fixtures on a weekly, monthly or less-frequent basis
- ad hoc cleaning of spills such as blood and bodily fluids, or chemical spills
- specific cleaning regimens for patients known or suspected to be infected with multi-resistant organism (MROs).

Although the OR is the main practice setting for aseptic procedures, it has the potential to be one of the most contaminated environments because of the high turnover of patients and the invasive nature of surgery. Furthermore, the presence of multiple disciplines in the OR module and their contribution to cleaning routines requires oversight and coordination to ensure that the cleaning of all necessary surfaces and equipment between patient care episodes has been completed.

Routine Cleaning of the OR

The following section focuses on cleaning the OR between patient care episodes and at the start of the day. Before the first patient is admitted to the OR, the perioperative team should inspect all surfaces and equipment in the OR to determine the need for spot cleaning (ACORN, 2020k). This is especially important when the OR module has been closed overnight, and nurses should check whether local facility policies require a routine damp cleaning of the OR module at the start of each day. Inspection should include all surfaces of the OR lights and OR table in the centre of the room, and then continue systematically outwards to include all of the equipment trolleys, tables and horizontal surfaces on the periphery of the room. This inspection and spot cleaning is also relevant for any additional equipment required from storage rooms and corridors. These items must be spot cleaned before they enter the OR, owing to the accumulation of dust and other particles during storage. Once the OR module has been deemed clean and ready for use, the specific resources and aseptic supplies for the first patient may be brought into the room and prepared for use.

Between each patient care episode, the perioperative team will need to clean the used equipment and surfaces in the OR and reset the room following the same

principles. All cleaning should be undertaken with an approved hospital cleaning agent, using lint-free cloths and mechanical friction to remove contamination and debris. High-touch surfaces in the OR, such as keyboards, telephone handsets or the handles on drawers and doors, are potential sites of high contamination which must also be cleaned as they may facilitate transfer of microbes between staff and patients (King & Spry, 2019; Livshiz-Riven, Borer, Nativ, Eskira, & Larson, 2015; Qureshi et al., 2020; White, 2017). In addition, equipment may need to be repositioned so that all discarded waste is removed, the OR floor can be cleaned and all waste bins are emptied. These practices have a secondary purpose beyond infection prevention and control, which is to ensure there are no discarded accountable items remaining in the OR that may be included incorrectly in the next patient's surgical count, leading to a count error (Butler, Ford, Boxer, & Sutherland-Fraser, 2010).

Terminal Cleaning of the OR

On completion of the day's surgical procedures or each regular 24-hour period, the OR should be terminally cleaned (ACORN, 2020k). Terminal cleaning specifically involves a thorough cleaning of the equipment, furniture and surfaces within the OR module, as well as the adjacent areas and corridors in the immediate vicinity. Depending on individual local operational work instruction, designated cleaning staff may be allocated to terminally clean the OR; however, perioperative nurses are responsible to ensure that the required cleaning regimen has been followed and the integrity of the room and equipment is maintained in readiness for the next day (ACORN, 2020k). After terminal cleaning when the OR floor and surfaces are dry, the perioperative nurses may be required to restock supplies and reposition the OR equipment. This is particularly relevant for OR readiness for obstetric and other emergencies, trauma surgery or disaster preparedness (King & Spry, 2019).

In addition to cleaning between procedures and terminal cleaning, each facility must maintain a schedule of periodic environmental cleaning and maintenance for fixtures and fittings such as air vents, walls and ceilings. Facilities should also maintain documentation verifying that the cleaning has been carried out according to hospital and infection prevention and control protocols (ACORN, 2020k).

WORKPLACE HEALTH AND SAFETY (WH&S) CONSIDERATIONS

The central principle of WH&S legislation is that all employees are responsible for identifying workplace hazards and the potential risk of harm for themselves and their co-workers (Commonwealth of Australia, 2011; New Zealand Government, 2015). A range of hazards exists within the workplace (Safe Work Australia, 2015). Not only is it important for staff to be aware of these hazards, but also recommended practices require that nurses use risk minimisation strategies to protect themselves and their co-workers as well as the patients in their care (ACORN, 2020l; ACSQHC/the Commission, 2017b).

Before workplace hazards can be managed or controlled, they should first be assessed and categorised according to the level of risk. This process is a mandatory requirement when managing certain risks under WH&S legislation and is supported by the **hierarchy of control measures** (Safe Work Australia, 2018a). The top of the hierarchy and most effective control measure is to eliminate the hazards and risks (Fig. 5.8). If elimination is not possible, the risk must be managed by working down the lower levels of protection and reliability, namely: reducing the risk (requiring substitution, isolation or engineering controls), reducing exposure

(requiring administrative controls to change the way people work) and, finally, protective controls (requiring protective equipment). The lower levels in the hierarchy of control will always be less effective than elimination and often depend upon high rates of worker compliance and supervision (Safe Work Australia, 2018a).

WH&S hazards in the perioperative environment have been grouped into five categories:

- manual handling
- electrical equipment (encompassing electrosurgery, surgical lasers, surgical plume and the prevention of fires and explosions)
- sensitivities or allergic reactions
- occupational exposures (encompassing waste anaesthetic gases, radiation and chemicals as well as exposure to biohazards and the management of splashes and sharps injuries)
- impacts on performance and well-being (encompassing noise, technology stress, fatigue and workplace stress, workplace bullying and harassment, and aggression).

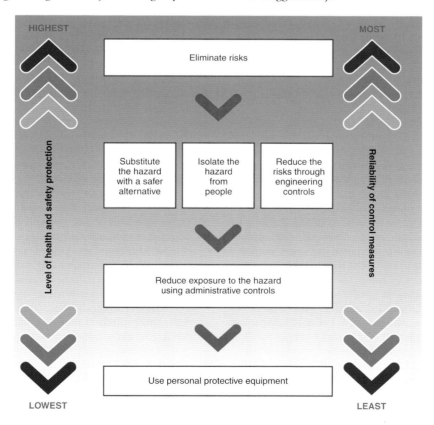

FIG. 5.8 The hierarchy of control measures. (Source: Safe Work Australia. (2018a). *The model Code of Practice: how to manage work health and safety risks*. 4.1, Figure 2.)

The following section provides a description of each of these workplace hazards and discusses the recommended practices for perioperative nurses to manage the risk of harm.

Manual Handling

As the average age of the health workforce increases, so too does the range of work- and age-related challenges (McCarthy, Wills, & Crowley, 2018). In Australia, there are almost as many nurses in the 25- to 45-year age group (enrolled and registered nurses combined) as there are in the 45 years and over age group (Nursing and Midwifery Board of Australia [NMBA], 2018a). National WH&S data show that the likelihood of workplace injuries also increases with age. For example, Australian data for the period from 2012 to 2016 show that the highest frequency rate for serious injury or illness in the healthcare and social assistance industry was in the age group 55–64 years (Safe Work Australia, 2018b). Nearly half of the work-related injuries (43%) occurring in hospitals were described as muscular stress while either handling, lifting, carrying or putting down objects (Safe Work Australia, 2018b). Perioperative nurses are exposed to many high-risk manual handling activities, such as assisting in the transfer of patients on and off OR beds, holding patients' limbs while prepping and draping, standing for long periods of time, moving large and heavy equipment, and maintaining awkward positions while scrubbed (ACORN, 2020m).

Compliance with WH&S legislation and industry codes requires that healthcare facilities demonstrate and provide evidence that manual handling risks in the workplace are identified and minimised (Commonwealth of Australia, 2011). Studies of the physical demands of the nursing workforce have found that keeping a personal level of health and fitness may help prevent workplace injuries (McCarthy, Wills, & Crowley, 2018). Training in manual handling techniques, plus having the specialised equipment available and prepared for each patient's needs, may also reduce the risk of workplace injuries and are important aspects of safe patient handling (Australian Nursing and Midwifery Federation [ANMF], 2018a; Smith, 2019). Recommended practices for perioperative nurses require that activities such as patient transfers and positioning are conducted by a team of people working in a coordinated manner to ensure everyone's safety (ACORN, 2020m). Devices such as slide sheets, patient transfer boards and air-assisted lateral transfer devices are also recommended when transferring patients (ACORN, 2020m). (See Chapter 9 for further information on patient positioning and the obese patient.) In addition, Australia and New Zealand have set a maximum weight restriction of 7 kg for instrument crates (Safe Work Australia, 2011; Standards Australia, 2014.)

Electrical Equipment

Australian and New Zealand healthcare facilities are guided by the same standard on the safe use of electricity in patient care areas (Standards Australia, 2004). All electrical equipment must be checked by the facility's biomedical engineering department prior to installation and thereafter at regular intervals to ensure safe function and compliance with standards. It is a recommended practice for perioperative nurses to check each piece of electrical equipment, including inspecting electrical cords for any damage prior to use to ensure correct functioning and patient safety (ACORN, 2020n). It is the responsibility of all staff to remove faulty equipment from use immediately (Ministry of Health, NSW, 2018a; South Eastern Sydney Local Health District [SESLHD], 2017).

The large amount of electrical equipment used in the OR places both staff and patients at potential risk of electrocution should equipment become faulty or be mishandled by staff. However, a range of safety features are incorporated into the design of ORs to reduce this risk. These include devices such as line-isolation monitoring (LIM) panels and, within each OR, residual current devices (RCD), which indicate faulty equipment or leakage of electrical current by initiating an audible alarm. In addition, an electrical fault will activate warning lights on the LIM panel and initiate the associated circuit breakers, subsequently interrupting the electrical supply to the RCD. Extension cords are not used within ORs owing to the risk of accidental dislodgement and because poor placement of these cords may present a trip hazard for staff (Standards Australia, 2004).

There are two main types of electrical shock against which staff and patients must be protected:

- *Macroshock.* This occurs when the body inadvertently becomes a conductor of electrical current when in contact with faulty equipment or leakage of current occurs. A person experiencing macroshock may exhibit muscle contractions, breathing difficulties and extreme pain. Normally, the skin provides resistance to electrical current; however, during surgical procedures this protection may be breached by the application of electrocardiograph (ECG) monitoring pads and/or electroconductive gel. Ventricular fibrillation may occur as a result of the shock, depending on the part of the body in contact with the current and the magnitude of the current. Line-isolation monitors are the first line of defence against macroshock, and areas with this protection are termed 'body protected', using the symbol shown in Fig. 5.9

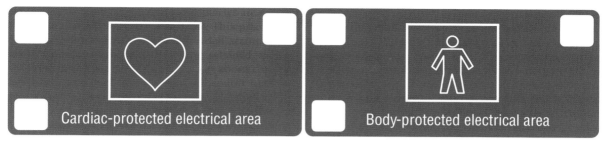

FIG. 5.9 Signage used to denote body- and cardiac-protected electrical areas.

(Standards Australia, 2004). Macroshock is the most common type of electrical shock.

- *Microshock.* In procedures where arterial catheters, pacing wires or other devices have direct connection to the heart, there is danger of a microshock, which may cause a fatal ventricular fibrillation. Only very small amounts of electrical current are needed to induce fibrillation when it is transmitted directly to myocardial tissue and there may be no external signs that the patient has suffered microshock. The line-isolation monitors that protect against macroshock incorporate supplementary special earthing devices, which alert staff to current leakage well below the level that would cause microshock (Standards Australia, 2004). Areas that incorporate these special earthing devices are termed 'cardiac protected' and are identified using the symbol shown in Fig. 5.9.

Electrosurgery

The perioperative environment includes a range of electrosurgical equipment that converts energy from a high-frequency electrical current into heat that can cut and cauterise tissue. All of these devices have the potential to interfere with implantable devices, cause thermal injuries, produce harmful surgical plume and ignite fires (Jones, Black, Robinson, & Jones, 2019), imposing risks for patients as well as members of the perioperative team. The **electrosurgical unit** (ESU, or diathermy machine) is a commonly used electrical device within the OR. The ESU generates an electrical current at extremely high frequency, which cuts or coagulates tissue (as well as variations of the latter, such as tissue desiccation or fulguration), controlling blood loss in the surgical field (Aminimoghaddam, Pahlevani, & Kazemi, 2018; Golpaygani, Movahedi, & Reza, 2016). There are two main types of electrosurgery: monopolar and bipolar. Recommended practices for electrosurgery are described in more detail with other examples of surgical interventions in Chapter 10.

Hazards of electrosurgery. There is a risk of thermal injuries such as burns or electrocution during electrosurgery if the patient return electrode has insufficient contact with the patient's skin (Golpaygani et al., 2016). If the electrical current finds an alternative pathway back to earth, for example through faulty leads, electrodes or cables, or some other contact of the patient's skin with metal (e.g. a hand touching the frame of the operating table), the patient may suffer thermal injuries (Bifulco et al., 2013). Wet drapes on the surgical field can also present a hazardous situation when electrosurgical devices or lasers are in use. Any damage to the patient's skin must be treated, reported, documented and investigated (ACORN, 2020n; NMBA, 2018b). Devices that may have caused patient harm must be removed from use and checked by a biomedical engineer (SESLHD, 2017).

Burns to surgical or nursing staff may also occur if the current used finds an alternative pathway back to the ESU (e.g. through a hole in the glove of the person applying the active electrode, or in cases where the insulation on endoscopic forceps is faulty). All ESUs have inbuilt alarm systems to disable faulty equipment and alert staff to situations where the patient return electrode has become detached from the patient (Standards Australia, 2004) (see also Chapter 10). Surgical plume is another hazard associated with electrosurgery, and plume evacuation equipment that is compatible with the surgical procedure and instrumentation should always be used during surgery (ACORN, 2020o). The specific occupational exposure hazards of surgical plume are discussed below.

Surgical lasers

The term **laser** is an acronym for 'light amplification by stimulated emission of radiation'. Laser is a unique form of light energy that is concentrated into a narrow beam of a single wavelength, with specific characteristics that allow it to cut, coagulate, vaporise or disrupt tissue. The effects of the laser on tissue depend on its wavelength; its absorption in water, melanin or haemoglobin; power output, focal length and size of the beam; as well as the type of device used to deliver the energy to the surgical field. Laser beams can travel over distance, in one single direction, sometimes beyond the intended operative site – with the potential to cause injury to the patient and members of the perioperative team. The nature of the potential hazards and the degree of risk for exposure to the hazards determine what control measures are necessary (ARPANSA, n.d.a).

Laser hazard classifications are found in the International Electrotechnical Commission (IEC, 2017) standards and have been adopted by Australian/New Zealand standards (Standards Australia, 2018a) and ARPANSA (2015).

Three different classes of laser are suitable for use within healthcare facilities: Class 1, Class 3b and Class 4.

- Class 1 lasers generally emit very low powers and require no specific control measures. These lasers are used for physiotherapy.
- Class 3b lasers are also considered low power; however, the laser outputs are high enough to require control measures. These lasers are used for ophthalmology and dermatology.
- Class 4 lasers are high powered and require a full range of control measures. These lasers are used in many different surgical specialties, including gynaecology, neurosurgery and plastic, cardiothoracic, ENT and otorhinolaryngology, orthopaedic, general, urology and laparoscopic surgery (Khalkhal, Rezaei-Tavirani, Zali, & Akbari, 2019).

Laser surgery generates a number of potential hazards and risks of exposure to anyone present in the OR. Compliance with facility policies, which should reflect international and national standards and general WH&S precautions, can minimise the risks of exposure for personnel (Ministry of Health, NSW, 2015; Smalley, 2011).

Surgical laser safety. Class 3b and 4 lasers have the potential to cause injury to the patient and anyone present in the room where these lasers will be used. Laser safety is the responsibility of everyone in the OR (ACORN, 2020p). Additionally, it is the specific responsibility of the laser safety officer (LSO) to ensure that all safety measures are in place and that the clinicians involved with the use, storage and management of lasers are able to comply with evidence-based standards of practice so as to minimise the risk of harm (Smalley, 2011; Standards Australia, 2011a, 2011b). The LSO is also required to conduct a hazard assessment of each laser prior to its first use. Once completed, the LSO will determine which control measures need to be followed

when the laser is required for clinical use. Routinely, the entire room will be considered a laser hazard area and, while the laser is in use, everyone in that room will need to adhere to the laser safety procedures (ACORN, 2020p). Health facility laser safety policies and procedures should also refer to the required hazard control measures: administrative controls, engineering controls and procedural controls (Standards Australia, 2011a).

- **Administrative controls** are the foundation for laser safety. These controls include:
  - appointment of a laser safety officer LSO and deputy LSO
  - requirements for initial and continuing education and training
  - documentation of laser use
  - criteria for laser user credentialling and certification
  - establishment of a laser safety committee to oversee audit processes, equipment selection, installation, service and maintenance. Another important role for the committee is verification that only personnel who have completed a recognised laser safety course and are familiar with the features, operation and specific safety requirements should be allowed to operate the laser. Surgeons wishing to use lasers must first complete all of the safety training and education required by the standards and any other as determined by local facility policy, to be confirmed as a qualified and approved laser user. Surgical registrars may operate lasers only under the direct supervision of surgeon who is a qualified and approved laser user. Medical and nursing staff expecting to work in rooms where lasers will be used must first complete the required safety training and education (Smalley, 2011; Standards Australia, 2011b).
- **Engineering controls** are safety features built in by the manufacturer. These features control the laser energy and include:
  - the standby and ready switches
  - the emergency stop button
  - mechanical and electrical shutters
  - the cover guard over the footswitch.
- **Procedural controls** are the safety practices that must be adhered to by all laser surgery team members. These controls include:
  - a secure laser key system
  - discussing the use of laser during team 'Time Out'
  - a preoperative equipment set-up and testing checklist
  - surgical plume management
  - the use of laser protective eyewear (Fig. 5.10)
  - danger signage indicating the class of laser in use and safety requirements for protective eyewear

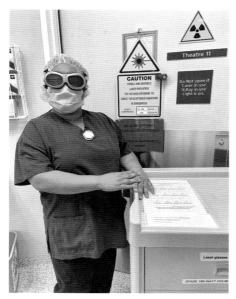

FIG. 5.10 Warning signs and laser protective eyewear outside the door to the controlled area. (Source: Taken by B. Lockwood).

posted on all doors with access into the laser room; this signage aims to control access into a designated nominal ocular hazard area (NOHA) (Standards Australia, 2018a)

- window barriers suitable for the laser wavelength to be used
- appropriate measures for fire prevention and emergency response
- patient protection.

There is a risk of damage to tissue, burns, fire, or eye injury caused by reflection of the laser beam off of a specular surface (instruments or curved tissue planes). This risk is minimised by using non-reflective instrumentation in the laser's path or close to the tissue being treated. Fibre breakage within the equipment can also result in damage from stray or reflected laser beams. Instrument nurses should examine fibreoptic cables and delivery systems prior to handing them off to be connected to the laser system, in order to verify their integrity (Standards Australia, 2011b). Health facility laser safety procedures should highlight the need for ongoing education for laser safety staff (Smalley, 2011) and must identify the endorsed laser-safe practices that align with the standards (Standards Australia, 2011b).

Surgical plume

Surgical plume is produced when biological tissue is disrupted or vaporised by energy-based surgical equipment such as electrosurgical and ultrasonic devices, lasers (Smalley, 2019; Tan & Russell, 2017) and high-speed surgical drills and saws (Ministry of Health, NSW, 2015). Surgical plume is made up of 95% water (steam) and 5% cellular debris, and includes visible and non-visible particles (Ministry of Health, NSW, 2015). This cellular debris has been shown to contain a number of dangerous toxins and gases, chemicals, carcinogens, blood and tissue particles, bacteria and viruses (Addley & Quinn, 2019; Harkavy & Novak, 2014; Ministry of Health, NSW, 2015). All personnel in the OR are at risk of exposure to the hazards of surgical plume inhalation (Brandon & LeRoy Young, 1997).

Numerous studies conducted over the past four decades have identified the potential diseases caused by exposure to surgical plume (Baggish, Poiesz, Joret, Williamson, & Refai, 1991; Lewin, Brauer, & Ostad, 2011; Rioux, Garland, Webster, & Reardon, 2013; Sawchuk, Weber, Lowy, & Dzubow, 1989), with increasing evidence showing a link between surgical plume exposure and resultant disease (Box 5.2 and Fig. 5.11). Furthermore, a small percentage of the population may carry the human papilloma virus (HPV) in their tissues without symptoms (Braggish et al., 1991; Garden et al., 1988; Neumann, Cavalar, Rody, Friemert, & Beyer, 2018). Since HPV is known to transmit in surgical plume, it is important to protect against this risk during all surgical procedures, regardless of the patient's HPV status. These risks may apply to other viruses and there are concerns for the potential of viral transmission of SARS-CoV-2, which causes COVID-19 from inhaled surgical plume (Pavlinec & Su, 2020; Vourtzoumis, Alkhamesi, Elnahas, Hawel, & Schlachta, 2020).

Surgical plume evacuation units extract, capture and filter the plume via an array of systems, each designed to be compatible with a variety of surgical procedures and instrumentation (see Chapter 10). A dedicated plume evacuation system that meets the latest International Organization for Standardization (ISO) standards or AS/NZS standards contributes to the first line of defence against occupational exposure to surgical plume. Surgical face masks are not designed to protect against the specific hazards of surgical plume and the ultrafine particles it contains; hence international or national standards make no recommendations about the use of surgical face masks as protection against surgical plume.

Prevention of fires or explosions

While reports of fires involving patients in Australasian hospitals are infrequent, these incidents are catastrophic (Waitemata District Health Board [WDHB], 2002) and have resulted in patient deaths when the patient's airway was involved (Victorian Surgical Consultative Council

BOX 5.2
International Council on Surgical Plume

The Australian College of Perioperative Nurses (ACORN) is a founding member of the International Council on Surgical Plume (ICSP), a not-for-profit clinical advocacy organisation established in 2015 to eliminate surgical plume from the perioperative environment (Smalley & Cubitt, 2015). The Perioperative Nurses College of the New Zealand Nurses Organisation (PNC NZNO) is also a member of ICSP, along with the Association of periOperative Registered Nurses (AORN), the Californian Nurses Association and the International Federation of Perioperative Nurses (IFPN). The ICSP has a strong commitment to eliminating surgical plume, and works towards this goal by:

- working with government leaders and agencies
- advocating for regulatory mandates for plume-free environments
- encouraging organisations worldwide to adopt standards, guidelines and policies
- partnering with international workplace health and safety agencies which manage workplace risks.
  ICSP aims to provide education on the hazards of surgical plume, disseminate literature and research findings and support the development of clinically relevant international standards. To learn more about the ICSP, visit https://www.plumecouncil.com.

(Source: International Council on Surgical Plume website https://www.plumecouncil.com.)

[VSCC], 2014). In the US, the number of serious fire-related incidents occurring in perioperative environments annually is decreasing (Burley, Arnold, Finley, Deutsch, & Treadwell, 2018; Ehrenwerth, 2019). The Emergency Care Research Institute (ECRI) estimated that fewer than 100 OR fires occurred in 2018, while up to 240 OR fires occurred in 2012 (Ehrenwerth, 2019). The risks of fire and explosion are high in the perioperative environment because oxygen and other flammable gases are in abundant supply (Box 5.3). Many flammable materials such as drapes, sponges and packaging are present and provide fuel for a fire, or have the potential to be ignited by electrosurgical or laser equipment in use (Jones et al., 2019; Rodger, 2020). Also, when alcoholic skin preparations or bone cement are in use, special care must be taken, as these are fire accelerants (Blazquez & Thorn, 2010; Jones et al., 2017). When skin preparations are in use, the perioperative nurses must ensure that the prepared operative area is allowed to dry for the length of time recommended by the manufacturer before the team applies the drapes (ACORN, 2020q). The nurse's specific attention is also required to ensure that the skin preparation does not accumulate in pools, or soak into the patient's hair or the surrounding padding (ACORN, 2020q; WDHB, 2002). Although rare, the potential exists for explosion when diathermy is used on hollow organs containing flammable gases, such as the bowel (Blazquez & Thorn, 2010; Standards Australia, 2004).

Acetonitrile furfural (aldehyde) Acetylene hexadecanoic acid Acroloin hydrogen cyanide Acrylonitrile indole (amine) Alkyl benzene isobutene	Benzaldeyde methane Benzene 3_methyl butenal (aldehyde) Benonitrile 6_methyl indole (amine) Butadiene 4-methyl phenol Butene 2-methyl propanol (aldehyde) 3-butenenitrile methyl pyrazine
Surgical plume	
Carbon monoxide phenol Creosol propene 1-decene (hydrocarbon) 2-propylene nitrile 2,3-dihydro indene pyridine	Ethane pyrrole (amine) Ethene styrene Ethylene toluene (hydrocarbon) Ethyl benzene 1-undecene (hydrocarbon) Ethynyl benzene xylene Formaldehyde

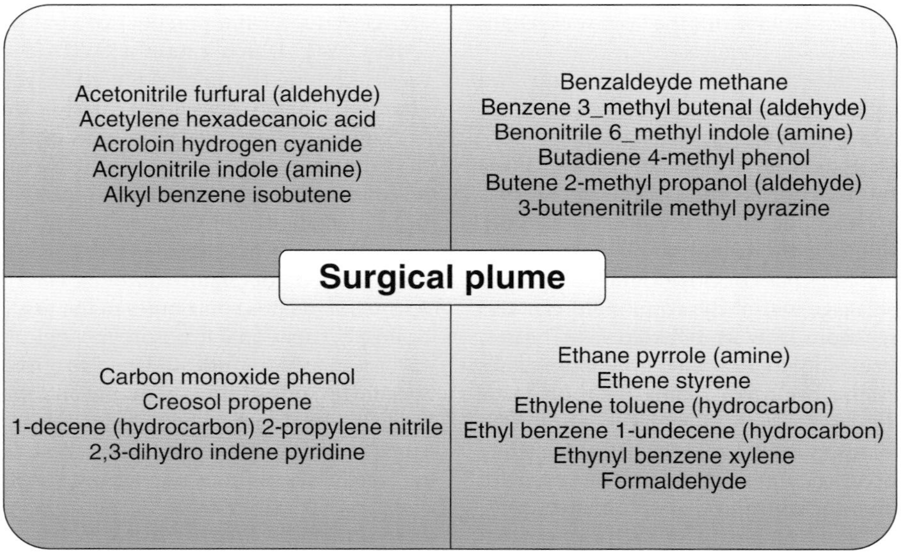

FIG. 5.11 Chemicals identified in surgical plume. (Source: Based on Hill, D., O'Neill, J., Powell, R., & Oliver, D. (2012) Surgical smoke – a health hazard in the operating theatre. A study to quantify exposure and a survey of the use of smoke extractor systems in UK plastic surgery units. *Journal of Plastic, Reconstructive and Aesthetic Surgery*, 65(7), Fig. 1.)

BOX 5.3
Fires in the Perioperative Environment

The following equipment and materials used in the perioperative environment are recognised as potential elements of the fire triangle (Jones et al., 2019):

Ignition Source	Oxidisers	Fuels
Electrosurgical devices	Oxygen Nitrous oxide	The OR environment:
Lasers		Fluids: alcohol-based skin preps and tissue glues
Fibreoptic light sources		Materials: endotracheal tubes (ETT), laryngeal masks, nasal canulae, linen, drapes gauzes and dressings
Power tools		The patient: hair and other tissues, intestinal gases

The Victorian Surgical Consultative Council (VSCC) reported the most common scenarios for airway fires are as follows:

Tracheostomy. When electrosurgery (ignition) is used for the tracheal incision and there is a high oxygen saturation (oxidiser), the ETT or vaporised tissue can become the fuel for an airway fire.

Tonsillectomy. During electrosurgery (ignition), when there is a high oxygen leak (oxidiser), the mask or uncuffed ETT (fuel) may be ignited with other dry materials such as packs, gauze or drapes (fuel) (VSCC, 2014).

The following links provide access to fire safety and risk assessment resources including posters, videos, interviews and re-enactments, reports and news media on catastrophic fires, which may be useful continuing education resources for those working in perioperative environments:

American Association of Nurse Anesthetists (AANA). (2020). Surgical fires [webpage] https://www.aana.com/practice/clinical-practice-resources/surgical-firesb

Anesthesia Patient Safety Foundation (APSF). (n.d.). Operating room fire safety video: prevention and management of operating room fires [webpage]. https://www.apsf.org/videos/or-fire-safety-video/

Association of periOperative Room Nurses (AORN). (2020). Fire safety tool kit [webpage] https://www.aorn.org/guidelines/clinical-resources/tool-kits/fire-safety-tool-kit

Council on Surgical and Perioperative Safety (CSPS). (2017). Resources and tools for preventing surgical fires [webpage] https://www.cspsteam.org/resources-and-tools-for-preventing-surgical-fires

Infonews.co.nz (2011). Fire evacuation in operating theatre [webpage] https://infonews.co.nz/news.cfm?id=70697

This news site reviews a DVD called *I smell smoke*, which re-enacts the events surrounding an OR fire in New Zealand that started in the plantroom above the operating theatres. The air-handling system collected the smoke and directed it into the theatre below, where a patient was undergoing laparoscopic surgery. It took two teams 10 minutes to evacuate the patient without serious injury; however, the staff were affected by smoke inhalation.

Waitemata District Health Board (2002). Report into the operating theatre fire accident 17 August 2002, Waitakere Hospital. https://www.medsafe.govt.nz/downloads/alertWaitemata.pdf.

Recommended practices require that nurses must position any devices with the potential to ignite flammable or combustible substances in a holster or place such devices in 'stand-by' mode so as to minimise the risk of inadvertent activation (ACORN, 2020q).

Medical and safety protocols must also be established for preparation and management of the patient's airway whenever a laser or ESU device is used in the presence of an endotracheal (ET) tube (Akhtar, Ansar, Baig, & Abbas, 2016; Roy & Smith, 2019). Everyone in the OR must be familiar with emergency response to this type of fire, as patients can suffer serious or mortal injury in a matter of minutes (Jones et al., 2019; Rodger, 2020). The protocol should be developed by anaesthetists, surgeons and perioperative nurses, and should include the selection of the

appropriate ET tube, levels of gases to be used, counting and packing of sponges around an inflated cuff to prevent an oxygen leak, instruments and medications needed, and a clear set of steps to take in case of fire (see also Box 5.3).

Storage of supplies and engineering controls are also important factors to consider in the perioperative environment (Standards Australia, 2004) as they can mitigate the risk of fire and/or explosion. For example, it is important to follow up and identify bulk storage limits of flammable/combustible substances and correlate these to the size of storage area. When the identified capacity exceeds these limits, a designated flameproof cabinet is required (Standards Australia, 2004). Likewise, gas cylinders or bottles, which are recognised as fire accelerants, require monitoring and strict controls. In compliance with Australian Standard 2030.1-2009 and guidelines, gas bottles are required to be stored vertically and secured within a well-ventilated area (British Oxygen Company [BOC], 2012). Furthermore, BOC (2012) specifies that gas cylinders higher than waist height should be transported on a cylinder trolley. Full and empty gas cylinders must be stored separately to avoid confusion (BOC, 2012).

PATIENT SCENARIOS

SCENARIO 5.2: FIRE IN THE OR

Consider the components of the fire triangle, which may be present in the OR.

> **Critical Thinking Question**
>
> - Identify the potential risks for a fire igniting while Mr Collins is in the OR undergoing his TKR surgery. Refer to the resources listed in Box 5.3 including the fire triangle and the fire risk assessment tool (Jones et al., 2019) when preparing your answer.

Sensitivities and Allergic Reactions

All healthcare workers can expect to encounter patients with sensitivities or allergic reactions to a range of common foods such as eggs and gluten, and to some common medications such as antibiotics, non-steroidal anti-inflammatory drugs (NSAIDs) and analgesics, neuromuscular blocking agents, or dyes and radio-contrast media, as well as blood and blood products. Other materials commonly used in hospitals such as natural rubber latex, some chemicals and skin-cleansing products such as chlorhexidine also contain potential allergens (Simons et al., 2015). An essential component of the patient's health record is the medical history of allergies, which should be checked for recency and accuracy during every admission, including a description of the previous reaction (see also Chapter 7 for pre-admission processes).

It is not only patients with sensitivities and allergic reactions to such products; individual healthcare workers are also susceptible and should be aware of the risks of exposure for themselves or for their colleagues. Many of these products and substances are used therapeutically in the perioperative environment, so it is important for perioperative nurses to use a risk management approach and to recognise the early signs and symptoms of sensitivities and allergic reactions that may develop. Guidelines published by the World Allergy Organization (WAO) report a continuing increase in hospital admissions due to anaphylaxis (Simons et al., 2015), so perioperative nurses should also understand the management of anaphylaxis. The following section focuses on the management of risks associated with latex and chlorhexidine, while Chapter 8 describes the management of anaphylaxis.

Latex

Latex is the milky-white sap produced by the rubber tree (*Hevea brasiliensis*). This natural product is manufactured under heat with the addition of chemicals and preservatives. One such additive is cornstarch powder, used as a dry lubricant to prevent the rubber from sticking to itself (Australasian Society of Clinical Immunology and Allergy [ASCIA], 2019a). Latex is a component of many common products, including elastic bands, rubber toys, teats on baby bottles and dummies, clothing, balloons and condoms. Historically, latex has also been a component in the manufacture of many products used in healthcare, including surgical gloves, bandages, drains, tubing and catheters (Hohler, 2015). It is now well recognised that the cumulative effect of allergens present within latex products predisposes patients and healthcare workers to a latex sensitivity or allergy, and the range and use of latex products in healthcare has consequently decreased (ASCIA, 2019a). International standards now require clear labelling of products containing latex (Hohler, 2015), it is a recommended practice for patients to be risk assessed, and healthcare workers must be prepared to respond to signs of reaction promptly and appropriately (ACORN, 2020r).

Types of allergic reactions to latex. There are three types of reactions listed below in order of severity:

1. *Immediate allergic reaction to latex (Type I).* This is the most serious allergic reaction. It is also known as an IgE antibody-mediated reaction, which occurs when a latex-sensitive person comes into contact with latex products or inhales latex proteins. Reactions are characterised by the body's release of histamine, which is responsible for a range of symptoms, including itching, tears or runny eyes and nose (allergic rhinitis or hay fever), hives and angioedema (swelling). Severe respiratory distress and a sudden drop in blood pressure are signs of anaphylaxis which may develop when latex is absorbed internally via moist mucous membranes, such as those in oral or nasal cavities, the genitourinary tract, vagina or rectum.

2. *Allergic contact dermatitis (Type IV).* This is the most common immune allergic reaction to latex. Unlike a Type I reaction, which is immediate, this is a delayed-onset hypersensitivity which develops 6–48 hours after

exposure to latex. Allergic contact dermatitis generally presents as an inflammatory reaction such as a rash, which may be rough and scaly or moist and weeping. Early recognition of this reaction is an important step in reducing the person's exposure to the allergen and can minimise the risk of a more serious Type I reaction.

3. *Irritant dermatitis (contact dermatitis).* This is the most common response to latex exposure. While the symptoms are similar in appearance to allergic contact dermatitis, irritant dermatitis is not a true allergic reaction. It develops as a localised area of irritation, which may present as redness, dryness, scaling, blistering or cracking. These symptoms may be exacerbated by sweating, glove irritation or frequent hand washing. As with all responses, early recognition can reduce the person's exposure to the specific irritant and this may prevent the person from going on to develop a latex allergy (ASCIA, 2019a).

(See also Box 5.4 and Feature box 5.2.)

Chlorhexidine

Chlorhexidine is a commonly used antiseptic in healthcare settings because of its persistent effect and broad-spectrum efficacy (Rose, Garcez, Savic, & Garvey, 2019). As chlorhexidine's usage has increased in recent years, so too have the reports of allergies associated with its use (ANZCA, 2016), with the first case being reported in 1989 (Mertes et al., 2019).

Common products which may contain chlorhexidine include:

- surface sprays and cleaning solutions
- antiseptic skin wipes
- topical skin antiseptic fluids used on wounds or as part of preoperative skin antisepsis
- lubricants and gels used on mucous membranes (e.g. urethral catheterisation, dental procedures)
- surgical dressings and mesh
- hidden impregnated coatings on devices such as urethral catheters and central venous catheters (CVC).

The most common cause of reaction in patients is the exposure on mucosal surfaces, which is associated with chlorhexidine-impregnated urethral catheters or chlorhexidine lubricants such as lubricant jelly (ASCIA, 2019b; Rose et al., 2019). The risk of allergic reaction to chlorhexidine applies not only to patients (Feature box 5.3), but also to perioperative nurses and other healthcare workers.

The potential source of exposure for perioperative nurses is through hand disinfectants and soaps containing chlorhexidine, which can cause localised contact dermatitis and hives or respiratory symptoms such as rhinitis, sneezing or asthma. Labelling on some of these antiseptic products may not state the full word 'chlorhexidine', or may use abbreviations such as CHG (e.g. in dressings) or AGB (e.g. on vascular devices) (ASCIA, 2019b). Currently, there is no designated symbol for chlorhexidine and no product registry, so perioperative nurses should always make time for careful examination of the product before selecting it for use. If perioperative nurses do have a reaction, they should have further tests to avoid repeated unnecessary exposure and possible future more severe reactions (Rose et al., 2019).

BOX 5.4
Precautions for Latex-sensitive Staff

The Australasian Society of Clinical Immunology and Allergy (ASCIA) is the peak professional body of clinical immunology and allergy in Australia and New Zealand. ASCIA recommends a common-sense approach by healthcare workers, including the following practices to minimise the risk of latex sensitisation in the course of their employment:

- Use appropriate work practices to reduce the chance of latex reactions.
- Use appropriate barrier protection such as wearing synthetic gloves when handling infectious material. If you choose to wear latex gloves:
  - Use powder-free gloves with reduced protein content: such gloves reduce exposures to latex protein and thus reduce the risk of latex allergy (note that symptoms may still occur in some workers).
  - Do not use oil-based hand creams or lotions unless they have been shown to reduce latex problems.

- Wash hands and dry thoroughly after removing latex gloves.
- Take advantage of all latex allergy education and training provided by your employer and learn to recognise the symptoms of latex allergy (refer to the ASCIA eTraining portal https://etraininghp.ascia.org.au).
- If you develop symptoms, avoid direct contact with latex products and see a physician experienced in latex allergy. Carefully follow your physician's instructions for dealing with allergic reactions to latex.
- If you are latex sensitive or have tested positive for an allergy to latex, avoid contact with latex products, avoid areas where you might inhale powder from latex gloves worn by others, tell your employer that you have a latex allergy and wear a medic-alert bracelet. It must be stressed that it is best to treat early to prevent the sensitisation to latex becoming too severe. See also Types of allergic reactions to latex.

(Source: Australasian Society of Clinical Immunology and Allergy. (2010a). ASCIA latex allergic information for new employees [webpage].)

FEATURE BOX 5.2
Precautions for Latex-sensitive Patients

Perioperative patients with latex sensitivity must be cared for in an environment free from contact with latex products. The growing range and wider availability of latex-free products, as well as improved labelling, have made it easier for operating suites to source and use latex-free products, supplies and equipment in latex-free environments.

General requirements for caring for the latex-sensitive patient are:

- Use synthetic gloves.
- Where required, perioperative staff should remove or replace any items of attire that may contain latex (e.g. some elastics contain latex).
- Discuss the patient's latex sensitivity and any required practice changes in all team briefings.
- Place signs on external doors denoting a latex-free environment.
- Protect the patient from anything that may contain latex (e.g. arm boards and OR tables, tourniquet cuffs or other equipment that may contain latex should be fully covered to prevent direct contact with the patient).

In facilities where latex products may still be in use, operating suites should have designated latex-free kits containing all the equipment necessary to care for a latex-sensitive patient. Additional requirements in ORs where powdered latex gloves are used:

- Schedule the latex-sensitive patient first on the list.
- Ensure the OR has been free of powdered latex gloves for at least 3 hours before the patient enters.
- Use this time to wash down all surfaces including furniture and equipment to remove any latex powder.
- Use products from the latex-free kit.
- Prevent inadvertent latex powder contamination from adjacent rooms.
- Limit the movement of staff who may have been in contact with powdered latex gloves.
- The patient may need to be transferred directly to the OR for anaesthetic induction and remain for postoperative recovery.
- Set up aseptic fields within the confines of the OR (ASCIA, 2010b).

PATIENT SCENARIOS

SCENARIO 5.3: SENSITIVITIES AND ALLERGIC REACTIONS

Mrs Patricia Peterson has just been transferred into the anaesthetic room from the holding bay. Her medical history includes a possible sensitivity to chlorhexidine. Thinking about your workplace now, investigate the systems that are in place to alert perioperative team members to patients with chlorhexidine sensitivities/allergies.

Critical Thinking Questions

- Identify the nursing actions which can minimise the risks for Mrs Peterson while she is in the department, including:
  - preparation of the environment by EN Marcus Macedo in the anaesthetic room
  - team communications and clinical handover between RN Rob Cohen and RN Jenny Sang (in PACU)
- Identify any additional practices that would be required to mitigate the risks for Mrs Peterson if her sensitivity were to latex instead of chlorhexidine.

Occupational Exposures

This section discusses the recommended practices for perioperative nurses to manage the risk of harm from occupational exposures in the perioperative environment. Potential exposures include anaesthetic waste gases, radiation, surgical products, cytotoxic substances and chemicals. This section also includes occupational exposure to blood and body substances and the management of splashes and sharps injuries (see Chapter 6 for more information on biohazards).

Waste anaesthetic gases

The anaesthetic team is responsible for the safe management of all wastes produced during the anaesthetic episode, including the emission of anaesthetic gases (ACORN, 2020s). Vapours and gases emitted from anaesthetic equipment or from anaesthetic techniques may accumulate in the perioperative environment when anaesthetic gas-scavenging systems are not in use or not used correctly (Lucio, Braz, do Nascimento Jr, Braz, & Braz, 2018). The potential risks for healthcare workers from exposure to accumulated waste anaesthetic gases (WAGs) have been studied since Vaisman's seminal paper was published in 1967 (Boiano & Steege, 2016; Lucio

---

FEATURE BOX 5.3
Precautions for Patients With a Known Allergy to Chlorhexidine

The most common source of exposure for patients is via mucosal surfaces associated with chlorhexidine-impregnated urethral catheters or chlorhexidine lubricants (Rose et al., 2019). Other mucosal areas such as the rectum, vagina, ophthalmic region or oral cavity are also potential sources of chlorhexidine entry into the body's system. Because the rate of chlorhexidine absorption through mucosal tissue is slow, it may not be discovered as the source of the allergic reaction. It takes time for chlorhexidine to reach the vascular system, and often the healthcare team mistakenly identifies systemic administration of a drug as the likely trigger to the allergic reaction (Rose et al., 2019).

Signs and symptoms of a chlorhexidine allergic reaction can vary from a mild skin irritation to anaphylaxis. Patients who experience itching, hives and/or swelling are showing signs of histamine release as part of an immediate reaction to chlorhexidine (ASCIA, 2019b). Typically, patients who experience a more severe reaction or anaphylaxis will have difficulty breathing, may feel dizzy and may show signs of hypotension, suggestive of an imminent systemic collapse (ASCIA, 2019b). While anaphylaxis is rare, the growing number of reactions reported worldwide suggests chlorhexidine has become one of the most common allergens in the perioperative environment (Rose et al., 2019). In light of this, perioperative nurses should always consider chlorhexidine as the potential trigger when a patient has an allergic reaction.

The recommended practices for the patient's perioperative journey begin with risk assessment. This should be undertaken during preoperative screening for any patient suspected to have any level of chlorhexidine allergy (see also Chapter 7). If required, allergy testing should be performed prior to hospital admission.

The following practices are recommended for patients with a known allergy to chlorhexidine:

- Documentation – chlorhexidine allergy should be documented in the patient's health record and included in clinical handover by all healthcare workers caring for that patient.
- Surgical safety – chlorhexidine allergy and potential supportive therapies should be discussed, and alternative products should be confirmed for use.
- Alerts – signage should be placed on each entry door to the OR. All personnel should be alert for signs of reaction to chlorhexidine and able to implement supportive therapy or resuscitation in the event of anaphylaxis.
- Product selection – any products labelled with chlorhexidine or considered likely to have chlorhexidine as an ingredient should be avoided and an alternative product sourced.
- Education – the patient should be educated to avoid chlorhexidine for life and to notify anyone looking after them of their allergy status. In the perioperative setting, all team members have this responsibility as the patient advocate, especially when the patient is unconscious.

(ANZCA, 2016; ASCIA, 2019b; Rose et al., 2019)

---

et al., 2018). More recent studies have focused on a number of settings including the OR (Kapoor, 2017), as well as the PACU (Hiller, Altamirano, Cai, Tran, & Williams, 2015), where patients emerge from anaesthesia and continue to exhale these gases (Clifford, 2014).

One of the most effective methods to remove WAGs from the environment is the scavenging of gases at their point of origin, and such scavenging systems are required by professional colleges and national standards (ANZCA, 2014; Standards Australia, 2005). Additional practices to manage WAGs and reduce the risk of staff exposure include effective air-handling systems in the OR, protocols for staff to identify and correct leaks within the anaesthetic equipment (including masks, airways, circuits and machines) and compliance with a regular maintenance program for anaesthetic equipment (Smith, 2010).

Radiation
The use of ionising radiation is an integral diagnostic and/or therapeutic component of modern healthcare.

This technology has the ability to improve patient outcomes; however, perioperative nurses must also manage the risks for patients by providing additional shielding for adjacent areas of anatomy. The Australian Radiation Protection and Nuclear Safety Agency publishes industry codes and standards of practice for the use of ionising radiation, with the purpose of promoting **radiation safety** for the public and clinicians (ARPANSA, 2014, 2020). Each facility must ensure that its practices align with the legislative requirements for storage, use and monitoring of compliance with these codes and national standards (Queensland Government, 2010).

Perioperative staff exposure to ionising radiation has been increasing with advancements in surgical techniques and technology such as hybrid ORs (Schuetze et al., 2019). Some level of exposure may be unavoidable when image intensification (II) or mobile radiography units are used to check anatomical alignment or the position of equipment. Because the effects of ionising radiation are cumulative but cannot be seen or felt, a risk management approach with constant vigilance is required to minimise occupational exposure. The single most effective protection against exposure is avoidance (i.e. leaving the vicinity of the radiation source or increasing the distance from the source) (Spruce, 2017). If it is not possible to avoid exposure, then staff should use one or all of the defences against radiation: time, distance and shielding. Appropriate shielding can be achieved by standing behind mobile lead barriers or by donning the radiation PPE recommended by standards (State of NSW and Environment Protection Authority [EPA], 2018; Standards Australia, 2000), which includes gowns, thyroid and lower limb shields, goggles and gloves (Fig. 5.12).

When PPE such as a gown, shield or thyroid protector is removed, it should be hung on a special gown hanger or laid out flat to avoid folds that can crack the protective barrier and render it ineffective (Fig. 5.13). Protective equipment must undergo regular checks to ensure its integrity has been maintained (Standards Australia, 2000). Staff who work in proximity to ionising radiation devices are required to wear a monitoring device, such as a dose meter badge, that is regularly checked to monitor occupational exposure limits (ARPANSA, 2014). In addition, a

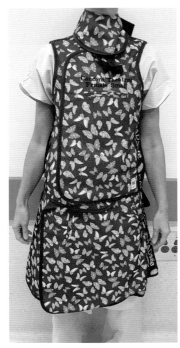

FIG. 5.12 Healthcare worker wearing X-ray protection. (Source: Reproduced with permission of Concord Repatriation General Hospital, Sydney.)

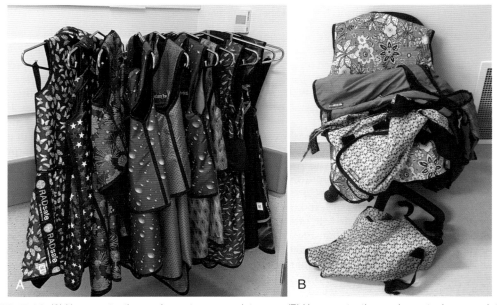

FIG. 5.13 (**A**) X-ray protective equipment – appropriate care. (**B**) X-ray protective equipment – inappropriate care. (Source: Reproduced with permission of Concord Repatriation Hospital.)

radiation warning sign must be posted at the entrance to rooms where radiation is used, and illuminating signs must be present at all entrances to rooms where fixed X-ray generators are housed (Queensland Government, 2010).

The intent of radiological PPE is to protect the clinician from radiation exposure; however, occupational-related injuries such as spinal and joint issues have also been attributed to the additional weight of wearing the lead gowns and protectors (Klein et al., 2009). Radiological PPE is evolving, and new designs include two weights: lead lined or a comparatively lightweight construction made of a composite material. It is always important to know the local requirements, as some states and territories do not support the use of lightweight PPE aprons when fluroscopy is used (ARPANSA, 2014).

Pregnancy should not prevent staff members working in the OR where radiation is used; however, appropriate protection and specific work practices must be applied. Employers are also required to consider the need for additional protection for the unborn child: *'The working conditions of a pregnant worker, after the declaration of pregnancy, should be as such to make it unlikely that the additional dose to the unborn child will exceed about 1 mSv during the remainder of pregnancy'* (ARPANSA, n.d.b).

Chemicals

Many chemicals are used prior to and during the provision of care within the OR. For example, detergents are used during environmental cleaning before and after surgical procedures, while enzymatic instrument cleaners, high-grade disinfectants and chemical sterilising products such as peracetic acid are used in the preparation and reprocessing of surgical instrumentation. Toxic chemicals and drugs such as bone cement and cytotoxic agents are adjunct therapies supporting the surgical intervention, while chemicals such as formaldehyde are used as fixatives for pathology specimens.

The most common route of exposure to chemicals is by inhalation (Monash University, 2019). In the perioperative environment, there are several other potential routes of exposure such as absorption via contact with exposed skin and splashes to unprotected mucosa, as well as injection and sharps injury. The following principles will help all members of the perioperative team to maintain a safe work environment and reduce the risk of exposure to hazards when handling chemical agents:

- Staff using chemicals and cytotoxic agents should be educated on safe use and handling, as well as management in the event of an accidental exposure, including where spill kits and other items required are stored.
- All staff should know where to access the safety data sheets (SDS), which describe the physical, chemical and toxicological properties and precautions for safe handling.
- All chemicals should be stored, used and disposed of according to the manufacturer's recommendations and state/territory or national guidelines.
- Pregnant staff can refer to container labels about the potential effects on the unborn child, including embryotoxic (toxic to the embryo), fetotoxic (toxic to the fetus) and teratogenic effects (induces developmental abnormalities in the fetus) (Monash University, 2017).
- Staff must don PPE to minimise exposure. Diligent use of PPE is effective in protecting staff from the potential risks associated with chemical agents in the perioperative environment (Downes, Rauk, & Van Heest, 2014), although the effectiveness is reliant on the user/wearer complying with the manufacturer's guidelines. PPE will vary depending on the chemical agent present but may include the following:
  - gloves, eye protection and sometimes long-sleeved impervious gowns and gauntlets
  - respirator masks may be included in chemical spill kits, while fume cabinets may also be provided in specimen-handling areas to remove fixative fumes from the environment.
- A number of chemicals emit vapours that cumulatively could be detrimental to the perioperative team's well-being, so specialised equipment has been engineered, such as orthopaedic helmet/hood systems and prepacked vacuum mixing systems to minimise exposure to bone cement fumes (Hines, 2018) (see also Box 5.5).
- Additional safety measures are required for staff handling cytotoxic substances, including confinement and separation of cytotoxic contaminated RMDs from other equipment and RMDs, record keeping for staff training and individual staff exposure (Eisenberg & Pacheco, 2018; State of Queensland, 2018).
- Personnel should also refer to local policies describing the safe management of patients' cytotoxic waste, including potentially contaminated fluids and linen (see also the waste management section of this chapter).

BOX 5.5
Safe Handling of Bone Cement

Staff education and procedures outlining endorsed practices are required when methyl methacrylate (MMA), a component of bone cement, is in use in the perioperative environment. Bone cement can be hazardous not only to the staff preparing the cement but also to anyone within the immediate area with major concerns about the vapours, skin contact and nervous and reproductive systems (Hines, 2018). The following safe practices are recommended when bone cement is used in the OR:

- Pregnant women should avoid exposure to bone cement because of research showing birth defects in animal studies (Downes, Rauk, & Van Heest, 2014).
- Contact lens wearers should also avoid exposure to bone cement because MMA is known to cause irritation of the eye.

- Where possible, MMA vapours should be controlled by the use of a closed system such as a bone cement vacuum mixing system and should occur only in rooms with air-handling and ventilation systems and appropriate air changes.
- Two pairs of surgical gloves are recommended when mixing and handling the bone cement because of the toxicity of MMA to skin.
- Contact with the bone cement should be avoided until it has reached a dough-like consistency.
- Any spills of bone cement should be isolated and ignition sources removed from the area because the liquid form of MMA is highly flammable (Hines, 2018).

PATIENT SCENARIOS

SCENARIO 5.4: WORK HEALTH AND SAFETY

You have now read about many of the WH&S risks for patients and staff working in the perioperative environment. Consider the staff working in the OR during Mr Collins' TKR surgery.

Critical Thinking Questions

- Describe how the perioperative team caring for Mr Collins can safely manage the generation of surgical plume, including:
  - preparation of equipment
  - intraoperative practices
  - postoperative disposal.
- List at least three other WH&S measures that would be relevant for the perioperative team caring for Mr Collins. Explain why each of those safety measures is important.

Noise

Environmental noise may be hazardous to the perioperative team, affecting concentration and/or communication. The impact of noise on team communication and performance is explained in more detail in Chapter 2.

The WHO recommends that noise levels in the OR remain below 35 decibels (dB). ORs can exceed the maximum noise pollution levels of 55 dB for mental concentration, with some noises avoidable such as loud conversations (Keller et al., 2018; Wright, 2016). Wright suggests that a 'No Interruption Zone' is created in which perioperative team members eliminate non-essential conversations during critical phases, which include surgical briefings, surgical counts, patient identification, induction, emergence and specimen management or any other complex tasks. The verbal communication that occurs regularly between team members is not always essential or patient related (Ford, 2015). The perioperative nurse should be alert to the negative impact of noise levels on patients and the team, and should limit noises and other non-essential communication, particularly during induction or the performance of surgical protocols such as the SSC or surgical count (Ford, 2015). An increase in adverse events, such as mental lapses, impaired thought processes and diversion of tasks, can occur because of high noise levels (Wright, 2016). A systematic review of 18 studies conducted between 2009 and 2018 on the effects of music on surgeons' task performance also noted some negative effects; however, these were far outweighed by the positive effects of classical music played at low volumes during surgical procedures (Boghdady & Ewalds-Kvist, 2020). There are other areas within the perioperative environment which may also have noisy equipment – for example, cleaning and reprocessing rooms. Where staff members find noise levels are disruptive to themselves or to their patients, they can manage these risks by following the WH&S hazard-reporting processes in their facility. This may include such steps as requesting that audiology testing be conducted on occupational sound levels (see also Box 5.6 and Feature box 5.4).

BOX 5.6
The Impact of the Perioperative Environment on Staff

There are a number of environmental conditions which have the potential to adversely affect the performance of perioperative staff (Byrne, Ludington-Hoe, & Voss, 2020). For example, staff members who are exposed to a range of extreme temperatures may suffer from a diminished performance and may need to exert additional energy to perform their tasks. Byrne and colleagues' (2020) integrative review included a study of foundry workers who reported higher cortisol levels and altered reaction times when exposed to higher ambient temperatures. Working in a heated environment, such as an OR for burns surgery, can affect the mathematical, perceptual and attentional tasks undertaken by staff (Katz, 2017). Working in a cold environment can negatively affect the staff members' learning, memory and reasoning skills. The severity of these negative impacts is influenced by the length of time a staff member is exposed to extreme conditions and the task being undertaken at the time (Katz, 2017).

Scrubbed surgical team members are most affected by the greater ambient temperatures because of the gown and the heat from the overhead surgical lights. One study examined the effect upon surgical residents performing minimally invasive surgery (MIS) in an OR with an ambient temperature of 26°C. Results indicated no negative impact upon the surgical tasks performed; however, an increase in physical demand was noted (sweating, which can compromise the aseptic field) and a feeling of being distracted (Katz, 2017).

Disruptions or delays to routines may also adversely affect the performance of perioperative staff. These disruptions can include malfunctioning equipment, the number of door openings in the OR, alarms and loud noises, breakdowns in communication and irrelevant conversations, environmental clutter and working in constrained spaces (Joseph et al., 2019; Loison et al., 2017). Joseph and colleagues (2018) identified that over 30% of flow disruptions were caused by non-essential staff entering the OR, equipment that had been spilled, and dropped or missing items that required a staff member to search for them within the OR.

FEATURE BOX 5.4
Impact of the Perioperative Environment on the Patient

Patients may feel anxious when they enter the unknown environment of the OR (Kömürcü et al., 2015). It is an intimidating and stressful environment because of the cool temperature, narrow operating table, surgical attire, sounds from technical equipment, and sight and sounds of the surgical instrumentation being unpacked and prepared (Katz, 2017). Perioperative team members should work together to prevent the patient from seeing or hearing things that may increase their anxiety before surgery. This could be achieved by opening surgical supplies out of the patient's view, placing drapes in front of the patient, quietly performing the surgical count while the anaesthetic nurse interacts with the patient and ensuring that all team members are wearing clean perioperative attire and shoes (Kömürcü et al., 2015).

Bone cement and electrosurgery can produce unwelcome smells during surgery (Kömürcü et al., 2015; Weinberg, Saleh, & Sinha, 2015). Patients under regional anaesthesia may also be able to hear when surgical saws, drills or other powered tools are in use. Reducing the potential triggers for patient anxiety can be achieved with distraction techniques using patient headphones and portable devices. One study found that, during arthroscopy procedures, patient anxiety was managed when patients watched their procedure on monitors (Kömürcü et al., 2015).

The layout of the OR has been the subject of much research. For example, the work of Joseph and colleagues (2018, 2019) and the Realizing Improved Patient Care through Human Centered Design in the OR (RIPCHD.OR) project found that a triangular workspace (with the OR table rotated from its central axis) could improve some staff movements and was beneficial for the anaesthetic team. The reduction of clutter can enhance patient safety, while mobile workstations for the circulating nurse and digital displays positioned high inside the OR were able to facilitate better visualisation of the surgery in most ORs studied.

Biohazards

Healthcare workers can be exposed to blood, fluids, tissue or other bodily substances during their daily work (Commonwealth of Australia, 2008), which increases the risk of contracting blood-borne virus infections (Queensland Health, 2017c). This may be a mucosal exposure from direct contact of the substance with non-intact skin, a splash to mucous membranes such as the eyes, nose or mouth (Murphy, 2014), or a percutaneous exposure from penetrating injuries with needles, scalpel blades or other sharps (Queensland Health, 2017c). Regardless of the exact mechanism, these workplace incidents are known collectively as occupational exposures (Ministry of Health, NSW, 2018b), and each exposure needs to be managed and reported according to the relevant WH&S legislation.

Occupational exposures may occur at any stage during the perioperative patient journey (ACORN, 2020t) – for example, managing an aggressive patient or during resuscitation procedures.

Perioperative nurses should take precautions to prevent occupational exposure, not only for themselves, but also for their colleagues. There is a range of standard measures that may be taken to avoid injury, beginning with an awareness of the potential risks.

High-risk situations with a potential for *mucosal exposure* during perioperative patient care include:

- intubation and extubation, suctioning or catheterisation, vascular access procedures or as a consequence of postoperative nausea and vomiting (PONV)
- surgical incision, dissection, debridement, irrigation or control of haemostasis, or during transfer and processing of specimens, etc.

High-risk situations with potential for *percutaneous injury* during perioperative patient care include:

- inserting or withdrawing needles into IV lines, for example, or from contact with sharp ampoules, cannulas or vascular access guidewires, etc.
- handling or passing surgical scalpels and trocars, dissecting instruments, power tools, prostheses such as screws and pins, suture needles and staples, as well as sharp ampoules and hypodermic needles, etc. (Centers for Disease Control and Prevention [CDC], 2015).

Other high-risk situations when occupational exposures may occur after perioperative patient care include environmental cleaning when contaminated fluids may be present, or separation of waste and equipment for reuse or disposal, or due to sharps remaining on working surfaces or on beds, in linen, around waste containers or on floors (ACSQHC/the Commission, 2017a; CDC, 2015).

Surgical procedures may be categorised as either non-exposure-prone procedures or exposure-prone procedures (Commonwealth of Australia, 2017), with different inherent risks to healthcare workers:

- *Non-exposure-prone procedures* (non-EPPs) are procedures where the hands and fingers of the healthcare worker (HCW) are visible and outside of the body at all times and in all procedures, or internal examinations that do not involve possible injury to the HCW's hands by sharp instruments and/or tissues,

provided routine infection prevention and control procedures are adhered to at all times.

- *Exposure-prone procedures* (EPPs) are procedures where there is a risk of injury to the HCW resulting in exposure of the patient's open tissues to the blood of the HCW. These procedures include those where the HCW's hands (whether gloved or not) may be in contact with sharp instruments, needle tips or sharp tissues (spicules of bone or teeth) inside a patient's open body cavity, wound or confined anatomical space where the hands or fingertips may not be completely visible at all times (CDC, 2015).

The following section describes sharps safety measures and the management of occupational exposures. Chapter 6 describes the most important standard measures for staff to avoid occupational exposures, including the use of PPE and additional infection prevention practices.

Standard sharps safety measures

In addition to the use of PPE, the general principles that may reduce perioperative nurses' overall risk of percutaneous injuries are to eliminate or reduce the use of sharps, to minimise the handling of sharps, and to isolate sharps wherever possible. These practices are outlined in Box 5.7.

Instrument nurses may have increased risk of sharps injury owing to the requirement to handle a range of sharps on the aseptic field. Chapter 10 describes the specific sharps safety practices recommended for instrument nurses during invasive and aseptic procedures. Double gloving is a recommended practice in Australia and, where the duration of procedures is extended, it is suggested that the outer glove should be examined and changed routinely (ACORN, 2020u; NHMRC, 2019). Mischke and colleagues' (2014) systematic review on the efficacy of surgical gloves to protect against sharps injury examined the evidence from 34 studies, including those which examined the use of thicker gloves and the practices of double gloving with or without indicator gloves. The review found that surgical staff can reduce the risk of glove perforation, and thereby the risk of occupational exposure to harmful pathogens, by wearing two pairs of gloves. Despite such measures, perioperative nurses should know how to respond when occupational exposures occur to themselves or another member of the perioperative team. Feature box 5.5 describes the immediate care of the healthcare worker following an occupational exposure. Such incidents require prompt assessment and management (Queensland Health, 2017c).

BOX 5.7
Sharps Safety Measures

Before using sharps – preparation:

- Learn about new sharps safety devices before using.
- Ensure adequate lighting in areas where sharps will be in use.
- Assess the need for sharps passing devices and sharps disposal containers (e.g. correct shapes and capacities for passing devices and sharps disposal containers, replace full containers before commencing procedures.
- Prepare your environment to ensure easy access to sharps disposal containers.
- Assess each individual risk before handling sharps.

When using sharps – awareness:

- Keep sharps in view.
- Work with deliberate care and without haste; stay focused on actions to avoid distractions.
- Be aware of others in close proximity and use verbal alerts when moving sharps.
- Reduce the likelihood of sharps passed hand to hand by using a puncture-proof container.

- Use safety-engineered sharps devices (SESDs) designed to prevent exposure to sharps during their use (and disposal).
- Use instruments, not fingers, to grasp needles, retract tissue and load/unload needles and scalpels.
- Separate reusable sharps from other instruments and equipment before cleaning and reprocessing.
- Wear two layers of surgical gloves (Mischke et al., 2014).

After using sharps – disposal:

- Everyone has responsibility for the safe management and disposal of the sharps they generate for use when using SESDs.
- Activate safety features after use.
- Dispose of single-use devices in rigid sharps containers; do not overfill containers.
- Keep fingers away from the opening of sharps containers.
- Anticipate risks including sharps unseen in linen, beds, on the floor or around waste containers (ACORN, 2020u; CDC, 2015; Ministry of Health, NSW, 2018a).

FEATURE BOX 5.5
The Immediate Care of the Healthcare Worker Following an Occupational Exposure

Immediately following exposure to blood or body fluids, it is recommended that the exposed person undertakes the following steps as soon as possible:

- Wash wounds and skin sites that have been in contact with blood or body fluids with soap and water.[a]
- Apply a sterile dressing as necessary, and apply pressure through the dressing if bleeding is still occurring.
- Do not squeeze or rub the injury site.[b]
- If blood gets on the skin, irrespective of whether there are cuts or abrasions, wash well with soap and water.
- Irrigate mucous membranes and eyes (remove contact lenses) with water or normal saline.[c]
- If eyes are contaminated, rinse while they are open, gently but thoroughly (for at least 30 seconds) with water or normal saline.[d]

- If blood or body fluids get in the mouth, spit them out and then rinse the mouth with water several times.[d]
- If clothing is contaminated, remove clothing and shower if necessary.[d]

When water is not available, use of non-water cleanser or antiseptic should replace the use of soap and water for washing cuts or punctures of the skin or intact skin. The application of strong solutions (e.g. bleach or iodine) to wounds or skin sites is not recommended.[e]

The exposed person should inform an appropriate person (e.g. a supervisor or manager) as soon as possible after the exposure so assessment and follow-up can be undertaken in a timely manner. After reporting the incident, the worker should be released from duty so that an immediate risk assessment can be performed.

(Sources: Verbatim excerpt from 4.2 Immediate care of the exposed person. In Queensland Health (2017c). *Management of occupational exposure to blood and body fluids*. Retrieved from https://www.health.qld.gov.au/__data/assets/pdf_file/0016/151162/qh-gdl-321-8.pdf.
a. Centers for Disease Prevention and Control. (n.d.). *Bloodborne infectious diseases: HIV/AIDS, hepatitis B, hepatitis C: emergency sharps information* [webpage]. Retrieved from https://www.cdc.gov/niosh/topics/bbp/emergnedl.html.
b. Centers for Disease Prevention and Control. (2001). Updated US Public Health Service guidelines for the management of occupational exposures to HBV, HCV, and HIV and recommendations for post exposure prophylaxis. *MMWR, 50*(RR-11), 1–42.
c. Australian Society for HIV Medicine (ASHM). (2016). *Australian national guidelines for post-exposure prophylaxis after non-occupational and occupational exposure to HIV* (2nd ed.). Retrieved from https://www.ashm.org.au/products/product/978-1-920773-47-2.
d. Department of Health, NSW. (2017). *HIV, hepatitis B and hepatitis C – management of health care workers potentially exposed*. Retrieved from https://www1.health.nsw.gov.au/pds/ActivePDSDocuments/PD2017_010.pdf.
e. Centers for Disease Prevention and Control. (2005). Updated US Public Health Service guidelines for the management of occupational exposures to HIV and recommendations for post exposure prophylaxis. *MMWR, 54*(RR-09), 1–17.)

Impacts on Performance and Well-being

The perioperative environment can be a fast-paced workplace with changeable, physically demanding workloads. Newly formed teams may be required to work long and unsocial hours and may encounter patients suffering significant physical trauma. Any of these factors may affect staff performance and well-being. The impact of the perioperative environment on staff performance and well-being has been the subject of research over several decades (Lizarondo, 2019). Studies in Australian settings have explored work-related trauma (Michael, 2001a, 2001b; Michael & Jenkins, 2001), workplace stress and technology stress (Gillespie & Kermode, 2003; Jacob, 2015; Luck & Gillespie, 2017; Smith & Palesy, 2018). Other subjects of research include nurses' attitudes towards transplantation (Regehr, Kjerulf, Popova, & Baker, 2004), negative and disruptive intraoperative behaviours (Gilmour & Hamlin, 2003, Philippon, 2016; Villafranca, Hamlin, Enns, & Jacobsohn, 2017) and perioperative nurses' resilience (Gillespie, 2007).

Professional colleges, employers and industrial associations recognise these factors and the potential harms in the workplace. Policies and position statements address such impacts as fatigue, incivility, bullying and harassment, occupational violence and sexual harassment (ANMF, 2018b; 2018c, 2019a; ANZCA, 2019; Royal Australasian College of Surgeons [RACS], 2017), and promote strategies for staff well-being and the prevention of workplace stress (ACORN, 2020v; ANMF, 2019b; AORN, 2015). (See also Research boxes 5.3 and 5.4.)

RESEARCH BOX 5.4
The Impact of Technology Stress on Perioperative Nurses

Over the past two decades, Australian researchers have reported a range of challenges that emerging technologies are creating for perioperative nurses, notably the ongoing struggle between the caring and nurturing aspect of nursing and the legitimate need to be competent technicians (Johnson, 2000; Luck & Gillespie, 2017; Richardson-Tench, 2007; Smith & Palesy, 2018).

Smith and Palesy (2018) also write about the ambiguity and confusion around the roles and responsibilities of perioperative nurses using technology, while Luck and Gillespie (2017) write about the specific demands of robotic-assisted surgery (RAS) and perioperative nurses' increasingly technocentric roles. These challenges can lead to the development of 'technology stress' (Smith & Palesy, 2018), with evidence that this has a significant impact on nurses' well-being, health, job satisfaction and retention (Catalano & Fickenscher, 2007; Johnson, 2000; Richardson-Tench, 2007).

Smith and Palesy (2018) believe that targeted strategies should be identified to assist perioperative nurses to manage work-related technology stress, with further research also needed to understand the impact of technology on perioperative nurses and the patients in their care.

RESEARCH BOX 5.3
Transition Shock

The notion of transition shock has been described by Duchscher (2009, in Wakefield, 2018) as a type of workplace stress that graduate nurses may experience during the first few months of professional practice. Undergraduate placements in the operating suite may not be adequate preparation for graduates' transition, so it is important that perioperative managers consider the skill mix when rostering and allow adequate supernumerary time (ACORN, 2020w). Educators and preceptors must set realistic expectations and timeframes for graduates' skill development (Wakefield, 2018), while more experienced colleagues can be positive role models and share strategies that will help the graduate manage the physical and psychological demands of the perioperative environment.

PREPARATION OF THE OPERATING ROOM

Prior to commencing the daily work scheduled within the OR, the assigned nurses must carry out a full check of the environment to identify and mitigate WH&S risks for the perioperative staff and patients. The assigned nurses must also ensure that all essential items are present, clean and in working order and that horizontal surfaces are dusted with facility-approved neutral detergent. These items include, but may not be limited to, the ceiling-mounted operating lights and OR table in the centre of the room, assembled instrument trolleys, ESU, suction equipment, positioning aids, linen skips and rubbish bags on the periphery of the room, and the anaesthetic machine and associated supplies at the head of the room. If any item is not clean, or is found to be missing or faulty, the perioperative nurses must take corrective action before the patient enters the OR (ACORN, 2020k). It is also recommended practice for the perioperative team to ensure that all rubbish and linen receptacles are empty before admitting a patient to the OR. This practice is designed to prevent the risk of discarded accountable items from previous patients being retained in the room, with the potential for confusion about correctness and completeness of the surgical counts for subsequent patients (ACORN, 2020x).

Once the room has been checked and considered clean, the perioperative team should collaborate on the placement of equipment, taking care to avoid congested workspaces and trip hazards associated with poorly placed equipment, leads and power cords. It is also very important to consider both the anaesthetic and the surgical approaches when setting up the OR and positioning equipment at the beginning of the list. This is not only for WH&S reasons and ergonomics; it is because some procedures may require specific lateral or bilateral access, head or foot of the bed access, while other procedures may be conducted according to various surgeons' preferences.

The anaesthetic, circulating and instrument nurses should also discuss any specific requirements for the patients on the operating list with the anaesthetic and surgical teams and support staff during team briefings, or as part of team 'Time Out' on the surgical safety checklist (SSC) (ACORN, 2020y). Any change in position of equipment or the need for additional equipment (e.g. PPE such as laser safety goggles and signage, cytotoxic waste receptacles, additional positioning equipment, tourniquets, power tools, head lights, microscopes and so forth) must be identified, collected and checked for cleanliness and functionality as part of the preparation of the OR. These checks will depend on the specific equipment, but are likely to include the following examples:

- running diagnostic cycles
- testing of alarms including volume levels to ensure these are audible
- correction of power settings to safe minimum limits
- confirmation of adequate supplies, volumes of fluids or gases, etc.
- confirmation of adequate power supply or battery charge
- testing of back-up systems such as spare lights
- estimation of reach required for power cords, lead length, tubing length, etc.

A final check of the room is recommended in terms of risk management for staff and to minimise the potential hazards for the patient (ACORN, 2020l; ACSQHC/the Commission, 2017c).

PATIENT SCENARIOS

SCENARIO 5.5: PREPARATION OF THE OR

Select one of the patients in our scenarios and draw a diagram to show the placement of the anaesthetic and surgical equipment in the OR, as well as any patient-positioning devices which you deem necessary for this patient's surgical procedure. Your diagram should also indicate the most likely positions of the perioperative team members around the OR table.

VISITORS TO THE PERIOPERATIVE ENVIRONMENT

In addition to regular nursing staff, medical staff, technicians and healthcare assistants, there are other personnel who may be required temporarily as visitors to the perioperative environment. For example, radiographers are required so often in the OR that many larger facilities base a team of radiographers inside the perioperative environment to be readily available for patient care. Other hospital personnel include midwives, paediatricians and/or neonatologists to care for the newborn infant born during obstetric surgery, or during some types of cancer surgery, such as brachytherapy, scientists and radiation physicists are required to provide expertise to the surgical team. Biomedical staff members are also commonly seen in the perioperative environment, undertaking maintenance and repairs on equipment.

Visitors must have a valid reason to be present during surgery so as not to compromise the rights of the patient and to ensure that patient safety is not compromised (Queensland Health, 2017d). Patient consent should always be obtained, either verbally or documented in the medical record (Queensland Health, 2017d). Complete or partial perioperative attire may need to be worn by visitors, depending upon the local policy and the areas of the environment the visitors will need to access during the visit. Visible identification such as a name badge or security pass may also be a requirement of local policy and for compliance with national standards.

Examples of visitors include the following:

- A patient support person (PSP) may include a parent accompanying their child to the OR, or a partner supporting a pregnant woman coming in for a lower-segment caesarean section (LSCS). It is a recommended practice for the PSP to be supervised and supported at all times by a member of the multidisciplinary team (ACORN, 2020c).

- Nursing, medical and allied health students may come to observe surgery and/or undertake clinical practice within the operating suite. It is a recommended practice that students are under the direct/indirect supervision of a member of the multidisciplinary team and have received appropriate instruction and training to ensure the safety of the patient, themselves and other staff (ACORN, 2020c).

- A medical company representative (MCR) can be present during surgery to assist the team members by providing technical guidance and support with new consumables, equipment and/or instrumentation. It is a recommended practice that MCRs work under the direct supervision of a member of the multidisciplinary team and have received appropriate instruction and training to ensure the safety of the patient, themselves and other staff (ACORN,

2020c). Documentation of such training may be required, depending upon the local policy.

- MCRs should not participate in direct patient care such as patient transfers, holding limbs for skin preparation or opening of sterile supplies. If the surgical technology requires intraoperative adjustment by the MCR, for example during brain stimulation surgery, this should be addressed through local policy development. Governance of any such exceptions is important to ensure appropriate assessment of risk and facility approval for the MCR role and responsibilities.

- Other visitors to the environment may include visiting medical staff, media personnel, police and custodial officers and volunteers (Queensland Health, 2017d). Governance in facilities where these groups are frequently present in the department would include development of local policy outlining roles and responsibilities, as well as lines of communication.

PATIENT SCENARIOS

SCENARIO 5.6: VISITORS TO THE PERIOPERATIVE ENVIRONMENT

Consider the new information regarding the patients below, and in particular the diverse needs of these visitors. During Mr James Collins' TKR surgery, Silvana Perez, a medical company representative (MCR), is present in the OR to support the surgical staff. Silvana's face and neck are splashed with blood in the early stages of the surgery. She tells RN Ben Lumby that she is wearing contact lenses and thinks the blood may have got into her eyes.

Critical Thinking Questions

- What immediate actions should Silvana take to manage this potential exposure?
- Name another precaution that Silvana may need to take during this procedure, in light of wearing contact lenses.

  Mrs Janine Clark's partner, Ari, will be allowed to come into the OR during her LSCS as her support person.

- Identify at least three potential environmental impacts Ari may encounter during this surgical procedure.
- Describe what the perioperative nurses can do to minimise each of these impacts.

  Master Thanh Nguyen will be accompanied briefly by one of his parents for his induction in the anaesthetic

room until he falls asleep. Following Thanh's operation, his parent will be allowed to enter the PACU.

- Identify the operating suite zone or zones that Thanh's parent will be visiting.
- Describe the perioperative attire that Thanh's parent be required to wear during their two visits to the perioperative environment.

  You should refer to your local policy and may need to review several sections of this chapter in preparing your answers.

CONCLUSION

The perioperative environment is complex and challenging, with many risks for patients and staff from environmental hazards and potentially hazardous substances. This chapter has described design features and work practices that can reduce the risk of injury and create a safe patient care environment and safe workplace for staff. These design features begin with a well-planned physical environment. In the operating suite, there are designated zones and coordinated traffic patterns for patients, staff and equipment. These are supported by environmental controls such as air handling and ventilation, recommended practices covering perioperative attire and PPE, as well as the storage of supplies, waste management and cleaning regimens. This chapter has presented strategies that all staff can use to incorporate sustainable waste management practices in all areas of the perioperative environment. The perioperative environment, and the operating suite in particular, place the staff at risk owing to the many WH&S issues and hazards present on each day. All members of the perioperative team require an understanding of how, when and why equipment, devices and supplies are used to minimise risk of injury and to ensure safe patient care.

RESOURCES

ASCIA eTraining portal
https://etraininghp.ascia.org.au
Association of periOperative Registered Nurses (AORN)
https://www.aorn.org
Australasian Healthcare Facility Guidelines (AHFG)
https://www.healthfacilityguidelines.com.au
Australasian Society of Clinical Immunology and Allergy (ASCIA)
https://www.allergy.org.au
https://www.allergy.org.au/hp/papers/management-of-latex-allergic-patients
Australian College of Operating Room Nurses (ACORN)
https://www.acorn.org.au
Australian Department of Health
https://www.health.gov.au
Australian Government WH&S Acts, regulations and code of practice
https://www.business.gov.au/Risk-management/Health-and-safety/Work-health-and-safety
Australian Radiation Protection and Nuclear Safety Agency (ARPANSA)
https://www.arpansa.gov.au
Centers for Disease Control and Prevention (CDC)
https://www.cdc.gov/niosh/topics/healthcare
Council on Surgical & Perioperative Safety (CSP)
https://www.cspsteam.org/resources-and-tools-for-preventing-surgical-fires
Emergency Care Research Institute (ECRI)
https://www.ecri.org
Infection Prevention and Control Nurses College
https://www.infectioncontrol.co.nz
International Council on Surgical Plume (ICSP)
https://www.plumecouncil.com/about.html
National Institute for Occupational Safety and Health (NIOSH)
https://www.cdc.gov/niosh/
Perioperative Nurses College of New Zealand Nurses Organisation (PNC NZNO)
https://www.nzno.org.nz/groups/colleges/perioperative_nurses_college
Standards Australia
https://www.standards.org.au

REFERENCES

Addley, S., & Quinn, D. (2019). Surgical smoke – what are the risks? *The Obstetrician and Gynaecologist, 21*, 102–106. https://dx.doi.org/10.1111/tog.12552

Ahmad, N., Hussein, A. A., Cavuoto, L., Sharif, M., Allers, J.C, Hinata, N., … Guru, K. A. (2016). Ambulatory movements, team dynamics and interactions during robot-assisted surgery. *BJU International, 118*(1), 132–139. https://dx.doi.org/10.1111/bju.13426

Akhtar, N., Ansar, F., Baig, M. S., & Abbas, A. (2016). Airway fires during surgery: management and prevention. *Journal of Anaesthesiology, Clinical Pharmacology, 32*(1), 109–111. https://dx.doi.org/10.4103/0970-9185.175710

Aminimoghaddam, S., Pahlevani, R., & Kazemi, M. (2018). Electrosurgery and clinical applications of electrosurgical devices in gynecologic procedures. *Medical Journal of the Islamic Republic of Iran, 32*, 90. https://dx.doi.org/10.14196/mjiri.32.90

Armellino, D. (2016). Optimal infection control practices in the OR environment. *AORN Journal, 104*(6), 516–522. https://dx.doi.org/10.1016/j.aorn.2016.09.019

Association of periOperative Registered Nurses (AORN). (2015). Position statement on a healthy perioperative practice environment. Retrieved from <https://www.aorn.org/guidelines/clinical-resources/position-statements>.

Australasian Health Infrastructure Alliance (AHIA). (2016a, March). Australasian Health Facility Guidelines. Part B: Health Facility Briefing and Planning 0080 – General Requirements. Version 6. Retrieved from <https://healthfacilityguidelines.com.au/health-planning-units>.

Australasian Health Infrastructure Alliance (AHIA). (2016b, March). Australasian healthcare facility guidelines. Part D: Infection prevention and control, Version 7. Retrieved from <https://healthfacilityguidelines.com.au/part/part-d-infection-prevention-and-control-0>.

Australasian Health Infrastructure Alliance (AHIA). (2016c, May). Australasian Health Facility Guidelines. Part B: Health Facility Briefing and Planning 0190 – Sterilising Services Unit. Version 6. Retrieved from <https://healthfacilityguidelines.com.au/health-planning-units>.

Australasian Health Infrastructure Alliance (AHIA). (2016d, June). Australasian Health Facility Guidelines. Part B: Health Facility Briefing and Planning 0270 – Day Surgery Procedure Unit. Version 6. Retrieved from <https://healthfacilityguidelines.com.au/health-planning-units>.

Australasian Health Infrastructure Alliance (AHIA). (2018a, July). Australasian Health Facility Guidelines. Part B: Health Facility Briefing and Planning 0520 – Operating Unit. Version 6. Retrieved from <https://healthfacilityguidelines.com.au/health-planning-units>.

Australasian Health Infrastructure Alliance (AHIA). (2018b, September). Australasian Health Facility Guidelines. Part C – Design for Access, Mobility, Safety and Security. Version 6. Retrieved from <https://healthfacilityguidelines.com.au/part/part-c-design-access-mobility-safety-and-security>.

Australasian Society of Clinical Immunology and Allergy (ASCIA). (2010a). Latex allergy information for new employees [webpage]. Retrieved from <https://www.allergy.org.au/hp/papers/management-of-latex-allergic-patients/latex-information-for-employees>.

Australasian Society of Clinical Immunology and Allergy (ASCIA). (2010b). Operating suite guidelines for latex allergic patients [webpage]. Retrieved from <https://www.allergy.org.au/hp/papers/management-of-latex-allergic-patients/operating-suite>.

Australasian Society of Clinical Immunology and Allergy (ASCIA). (2019a). Information for patients, carers and consumers PCC latex allergy. Retrieved from <https://www.allergy.org.au/patients/other-allergy/latex-allergy>.

Australasian Society of Clinical Immunology and Allergy (ASCIA). (2019b). Information for patients, carers and consumers PCC chlorhexidine allergy. Retrieved from <https://www.allergy.org.au/patients/drug-allergy/chlorhexidine-allergy>.

Australian and New Zealand College of Anaesthetists (ANZCA). (2014). PS31 Guidelines on checking anaesthesia delivery systems. Retrieved from <https://www.anzca.edu.au/resources/professional-documents>.

Australian and New Zealand College of Anaesthetists (ANZCA). (2016). PS60 Guidelines on the perioperative management of patients with suspected or proven hypersensitivity to chlorhexidine. Retrieved from <https://www.anzca.edu.au/resources/professional-documents>.

Australian and New Zealand College of Anaesthetists (ANZCA). (2018a). PS04BP Statement on the post-anaesthesia care unit. Retrieved from <https://www.anzca.edu.au/resources/professional-documents>.

Australian and New Zealand College of Anaesthetists (ANZCA). (2018b). PS15 Guidelines for the perioperative care of patients selected for day stay procedures. Retrieved from <https://www.anzca.edu.au/resources/professional-documents>.

Australian and New Zealand College of Anaesthetists (ANZCA). (2019). PS43 Guideline on fatigue risk management in anaesthesia practice. Retrieved from <https://www.anzca.edu.au/resources/professional-documents>.

Australian and New Zealand College of Anaesthetists (ANZCA). (2020). PS66 Guideline on the role of the anaesthetist in commissioning medical gas pipelines. Retrieved from <https://www.anzca.edu.au/resources/professional-documents>.

Australian and New Zealand College of Anaesthetists (ANZCA). (2021). PS54 Statement on the minimum safety requirements for anaesthetic machines and workstations for clinical practice. Retrieved from <https://www.anzca.edu.au/resources/professional-documents>.

Australian and New Zealand Society of Cardiac and Thoracic Surgeons (ANZSCTS). (2014). Guidelines for the establishment of an adult cardiac surgery unit. Retrieved from <https://anzscts.org/anzscts-guidelines-for-establishment-of-an-adult-cardiac-surgery-unit/>.

Australian College of Perioperative Nurses (ACORN). (2020a). Planning and design of the perioperative environment. In *ACORN standards for perioperative nursing in Australia* (16th ed., Vol. 1). Adelaide: Author.

Australian College of Perioperative Nurses (ACORN). (2020b). Perioperative attire. In *ACORN standards for perioperative nursing in Australia* (16th ed., Vol. 1). Adelaide: Author.

Australian College of Perioperative Nurses (ACORN). (2020c). Visitors to the perioperative environment. In *ACORN standards for perioperative nursing in Australia* (16th ed., Vol. 1). Adelaide: Author.

Australian College of Perioperative Nurses (ACORN). (2020d). Staffing for safety. In *ACORN standards for perioperative nursing in Australia* (16th ed., Vol. 2). Adelaide: Author.

Australian College of Perioperative Nurses (ACORN). (2020e). Reprocessing of RMDs. In *ACORN standards for perioperative nursing in Australia* (16th ed., Vol. 1). Adelaide: Author.

Australian College of Perioperative Nurses (ACORN). (2020f). Fatigue. In *ACORN standards for perioperative nursing in Australia* (16th ed., Vol. 1). Adelaide: Author.

Australian College of Perioperative Nurses (ACORN). (2020g). Loan sets. In *ACORN standards for perioperative nursing in Australia* (16th ed., Vol. 1). Adelaide: Author.

Australian College of Perioperative Nurses (ACORN). (2020h). Asepsis. In *ACORN standards for perioperative nursing in Australia* (16th ed., Vol. 1). Adelaide: Author.

Australian College of Perioperative Nurses (ACORN). (2020i). Environmentally sustainable practices. In *ACORN standards for perioperative nursing in Australia* (16th ed., Vol. 1). Adelaide: Author.

Australian College of Perioperative Nurses (ACORN). (2020j). Infection prevention. In *ACORN standards for perioperative nursing in Australia* (16th ed., Vol. 1). Adelaide: Author.

Australian College of Perioperative Nurses (ACORN). (2020k). Cleaning and maintaining the perioperative environment. In *ACORN standards for perioperative nursing in Australia* (16th ed., Vol. 1). Adelaide: Author.

Australian College of Perioperative Nurses (ACORN). (2020l). Risk management. In *ACORN standards for perioperative nursing in Australia* (16th ed., Vol. 2). Adelaide: Author.

Australian College of Perioperative Nurses (ACORN). (2020m). Manual handling. In *ACORN standards for perioperative nursing in Australia* (16th ed., Vol. 1). Adelaide: Author.

Australian College of Perioperative Nurses (ACORN). (2020n). Electrosurgical equipment. In *ACORN standards for perioperative nursing in Australia* (16th ed., Vol. 1). Adelaide: Author.

Australian College of Perioperative Nurses (ACORN). (2020o). Surgical plume. In *ACORN standards for perioperative nursing in Australia* (16th ed., Vol. 1). Adelaide: Author.

Australian College of Perioperative Nurses (ACORN). (2020p). Laser safety. In *ACORN standards for perioperative nursing in Australia* (16th ed., Vol. 1). Adelaide: Author.

Australian College of Perioperative Nurses (ACORN). (2020q). Fire safety. In *ACORN standards for perioperative nursing in Australia* (16th ed., Vol. 1). Adelaide: Author.

Australian College of Perioperative Nurses (ACORN). (2020r). Latex sensitivity. In *ACORN standards for perioperative nursing in Australia* (16th ed., Vol. 1). Adelaide: Author.

Australian College of Perioperative Nurses (ACORN). (2020s). Anaesthetic gas pollution. In *ACORN standards for perioperative nursing in Australia* (16th ed., Vol. 1). Adelaide: Author.

Australian College of Perioperative Nurses (ACORN). (2020t). Sharps and preventing sharp related injuries. In *ACORN standards for perioperative nursing in Australia* (16th ed., Vol. 1). Adelaide: Author.

Australian College of Perioperative Nurses (ACORN). (2020u). Surgical hand antisepsis, gowning and gloving. In *ACORN standards for perioperative nursing in Australia* (16th ed., Vol. 1). Adelaide: Author.

Australian College of Perioperative Nurses (ACORN). (2020v). Bullying and harassment, Emotional support for personnel and wellbeing. In *ACORN standards for perioperative nursing in Australia* (16th ed., Vol. 2). Adelaide: Author.

Australian College of Perioperative Nurses (ACORN). (2020w). Staffing for safety, undergraduate nursing students. In *ACORN standards for perioperative nursing in Australia* (16th ed., Vol. 2). Adelaide: Author.

Australian College of Perioperative Nurses (ACORN). (2020x). Accountable items. In *ACORN standards for perioperative nursing in Australia* (16th ed., Vol. 1). Adelaide: Author.

Australian College of Perioperative Nurses (ACORN). (2020y). Surgical safety. In *ACORN standards for perioperative nursing in Australia* (16th ed., Vol. 1). Adelaide: Author.

Australian Commission on Safety and Quality in Healthcare (ACSQHC/the Commission). (2017a). *Preventing and controlling healthcare-associated infection standard. Infection prevention and control systems*. Sydney: Author. Retrieved from <https://www.safetyandquality.gov.au/standards/nsqhs-standards/preventing-and-controlling-healthcare-associated-infection-standard/infection-prevention-and-control-systems>.

Australian Commission on Safety and Quality in Healthcare (ACSQHC/the Commission). (2017b). *Comprehensive care standard. Safe environment for the delivery of care*. Sydney: Author. Retrieved from <https://www.safetyandquality.gov.au/standards/nsqhs-standards/clinical-governance-standard/safe-environment-delivery-care>.

Australian Commission on Safety and Quality in Healthcare (ACSQHC/the Commission). (2017c). *Comprehensive care standard. Minimising harm*. Sydney: Author. Retrieved from <https://www.safetyandquality.gov.au/standards/nsqhs-standards/comprehensive-care-standard/minimising-patient-harm>.

Australian Commission on Safety and Quality in Health Care (ACSQHC/the Commission). (2020a). *AS18/07: Reprocessing of reusable medical devices in health service organisations*. Sydney: Author. Retrieved from <https://www.safetyandquality.gov.au/publications-and-resources/resource-library/as1807-reprocessing-reusable-medical-devices-health-service-organisations>.

Australian Commission on Safety and Quality in Health Care (ACSQHC/the Commission). (2020b). *Principles of environmental cleaning: product selection* [fact sheet]. Sydney: Author. Retrieved from <https://www.safetyandquality.gov.au/publications-and-resources/resource-library/principles-environmental-cleaning-product-selection-july-2020-fact-sheet>.

Australian Nursing and Midwifery Federation (ANMF). (2018a). ANMF Policy Safe patient handling. Retrieved from <https://anmf.org.au/pages/anmf-policies>.

Australian Nursing and Midwifery Federation (ANMF). (2018b). ANMF Policy Bullying in the workplace. Prevention. Retrieved from <https://anmf.org.au/pages/anmf-policies>.

Australian Nursing and Midwifery Federation (ANMF). (2018c). ANMF Policy Prevention of occupational violence and aggression in the workplace. Retrieved from <https://anmf.org.au/pages/anmf-policies>.

Australian Nursing and Midwifery Federation (ANMF). (2019a). ANMF policy fatigue prevention. Retrieved from <https://anmf.org.au/pages/anmf-policies>.

Australian Nursing and Midwifery Federation (ANMF). (2019b). ANMF Policy Workplace stress prevention. Retrieved from <https://anmf.org.au/pages/anmf-policies>.

Australian Radiation Protection and Nuclear Safety Agency (ARPANSA). (2014). *Fundamentals for protection against ionizing radiation. Radiation Protection Series F-1*. Yallambi: Author. Retrieved from <https://www.arpansa.gov.au/Publications/Codes/rpsF-1.cfm>.

Australian Radiation Protection and Nuclear Safety Agency (ARPANSA). (2015). *Lasers and intense pulsed light (IPL) sources used for cosmetic purposes [fact sheet]*. Yallambi: Author. Retrieved from <https://www.arpansa.gov.au/radiationprotection/Factsheets/index.cfm>.

Australian Radiation Protection and Nuclear Safety Agency (ARPANSA). (2020). *Occupational exposure: management of pregnant workers. Code for radiation protection in planned exposure situations. Radiation protection series C-1 (Rev. 1)*. Yallambi: Author. Retrieved from <https://www.arpansa.gov.au/sites/default/files/rps_c-1_rev_1.pdf>.

Australian Radiation Protection and Nuclear Safety Agency (ARPANSA). (n.d.a). *Lasers* [webpage]. Yallambi: Author. Retrieved from <https://www.arpansa.gov.au/understanding-radiation/what-is-radiation/non-ionising-radiation/laser>.

Australian Radiation Protection and Nuclear Safety Agency (ARPANSA). (n.d.b). *Occupational exposure: management of pregnant workers*. Yallambi: Author. Retrieved from <https://www.arpansa.gov.au/understanding-radiation/sources-radiation/occupational-exposure/occupational-exposure-management>.

Baggish, M. S., Poiesz, B. J., Joret, D., Williamson, P., & Refai, A. (1991). Presence of human immunodeficiency virus DNA in laser smoke. *Lasers in Surgery and Medicine, 11*, 197–203.

Bashaw, M. A., & Keister, K. J. (2019). Perioperative strategies for surgical site infection prevention. *AORN Journal, 109*(1), 68–78. https://dx.doi.org/10.1002/aorn.12451

Bifulco, P., Massa, R., Cesarelli, M., Romano, M., Fratini, A., Gargiulo, G. D., & McEwan, A. L. (2013). Investigating the role of capacitive coupling between the operating table and the return electrode of an electrosurgery unit in the modification of the current density distribution within the patients' body. *Biomedical Engineering Online, 12*, 80. Retrieved from <https://www.biomedical-engineering-online.com/content/12/1/80>.

Bischoff, P., Zeynep Kubilay, N., Allegranzi, B., Egger, M., & Gastmeier, P. (2017). Effect of laminar airflow ventilation on surgical site infections: a systematic review and meta-analysis. *Lancet Infectious Diseases, 17*(5), 553–561. https://dx.doi.org/10.1016/S1473-3099(17)30059-2

Blazquez, E., & Thorn, C. (2010). Fires and explosions. *Anaesthesia and Intensive Care Medicine, 11*(11), 455–457.

Blocker, R. C., Forsyth, K. L., Branaghan, R. J., & Hallbeck, M. S. (2017). Operative traffic in orthopedics: a glimpse into surgical team transformations. *Perioperative Care and Operating Room Management*, 8, 29–32. https://dx.doi.org/10.1016/j.pcorm.2017.07.004

Boghdady, E., & Ewalds-Kvist, M. A. (2020). The influence of music on the surgical task performance: a systematic review. *International Journal of Surgery*, 73, 101–112. https://dx.doi.org/10.1016/j.ijsu.2019.11.012

Boiano, J. M., & Steege, A. L. (2016). Precautionary practices for administering anesthetic gases: a survey of physician anesthesiologists, nurse anesthetists and anesthesiologist assistants. *Journal of Occupational and Environmental Hygiene*, 13(10), 782–793. https://dx.doi.org/10.1080/15459624.2016.1177650

Brandon, H. J., & LeRoy Young V. (1997). Characterization and removal of surgical smoke. *Surgical Services Management*, 3(3), 14–16.

British Oxygen Company (BOC). (2012). Guidelines for gas cylinder safety. Retrieved from <https://www.boc-gas.com.au/en/index.html>.

Burley, M. E., Arnold, T. V., Finley, E., Deutsch, E. S., & Treadwell, J. R. (2018). Surgical fires: decreasing incidence relies on continued prevention efforts. *PA Patient Safety Advisor*, 15(2), 1–13. Retrieved from <https://patientsafety.pa.gov/ADVISORIES/Pages/201806_SurgicalFires.aspx>.

Butler, M., Ford, R., Boxer, E., & Sutherland-Fraser, S. (2010). Lessons from the field: an examination of count errors in the operating theatre [online]. *ACORN Journal*, 23(3), 6–16.

Byrne, J., Ludington-Hoe, S. M., & Voss, J. G. (2020), Occupational heat stress, thermal comfort, and cognitive performance in the OR: an integrative review. *AORN Journal*, 111, 536–545. https://dx.doi.org/10.1002/aorn.13009

Canterbury District Health Board (CDHB). (2016). Returning of tissue/body parts to patients. Retrieved from <https://www.cdhb.health.nz/Hospitals-Services/Health-Professionals/CDHB-Policies/Clinical-Manual/Pages/default.aspx>.

Casar Berazaluce, A. M., Hanke, R. E., von Allmen, D., & Racadio, J. M. (2019). The state of the hybrid operating room: technological acceleration at the pinnacle of collaboration. *Current Surgery Reports*, 7, 7. https://dx.doi.org/10.1007/s40137-019-0229-x

Catalano, K., & Fickenscher, K. (2007). Emerging technologies in the OR and their effect on perioperative professionals. *AORN Journal*, 86(6), 958–968.

Centers for Disease Control and Prevention (CDC). (2015). Sharps safety for healthcare settings [webpage]. Retrieved from <https://www.cdc.gov/sharpssafety/>.

Clifford, T. (2014). Environmental hazards: waste anesthesia gases. *Journal of PeriAnesthesia Nursing*, 29(4), 330–331. https://dx.doi.org/10.1016/j.jopan.2014.05.007

Clinical Excellence Commission (CEC) (n.d.). *Environmental cleaning standard operating procedures*. Sydney: Author. Retrieved from <https://www.cec.health.nsw.gov.au/keep-patients-safe/infection-prevention-and-control/cleaning-and-reprocessing>.

Collins, S., Budds, M., Raines, C., & Hooper, V. (2019). Risk factors for perioperative hypothermia: a literature review. *Journal of PeriAnesthesia Nursing*, 34(2), 338–346.

Commonwealth of Australia. (2008). Occupational health and safety risk factors for rural and metropolitan nurses: comparative results from a national nurses' survey. Australian Safety and Compensation Council (ASCC). Retrieved from <https://www.safeworkaustralia.gov.au/resources-publications/reports?combine=occupational+exposure&sort_by=field_publication_date_value&sort_order=DESC>.

Commonwealth of Australia. (2011). Work Health and Safety Act 2011. Select Legislative Instrument 2011, No. 262. Compilation date: 1 December 2019. Retrieved from <https://www.legislation.gov.au/Details/F2019C00898>.

Commonwealth of Australia. (2017). Guidance on classification of exposure prone and non-exposure prone procedures in Australia 2017. Communicable Diseases Network Australia (CDNA). Retrieved from <https://www1.health.gov.au/internet/main/publishing.nsf/content/cda-cdna-blood-borne.htm>.

Corrin, T., Lin, J., MacNaughton, C., Mahato, S., & Rajendiran, A. (2016). The role of mobile communication devices in the spread of infections within a clinical setting. *Environmental Health Review*, 59(2), 63–70. https://dx.doi.org/10.5864/d2016-014

Downes, J., Rauk, P. N., & Van Heest, A. E. (2014). Occupational hazards for pregnant or lactating women in the orthopaedic operating room. *Journal of the American Academy of Orthopaedic Surgeons*, 22(5), 326–332. https://dx.doi.org/10.5435/JAAOS-22-05-326

Ehrenwerth, J. (2019). Operating room fires: comment. *Anesthesiology*, 131(4), 946–947. https://dx.doi.org/10.1097/ALN.0000000000002922

Eisenberg, S., & Pacheco, L. (2018). Applying hazardous drug standards to antineoplastics used for ophthalmology surgery. *AORN Journal*, 107(2), 200–210. https://dx.doi.org/10.1002/aorn.12022

Ford, D. (2015). Speaking up to reduce noise in the OR. *AORN Journal*, 102(1), 85–88. https://dx.doi.org/10.1016/j.aorn.2015.04.019

Garden, J. M., O'Banion, M. K., Shelnitz, L. S., Pinski, K. S., Bakus, A. D., Reichmann, M. E., & Sundberg, J. P. (1988). Papillomavirus in the vapor of carbon dioxide laser-treated verrucae. *Journal of the American Medical Association*, 259, 1199–1202.

Gillespie, B. M. (2007). *The predictors of resilience in operating room nurses* [thesis]. Brisbane: Faculty of Health, Griffith University. Retrieved from <https://hdl.handle.net/10072/365391>.

Gillespie, B. M., & Kermode, S. (2003). How do perioperative nurses cope with stress? *Contemporary Nurse*, 8(16), 24–33.

Gilmour, D., & Hamlin, L. (2003). Bullying and harassment in perioperative settings. *British Journal of Perioperative Nursing (United Kingdom)*, 13(2), 79–85. https://dx.doi.org/10.1177/175045890301300203

Global Green and Healthy Hospitals (GGHH). (n.d.). Case studies from GGHH members. Retrieved from <https://www.greenhospitals.net/case-studies-waste/>.

Golpaygani, A. T., Movahedi, M. M., & Reza, M. (2016). A study on performance and safety tests of electrosurgical equipment. *Journal of Biomedical Physics & Engineering*, 6(3), 175–182.

Government of South Australia. (2015). *Cytotoxic drugs and related waste. A risk management guide for South Australian health services*. Adelaide: South Australia Health. Retrieved from <https://www.sahealth.sa.gov.au/wps/wcm/connect/public+content/sa+health+internet/clinical+resources/clinical+programs+and+practice+guidelines/medicines+and+drugs/hazardous+drugs>.

Government of South Australia. (2017). *Cleaning standards for healthcare facilities*. Adelaide: Department for Health and Ageing. Retrieved from <https://www.sahealth.sa.gov.au/wps/wcm/connect/public+content/sa+health+internet/clinical+resources>.

Guetter, C. R., Williams, B. J., Slama, E., Arrington, A., Henry, M. C., Möller, M. G., … Crandall, M. (2018). Greening the operating room. *American Journal of Surgery, 216*(4), 683–688. https://dx.doi.org/10.1016/j.amjsurg.2018.07.021

Guillou, M., Maurel, B., Necib, H., Vent, P. A., Costargent, A., Chaillou, P., Gouëffic, Y., & Kaladji, A. (2018). Comparison of radiation exposure during endovascular treatment of peripheral arterial disease with flat-panel detectors on mobile c-arm versus fixed systems. *Annals of Vascular Surgery, 47*, 104–113. https://dx.doi.org/10.1016/j.avsg.2017.08.036

Harkavy, L. M., & Novak, D. A. (2014). Clearing the air: surgical smoke and workplace safety practices. *Operating Room Nurse, 8*(6), 1–7.

Hill, D., O'Neill, J., Powell, R., & Oliver, D. (2012). Surgical smoke: a health hazard in the operating theatre. A study to quantify exposure and a survey of the use of smoke extractor systems in UK plastic surgery units. *Journal of Plastic, Reconstructive and Aesthetic Surgery, 65*(7), 911–916. https://dx.doi.org/10.1016/j.bjps.2012.02.012

Hiller, K. N., Altamirano, A. V., Cai, C., Tran, S. F., & Williams, G. W. (2015). Evaluation of waste anesthetic gas in the postanesthesia care unit within the patient breathing zone. *Anesthesiology Research and Practice, 2015*, 354184. https://dx.doi.org/10.1155/2015/354184

Hines, C. B. (2018). Understanding bone cement implantation syndrome. *Journal of American Association of Nurse Anesthetists, 86*(6), 433–441.

Hohler, S. (2015). Latex allergies: protecting patients and staff. *OR Nurse Journal, 9*(1), 12–18. https://dx.doi.org/10.1097/01.ORN.0000457107.47873.aa

Hubbard, R. H., Hayanga, J. A., Quinlan, J. J., Soltez, A. K., & Hayanga, H. K. (2017). Optimizing anesthesia-related waste disposal in the operating room: a brief report. *Anesthesia and Analgesia, 125*(4), 1289–1291. https://dx.doi.org/10.1213/ANE.0000000000001932

International Council of Nurses (ICN). (2018). *Nurses, climate change and health*. Position statement. Geneva: Author.

International Electrotechnical Commission (IEC). (2017). Safety of laser products part 1: Equipment classification and requirements interpretation sheet 1 (IEC60825:2017). Retrieved from <https://webstore.iec.ch/publication/61058>.

Jacob, J. (2015). Occupational stress of scrub/scout practitioner: overview of selected literature [online]. *ACORN Journal, 28*(3), 15–21.

Johnson, L. (2000). 1990s surgical technologies implicated in role conflict – inducing stress amongst instrument and circulating nurses. *ACORN Journal, 13*(1), 19–27.

Jones, E. L., Overbey, D. M., Chapman, B. C., Jones, T. S., Hilton, S. A., Moore, J. T., & Robinson, T. N. (2017). Operating room fires and surgical skin preparation. *Journal of the American College of Surgeons, 225*(1), 160. https://dx.doi.org/10.1016/j.jamcollsurg.2017.01.058

Jones, T. S., Black, I. H., Robinson, T. N., & Jones, E. L. (2019). Operating room fires. *Anesthesiology, 130*, 492–501.

Joseph, A., Joshi, R., & Allison, D. (2018). Realizing improved patient care through human-centered design in the OR. *(RIPCHD.OR), 2*, 2016–2017 – ISSUU Publication. Retrieved from <https://www.clemson.edu/centers-institutes/health-facilities-design-testing/projects/publications.html>.

Joseph, A., Khoshkenar, A., Taaffe, K. M., Catchpole, K., Machry, H., Bayramzadeh, S., & RIPCHD.OR study group. (2019). Minor flow disruptions, traffic-related factors and their effect on major flow disruptions in the operating room. *British Medical Journal of Quality and Safety, 28*(4), 276–283. https://dx.dx.doi.org/10.1136/bmjqs-2018-008670

Kagoma, Y. K, Stall, N., Rubinstein, E., & Naudie, D. (2012). People, planet and profits: the case for greening operating rooms. *Canadian Medical Association Journal, 184*(17), 1905–1911. https://dx.doi.org/10.1503/cmaj.112139

Kaneko, T., & Davidson, M. (2014). Use of the hybrid operating room in cardiovascular medicine. *Circulation, 130*, 910–917. https://dx.doi.org/10.1161/circulationaha.114.006510

Kapoor, M. C. (2017). Atmospheric pollution in cardiac operating rooms. *Annals of Cardiac Anaesthesia, 20*(4), 391–392. https://dx.doi.org/10.4103/aca.aca_126_17

Katz, J. D. (2017). Control of the environment in the operating room. *Anesthesia and Analgesia, 125*(4), 1214–1218. https://dx.doi.org/10.1213/ANE.0000000000001626

Keller, S., Tschan, F., Semmer, N. K., Holzer, E., Candinas, D., Brink, M., & Beldi, G. (2018). Noise in the operating room distracts members of the surgical team: an observational study. *World Journal of Surgery, 42*, 3880–3887. https://dx.doi.org/10.1007/s00268-018-4730-7

Kenters, N., Gottlieb, T., Hopman, J., Mehtar, S., Schweizer, M. L., Tartari, E., … Voss, A. (2018). An international survey of cleaning and disinfection practices in the healthcare environment. *Journal of Hospital Infection, 100*(2), 236–241. https://dx.doi.org/10.1016/j.jhin.2018.05.008

Khalkhal, E., Rezaei-Tavirani, M., Zali, M. R., & Akbari, Z. (2019). The evaluation of laser application in surgery: a review article. *Journal of Lasers in Medical Sciences, 10*(Suppl. 1), S104–S111. https://dx.doi.org/10.15171/jlms.2019.S18

Khankari, K. (2018). Computational fluid dynamics (CFD) analysis of hospital operating room ventilation systems, part I: analysis of air change rates. *ASHRAE Journal, 60*(6). Retrieved from <https://www.ashrae.org/technical-resources/ashrae-journal/featured-articles/computational-fluid-dynamics-cfd-analysis-of-hospital-operating-room-ventilation-systems-part-i-analysis-of-air-change-rates>.

King, C. A., & Spry, C. (2019). Infection prevention and control. In J. C. Rothrock & D. L McEwen (Eds.), *Alexander's care of the patient in surgery* (16th ed., pp. 54–106). St. Louis, MO: Elsevier.

Klein, L., Miller, D., Balter, S., Laskey, W., Haines, D., Norbash, A., … Goldstein, J. A. (2009). Occupational health hazards in interventional laboratory: time for a safer environment. *Radiology*, *250*(2), 538–544.

Knulst, A., & Dankelman, J. (2017). Surgical lighting [Unpublished thesis]. 10.4233/uuid:19182ec3-bffe-4b2c-a366-ef58c11d2e4f. Retrieved from <https://www.researchgate.net/publication/320195804_Surgical_Lighting>.

Kömürcü, E., Kiraz, H. A., Kaymaz, B., Gölge, U. H., Nusran, G., Göksel, F., … Hanci, V. (2015). The effect of intraoperative sounds of saw and hammer on psychological condition in patients with total knee arthroplasty: prospective randomized study. *The Scientific World Journal*, Article ID 690569. https://dx.doi.org/10.1155/2015/690569

Külpmann, R., Christiansen, B., Kramer, A., Lüderitz, P., Pitten, F. A., Wille, F., … Halabi, M. (2016). Hygiene guideline for the planning, installation, and operation of ventilation and air-conditioning systems in health-care settings – Guideline of the German Society for Hospital Hygiene (DGKH). *GMS Hygiene and Infection Control*, *11*, 2196–5226. https://dx.doi.org/10.3205/dgkh000263

Lewin, J. M., Brauer, J. A., & Ostad, A. (2011). Surgical smoke and the dermatologist. *Journal of the American Academy of Dermatology*, *65*(3), 636–641. https://dx.doi.org/10.1016/j.jaad.2010.11.017

Link, T. (2019). Guideline implementation: design and maintenance of the surgical suite. *AORN Journal*, *109*(4), 479–491. https://dx.doi.org/10.1002/aorn.12628

Livshiz-Riven, I., Borer, A., Nativ, R., Eskira, S., & Larson, E. (2015). Relationship between shared patient care items and healthcare-associated infections: a systematic review. *International Journal of Nursing Studies*, *52*(1), 380–392. https://dx.doi.org/10.1016/j.ijnurstu.2014.06.001

Lizarondo, L. (2019). *Evidence summary: ensuring perioperative nurses' well-being and mental health*. Adelaide: Joanna Briggs Institute.

Loison, G., Troughton, R., Raymond, F., Lepelletier, D., Lucet, J. C., Avril, C., & Birgand, G. (2017). Dress code and traffic flow in the operating room: a multicentre study of staff discipline during surgical procedures. *Journal of Hospital Infection*, *96*(3). https://dx.doi.org/10.1016/j.jhin.2017.03.026

Lucio, L. M. C., Braz, M. G., do Nascimento Jr, P., Braz, J. C., & Braz, L .G. (2018). Occupational hazards, DNA damage, and oxidative stress on exposure to waste anesthetic gases. *Brazilian Journal of Anesthesiology (English ed.)*, *68*(1), 33–41. Retrieved from <https://creativecommons.org/licenses/by-nc-nd/4.0/>.

Luck, E. S., & Gillespie, B. M. (2017). Technological advancements in the OR: do we need to redefine intraoperative nursing roles? *AORN Journal*, *106*(4), 4279–4281. https://dx.doi.org/10.1016/j.aorn.2017.08.012

Malik, A., Lenzen, M., McAlister, M., & McGain, F. (2018). The carbon footprint of Australian health care. *Lancet Planet Health*, *2*, e27–e35. https://dx.doi.org/10.1016/S2542-5196(17)30180-8

Mangeshikar, P., & Mangeshikar, A. P. (2018). Uterine manipulators for total laparoscopic hysterectomy. In I. Alkatout & L. Mettler (Eds.), *Hysterectomy: a comprehensive surgical approach* (pp. 359–368). Champaign, IL: Springer.

McCarthy, V. J. C., Wills, T., & Crowley, S. (2018). Nurses, age, job demands and physical activity at work and at leisure: a cross-sectional study. *Applied Nursing Research*, *40*, 116–121. https://dx.doi.org/10.1016/j.apnr.2018.01.010

Mertes, P. M., Ebo, D., Garcez, T., Rose, M., Sabato, V., Takazawa, T., … Voltolini, S. (2019). Comparative epidemiology of suspected perioperative hypersensitivity reactions. *British Journal of Anaesthesia*, *123*(1), e16–e28. https://dx.doi.org/10.1016/j.bja.2019.01.027

Michael, R. (2001a). When the specialty becomes a nightmare: workplace traumatic experiences amongst perioperative nurses. *ACORN Journal*, *14*(3), 11–15.

Michael, R. (2001b). Survive or thrive? The impact of workplace trauma on perioperative nurses: part 2. *ACORN Journal*, *14*(4), 10–14.

Michael, R., & Jenkins, H. (2001). Work related trauma: the experiences of perioperative nurses. *Collegian (Royal College of Nursing, Australia)*, *8*(1), 19–25. https://dx.doi.org/10.1016/s1322-7696(08)60398-4

Ministry of Health, New South Wales (NSW). (2015). *GL2015_002. Work health and safety – controlling exposure to surgical plume*. Sydney: Author. Retrieved from <https://www1.health.nsw.gov.au/pds/ActivePDSDocuments/GL2015_002.pdf>.

Ministry of Health, New South Wales (NSW). (2016). GL2016_020. *Engineering services guidelines*. Sydney: Author. Retrieved from <https://www1.health.nsw.gov.au/pds/Pages/doc.aspx?dn=GL2016_020>.

Ministry of Health, New South Wales (NSW). (2017a). Duress alarm systems. In *Protecting people and property NSW health policy and standards for security risk management in NSW health agencies, June 2013* (Ch. 11). Retrieved from <https://www.health.nsw.gov.au/policies/manuals/Documents/prot-people-prop.pdf>.

Ministry of Health, New South Wales (NSW). (2017b). *PD2017_026 Clinical and related waste management for health services*. Sydney: Author. Retrieved from <https://www1.health.nsw.gov.au/pds/Pages/doc.aspx?dn=PD2017_026>.

Ministry of Health, New South Wales (NSW). (2018a). *PD2018_013 Work health and safety: better practice procedures*. Sydney: Author. Retrieved from <https://www1.health.nsw.gov.au/pds/Pages/doc.aspx?dn=PD2018_013>.

Ministry of Health, New South Wales (NSW). (2018b). *GL2018_013 Work health and safety – blood and body substances occupational exposure prevention*. Sydney: Author. Retrieved from <https://www1.health.nsw.gov.au/pds/ActivePDSDocuments/GL2018_013.pdf>.

Ministry of Health, New South Wales (NSW). (2020). *PD2020_022 Cleaning of the healthcare environment*. Sydney: Author. Retrieved from <https://www1.health.nsw.gov.au/pds/Pages/doc.aspx?dn=PD2020_022>.

Mischke, C., Verbeek, J. H., Saarto, A., Lavoie, M. C., Pahwa, M., & Ijaz, S. (2014). Gloves, extra gloves or special types of gloves for preventing percutaneous exposure injuries in healthcare personnel. *Cochrane Database of Systematic Reviews*, 3, CD009573. https://dx.doi.org/10.1002/14651858. CD009573.pub2

Monash University. (2017). Protecting unborn and breast-fed children from the effects of maternal exposure to chemicals, biologicals, animals and radiation [procedure]. Retrieved from <https://www.monash.edu/__data/assets/pdf_file/0005/147155/unborn-child.pdf>.

Monash University. (2019). Pregnancy and work [webpage]. Retrieved from <https://www.monash.edu/ohs/info-docs/safety-topics/events-and-people/pregnancy-and-work>.

Murphy, C. L. (2014). The serious and ongoing issue of needle-stick in Australian healthcare settings. *Collegian*, *21*(4), 295–299. https://dx.doi.org/10.1016/j.colegn.2013.06.003

National Health and Medical Research Council (NHMRC). (2019). Australian guidelines for the prevention and control of infection in healthcare. Retrieved from <https://www.nhmrc.gov.au/about-us/publications/australian-guidelines-prevention-and-control-infection-healthcare-2019>.

Neumann, K., Cavalar, M., Rody, A., Friemert, L., & Beyer, D. A. (2018). Is surgical plume developing during routine LEEPs contaminated with high-risk HPV? A pilot series of experiments. *Archives of Gynecology and Obstetrics*, *297*, 421–424. https://dx.doi.org/10.1007/s00404-017-4615-2

New Zealand Government. (2015). Health and Safety at Work Act 2015. Retrieved from <https://www.legislation.govt.nz/act/public/2015/0070/latest/DLM5976660.html>.

Nursing and Midwifery Board of Australia (NMBA). (2018a). *Registrant data 1 July 2018–30 September 2018*. Melbourne: AHPRA. Retrieved from <https://www.nursingmidwiferyboard.gov.au/About/Statistics.aspx>.

Nursing and Midwifery Board of Australia (NMBA). (2018b). *Code of conduct for nurses*. Melbourne: Author. Retrieved from <https://www.nursingmidwiferyboard.gov.au/Codes-Guidelines-Statements/Professional-standards.aspx>.

Pavlinec, J., & Su, L. M. (2020). Surgical smoke in the era of the COVID-19 pandemic – is it time to reconsider policies on smoke evacuation? *Journal of Urology*, *204*, 1–3. https://dx.doi.org/10.1097/JU.0000000000001142

Philippon, J. (2016). Hazardous intraoperative behaviors: What's at risk? *American Association of Nurse Anesthetists Journal*, *84*(3), 155–156. Retrieved from <https://search.proquest.com.acs.hcn.com.au/docview/1812275953/1DC7D62D918943A4PQ/3?accountid=130851>.

Phillips, N. (2017). *Berry & Kohn's operating room technique* (13th ed.). St. Louis, MO: Elsevier, Mosby.

Queensland Government. (2010). PR100: 2010. Standard for premises – ionising radiation sources. Retrieved from <https://www.health.qld.gov.au/system-governance/licences/radiation-licensing/regulation-compliance/safety-standards>.

Queensland Government. (2019). Guideline: clinical and related waste. Retrieved from <https://environment.des.qld.gov.au/__data/assets/pdf_file/0029/89147/pr-gl-clinical-and-related-waste.pdf>.

Queensland Health. (2017a). *Capital infrastructure requirements* (3rd ed.). Volume 4: Engineering and infrastructure.

Section 3: Specifications. Brisbane: Author. Retrieved from <https://www.health.qld.gov.au/__data/assets/pdf_file/0035/397466/qh-gdl-374-4-1.pdf>.

Queensland Health. (2017b). *Capital infrastructure requirements* (3rd ed.). Volume 3: Architecture and health facility design. Section 2: Manual. Brisbane: Author. Retrieved from <https://www.health.qld.gov.au/__data/assets/pdf_file/0031/397282/qh-gdl-374-3-2.pdf>.

Queensland Health. (2017c). Management of occupational exposure to blood and body fluids. Retrieved from <https://www.health.qld.gov.au/__data/assets/pdf_file/0016/151162/qh-gdl-321-8.pdf>.

Queensland Health. (2017d). *Guide to informed decision-making in healthcare* (2nd ed). Brisbane: Author. Retrieved from <https://www.health.qld.gov.au/consent/documents/ic-guide.pdf>.

Qureshi, N. Q., Mufarrih, S. H., Irfan, S., Rashid, R. H., Zubairi, A. J., Sadruddin, A., … Noordin, S. (2020). Mobile phones in the orthopedic operating room: microbial colonization and antimicrobial resistance. *World Journal of Orthopedics*, *11*(5), 252–264. https://dx.doi.org/10.5312/wjo.v11.i5.252

Regehr, C., Kjerulf, M., Popova, S. R., & Baker, A. J. (2004). Trauma and tribulation: the experiences and attitudes of operating room nurses working with organ donors. *Journal of Clinical Nursing*, *13*(4), 430–437. https://dx.doi.org/10.1111/j.1365-2702.2004.00905.x

Richardson-Tench, M. (2007). Technician or nurturer: discourse within the OR. *ACORN Journal*, *20*(3), 12–15.

Rioux, M., Garland, A., Webster, D., & Reardon, E. (2013). HPV positive tonsillar cancer in two laser surgeons: case reports. *Journal of Otolaryngology – Head & Neck Surgery*, *42*, 54. https://dx.doi.org/10.1186/1916-0216-42-54

Rodger, D. (2020). Surgical fires: still a burning issue in England and Wales. *Journal of Perioperative Practice*, *30*(5), 135–140. https://dx.doi.org/10.1177/1750458919861906

Rose, M. A., Garcez, T., Savic, S., & Garvey, L. H. (2019). Chlorhexidine allergy in the perioperative setting: a narrative review. *British Journal of Anaesthesia*, *123*(1), e95–e103. https://dx.doi.org/10.1016/j.bja.2019.01.033

Rovaldi, C. J., & King, P. J. (2015). The effect of an interdisciplinary QI project to reduce OR foot traffic. *AORN Journal*, *101*, 667–678. https://dx.doi.org/10.1016/j.aorn.2015.03.011

Roy, S., & Smith, L. P. (2019). Preventing and managing operating room fires in otolaryngology-head and neck surgery. *Otolaryngologic Clinics of North America*, *52*(1), 163–171. https://dx.doi.org/10.1016/j.otc.2018.08.011

Royal Australasian College of Surgeons (RACS). (2017). *Discrimination, bullying and sexual harassment, Policy Reference: REL-GOV-028*. Royal Australasian College of Surgeons. Retrieved from <https://www.surgeons.org/about-racs/policies>.

Rychetnik, L., Sainsbury, P., & Stewart, G. (2018). How local health districts can prepare for the effects of climate change: an adaptation model applied to metropolitan Sydney. *Australian Health Review*, *43*, 601–610. https://dx.doi.org/10.1071/AH18153. Retrieved from <https://www.publish.csiro.au/AH/AH18153>.

Safe Work Australia. (2011). Design and handling of surgical instrument transport cases: a guide on health and safety standards. Retrieved from <https://www.safework.nsw.gov.au/resource-library/health-care-and-social-assistance/design-and-handling-of-surgical-instrument-transport-cases-guide-on-health-and-safety-standards>.

Safe Work Australia. (2013). Guide for managing the risk of fatigue at work. Retrieved from <https://www.safeworkaustralia.gov.au/system/files/documents/1702/managing-the-risk-of-fatigue.pdf>.

Safe Work Australia. (2015). Exposure to multiple hazards among Australian workers. Canberra: Author. Retrieved from <https://www.safeworkaustralia.gov.au/system/files/documents/1702/exposure-to-multiple-hazards-report.pdf>.

Safe Work Australia. (2018a). *The model code of practice: How to manage work health and safety risks*. Canberra: Author. Retrieved from <https://www.safeworkaustralia.gov.au/book/model-code-practice-how-manage-work-health-and-safety-risks#41-the-hierarchy-of-control-measures>.

Safe Work Australia. (2018b). Priority industry snapshot: Health care and social assistance. Retrieved from <https://www.safeworkaustralia.gov.au/collection/priority-industry-snapshots-2018>.

Safe Work New South Wales (NSW). (2017). Cytotoxic drugs and related waste – risk management. Catalogue no. SW08559. Retrieved from <https://www.safework.nsw.gov.au/__data/assets/pdf_file/0005/287042/SW08559-Cytotoxic-drugs-and-related-risk-management-guide.pdf>.

Sawchuk, W. S., Weber, P. J., Lowy, D. R., & Dzubow, L. M. (1989). Infectious papillomavirus in the vapor of warts treated with carbon dioxide laser or electrocoagulation: detection and protection. *Journal of the American Academy of Dermatology*, 21, 41–49. https://dx.doi.org/10.1016/s0190-9622(89)70146-8

Schuetze, K., Eickhoff, A., Dehner, C., Schultheiss, M., Gebhard, F., & Richter, P. H. (2019). Radiation exposure for the surgical team in a hybrid-operating room. *Journal of Robotic Surgery*, 13, 91–98. https://dx.doi.org/10.1007/s11701-018-0821-6

Simons, F. E. R., Ebisawa, M., Sanchez-Borges, M., Thong, B. Y., Worm, M., Tanno, L. K., … Sheikh, A. (2015). 2015 update of the evidence base: World Allergy Organization anaphylaxis guidelines. *World Allergy Organization Journal*, 8(1), 32. https://dx.doi.org/10.1186/s40413-015-0080-1

Singh, S., Reddy, S., & Shrivastava, R. (2017). Does laminar airflow make a difference to the infection rates for lower limb arthroplasty: a study using the National Joint Registry and local surgical site infection data for two hospitals with and without laminar airflow. *European Journal of Orthopaedic Surgery & Traumatology*, 27(2), 261–265. https://dx.doi.org/10.1007/s00590-016-1852-1

Smalley, P. (2011). Laser safety: risks, hazards, and control measures. *Laser Safety*, 20(2), 95–106.

Smalley, P. (2019). Are you ready to take control of surgical plume? Unpublished conference paper. The 9th Conference of the European Operating Room Nurses Association, 16–19 May 2019. The Hague, The Netherlands.

Smalley, P., & Cubitt, J. (2015). Clean air in surgery: a new ACORN initiative. *ACORN Journal*, 28(3), 38–39.

Smith, C. E. (2019). Workplace issues and staff safety. In J. C. Rothrock & D. L McEwen (Eds.), *Alexander's care of the patient in surgery* (16th ed., pp. 37–53). St. Louis, MO: Elsevier.

Smith, F. D. (2010). Management of exposure to waste anesthetic gases. *AORN Journal*, 91, 482–494. https://dx.doi.org/10.1016/j.aorn.2009.10.022

Smith, J., & Palesy, D. (2018). Technology stress in perioperative nursing: an ongoing concern. *ACORN Journal*, 31(2), 25–28.

South Eastern Sydney Local Health District (SESLHD). (2017). SESLHNPR/268, Work health and safety – electrical risks management procedure. Sydney: Author. Retrieved from <https://www.seslhd.health.nsw.gov.au/sites/default/files/documents/SESLHDPR268.pdf>.

Spruce, L. (2017). Back to basics: radiation safety. *AORN Journal*, 106(1), 42–49. https://dx.doi.org/10.1016/j.aorn.2017.05.001

St George Hospital and Community Health Service. (2019). Management of cytotoxic waste in the operating room. In *The St George Hospital and Community Health Service Perioperative Unit Workplace Instruction Manual*. (pp. 1–5). Sydney: Author.

Standards Australia. (2000). *AS/NZS 4543.3.2000 Protective devices against diagnostic medical X-radiation*. Part 3: Protective clothing and protective devices for gonads. Sydney: Author.

Standards Australia. (2004). *AS/NZS 2500 Guide to the safe use of electricity in patient care*. Sydney: Author.

Standards Australia. (2005). *AS/NZS 3200.2.13-2005. Guide to the safe use of medical electrical equipment – particular requirements for safety – anaesthetic systems* (2nd ed.). Sydney: Author.

Standards Australia. (2011a). *AS/NZS IEC 60825.1:2011 Safety of laser products: equipment classification and requirements*. Sydney: Author.

Standards Australia. (2011b). *AS/NZS IEC 60825.14:2011 Safety of laser products: a user guide*. Sydney: Author.

Standards Australia. (2012). *AS1668.2 The use of ventilation and air conditioning in buildings. Part 2: Mechanical ventilation in buildings*. Sydney: Author.

Standards Australia. (2014). *AS/NZS 4187 Reprocessing of reusable medical devices in health service organizations*. Sydney: Author.

Standards Australia. (2018a). *Safe use of lasers and intense light sources in healthcare*. Sydney: Author.

Standards Australia. (2018b). *AS 3816:2018 Management of clinical and related wastes*. Sydney: Author.

State of NSW and Environment Protection Authority (EPA). (2018). Radiation guideline 4 Compliance requirements for x-ray protective clothing. Retrieved from <https://www.epa.nsw.gov.au/-/media/epa/corporate-site/resources/radiation/18p0695-radiation-guideline4-xray-clothing.pdf>.

State of Queensland. (2018). Guide for handling cytotoxic drugs and related waste. Office of Industrial Relations. Workplace Health and Safety Queensland. Retrieved from <https://www.worksafe.qld.gov.au/__data/assets/pdf_file/0006/88710/guide-handling-cytoxic-drugs-related-waste.pdf>.

State of Victoria. (2018). Waste education in healthcare. Summary report. Department of Health and Human Services.

Retrieved from <https://www2.health.vic.gov.au/hospitals-and-health-services/planning-infrastructure/sustainability/waste>.

State of Victoria. (2020). Clinical and related waste guidance – supplement for healthcare staff. Victorian Health and Human Services Building Authority. Retrieved from <https://www2.health.vic.gov.au/about/publications/policiesand guidelines/clinical-related-waste-guidance>.

Tan, E., & Russell, K. P. (2017). Surgical plume and its implications: a review of the risk and barriers to a safe work place. *Journal of Perioperative Nursing, 30*(4), 2.

Thomas, A. M., & Simmons, M. J. (2018). The effectiveness of ultra-clean air operating theatres in the prevention of deep infection in joint arthroplasty surgery. *Bone & Joint Journal, 100-B*(10), 1264–1269. https://dx.doi.org/10.1302/0301-620X.100B10

Vaisman, A. I. (1967). Working conditions in the operating room and their effect on the health of anesthetists. *Experimental Surgery and Anesthesiology [Eksp Khir Anesteziol – Russian], 12*, 44–49.

Victorian Surgical Consultative Council (VSCC). (2014). Victorian surgical consultative council triennial report 2011–2013. Retrieved from <https://www2.health.vic.gov.au/about/publications/annualreports/Victorian%20Surgical%20Consultative%20Council%20Triennial%20Report%202011-2013>.

Villafranca, A., Hamlin, C., Enns, S., & Jacobsohn, E. (2017). Disruptive behaviour in the perioperative setting: a contemporary review. *Canadian Journal of Anaesthesia, 64*(2), 128–140. https://dx.doi.org/10.1007/s12630-016-0784-x

Vourtzoumis, P., Alkhamesi, N., Elnahas, A., Hawel, J. E., & Schlachta, C. (2020). Operating during COVID-19: is there a risk of viral transmission from surgical smoke during surgery? *Canadian Journal of Surgery, 63*(3), E299–E301. https://dx.doi.org/10.1503/cjs.007020

Waitemata District Health Board (WDHB). (2002). Report into the operating fire incident. Retrieved from <https://www.medsafe.govt.nz/downloads/alertWaitemata.pdf>.

Wakefield, E. (2018). Is your graduate nurse suffering from transition shock? *Journal of Perioperative Nursing, 31*(1), Article 5. Retrieved from <https://dx.doi.org/10.26550/2209-1092.1024>.

Weinberg, D., Saleh, M., & Sinha, Y. (2015). Twelve tips for medical students to maximise learning in theatre. *Medical Teacher, 37*, 34–40. https://dx.doi.org/10.3109/0142159X.2014.932899

Weinstein, R. A., & Bonten, M. J. M. (2017). Laminar airflow and surgical site infections: the evidence is blowing in the wind. *Lancet Infectious Diseases, 17*(5), 472–473. https://dx.doi.org/10.1016/S1473-3099(17)30060-9

Weiss, A., Hollandsworth, H. M, Alseidi, A., Scovel, L., French, C., Derrick, E. L., & Klaristenfeld, D. (2016). Environmentalism in surgical practice. *Current Problems in Surgery, 53*(4), 165–205. https://dx.doi.org/10.1067/j.cpsurg.2016.02.001.

Western Australia Department of Health. (2018, April). Building guidelines. In *Western Australia health facility guidelines for architectural requirements*. Retrieved from <https://ww2.health.wa.gov.au/,/media/Files/Corporate/general%20documents/Licensing/PDF/standards/building-guidelines-architectural-requirements.pdf>.

White, S. A. (2017). Determination of the infection risks posed by the use of mobile technology in healthcare settings [thesis], University of Huddersfield, UK. Retrieved from <https://eprints.hud.ac.uk/id/eprint/32623/1/FINAL%20THESIS%20-%20WHITE.pdf>.

Wong, S. W., Smith, R., & Crowe, P. (2010). Optimizing the operating theatre environment. *Australia and New Zealand Journal of Surgery, 80*, 917–924. https://dx.doi.org/10.1111/j1445-2197.2010.05526x

World Health Organization (WHO). (2019). Building climate-resilient health systems [Fact sheet: August]. WPR/2019/RDO/005. WHO Western Pacific Region. Retrieved from <https://iris.wpro.who.int/bitstream/handle/10665.1/14390/WPR-2019-RDO-005-eng.pdf>.

Wright, M. I. (2016). Implementing no interruption zones in the perioperative environment. *AORN Journal, 104*(6), 536–540. https://dx.doi.org/10.1016/j.aorn.2016.09.018

Wyssusek, K. H., Foong, W. M., Steel, C., & Gillespie, B. M. (2016). The gold in garbage: implementing a waste segregation and recycling initiative. *AORN Journal, 103*(3), 316.e1–8. https://dx.doi.org/10.1016/j.aorn.2016.01.014

Xie, A., & Carayon, P. (2015). A systematic review of human factors and ergonomics (HFE) based healthcare system redesign for quality of care and patient safety. *Ergonomics, 58*(1), 33–49. https://dx.doi.org/10.1080/00140139.2014.959070

Zabihirad, J., Mojdeh, S., & Shahriari, M. (2019). Nurse's perioperative care errors and related factors in the operating room. *Electronic Journal of General Medicine, 16*(2), em132. https://dx.doi.org/10.29333/ejgm/94220

FURTHER READING

American Society of Anesthesiologists (ASA). (2013). Practice advisory for the prevention and management of operating room fires: an updated report by the American Society of Anesthesiologists task force on operating room fires. *Anesthesiology, 118*(2), 271–290. https://dx.doi.org/10.1097/ALN.0b013e31827773d2

Australian College of Perioperative Nurses (ACORN). (2020). *ACORN standards for perioperative nursing* (16th ed., Vols. 1–2). Adelaide: Author.

Brown, C., & Owen, S. L. F. (2019). An exploration on the relationship between traffic flow and the rate of surgical site infections: a literature review. *Journal of Perioperative Practice, 29*(5), 135–139. https://dx.doi.org/10.1177/1750458918815550

Centers for Disease Control and Prevention (CDC) and the Infection Control Africa Network (ICAN). (2019). *Best practices for environmental cleaning in healthcare facilities in resource-limited settings*. Atlanta, GA: US Department of Health and Human Services, CDC. Retrieved from <https://www.cdc.gov/hai/prevent/resource-limited/index.html>.

Otter, J. A., Yezli, S., & French, G. L. (2011). The role played by contaminated surfaces in the transmission of nosocomial pathogens. *Infection Control and Hospital Epidemiology*, *32*(7), 687–699. https://dx.doi.org/10.1086/660363

Royal Children's Hospital, Melbourne. (n.d.). Biomedical engineering electrical safety. Retrieved from <https://www.rch.org.au/bme_rch/electrical_safety>.

Society for Healthcare Epidemiology of America (SHEA). (2014). Strategies to prevent surgical site infections in acute care hospitals. *Infection Control and Hospital Epidemiology*, *35*(6), 605–627. https://dx.doi.org/10.1086/676022

State of Victoria. (2018). Victorian Surgical Consultative Council (VSCC) chairperson's triennial report 2015–2017. Department of Health and Human Services. Retrieved from <https://www.bettersafercare.vic.gov.au/reports-and-publications/victorian-surgical-consultative-council-report>.

State of Victoria. (n.d.). Managing exposures to blood and body fluids or substances. Retrieved from <https://www2.health.vic.gov.au/public-health/infectious-diseases/infection-control-guidelines/manage-exposure-blood-body-fluids-substances>.

University of South Australia. (2017). *What is the impact of chlorhexidine use on the incidence of anaphylaxis? Literature review – commissioned by the National Health and Medical Research Council (NHMRC)*. Adelaide: University of South Australia. Division of Health Sciences. Retrieved from <https://www.nhmrc.gov.au/about-us/publications/australian-guidelines-prevention-and-control-infection-health-care-2019>.

CHAPTER 6

Infection Prevention and Control

JANNELLE CARLILE • TIM COLE
EDITOR: MENNA DAVIES

LEARNING OUTCOMES

- Differentiate between microorganisms and their pathogenicity
- Discuss the human body's defence mechanisms against infection
- Explore measures to minimise the transmission of pathogens in the perioperative environment
- Identify the principles of standard and transmission-based precautions
- Apply the principles of aseptic technique in perioperative practice
- Discuss the practices used in reprocessing, sterilisation and disinfection of reusable medical devices (RMDs)

KEY TERMS

asepsis	healthcare-associated infections
aseptic field	microorganisms
aseptic technique	personal protective equipment
biofilms	scrubbing
biological indicators	skin antisepsis
disinfection	sterile
double gloving	sterilisation
gowning	surgical/professional conscience

INTRODUCTION

This chapter presents fundamental aspects of infection prevention and control and the application of the principles of asepsis, which are the cornerstone of perioperative nursing practice. The infective process is discussed along with modes of transmission and how the body combats pathogenic microorganisms. Environmental controls enacted to reduce the spread of infection, along with standard and transmission-based precautions, are described and their practical application discussed. The principles of asepsis, the practical application of aseptic technique and the concept of surgical conscience are examined; also addressed is the surgical scrub, and the methods of prepping and draping the surgical patient and creating an aseptic field. Infection control as an adverse event is briefly explored. A description of practices used to reprocess, sterilise and disinfect reusable medical devices completes this chapter.

The critical thinking questions in this chapter will relate to the infection prevention and aseptic practices of the following surgical team:
- RN Sandy Pereira and RN Rob Cohen – instrument and circulating nurses
- Dr Patrick Slattery and Dr Ivy West – consultant surgeon and registrar
- Dr Marion Thomas and Dr Vince De Silva – consultant anaesthetist and registrar
- EN Marcus Macedo – anesthetic nurse
- Student Nurse Rose Cheng – on clinical rotation
- Jimmy Montano – theatre orderly.

A brief description of the healthcare setting and full history of the patient, Mrs Peterson, in this unfolding scenario is provided in the Introduction at the front of the book for readers to review when answering the questions.

CLASSIFICATION AND TYPES OF MICROORGANISMS

In order to understand the infective process and the measures taken to prevent transmission of **microorganisms**, it is necessary to review aspects of microbiology. It is beyond the scope of this text to explore microbiology in depth, but a brief examination of the particular organisms of concern, in relation to the care of surgical patients, is presented. Two main classifications of microorganisms are described by Engelkirk, Fader and Duben-Engelkirk (2019):

- cellular (e.g. bacteria, algae, protozoa and fungi)
- acellular (e.g. viruses and prions).

Microorganisms of special interest to perioperative nurses include several types of bacteria, fungi, viruses and prions, which are outlined below; this does not include all microorganisms that may be found in the hospital setting.

Bacteria

Bacteria are simple, unicellular organisms containing internal structures such as a nucleus, cytoplasm, plasmids and ribosomes (Lee & Bishop, 2016). Even though there are thousands of types of bacteria, very few cause disease/infection. Bacteria are extremely adaptable and survive and grow in various environments, often multiplying rapidly. Bacteria are the most common cause of surgical site infections (SSIs), with staphylococci and streptococci being responsible for many of these (Lee & Bishop, 2016). Most bacteria found in the perioperative environment are shed from the skin of personnel, so hand hygiene is the most efficacious way of countering their spread (National Health and Medical Research Council [NHMRC], 2019).

Gram-positive cocci

Staphylococci. Staphylococci (e.g. *Staphylococcus aureus* and *Staphylococcus epidermidis*) are part of the normal flora found on the skin and mucous membranes of the nasopharynx, urethra and vagina. They can coexist in these areas without any adverse effect on the host, and those that live on the skin are termed *transient organisms*. Staphylococci can survive for long periods in the air, dust, bedding and clothing, making cleanliness of the perioperative environment paramount (King & Spry, 2019). In the perioperative setting, these bacteria can be transmitted from one patient to another on the hands of healthcare workers, where they can subsequently have significant negative effects. For example, they can enter the wound of a surgical patient, causing either a superficial or a deep infection; more seriously, exotoxins secreted by *S. aureus* can cause toxic shock syndrome, which can be fatal if left untreated (Lee & Bishop, 2016). Staphylococci are strongly associated with **healthcare-associated infections** (HAIs).

Streptococci. Streptococci are responsible for a wide range of diseases and infections. These include throat and wound infections, pneumonia, septicaemia and necrotising fasciitis. *Streptococcus pyogenes* is frequently implicated in SSIs. Streptococci tend to be more virulent than staphylococci; however, they are much more likely than the latter to be sensitive to penicillin. Streptococci can be a normal resident of the upper airway, vagina and anus and are spread via direct and indirect contact, causing infection and illness in susceptible populations (Lee & Bishop, 2016; Wilson, McNab, & Henderson, 2019).

Enterococci. Enterococci are bacteria normally found in the gastrointestinal tract and female genital tract. They cause infections such as SSIs and bloodstream infections (BSIs). They can be transmitted via the hands of a healthcare worker or contaminated equipment to susceptible, high-risk patients, including surgical patients. They are significant hospital pathogens because strains of enterococci have developed resistance to commonly used antibiotics, for example methicillin-resistant *S. aureus* (MRSA) and vancomycin-resistant *Enterococcus* (VRE) (Lee & Bishop, 2016).

Gram-positive rods. Clostridia are Gram-positive anaerobic bacteria that can cause serious illness owing to their ability to produce endospores, which can survive for many years in a dormant state and are highly resistant to drying, heat and routine disinfection procedures (King & Spry, 2019). Sterilisation processes must demonstrate their effectiveness against spore-forming microorganisms for a reusable medical device (RMD) to be considered sterile. Without these measures, the endospores germinate into new bacterial cells and can cause significant infections, which can be fatal (e.g. *Clostridium perfringens*, which can cause gas gangrene).

A more common and highly infectious bacterium is *Clostridium difficile*, which forms part of the normal flora of the large bowel. Disruption of the normal flora can occur in patients taking high doses of antibiotics, particularly over a prolonged period, allowing *C. difficile* to release toxins that can cause significant complications such as dehydration, kidney failure, toxic megacolon and bowel perforation. Patients are treated with antibiotics (e.g. metronidazole or vancomycin), combined with strict infection control measures (King & Spry, 2019; Stuart et al., 2019).

C. difficile is transmitted by contact with an infected person or objects and, due to its highly infectious nature, patients with *C. difficile* should not be admitted to the operating suite unless requiring urgent surgery. Management of patients with *C. difficile* in the perioperative environment requires strict infection prevention and control measures. Contact precautions should be followed. Hand washing using antimicrobial soap and water is preferred to alcoholic-based hand rub, as washing mechanically dislodges the organism, including spores, from skin surfaces. After the patient's procedure, the environment will require thorough cleaning. Once all visible contaminants have been removed using a neutral detergent, surfaces must be cleaned with a bleach-based solution, which is left in contact with surfaces for 10 minutes (NHMRC, 2019).

Gram-negative bacteria

Gram-negative bacteria have a complex outer cell wall which acts as a protective barrier, enabling them to withstand penetration by many substances including widely used antiseptics, disinfectants and antibiotics (Lee & Bishop, 2016, Wilson et al., 2019). It also enables some Gram-negative organisms to produce enzymes such as extended β-lactamases (ESBLs), which neutralise commonly used β-lactam antibiotics such as penicillins and cephlaosporins, rendering them ineffective. In more recent years, metallo β-lactamase enzymes (MBLs) have also developed the capability to pass on this resistant property to other closely related species that are now resistant to the carbapenum class of antibiotics, developing into what are colloquially termed 'superbugs' such as carbapenum-producing Enterobacterales (CPE) (Australian Commission on Safety and Quality in Health Care [ACSQHC/the Commission], 2017; Lee & Bishop, 2016). CPE are the newest in a long line of 'superbugs' and are a particular problem in hospital settings. CPE are (typically) resistant to nearly all known antibiotics; they increase patient morbidity and mortality and have the potential to spread and act as a reservoir of resistant genes for transmission to other organisms. Aggressive infection prevention measures, such as environmental cleaning, and prudent use of antibiotics are vital to combat this and potential emerging 'superbugs' (New Zealand [NZ] Ministry of Health, 2018).

Other Gram-negative bacteria of note are the Enterobacterales such as *Klebsiella, Serratia, Proteus* and *Yersinia,* which are naturally occurring bacteria found within the gastrointestinal tract. They can easily transmit beyond the gut to other areas within the body, causing serious infections such as urinary tract and surgical site infections (NSW Health, 2019). *Pseudomonas aeruginosa* is a biofilm-producing bacterium that is commonly found in soil and water and can become problematic within the hospital environment when it colonises the inside of sinks and taps (Lee & Bishop 2016). This opportunistic Gram-negative bacterium is commonly identified in SSIs.

Both Gram-positive and Gram-negative pathogens have the capacity to produce **biofilms**. Biofilms adhere to device surfaces (e.g. urinary catheters, orthopaedical implants) and act as a protective layer, encasing the organisms in a complex extracellular matrix. This layer protects the bacteria from the host's immune system and antibiotic therapy. Once a biofilm develops on a device it can be very challenging to remove and can lead in some cases to failure of the implant because of overwhelming infection (Schrank & Branch-Elliman, 2017). Treatment options include high-dose antibiotics. Prevention of biofilm formation can be achieved by the use strict aseptic technique and minimal handling of implants. Research is being carried out on coating devices with a protective layer to prevent bacteria attaching to the device, using natural and synthetic products (Khatoon, McTiernan, Suuronen, Mah, & Alarcon, 2018).

Fungi

There are two major types of fungi – yeast and moulds – and many are beneficial to humans; for example, moulds are a source of antibiotics (Lee & Bishop, 2016). They are often termed 'nature's original recyclers' because they secrete enzymes that decompose dead plant and animal matter, turning them into absorbable nutrients. Although of less significance within the perioperative setting, some fungal strains, such as *Candida albicans*, cause localised infections in the mouth and reproductive tract, which have the potential to become systemic infections. *Candida auris* is a newly emerging multiresistant strain of fungi reported to have a mortaility rate of up to 59% (South Australia Health, 2020). Fungi have been isolated in the nail beds of nurses who wear acrylic nails, even following normal surgical scrub techniques. This has led to policies prohibiting acrylic- and gel-coated nails within the operating suite owing to the danger of transmitting fungal infections to patients (Australian College of Perioperative Nurses [ACORN], 2020a; Clinical Excellence Commission [CEC], 2020a; NHMRC, 2019).

Aspergillus fumigatus is a fungus commonly found in the environment, and it may be liberated into the air in and around the perioperative environment during routine maintenance work and building renovations, and via air-conditioning vents. Strict infection prevention and control risk management practices must be implemented to minimise any potential outbreaks of *Aspergillosis* when any maintenance requiring entry into the roof space or building works within close proximity to the operating suite is being conducted. Such an infection can be lethal to immunosuppressed patients in particular (Patterson, 2019).

Viruses

A virus (from the Latin *virus*, meaning toxin or poison) is a microscopic organism. Viruses are among the smallest known infectious agents and are responsible for causing severe, often fatal infections (e.g. hepatitis C). Viruses replicate by invading a host cell and using its DNA/RNA, protein and other nutrients to survive and reproduce. In the process, they damage or destroy the host cell. The reproductive process concludes when the host cell bursts (cell lysis), spreading new viruses to nearby cells, where the process is repeated (Lee & Bishop, 2016). This process stimulates an antibody response in the infected person.

Hepatitis-causing viruses are among the most common viruses and there are nine identified viral strains: hepatitis A to I (Australian Society for HIV Medicine [ASHM], 2020; Bowden & Locarnini, 2018). The strains of most concern to perioperative nurses are hepatitis B and C viruses. These blood-borne pathogens, along with human immunodeficiency virus (HIV), can be transmitted through contact with blood and body fluids during invasive procedures. This may be through exposure to a sharps injury or via splashes into unprotected eyes or mucous membranes.

In 2020, the COVID-19 pandemic required healthcare professionals to re-examine infection prevention and control practices. Feature box 6.1 provides a summary of these practices as they relate to the perioperative environment.

FEATURE BOX 6.1
COVID-19 – Global Pandemic 2020

Coronavirus/COVID-19 (SARS-CoV-2 as it is now known), is closely related to the severe acute respiratory syndrome (SARS) and Middle East respiratory syndrome (MERS) that emerged in 2003 and 2015 respectively. As COVID-19 is an emerging disease in 2020–21, there is still much to be learnt. The impact of a COVID-19 patient (suspected or positive) within the operating suite centres on the protection of healthcare workers from exposure to a COVID-19 positive patient when they transition through the perioperative environment, and in particular during anaesthetic induction and intubation.

Basic principles of transmission-based precautions apply, with contact, droplet and airborne precautions to be applied in accordance with current national and state policy guidelines and managed under a risk management framework. As COVID-19 is an evolving situation, guidelines will change in accordance with the latest research.

Social distancing, cough etiquette, hand hygiene and wearing of masks when <1.5 m from a patient are currently recommended practices to reduce the transmission of COVID-19. Of particular importance is the fit testing of P2 and N95 masks for individual staff members to ensure maximum protection. These masks are recommended for all frontline staff caring for patients with diseases that are transmissible via airborne particles, such as measles, tuberculosis and COVID-19 (Centers for Disease Control and Prevention [CDC], 2021; CEC, 2020a).

Chapter 8 describes the precautions to be taken by the anaesthetic team when managing patients who are COVID-19 positive.

Instrument/Circulating Nurse Considerations When Managing COVID-19 Positive Patients

These include, but are not limited to, the following procedures, which are subject to local policies:

- wear appropriate PPE (i.e. N95/P2[a] masks and eye protection) – all donning and doffing should take place in the designated area and a 'buddy' system used to ensure donning/doffing is completed correctly
- use negative-pressure ORs where possible (this ensures that aerosols are not pushed out of the OR into surrounding areas)
- the minimum number of staff is to be within the OR
- remove or cover non-essential equipment
- use an outside 'runner', for example to obtain additional equipment or dispatch specimens as required, so that the inside circulating nurse does not leave the OR
- delay bringing instrument setups into the OR until all anaesthetic procedures have been completed, to allow any aerosol particles to disperse
- process reusable medical devices (RMDs) in the usual manner
- follow local policy for cleaning in between procedures and 'resting' the OR for at least 30 minutes/5 air changes (Agency for Clinical Innovation [ACI], 2020; CEC, 2020a).

[a]Fit testing uses specialised equipment to provide quantitative data on how well a P2/N95 mask/respirator seals against the wearer's face, thus ensuring maximum protection. Records must be kept of the staff member's details, overall fit factor; make, model, style and size of respirator used; and date tested. The staff member must ensure they don the mask/respirator of the correct fit factor and must be fit checked following donning to ensure the mask/respirator is properly applied (CEC, 2020a).

Prions

Prions are small infectious particles consisting of protein only, with no nucleic acid. They are implicated in unusual neurodegenerative disorders, including bovine spongiform encephalopathy (BSE) or 'mad cow disease' and, in humans, Creutzfeldt–Jakob disease (CJD) (Lee & Bishop, 2016). The latter is thought to be due to an intracellular accumulation of an abnormal form of a normal prion protein found throughout the body and brain, and appears to assist the neurons to communicate and transport minerals. The disease can have a long incubation period, sometimes lasting years, and is most often fatal (Lee & Bishop, 2016). Prions are unusually resistant to conventional chemical and physical sterilising methods; special protocols for managing instruments that have been used on infected or potentially infected patients are discussed later in this chapter (NHMRC, 2019; NSW Health, 2019). Table 6.1 summarises the common microorganisms found in the perioperative environment.

Development of Resistance to Antimicrobial Drugs

It is thought that the overuse and inappropriate use of antibiotics are major factors in the emergence of resistant pathogens such as CRE, ESBL and multidrug-resistant tuberculosis (MDR-TB). This, combined with a reduction in the discovery and development of new antibiotic agents, is placing patients at risk of prolonged recovery from infections – and in some cases patients will die from drug-resistant infections (Lee & Bishop, 2016).

Current and emerging resistant pathogens are frequently implicated in SSIs and pose serious ongoing threats to surgical patients (Lee & Bishop, 2016). Perioperative nurses are in the forefront of implementing infection prevention strategies to prevent the spread of these microorganisms and these will be discussed later in the chapter.

Antimicrobial Stewardship

Antimicrobial stewardship (AMS) is the term used to describe the activities, strategies and coordinated interventions designed to optimise antimicrobial use. AMS is used by hospitals and health organisations to promote quality use of antimicrobials with the aims of:
- using antimicrobials only when needed and avoiding use where there is no evidence of benefit
- selecting antimicrobials appropriately – using narrow-spectrum drugs where possible, and keeping broader-spectrum drugs in reserve

TABLE 6.1
Microorganisms Commonly Found in the Perioperative Environment

Microorganism	Source/Location	Mode of Transmission
Aspergillus fumigatus	Dust from maintenance work in proximity to OR	Airborne Direct contact
Clostridium difficile	Large bowel	Direct contact
Escherichia coli	Intestinal tract Urinary tract	Faeces Urine Direct contact
Hepatitis virus HIV	Blood Body fluids	Blood-borne Direct contact
Mycobacterium tuberculosis	Respiratory tract Urinary tract	Airborne Droplet Direct contact
Pseudomonas	Urinary tract Intestinal tract Water	Direct contact Urine Faeces
Staphylococci	Skin, hair, bedding Upper respiratory tract	Direct contact Airborne
Serratia marcescens	Urinary tract Respiratory tract	Direct contact Water
Streptococci	Oronasopharynx Skin, perianal area	Direct contact Airborne

(Source: Adapted from Phillips, N. (2017). Surgical microbiology and antimicrobial therapy. In *Berry & Kohn's operating theatre technique* (13th ed., Ch. 14). St Louis, MO: Mosby.)

- using safe and effective doses – using correct doses and limiting the duration of use to what is needed according to evidence (ACSQHC/the Commission, 2018a; CEC, 2020b).

Both Australia and New Zealand have government advisory groups to provide information and guidance and to coordinate surveillance programs (Health Quality and Safety Commission New Zealand, 2018a; NHMRC, 2019; NZ Ministry of Health, 2017).

RISK MANAGEMENT OF MICROORGANISMS

The process of infection can be likened to the links in a chain – break any of the links and infection can be prevented (VanMeter & Hubert, 2016). There are six links in the chain of infection:

1. infectious agent
2. reservoir
3. portal of exit
4. transmission
5. portal of entry
6. susceptible host.

Infectious Agent

An infection results from microorganisms invading and multiplying in the host. Pathogenic microorganisms in the form of bacteria, viruses and fungi are the causative agents in wound and systemic infections suffered by patients. The virulence and pathogenicity of the infective agent will determine the extent and severity of the infection that is produced (Shaban, Macbeth, Russo, Mitchell, & Potter, 2019).

Reservoir

The microorganisms responsible for the majority of HAIs originate from either the patient's own body flora (endogenous infections) or external (exogenous) sources such as other patients, staff or equipment. Some microorganisms exist harmlessly on patients' skin, in hair follicles, sweat glands (staphylococci) or within the bowel as normal flora (*Escherichia coli*). However, when these microorganisms enter another area of the body they can cause infection (e.g. *E. coli* can cause bladder infections and *S. aureus* causes SSIs). Both transient and resident microorganisms are found on the skin, and these can be transferred by direct contact between patients, healthcare workers, visitors and equipment, or by transfer to other body sites within the same patient where infection can subsequently develop. Transient microorganisms are easily removed by good hand hygiene (Shaban et al., 2019).

Portal of Exit

For microorganisms to continue infecting other hosts, they must have a means of leaving the body. The microorganism may exit via the same portal through which it entered the body, or it may be excreted through blood or other body fluids, faeces or droplets from the respiratory tract (Shaban et al., 2019; VanMeter & Hubert, 2016).

Transmission

The main modes of transmission within a hospital setting are via contact (including blood-borne), airborne microorganisms or larger droplets. With the exception of airborne microorganisms, the transmission of microorganisms cannot occur unassisted. In the hospital setting, the most common mode of transmission is through contact – mainly via the hands of healthcare workers, other patients or visitors, either *directly* touching the patient or *indirectly* through contact with contaminated objects (NHMRC, 2019). Vigilance in cough etiquette, hand hygiene and the use of **aseptic technique** is the most efficient method of preventing the transmission of microorganisms. Understanding the routes and sources of transmission is vital if this link in the chain is to be broken (Shaban et al., 2019).

Portal of Entry

The majority of pathogens have a preferred portal of entry as this provides the ideal environment for growth and spread. *Streptococcus* and *Staphylococcus* have adapted to several portals of entry (e.g. skin, urogenital and respiratory tracts). The main points of entry are via the skin through trauma, planned surgery or sharps injury, or via the mucous membranes of the respiratory (whooping cough), gastrointestinal (*Salmonella*) and genitorurinary tracts (*C. albicans*) (VanMeter & Hubert, 2016).

Susceptible Host

Patients undergoing surgery become susceptible hosts when their skin barrier is breached by a surgical incision. Their immune system is also compromised, further increasing their susceptibility to infection. Others who have increased susceptibility include those:

- who are very young or in the older group
- with poor nutritional status
- with underlying conditions, such diabetes, vascular disease, or chronic renal or liver failure
- who are immunocompromised (e.g. patients receiving chemotherapy) (NHMRC, 2019; Schrank & Branch-Elliman, 2017).

Healthcare workers are also susceptible hosts who may be exposed to pathogenic microorganisms from

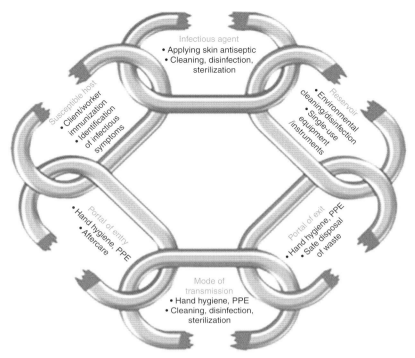

FIG. 6.1 Prevention strategies that break the chain of infection. (Source: Public Health Ontario (2019) Guide to infection prevention and control in personal service settings (3rd ed). Public Health Ontario https://www.publichealthontario.ca/-/media/documents/G/2019/guide-ipac-personal-service-settings.pdf?la=en.)

infected patients, instruments or equipment (Shaban et al., 2019).

Fig. 6.1 demonstrates how implementing prevention strategies can break a link in the chain of transmission and safeguard the patient.

NORMAL BODY DEFENCES

Whether or not a person develops an infection as a result of invasion by microorganisms will depend on the susceptibility of that person (the host) and the virulence of the microorganism. It will also depend on the body's ability to defend itself against the invading pathogens.

External Barriers

External barriers include the skin, mucous membranes and their respective secretions; these are the body's first line of defence in preventing infection. The epidermal layer of the skin contains a protein, keratin, which provides substantial resistance to bacterial enzymes and toxins. The dermal layer of skin contains sebum-secreting sebaceous glands, which lower the pH of the skin, inhibiting the growth of some bacteria and fungi (Shaban et al., 2019).

Mucous membranes heal quickly despite much wear and tear, and their sticky, mucous secretions trap foreign particles and microorganisms. Breaching the skin with a planned surgical incision bypasses this defence, increasing the risk of invasion by pathogenic organisms.

Inflammatory Response

The onset of inflammation is a non-specific defence and the body's response to tissue damage. It is evoked following any injury (e.g. physical, chemical, radiation) or invasion by microorganisms. The function of inflammation is to clear the injured site of cellular debris and any pathogens present, and to enable tissue repair to commence (Shaban et al., 2019).

Once the inflammatory response is evoked, several biochemical mediators are released, localised vasodilation occurs and plasma fluid (containing leucocytes and proteins) moves into the injured area. This causes the four outward signs of inflammation: redness, heat, swelling and pain (Shaban et al., 2019).

If the inflammatory response does not eliminate all organisms or foreign material, healing of the injury is delayed and chronic inflammation can result, which can persist for weeks or even months (Shaban et al., 2019).

See Chapter 11 for further information about wound healing.

Immune Response

The immune response, the third line of protection, is a specific body defence. Immunity is the capacity of the body's immune system to defend itself successfully against potentially infectious agents. Immunity is acquired in two ways.

- *Active immunity* is acquired when the body has been exposed to or suffered an infection; this is 'naturally acquired' immunity. Artificially acquired active immunity results from immunisation, such as with vaccines (e.g. diphtheria) given in childhood.
- *Passive immunity* may be natural and occurs when antibodies are transferred from a person with immunity to another who does not have immunity (e.g. from a mother to her fetus across the placental barrier), or it may be artificial and can be conferred with injections of immune globulins. For example, hepatitis B immunoglobulin injections may be given to a non-immune healthcare worker following a sharps injury and potential exposure to hepatitis B virus. Unlike active immunity, passive immunity is relatively short lived (Shaban et al., 2019).

INFECTION AS AN ADVERSE EVENT

Infection is one of the most frequent adverse events associated with surgical procedures and/or interventions. It is estimated that 165,000 HAIs occur in Australian hospitals each year, most of which are avoidable (NHMRC, 2019). The cost of HAIs can be measured in terms of increased morbidity and mortality, increased length of stay in hospital and an increase in both human and clinical resources (Gillespie et al., 2018). Worldwide, HAIs and the present threat from multidrug-resistant organisms (MROs) constitute one of medicine's greatest challenges. Healthcare facilities are implementing MRO-specific policies and strategies, such as the SSI bundle approach, which is discussed later in the chapter (NHMRC, 2019; NZ Ministry of Health, 2018). In 2016–17, 1502 cases of *S. aureus* bloodstream infections were reported in Australian public hospitals; such an infection has the potential to be a serious threat to patients' health (Australian Institute of Health and Welfare, 2017).

Surgical patients have a threefold greater risk of HAIs compared with other patients (ACSQHC/the

---

FEATURE BOX 6.2
Evacuation of Surgical Plume may Reduce SSIs

Surgical plume generated by electrosurgery or laser contains a cocktail of toxic gases, live viruses and bacteria (Hill, O'Neill, Powell, & Oliver, 2012). Evidence strongly suggests that, if inhaled by perioperative personnel, surgical plume can cause disease (Harkavy & Novak, 2014). A laboratory study by Schultz (2015) suggests that viable bacteria aerosolised in surgical plume could be reduced by using a surgical plume evacuator; in turn, this would reduce contamination of the surgical wound and SSIs. Further studies are required in a clinical environment to establish whether similar results can be replicated.

Commission, 2018b). Despite compelling evidence about the effectiveness of hand hygiene in reducing the spread of infection within healthcare facilities, compliance remains problematic. For a surgical patient, an HAI in the form of an SSI can be a serious postoperative complication, resulting in pain, delayed healing, longer hospital stay, prolonged use of antibiotics and, in some cases, even death. Every effort must be made both within the operating suite and in ward areas to reduce the risk of SSIs. A study by Schultz (2015) suggests that surgical plume generated by electrosurgical equipment may contain aerosolised viable bacteria and that evacuating plume can play a role in reducing SSIs (Feature box 6.2). For more information on surgical plume, see Chapter 5.

INFECTION PREVENTION AND CONTROL PRACTICES

Successful infection prevention and control practices focus on prevention; this involves identifying hazards and classifying associated risks. In turn, this requires healthcare facilities to develop infection prevention and control risk management plans, ideally within a clinical governance framework, to minimise the risk of preventable HAIs (NHMRC, 2019). Elements of successful infection prevention and control include quality and risk management policies, effective work practices and procedures, and adequate physical facilities and operational controls (NHMRC, 2019; NZ Ministry of Health, 2017). As many major infection risk factors can be found within the perioperative setting, specific requirements to prevent infection are needed (NHMRC, 2019).

FEATURE BOX 6.3
Terminology in Infection Control Practices

The use of accurate terminology used in describing infection control practices is important in order to clarify perioperative practice and avoid misunderstanding. Due to the naturally occurring organisms in the atmosphere within the perioperative environment, it is not possible to achieve a sterile technique. The commonly used term 'sterile technique' (i.e. the instruction to maintain sterility of equipment exposed to air) is obviously not possible and is often applied inaccurately. Items remain sterile as long as they are unopened in a sterilised, uncompromised package. Once opened and placed onto the surgical field, the item is exposed to airborne pathogens within the OR or procedural area and therefore cannot be accurately termed *sterile*. The more accurate term *aseptic* was adopted by ACORN in 2016 and is reflected in this book in terms such as *aseptic field* (instead of sterile field) and *aseptic technique* (instead of sterile technique).

An *aseptic technique* aims to prevent pathogenic organisms, in sufficient quantity to cause infection, from being introduced to susceptible sites by hands, surfaces and equipment.

Therefore, unlike sterile techniques, aseptic techniques are possible and can be achieved in typical hospital and community settings.

(Source: National Health and Medical Research Council. (2019). *Australian guidelines for the prevention and control of infection in healthcare*. https://www.nhmrc.gov.au/about-us/publications/australian-guidelines-prevention-and-control-infection-health-care-2019, p. 91.)

For nurses entering the perioperative environment for the first time, the array of rules and protocols can appear bewildering. While most policies are based on research evidence, some (particularly aseptic principles discussed later in the chapter) are based more on common sense, logic and rational thinking. Regardless of origin, policies and protocols provide perioperative personnel with boundaries within which they can apply infection prevention principles.

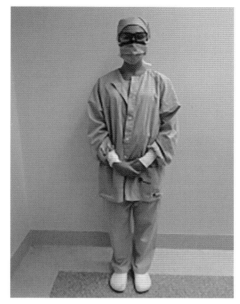

FIG. 6.2 Correct perioperative attire.

In Feature box 6.3 is a reminder of the current terminology used to guide infection prevention practices.

Environmental Controls

Chapter 5 discussed aspects of the perioperative environment, noting that many operating suite design features are necessary for effective infection prevention. These include the concept of the three zones of the perioperative environment. Personnel entering the semi-restricted and restricted zones of the operating suite must be correctly dressed in perioperative attire in order to minimise the entry of potentially pathogenic microorganisms found on the outside (street) clothing of personnel (King & Spry, 2019).

(See Fig. 6.2 and Table 6.2, which summarises correct perioperative attire.)

PATIENT SCENARIOS

SCENARIO 6.1: PERIOPERATIVE ATTIRE

RN Sandy Pereira and EN Pauline Noakes arrive at work with Student Nurse Rose Cheng and are preparing to change into perioperative attire.

Critical Thinking Question

- Describe the items of perioperative attire that the nurses will change into. Provide a rationale for each piece of attire they will wear.

TABLE 6.2
Perioperative Attire

Perioperative Attire	Rationale
Wear loose-fitting, tightly woven cotton pants and tops or dresses ('scrubs')	Friction and chafing caused by tight-fitting clothing causes dispersal of epithelial skin cells into the environment, which have the potential to contaminate aseptic fields
A fresh set of scrubs should be worn daily and changed if they become contaminated with blood/body fluids	Scrubs that have been worn or are contaminated increase the risk of cross-contamination
Perioperative attire should be changed on leaving and re-entering the suite	Scrubs worn in areas outside the perioperative environment can become contaminated, which increases the risk of cross-contamination if worn on return to the perioperative environment Long-sleeved cover gowns maybe worn when staff members leave the perioperative environment Local policies vary for this practice and should be followed in relation to use of cover gowns
Perioperative nurses who wear their own scrubs should not take them home to launder; all items worn within the perioperative environment should be laundered by the healthcare facility's laundry system	Studies have shown that microorganisms can live on fabrics which, when transported home, can place workers and their families at risk of infection Similarly, contamination from home can be brought back into the perioperative environment, as demonstrated in an early study by Neely and Maley (2000)
Street clothes should not be worn underneath perioperative attire	Street clothes harbour potentially pathogenic bacteria and should not be worn within restricted and semi-restricted areas
Within restricted areas, unscrubbed personnel should wear long-sleeved gowns fastened/tied at the back, or buttoned-up warm-up jackets with cuffed wrists	Wearing long-sleeved gown/jackets prevents the dispersal of epithelial skin cells from the arms and possible contamination of aseptic fields. Securely fastening the gowns/jackets prevents flapping and possible contamination of the aseptic field
Disposable caps or scarves that completely cover the hair should be worn and changed daily Beards require a balaclava-type headwear Perioperative staff may wear brightly coloured cotton headwear, which should comply with Australian Standards for healthcare textiles They should be laundered in an approved commercial laundry or by the healthcare facility	Hair is a significant source of microorganisms and should be completely covered. Although there is no conclusive evidence that hair covering prevents SSIs, there is evidence that hair contains potentially pathogenic bacteria and, as such, professional perioperative organisations (e.g. ACORN and AORN) recommend completely covering hair and ears when working in semi-restricted and restricted areas (ACORN, 2020a, 2020e; AORN, 2019; Spruce, 2017) Domestic washing machines are unsuitable as they do not reach the temperature required to destroy microorganisms (ACORN, 2020a)
Wear closed-toe, non-slip, low-heeled, well-fitting shoes dedicated for use within the perioperative environment NOTE: The use of shoe coverings for infection control reasons is not warranted, as no cause-and-effect relationship has been demonstrated between footwear and SSIs. Furthermore, there is an increased risk of hand contamination and cross-infection when the wearer touches the coverings to apply/remove them. It is highly recommended that staff wear shoes that are designated for wear only in the operating suite to avoid transmission of microorganisms to and from the home environment (ACORN, 2020a)	This type of footwear is easier to clean and made of material that reduces risk of penetration by sharps items and splashes from blood/body fluids Dedicated shoes that are only worn within theatres decrease the amount of outside bacteria brought into the perioperative environment (AORN, 2019; Society for Healthcare Epidemiology of America [SHEA], 2014)
Jewellery should not be worn with the operating suite; this includes wedding bands	Jewellery can harbour microorganisms and may be dislodged and drop onto the aseptic field. Wedding bands and wrist jewellery can interfere with techniques used to perform hand hygiene, resulting in higher total bacterial counts (ACSQHC/the Commission, 2020; NHMRC, 2019 p. 33; Royal Australasian College of Surgeons [RACS], 2015)
Nails should be kept short, 0.5 cm in length. All nail polish, false nails or extensions should be removed	Cracked nail polish can harbour microorganisms and cannot be cleaned effectively during routine or surgical hand washing. False nails and nail extensions can harbour fungal infections, which may be transmitted to the patient, so should be avoided (ACSQHC/the Commission, 2020; NHMRC, 2019, p. 33)
Lanyards should not be worn	Lanyards harbour bacteria, are rarely cleaned and pose a threat of transmission to patients. There is also a danger of them dangling from the wearer's neck, increasing the risk of contaminating aseptic fields (Murphy et al., 2017)
Personal items such as briefcases, handbags and backpacks should not be brought into the restricted areas of the operating theatre	Items brought from outside the perioperative environment are known to harbour potentially pathogenic bacteria (similar to outdoor clothing) and are a cross-contamination risk

Standard Precautions

Standard precautions are the first-tier approach to infection prevention and control and must be applied at all times. They are designed to reduce the transmission of microorganisms from both recognised and unrecognised sources. Standard precautions protect patients and healthcare workers, and apply when there is a risk of exposure to blood (including dried blood) and body substances, secretions and excretions (excluding sweat), regardless of whether or not they contain visible blood. Non-intact skin and mucous membranes (including the eyes) are portals of entry and must be protected. Standard precautions involve consistently applying safe work practices and protective barriers, regardless of the patient's known infectious status (ACORN, 2020b; NHMRC, 2019).

Hand hygiene

Hand hygiene is the single most important practice to reduce transmission of infectious agents in healthcare settings (ACSQHC/the Commission, 2020; Health Quality and Safety Commission New Zealand, 2018b; NHMRC, 2019; World Health Organization [WHO], 2009). The value of hand hygiene was first recognised by Semmelweis in the 19th century (Feature box 6.4). Alcohol-based hand rub containing chlorhexidine is superior in effectiveness to soap and water, but if hands are contaminated with blood or body fluids or are physically dirty then antimicrobial soap and water are required (ACSQHC/the Commission, 2020).

In 2009, WHO launched its global 'Save Lives: Clean Your Hands' program centred on the '5 moments of hand hygiene' (ACSQHC/the Commission, 2020; WHO, 2009). The '5 moments of hand hygiene' are performed:

1. before touching a patient
2. before commencing a procedure
3. after a procedure or body fluid risk exposure
4. after touching a patient
5. after touching the patient's surroundings.

While carrying out the '5 moments' may be straightforward in a ward setting, the nature of perioperative practice requires some modification to place them within the perioperative context and environment. Table 6.3 provides examples of perioperative application.

Personal protective equipment

Personal protective equipment (PPE) must be worn during activities when there is a risk of contact with blood or body fluids. PPE consists of the following items.

Non-sterile gloves. Non-sterile gloves provide an effective barrier when touching contaminated equipment, blood and body fluids. However, wearing gloves is no substitute for proper hand hygiene. Gloves should be removed after completing a task, the hands cleansed and a fresh set of gloves donned before engaging in further activities involving potentially contaminated items. Circulating nurses should not wear gloves when opening sterile supplies, answering telephones, entering data into the computer, documenting the count or leaving the OR to collect extra items from sterile stockroom. Wearing gloves during these activities risks contamination of the items touched and transmission of microorganisms (ACORN, 2020b).

FEATURE BOX 6.4
The Father of Infection Control

In May 1847 in Vienna, Ignaz Phillip Semmelweis (1818–65) provided evidence of the significance of hand washing to prevent the spread of puerperal sepsis. Semmelweis, an obstetrician, observed that the maternal mortality rate in women attended by doctors was 20%, which was four to five times greater than in women attended only by midwives.

Semmelweis identified that midwives did not attend the anatomical laboratories where autopsies were carried out. Following the death of a colleague who accidentally cut his finger during an autopsy and died a few days later, it was discovered at autopsy that he had died from the same causative microorganism responsible for puerperal sepsis. This finding moved Semmelweis to immediately implement a rigorous hand-washing policy using 4% chlorinated lime solution prior to the examination of women in labour. The results almost immediately lowered maternal mortality rates and a full year after the implementation of Semmelweis' hand-washing policy the mortality rate from puerperal sepsis had dropped to 1.2%.

However, these results were not published for another 14 years and, although Semmelweis had many who supported his findings, there were those who opposed the idea of the doctor being the cause of the spread of puerperal sepsis. Semmelweis was not recognised for his findings until after his death. Although Semmelweis' antiseptic practices were ultimately adopted by the medical community throughout the world, he was never given the recognition during his lifetime that he so richly deserved.

(Source: Best, M., & Neuhauser, D. (2004). Ignaz Semmelweis and the birth of infection control. *Quality Safety Health Care, 13*, 233–234.)

TABLE 6.3
'5 Moments of Hand Hygiene' in the Perioperative Environment

Moment	Example
1. Before touching a patient in any way, before any non-invasive treatment or observation	• Placing a theatre cap on the patient's head • Touching the patient's armband • Transferring the patient onto the operating table • Positioning or repositioning the patient • Touching any medical device connected to the patient (e.g. IV pump or anaesthetic machine[a]) • Applying calf compressors or tourniquet
2. Before a procedure	• Opening sterile items onto the aseptic field • Inserting intravenous access devices • Intubation • Inserting a urinary catheter • Prior to donning non-sterile gloves
3. After a procedure or body fluid exposure	• Following moment 2 • Removing gloves following contact with body tissue during surgery • Suctioning of airway • Extubating the patient • Contact with used specimen jars/pathology samples • Cleaning spills of blood, urine, faeces or vomit from the patient's surroundings, bag
4. After touching a patient	• After moment 1
5. After touching the patient's immediate surroundings when the patient has not been touched	• Cleaning the operating table • Positioning devices, linen, patient notes (transported with the patient on or under the patient's bed; thus become part of the patient zone) • Cleaning the anaesthetic bay and OR following the patient's departure

[a]The anaesthetic machine, including the touch screen, knobs and tubing, must be cleaned between patients, as this becomes part of the patient and is touched freely by the anaesthetist during the procedure.
(Source: Adapted from Australian Commission on Safety and Quality in Health Care. (2020). *National Hand Hygiene Initiative (NHHI). 5 moments of hand hygiene.* https://www.safetyandquality.gov.au/our-work/infection-prevention-and-control/national-hand-hygiene-initiative-nhhi/national-hand-hygiene-initiative-manual.)

In response to the high levels of inappropriate glove use when using transmission-based precautions, Jain and colleagues (2018) proposed deleting the use of gloves from the transmission-based precautions and relying on appropriate hand hygiene. They showed that healthcare workers are more compliant with appropriate hand hygiene when gloves are removed (Jain et al., 2018) (Research box 6.1).

Face masks. Face masks have been an important component of infection prevention practices for many years. Initially they were used to prevent the transmission of microorganisms from healthcare staff to patients. However, a number of research studies have cast doubt on the efficacy of face masks to protect patients and the focus has shifted to their current use predicated on the need to protect healthcare workers as part of PPE (Shaban et al., 2019; Webster et al., 2010). However, there is sufficient evidence to warrant the use of face masks to prevent the droplet spread of oropharyngeal flora during insertion of spinal or epidural anaesthesia, and this provides sufficient evidence to warrant their continued use during surgery (Australian and New Zealand College of Anaesthetists [ANZCA], 2015; King & Spry, 2019; Loveday et al., 2014). While local policy should be followed in relation to the wearing of masks and staff should make themselves aware of relevant research on this topic, the following practices are currently recommended:
• masks should be worn in the OR when open aseptic set-ups, supplies or scrubbed personnel are present

RESEARCH BOX 6.1
Modified Glove Use for Contact Precautions
Healthcare Workers' Perceptions and Acceptance

In an Australian study, Jain and colleagues (2018) trialled the removal of gloves from contact precaution guidelines where there was no contact with bodily fluids, in order to demonstrate improved hand hygiene compliance between multiple patient contacts. Gloves were noted to be associated with poor hand hygiene compliance, with nurses not changing gloves between patient contact, thereby increasing the risk of environmental transmission.

A qualitative study using pre- and post-trial focus groups, surveys, clinical trial and quantitative microbiology testing was carried out with 250 participants in total.

The outcome of the study showed success in promoting appropriate non-glove use when dry contact with patients with MRSA and VRE occurred. The results reinforced the need for a selective approach for glove use, clinical judgement and the performance of risk assessment for individual patients.

(Source: Jain, S., Clezy, K., & McLaws, M-L. (2018). Safe removal of gloves from contact precautions: the role of hand hygiene. *American Journal of Infection Control* 46 (7), 764–767.)

- masks should be combined with eye protection to protect the mucous membranes and conjunctiva of the wearer when exposure to body fluids may occur (NHMRC, 2019)
- masks should meet appropriate Australian and New Zealand standards and protect the wearer from potential splashes during operative or invasive procedures (ANZCA, 2015; NHMRC, 2019)
- ensure that the mask covers both the nose and the mouth, and tie it securely at the back of the head
- change masks frequently – at least every 2 hours to maintain effectiveness in preventing dispersal of flora from the wearer's oropharynx (Kelkar, Gogate, Kurpad, Gogate, & Deshpande, 2013)
- remove the mask by handling the ties only, to avoid contact with the area that has covered the nose and mouth. Perform hand hygiene after removing the mask
- do not wear the mask loosely or leave it around the neck (King & Spry, 2019).

Eye protection. Eye protection in the form of face shields, goggles and/or visors must be worn to protect the mucous membranes of the eyes, nose and mouth when performing aerosolisation-generating procedures and other instances where when there is a likelihood of sprays or splashes of blood or body fluids (ANZCA, 2015; NHMRC, 2019).

Sharps safety. All staff must take precautions to prevent sharps injuries not only to themselves, but also to their colleagues, by taking standard measures to avoid injury. Injuries can be caused by needles, scalpels and instruments used during procedures, when cleaning instruments and when disposing of used needles. Chapters 5 and 10 provide detailed information about sharps safety; however, examples of standard safety measures include:

- using instruments, rather than fingers, to grasp needles, retract tissue and load/unload needles and scalpels
- the instrument nurse letting members of the surgical team know when sharps are being passed
- avoiding hand-to-hand passing of sharp instruments by using a puncture-proof container and using a predetermined neutral zone
- using round-tipped scalpel blades instead of pointed sharp-tipped blades
- separating reusable sharps from other instruments and equipment before cleaning and reprocessing (NHMRC, 2019).

Wearing a second pair of surgical gloves, or '**double gloving**', may provide added protection against puncturing the inner gloves and minimising sharps injury. Members of the surgical team are advised to double glove for their own protection, particularly when scrubbed for puncture-prone procedures (e.g. orthopaedic surgery or long cases). In this instance, it is suggested that the outer glove should be changed routinely. Double gloving can also reduce the microbial load if the skin is broken. Inner gloves that change colour when punctured are available and provide a visual indication (ACORN, 2020c; Loveday et al., 2014; Murphy, 2018; NHRMC, 2019; Society for Healthcare Epidemiology of America [SHEA], 2014).

Respiratory hygiene and cough etiquette. Coughing and sneezing increase the risk of spreading potential infectious particles. Where possible, cough into the crook of the arm or sneeze into a tissue, then place the tissue immediately into a bin. Hand hygiene should be performed afterwards (NHMRC, 2019).

Food and drink in clinical areas. Eating and drinking should not occur in the operating suite, other than in designated staff rooms. There are risks that blood or body fluids may contaminate food that is then eaten by staff, or that work surfaces used for setting up sterile equipment will become contaminated by food and drink. Discarded food can also attract insects, which can lead to contamination of aseptic surfaces and equipment (ACORN, 2020b). Apart from the infection control risks, there are work health and safety concerns with spillage of hot liquids located in work areas (CEC, 2020a). Finally, from a patient sensitivity perspective, a patient who has been fasting for a number of hours is unlikely to appreciate seeing or smelling food or drink when they enter the operating suite.

Environmental cleaning

Following each procedure, all horizontal work surfaces (e.g. trolleys, operating table, bench tops) should be cleaned using neutral detergent. Floors should be cleaned using clean mop-heads and clean water for each OR. Rubbish and linen bins should be emptied and receptacles cleaned. Any visible blood or body substances on any surfaces should be cleaned as soon as practicable during the procedure, and areas such as operating lights, ceilings, walls and other fixtures should be inspected after each case. PPE should be worn by personnel carrying out environmental cleaning (ACORN, 2020d).

Current research has identified a number of adjunct environmental decontamination methods for the OR. Vaporised hydrogen peroxide, peracetic acid 'fogging' and continuous ultraviolet-emitting devices have shown to reduce microbial surface contamination. Despite some promising results, further research is required to ascertain their efficacy and cost effectiveness (Boyce, 2016; Murrell, Hamilton, Johnson, & Spencer, 2018). (See Chapter 5 for further information.)

Transmission-Based Precautions

Transmission-based precautions are the second-tier approach to infection prevention and control. These precautions are applied when standard precautions alone are not adequate to prevent airborne, droplet or contact transmission of microorganisms. On occasions, a combination of these transmission-based precautions will be required, such as when a patient has norovirus and is vomiting (ACORN, 2020b; NHMRC, 2019).

Airborne precautions

Airborne transmission of microorganisms occurs because the organisms are extremely small (less than 5 μm)

and they float in air currents or are disseminated in dust particles that are suspended in the air flow. Examples of infections requiring airborne precautions are TB, severe acute respiratory syndrome (SARS), COVID-19, measles and chickenpox. Maximum protection requires fit testing of P2 or N95 masks, to prevent the passage of microorganisms. In addition, face shields/goggles should also be worn (ACORN, 2020b; CEC, 2020a; King & Spry, 2019; NHMRC, 2019). See Feature box 6.1 for further information about fit testing of P2/N95 masks.

Droplet precautions

Droplet transmission involves larger particles generated when a person sneezes or coughs. Droplets are greater than 5 μm (e.g. influenza, meningococcal) and fall to the floor within 1 metre of the source. On occasions, procedures such as suctioning, diathermy and nebulisers may cause these droplets to become airborne, requiring airborne precautions. The P2 and N95 masks are effective in preventing transmission of droplet infections and face shields/goggles should also be worn (ACORN, 2020b; Agency for Clinical Innovation [ACI], 2020; CEC, 2020a; NHMRC, 2019). It is recommended that patients with airborne or droplet infections wear a surgical mask when being transported within the hospital to reduce the risk of infecting other people (NHMRC, 2019).

Contact precautions

Contact precautions are intended to prevent the transmission of MROs (e.g. MRSA, VRE or C. difficile) by direct or indirect contact with the patient or the patient's environment. Contact precautions are applied to patients known to be infected or colonised with these MROs. As these organisms may be present on the patient's skin, clothing, bedclothes and equipment, healthcare workers must wear aprons or gowns, gloves, protective eyewear and masks when participating in direct patient care activities. All items of protective equipment must be disposed of once contact with the patient has been completed and hand hygiene performed (King & Spry, 2019; NHMRC 2019). There should be restricted access to the OR, with only essential personnel present. Similarly, only essential equipment required for the procedure should be in the OR and, where possible, disposable equipment should be used. These measures will assist in reducing the risk of microorganisms being spread within the OR. Environmental cleaning must follow use of contact precautions (see below) (ACORN, 2020b).

Environmental Cleaning Following Use of Transmission Precautions

Due to the virulence of current and emerging MROs (including COVID-19) and the ease with which they can be spread through aerosolisation, direct or indirect contact, cleaning alone with neutral detergent is not sufficient. Meticulous cleaning regimens should be implemented using a two-step approach: environmental cleaning using neutral detergent on all surfaces, followed by cleaning with sodium hypochlorite or other solution approved by the Therapeutic Goods Authority (ACORN, 2020b; NHMRC, 2019). Staff should be familiar with the specific local policies in relation to environmental cleaning following the use of transmission precautions. See Feature box 6.1 for specific information on environmental cleaning for COVID-19 cases.

PATIENT SCENARIOS

SCENARIO 6.2: TRANSMISSION-BASED CONTACT PRECAUTIONS

The next patient on the operating list, Mrs Peterson, requires contact precautions. Jimmy Montano, the theatre orderly, asks RN Pereira what he needs to do for contact precautions.

Critical Thinking Question

• What instructions should RN Pereira give Jimmy Montano to assist him manage Mrs Peterson, protect himself and prepare the environment in the perioperative period? Give rationales for your answers.

Patient Considerations in Infection Prevention

The NHMRC (2019) advocates the use of a 'care bundle' approach to infection prevention. This is a critical set of evidence-based processes applied to patient care (Table 6.4). This approach is also supported by the WHO (2018) and provides a consistent, structured approach to infection prevention (NHMRC, 2019; SHEA, 2014; Vassello, 2016). The approach has been shown to have a significant effect in reducing SSIs when used in combination with other well-established infection prevention measures described in this chapter.

ASEPSIS AND ASEPTIC TECHNIQUE

Asepsis can be defined as the absence of pathogenic microorganisms on living tissue (King & Spry, 2019), while **sterile** means free from microorganisms. Items used in surgical procedures are wrapped and sterilised, remaining sterile until they are opened (ACORN, 2020e). **Aseptic technique** aims to prevent sufficient quantities of pathogenic microorganisms from being introduced to surgical sites by hands, surfaces and equipment. Therefore, unlike sterile technique, aseptic technique is achievable and must be strictly adhered to in order to minimise contamination of the wound and prevent infection, so aiding an uneventful postoperative recovery (King & Spry, 2019; NHMRC, 2019).

The patient is the centre of aseptic **field**, which comprises personnel wearing scrub attire and those areas of the patient, operating table, instrument trolleys and other furniture that are covered in sterile drapes. Aseptic practices guide perioperative nurses' actions – for example, when opening sterile supplies, moving in and around the aseptic field or setting up aseptic instrument trolleys. Application of the principles and practices of aseptic technique, which are necessary to create and maintain an aseptic field, rely on the perioperative nurse and other members of the surgical team exercising a **surgical conscience** (King & Spry, 2019). In some instances, the principles provide arbitrary boundaries only, but they assist the perioperative nurse to determine where aseptic areas start and end, hence contributing to safe practice. Aseptic technique utilises the principles of asepsis.

Standard and Surgical Aseptic Technique

Aseptic technique terminology is used to describe the type and complexity of the procedure being carried out.

• *Standard aseptic technique* is practised in perioperative and proceduralist settings for procedures that are simple, of short duration and involve only a few key parts (syringe hub or cannula) or sites (entry point to patient via a vein, which will require cleaning with antiseptic solution). Key parts and sites must be identified and protected from contact with unsterile items.

TABLE 6.4
Example of a 'Care Bundle' Approach to Preventing SSIs

Practice	Elements
Antimicrobial prophylaxis	• Antimicrobial stewardship is a key strategy in reducing MROs • The key principle is to administer appropriate antibiotics between 30 and 60 minutes prior to the incision; in patients undergoing extended surgery or when excessive bleeding occurs, consideration may be given to administering a second dose of antibiotics
Hair removal	• Body hair around the proposed surgical site can be a source of infection and may need to be removed prior to surgery • Hair removal, if required, should be carried out as close to the time of surgery as possible • Clippers or a depilatory agent should be used outside the OR (recommended practice, but may not always be possible in emergency situations)
Control blood glucose	• Glucose levels can affect wound healing • Hypo- and hyperglycaemia should be avoided by regular monitoring of at-risk patients
Maintain normothermia	• Body temperature should be maintained ≥36°C • Even mild hypothermia can increase SSI rates as it may directly impair neutrophil function or impair it indirectly by triggering subcutaneous vasoconstriction and subsequent tissue hypothermia (see Chapters 8 and 9 for further information)
Optimise tissue oxygenation	• Oxygen should be administered during and immediately following surgery
Skin preparation products	• Alcohol has highly bactericidal properties • Products combining an antimicrobial agent and alcohol may provide greater effectiveness at removing transient and resident microbial count (see section on skin preparation)
Use WHO Surgical Safety Checklist (WHO SSC)	• The WHO SSC reduces perioperative risks to patients and improves team communication (see Chapters 2 and 9 for further information)
Perform surveillance	• High-risk or high-volume procedures should be identified and monitored
Provide feedback on SSIs to staff	• Feedback improves performance and identifies areas for practice to be reviewed

MRO = multidrug-resistant organism; SSI = surgical site infection.
(Sources: Berrios-Torres, S. I., Umscheid, C. A., Bratzler, D. W., Leas, B., Stone , E. C., Kelz , R. R., ... Healthcare Infection Control Practices Advisory Committee. (2017). Centers for disease control and prevention guideline for the prevention of surgical site infection. *Journal of the American Medical Association Surgery, 152*(8), 784–791; National Health and Medical Research Council. (2019). *Australian guidelines for the prevention and control of infection in healthcare.* https://www.nhmrc.gov.au/about-us/publications/australian-guidelines-prevention-and-control-infection-healthcare-2019; Vassello, A. (2016). *Preventing surgical site infections with the SHEA bundle.* http://sdapic.org/wp-content/uploads/2016/09/Vassallo-Prev-SSI-w-the-SHEA-Bundle-Sept-2016.pdf.)

For standard aseptic technique, the aseptic field is termed 'general', usually requiring non-sterile gloves (e.g. insertion of IV cannulae or injection into an IV line/port) (NHMRC, 2019). Perioperative nurses may use standard aseptic techniques when inserting an IV or changing a dressing in PACU.
• *Surgical aseptic technique* is required when procedures are more complex and longer in duration, involving numerous key parts and key sites. The most obvious examples are surgical procedures where the instrument nurse and surgical team are involved. Anaesthetic nurses will also be required to set up a surgical aseptic field when the anaesthetist is inserting invasive monitoring or a spinal anaesthetic. For surgical aseptic technique, the aseptic field is termed 'critical' and requires the use of sterile drapes, instruments and equipment; additionally, all members of the surgical team must wear a sterile gown and gloves (NHMRC, 2019).

TABLE 6.5
Aseptic Principles and Practices for Unscrubbed Personnel (Anaesthetic Team, Circulating Nurse, Radiographers, Visitors, etc.)

Aseptic Principles and Practices	Rationales
Unscrubbed personnel must touch only non-sterile items	Contamination of sterile items, which will pose an infection risk to the patient, is avoided. If personnel are in doubt as to whether or not items are sterile, they should seek clarification. If a sterile item is accidently touched, personnel should inform a member of the surgical team immediately
All personnel moving around the aseptic field should do so in a manner that maintains the integrity of the aseptic field A distance of at least 30 cm away from the aseptic field should be maintained while always facing the aseptic field	Accidental contamination of the aseptic field is avoided by vigilant observation and careful movement
Unscrubbed personnel should not lean across the aseptic field	Skin squames are continually shed from the skin or from attire and may fall onto the aseptic field, thereby contaminating it.
Unscrubbed personnel should not walk between two aseptic fields as this can lead to contamination of the aseptic fields	Accidental contamination of the aseptic field is avoided by vigilant observation and careful movement within the OR Aseptic fields/trollies should be positioned within the OR in such a way as to reduce risk of contamination, while facilitating traffic flow around the room
Only the minimal number of personnel should be present in the OR during a procedure	The risk of transmitting airborne contaminants increases with the number of personnel in the room Each operating suite should have a policy in relation to the number of visitors permitted within each OR All visitors should observe infection control policies and be monitored for compliance
Talking should be kept to a minimum	Reduces droplet spread
Doors of the OR should be kept closed and opened only when required. All the requirements for the procedure should be placed in the OR prior to commencement to reduce the need to repeatedly exit and enter the OR to access equipment	Frequent opening and closing of doors creates air currents and alters the normally positive pressure air flow within the OR itself, further increasing the possibility of airborne contaminants (sourced from personnel, supplies and equipment) entering the wound By ensuring that all supplies required for the procedure are within the OR, the need to gather supplies and repeated exit/entry will be avoided

(Sources: Australian College of Perioperative Nurses (ACORN, 2020e). Asepsis. *Standards for perioperative nursing in Australia. Volume 1.* Adelaide: Author; Ban et al., (2017). American College of Surgeons and Surgical Infection Society surgical site infection guidelines, 2016 update. *Journal of the American College of Surgeons, 224*(1), 59–74; King, C., & Spry, C. (2019). Infection prevention and control. In J. Rothrock (Ed.), *Alexander's care of the patient in surgery* (16th ed., pp. 54–106). St Louis, MO: Elsevier; WHO, 2018.)

Putting Principles into Practice

Putting aseptic principles into practice can be daunting for the beginning perioperative nurse. However, practising techniques under supervision will ensure that skills and dexterity are developed. Tables 6.5 and 6.6 contain practical hints and demonstrations of aseptic techniques for both unscrubbed and scrubbed personnel.

Opening Sterile Supplies

The circulating nurse provides a link between the aseptic field and the sterile supplies required for a surgical procedure. The circulating nurse needs to be able to open and transfer sterile items safely onto the aseptic field (Table 6.7, Feature box 6.5). Hand hygiene must be carried out prior to opening a sterile item.

TABLE 6.6
Aseptic Principles and Practices for Scrubbed Personnel (Surgical Team, Instrument Nurse)

Aseptic Principles and Practices	Rationales
Items used within the aseptic field must be sterile	Sterile items free from all micro organisms and spores will minimise the patient's risk of infection
Aseptic fields should be prepared as close as possible to the time of use	Reduces risk of contamination by airborne particles containing microorganisms
For patients having multiple procedures sequentially, prepare one aseptic field for one patient at a time within the confines of the operating/procedure room Covering aseptic setups with sterile drapes is not currently supported by ACORN	Reduces risk of contamination by airborne particles containing microorganisms Risk of contaminating the aseptic field while removing drapes is considered too great
Receive sterile items transferred to the aseptic field by lifting them vertically or using a grasping instrument to retrieve the items (see Fig. 6.6)	Maintains sterility of item by minimising risk of contact with unscrubbed personnel or unsterile outer package
All personnel within the aseptic field must wear a sterile gown and gloves and touch only sterilised items (Fig. 6.3).	Wearing sterile gown and gloves will facilitate aseptic technique and minimises the patient's risk of exposure to potentially pathogenic organisms
Sterile drapes must be used to create an aseptic field around the proposed operative site	Although skin preparation solutions reduce resident and transient microorganisms around the proposed operative site, these cannot be eliminated and can increase the risk of SSIs. Sterile drapes strategically placed around the proposed operative site isolate the operative area from surrounding skin and patient gown and surrounding coverings (see 'Skin preparation of the patient')
Only the horizontal surfaces of tables draped with sterile drapes are considered aseptic; any item that hangs below table-top level is considered contaminated	Items that fall below the horizontal surface cannot be monitored for sterility and therefore should be discarded
The aseptic field must be monitored at all times and never left unattended	Aseptic fields can be accidently contaminated and if not reported increases the infection risk to the patient

(Sources: Australian College of Perioperative Nurses (ACORN, 2020e). Asepsis. *Standards for perioperative nursing in Australia. Volume 1.* Adelaide: Author; King, C., & Spry, C. (2019). Infection prevention and control. In J. Rothrock (Ed.), *Alexander's care of the patient in surgery* (16th ed., pp. 54–106). St Louis, MO: Elsevier.)

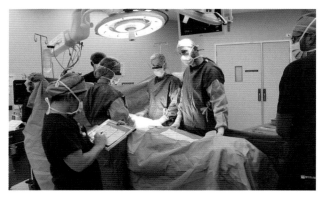

FIG. 6.3 Perioperative team in sterile gown and gloves. (Source: Dr Nicola Dean, Consultant Plastic and Reconstructive Surgeon, Flinders Medical Centre, South Australia, with permission.)

TABLE 6.7
Circulating Nurse – Management of Sterile Supplies and Fluids

Aseptic Principles and Practices	Rationales
OPENING STERILE SUPPLIES	
Examine the external sterility indicator	Indicates whether the item has been through a sterilisation process
Check the expiry date	Although an event (e.g. dropping a sterile item) rather than time is the determining factor, some companies place an expiry date on items
Inspect the item prior to opening to ensure it is securely sealed and its packaging is intact (no tears, etc.)	If the integrity of the sterile package has been compromised it cannot be considered sterile and must be discarded
Assess for watermarks or any dampness	Indicates strikethrough has occurred, and the item can no longer be considered sterile and must be discarded
All items introduced onto the aseptic field must be opened, dispensed and transferred by methods that maintain their sterility and integrity	Techniques to ensure safe transfer of items onto the aseptic field will maintain sterility and minimise infection risk to the patient
Commercial packaged items are designed to be peeled open and should not be torn	Tearing a package designed for peeling will compromise safe transfer to the aseptic field
To open a sterile bundle, open the first fold towards you (Fig. 6.4A), then move around to the opposite side of the bundle and open the second fold (Fig. 6.4B), to avoid leaning across the aseptic field	Technique will ensure item is not compromised during the opening process
Open a wrapped sterile article without your hands touching the inside wrapper (Fig. 6.5). Open the outer wrapper edge furthest away from you first and the nearest wrapper edge last. Secure all open wrapper edges to avoid contamination while making the item available to be retrieved by the scrubbed person (Fig. 6.6) See Feature box 6.5 and Fig. 6.7 for information on 'flipping' items onto the aseptic field	Technique will ensure item is not compromised during the opening process and is retrieved by the instrument nurse without compromising sterility
Wrapped/packaged sterile items dropped on the floor are no longer considered sterile and must be discarded; after picking articles up off the floor, the hands should be cleansed	Floors harbour microorganisms which may compromise the sterility of an item, regardless of type of packaging Hand washing after retrieving article from floor minimises transmission risk when handling subsequent articles
POURING LIQUIDS ONTO THE ASEPTIC FIELD	
Do not reach over the aseptic field – if container (e.g. jug) is not accessible, request the instrument nurse to move container close to edge of aseptic field Pour liquid carefully to prevent splashing or dripping of contents onto the aseptic field Pour the total contents of the bottle into a container such as a jug, which should then be labelled (see Fig. 6.8). Do not recap bottle for reuse	Skin squames are continually shed from the skin or from attire and may fall onto and therefore contaminate aseptic fields during pouring action Splashing/drips may compromise integrity of drapes on aseptic field Volume of fluid used can be recorded and minimises risk of contents being accidently used for subsequent patients Contamination may occur when recapping

(Sources: Australian College of Perioperative Nurses (ACORN, 2020e). Asepsis. *Standards for perioperative nursing in Australia. Volume 1.* Adelaide: Author; King, C., & Spry, C. (2019). Infection prevention and control. In J. Rothrock (Ed.), *Alexander's care of the patient in surgery* (16th ed., pp. 54–106). St Louis, MO: Elsevier.)

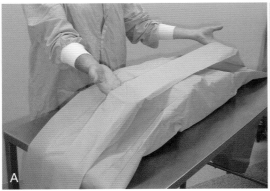
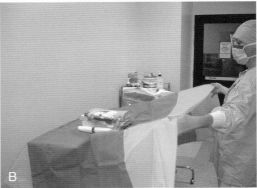

FIG. 6.4 (**A**, **B**) Opening a sterile bundle.

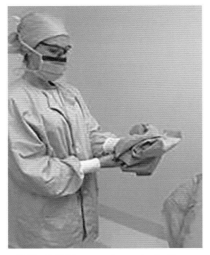

FIG. 6.5 Unwrapping a sterile item.

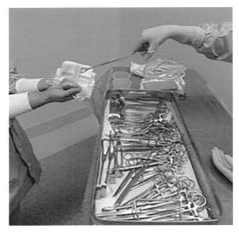

FIG. 6.6 The circulating nurse presenting a sterile item to the instrument nurse.

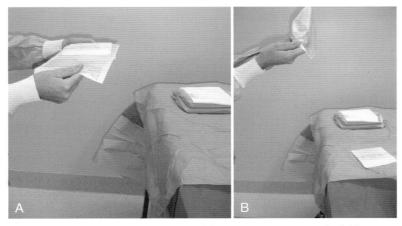

FIG. 6.7 (**A**, **B**) Demonstration of flipping items onto aseptic field.

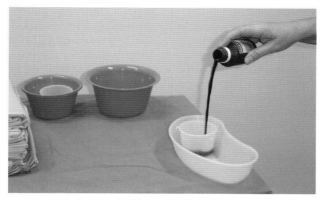

FIG. 6.8 Pouring fluid into a gallipot on an aseptic field.

FEATURE BOX 6.5
To Flip or Not to Flip: a Practice Issue for Discussion

'Flipping' refers to the practice of transferring the aseptic contents of small, sterilised packaged items onto the aseptic field (e.g. gauze swabs). It is a skill that most nurses will have practised in wards and other departments when setting up aseptic fields to undertake procedures such as dressing changes. It is used when the nurse is working without assistance and must open all supplies before washing hands and donning sterile gloves.

Flipping in the operating theatre/procedural rooms is not supported by professional standards and recommended practices, as the action can increase air turbulence, causing particles to land on the aseptic field and compromising sterility.

It is recommended that, when transferring sterile supplies to the aseptic field, the instrument nurse takes the aseptic item from the circulating nurse using forceps to reduce the possibility of contamination (ACORN, 2020e).

The need to flip items has been significantly reduced by the introduction of sterile 'custom packs'. These packs contain a wide range of disposable items previously opened individually and commonly transferred using the flipping technique onto the aseptic field.

Perioperative nurses are likely to witness flipping and this poses a dilemma, particularly for those new to the specialty. For example, prior to performing the surgical scrub, the instrument nurse and other members of the surgical team commonly use a flipping technique to transfer their sterile surgical gloves on the gown trolley. In emergency situations or when the instrument nurse is busy, the circulating nurse may be required to flip items such as gauze squares or sutures directly onto the aseptic field (see Fig. 6.7A and B).

Nurses should have regard for their professional standards and follow local policy regarding this issue. Where flipping is still practised, nurses should ensure that they receive adequate education and supervised practice of this technique so that they are confident and skilful when opening aseptic supplies in emergency situations.

PATIENT SCENARIOS

SCENARIO 6.3: ASEPTIC TECHNIQUE

EN Pauline Noakes is scrubbed for the next procedure. RN Pereira is the circulating nurse and is opening the sterile supplies with Student Nurse Rose Cheng.

Critical Thinking Questions

- Prior to opening sterile items for a procedure, what checks will RN Pereira and Student Nurse Cheng carry out to confirm that the item is sterile? Explain the reason for each check.
- While checking the packaging of a wrapped item, Student Nurse Cheng notices there is a small hole in the outer wrapper. She asks RN Pereira if it can still be used, as the inner wrapper is not compromised. What advice should RN Pereira give Student Nurse Rose Cheng? Provide rationales for your answer.

Surgical/Professional Conscience

A **surgical/professional conscience** is defined as an individual's professional honesty and inner morality system, which allows no compromise in practice whether a breach occurs within the team or when working alone. For example, if a member of the surgical team contaminates a glove or piece of equipment, the breach must be pointed out immediately to prevent any compromise to the patient's safety. The patient's well-being must be placed above any personal/professional embarrassment or fear of speaking up. The surgical team must share responsibility for monitoring and correcting the actions of team members if a breach of aseptic technique is noted (ACORN, 2020e; King & Spry, 2019).

Surgical Hand Antisepsis (Surgical Scrub)

Before the surgeon(s) and instrument nurse(s) can prepare or enter an aseptic field, they must perform a surgical hand antisepsis (a surgical scrub), followed by donning sterile gown and gloves according to local hospital policy. The practice of surgical **scrubbing** is integral to reducing SSIs and the procedure is carried out to eliminate transient flora and reduce resident flora from the hands and forearms, leaving residual antimicrobial agent on the skin to inhibit the growth of microorganisms. A broad-spectrum antimicrobial solution that is fast acting, persistent and has a cumulative effect is recommended (ACORN, 2020c) (e.g. aqueous antimicrobial solutions such as povidone-iodine and chlorhexidine). Recommendations from a number of organisations have seen the increased use of alcohol-based products for surgical hand antisepsis, with solutions containing 60%–80% alcohol found to be the most effective. While alcohol solutions do not have the same residual effect as aqueous solutions, they have a sublethal effect, slowing regrowth of bacteria. Alcohol also acts rapidly and has a broad-spectrum effect (King & Spry, 2019; NHMRC, 2019; SHEA, 2014; WHO, 2009).

Before the surgical scrub personnel should:

- be dressed in clean perioperative attire
- remove rings and confine/remove all other visible jewellery, such as earrings and neck chains (Royal Australasian College of Surgeons [RACS], 2015)
- remove nail polish or nail extensions
- don surgical mask and eye protection
- don radiation protective gowns and thyroid protection, if applicable
- perform an inspection of the hands, paying close attention to any breaks in the skin
- open a sterile gown pack and add sterile gloves to it.

Australian and New Zealand professional perioperative organisations provide detailed descriptions of the surgical scrub and each operating suite should display the technique for all staff to follow. Although the actual technique may differ between areas, the basic principles for surgical scrubbing remain the same.

- principles of scrub technique using aqueous antimicrobial solution:
  1. First scrub of the day is 5 minutes in length and includes use of sterile sponge and nail cleaner.
  2. Subsequent scrubs are 3 minutes as the cleaning of nails is not required.
  3. Prepare a sponge/nail cleaner, maintaining it in an aseptic manner until it is required.
  4. Turn tap on to an even flow to prevent splashing.
  5. Antimicrobial solution applied to hands and arms should remain in contact with the skin according to manufacturer's instructions. The solution selected for the first scrub of the day should be used for subsequent scrubs, as this will provide a cumulative and sustained effect (WHO, 2009).
  6. When applying solution, work from hands to the elbow, using a circular motion to move up the arms, and do not return to the hands.
  7. When rinsing hands and arms, water should flow from cleanest areas (the hands) to less clean areas (elbows) – that is, always keep hands above elbows (see Fig. 6.9).
  8. After completing the surgical scrub, hold hands above the waist and dry using a sterile towel, before donning a sterile gown (ACORN 2020c).

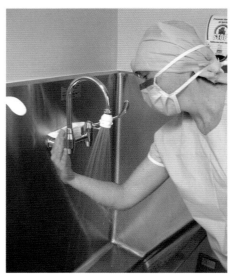

FIG. 6.9 Rinsing hands. Note the hands are higher than the elbows.

- principles of scrub technique using alcohol scrub solution:
  1. Prewash – wash and dry hands using a non-anti-microbial solution only if hands are visibly soiled
  2. Apply the correct amount of alcohol scrub solution (approximately 5 mL) to hands and arms in accordance with the manufacturer's instructions.
  3. The contact time of the scrub solution will depend on the type and percentage of alcohol within the solution and the presence of added antimicrobials.
  4. Subsequent alcohol scrubs require a social hand wash and careful drying if the hands are visibly dirty prior to the application of the alcohol solution (ACORN 2020c).
  5. Regardless of the solution used, it is important that correct technique is taught to all new staff and used consistently to ensure the effectiveness of the antimicrobial solutions and reduce the risk of SSIs.

Gowning

Sterile gowns are worn to provide a barrier to prevent the transfer of microorganisms to the patient during the surgical procedure. They should be made of a combustion-resistant material that provides an effective barrier between the wearer and the patient, minimising the passage of microorganisms, blood and fluid between unsterile and sterile areas. While reusable (linen) gowns are still used, single-use gowns are recommended owing to their superior impervious, protective barrier qualities. Regardless of the fabric used, all gowns must meet strict international standards, having undergone rigorous testing (International Organization for Standardization [ISO], 2018). Single-use gowns are available with differing levels of protection depending on the type of surgery being undertaken. For example, some gowns have reinforced sleeves and front panels as added protection for the wearer involved in procedures where there is likely to be a lot of blood or fluid (e.g. trauma or procedures using irrigation).

The main principles for **gowning** are as follows (Fig. 6.10):

- the gown must be folded in a manner that enables the inside of the gown to be handled with surgically clean hands
- minimise handling during donning procedure
- extend both arms into sleeves simultaneously
- do not extend hands through gown cuffs – this allows for closed gloving (see below)
- keep arms bent at the elbows and above the waist
- have an unscrubbed person secure the ties at the back of the gown.

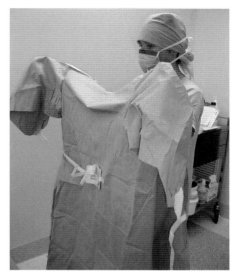

FIG. 6.10 Donning a sterile gown.

Gloving

Wearing sterile gloves provides a barrier between the wearer and the patient, protecting both against the transmission of infection. Glove perforation during the course of the procedure may cause contamination of the patient's surgical site and also puts the wearer at risk of exposure to blood-borne pathogens. Research by Guo and colleagues (2012) showed that the average time for a perforation to occur in operating theatres is 69.8 minutes. The rate increased when surgery lasted longer than 2 hours (Makama, Okeme, Makama, & Ameh, 2016).

To ensure the highest level of protection for the surgical team and the patient, Makama and colleagues (2016) recommend double gloving (wearing two pairs of gloves) for all surgical procedures, stating that wearing both an under glove and outer glove provides 98.83% protection. A Cochrane systematic review by Mischke and colleagues (2014) also supports the use of double gloving. Current NHMRC (2019) guidelines recommend double gloving for high-risk procedures such as orthopaedic surgery where drills and chisels are used. Gloves with properties that indicate when a perforation has occurred (an indicator glove) are recommended for wearing as the first pair of gloves donned, followed by a second pair. If a perforation occurs, both gloves should be changed. ACORN (2020c) recommends that gloves should be changed after a maximum 90–120 minutes of surgery.

Gloves should be powder-free latex or latex free, having regard for patient and staff sensitivities to latex products. Latex gloves have been associated with adverse reactions in patients (e.g. wound inflammation), as well as systemic allergic reactions and, in rare cases, anaphylaxis (King & Spry, 2019) (see Chapter 5).

Gloves with antimicrobial properties are available as a further strategy to prevent wound contamination if perforations occur, and current research results are promising (Murphy, 2018).

Closed gloving is the recommended method to don gloves as it reduces the risk of contaminating the sterile gloves by the bare hands. The procedure is as follows:

- with the hands remaining inside the cuffs, remove one glove from the packet with one hand
- with the palm of the other hand uppermost, place the glove onto the cuff with the fingers of the glove pointing towards the wrist, the thumb down and the folded edge of the glove flush against the edge of the cuff of the gown
- with both hands working inside the gown sleeves, use the thumbs to hold onto the edge of the glove cuffs
- using one motion, stretch the glove out and over the hand and insert the gown cuff into the glove
- grasp both the glove and the gown, manoeuvring the hand through the cuff into the glove (Fig. 6.11)
- repeat the procedure for the other hand. The second pair of gloves is then donned by sliding each gloved hand into the second pair.

Once both pairs of gloves are donned, there is one final action taken to complete gowning. There are side tapes on the front of the gown that require assistance from a scrubbed or unscrubbed person (depending on the type of gown) to turn the wearer so that the tapes are secured at the front of the gown. The effect of this manoeuvre is to close the back panel of the gown. It does not mean that the back is sterile, but it provides all-round protection to the wearer.

Once gowned and gloved, the areas considered aseptic are from the tips of the fingers to the elbows and from the nipples to the waist. This arbitrary boundary allows the wearer to monitor any obvious contamination by unscrubbed persons or equipment. Should contamination occur, then the gown or gloves or both, depending on the extent of the contamination, must be removed and replaced (ACORN, 2020c).

In *assisted (open) gloving*, one scrubbed person gloves another scrubbed person; this may occur should the wearer contaminate a glove intraoperatively. Closed gloving cannot be achieved because the cuffs should not be pulled back over the hands as they are now contaminated. Therefore, the safest method of donning a replacement glove is for another aseptic member of the team to assist with the gloving.

If both gown and gloves become contaminated, both must be removed and the donning procedure is carried out as previously described. Once gowned and gloved (Fig. 6.12), the scrubbed person must stay close to the aseptic field and not move out of the OR into semi-restricted or unrestricted areas as this will increase the risk of cross-infection.

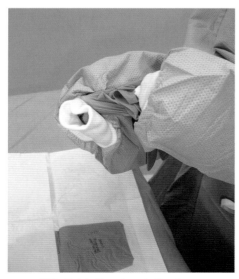

FIG. 6.11 Donning sterile gloves.

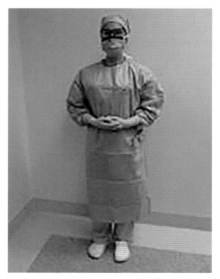

FIG. 6.12 Scrubbed person wearing sterile gown and gloves.

At the conclusion of the procedure, the outermost pair of gloves, which may be visibly contaminated, may be removed and discarded prior to applying the dressing. When removing gown and gloves, to avoid contamination of bare hands, the gown is removed first, rolled up so the inner surface is on the outside and discarded. This is followed by removal of the inner gloves, by gloved surface touching gloved surface to remove one glove and then placing a 'clean' finger inside the remaining glove, which is then pulled off. This method protects bare skin from the contaminated outer surface of the glove.

The surgical team must discard gowns, gloves and masks in a manner that confines and contains – that is, into designated waste containers within the OR, according to local policy. The mask should be removed by touching the strings only to prevent contamination of the hands from blood or body fluids that may have splashed onto the mask. The hands should be cleansed following removal of the gown, gloves, mask and visor (ACORN, 2020c).

Skin Preparation of the Patient

The patient's skin provides a defence against the entry of infection. The abundant resident and transient microorganisms that live on the skin can be a major source of pathogens, which can cause SSIs. As a patient's surgical outcome can be adversely affected by developing an SSI, preoperative **skin antisepsis** ('prepping') is undertaken just prior to the commencement of the procedure with the aim of removing soil and reducing the transient and resident microorganisms from the patient's skin to the lowest possible levels (ACORN, 2020f; Health Quality and Safety Commission New Zealand, 2014). This is achieved by using an antimicrobial agent which has a broad-spectrum, rapid and persistent effect. There are a number of commonly used antimicrobial skin antisepsis solutions available, including aqueous povidone-iodine or chlorhexidine solutions. The addition of alcohol to each of these solutions has shown to be more effective at rapidly killing bacteria and reducing the microbial count on the skin. The WHO (2016a) recommends the use of alcohol-based chlorhexidine solutions. The selection of which solution to use will be based on the type of surgery performed and surgeons' preference (e.g. orthopaedic surgeons generally prefer an alcohol-based solution to reduce risk of infection within joints; however, this solution cannot be used in eye surgery). Extreme care must be taken when selecting antimicrobial solutions, and a visual check of label by the instrument and circulating nurse must be carried out prior to transfer to the aseptic field to ensure the correct solution is used. Many solutions have a tint added to assist in visualising areas being 'prepped' and in identifying pooling of the solution (National Health Service [NHS], 2015).

Safe use of alcohol-based skin preparation solutions

Strict safety measures must be exercised when alcohol-based solutions are used in order to reduce the risk of ignition and fire when electrosurgery is in use (Ball, 2019). Care must be taken to ensure that the alcohol dries completely and all vapours have evaporated prior to the patient being draped and electrical equipment activated. The alcohol-based solution must not be kept in the OR and should be stored according to the manufacturer's and government guidelines. All staff must be trained in the use of alcohol-based solutions, with local policies in place to manage its safe use within the perioperative environment (Health Quality and Safety and Quality Commission New Zealand, 2014; NSW Health, 2011).

Prepping procedure

Following positioning of the patient and team 'Time Out', the patient should be 'prepped' using a suitable antimicrobial solution selected on the basis of avoiding patient allergies, suitability for the location and type of procedure to be carried out and the surgeon's preferences. Preparation of the operative site is carried out by the surgeon or instrument nurse using gauze swabs dipped in antimicrobial solution or a disposable, commercially produced preloaded purpose-built applicator, observing aseptic technique. Skin cleansing commences from the cleanest area, usually the proposed operative site, and proceeds in concentric circles or squares outwards to the least clean areas. Using a clean swab (no double dipping), this process is repeated several times, with the prepared area wide enough to allow extension of the incision if required (Fig. 6.13).

Areas that have a high microbial count (e.g. groin, umbilicus, body orifices, open wounds or stomas) should be prepared last using a separate swab. The preparation of these areas is also carried out in reverse; that is, the cleaner, peripheral areas are cleansed first prior to cleansing the more heavily contaminated areas, even though these may be the operative site. The surgical principle is to work from the cleanest to the least clean area (King & Spry, 2019).

The antimicrobial solution should **not** be allowed to pool under the patient as this can cause skin

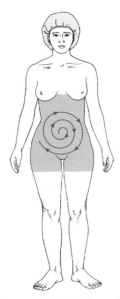

FIG. 6.13 Circular prepping technique. (Source: King, C., & Spry, C. (2019). Infection prevention and control. In J. Rothrock (Ed.), *Alexander's care of the patient in surgery* (16th ed., pp. 54–106). St Louis, MO: Mosby.)

maceration. Plastic-backed absorbent sheets can be placed under the patient to collect any excess solution. These sheets can then be removed prior to placing the sterile drapes on the patient, thereby minimising the risk of skin damage and potential fire if alcohol-based solutions are used (ACORN, 2020f; King & Spry, 2019).

Draping the Patient

An aseptic field within which surgery can be carried out is created using sterile drapes that are strategically placed on the patient in a manner that exposes only the operative site and isolates it from surrounding areas. Within this defined aseptic field, the surgical procedure takes place and all those involved must be dressed in sterile gowns, gloves and PPE. The drapes covering the patient's body provide an area on which instruments and equipment, such as suction tubing and the active diathermy electrode (handpiece), can be placed (King & Spry, 2019).

Reusable linen or synthetic single-use drapes used in the creation of the aseptic field should be made of materials that inhibit the migration of microbial particles and moisture. Drapes may be available as single items, or they may be packaged in predetermined configurations for specific surgical procedures. They are folded in such a manner as to facilitate easy opening and placement on the patient. Reusable drapes are held in place with towel clips or sutures, whereas single-use drapes have an adhesive section to secure them in place without slippage (King & Spry, 2019).

Points to consider when handling drapes are as follows:

- handle drapes as little as possible, as excessive movement can cause air currents and dispersal of dust particles
- hold the drapes above waist level and, once in place, do not move them. If a drape requires repositioning, it should be discarded and a new one used
- drape the incision site first and work towards the periphery, draping from aseptic to contaminated areas
- protect the gloved hands from contamination by 'cuffing' the drape over them during placement (King & Spry, 2019).

International standards recommend the use of disposable drapes as they provide a more efficient microbial and moisture barrier than reusable linen drapes. The passage of moisture through drapes can compromise the aseptic field (see below) and endanger the surgical team by exposing them to blood and body fluids (European Committee for Standardization [CEN], 2011; Kieser, Wyatt, Beswick, Kunutsor, & Hoopera, 2018). Disposable drapes can be incorporated into custom packs and reduce the amount of debris liberated into the environment when compared with traditional linen drapes.

Strikethrough

Gowns and drapes act as barriers to prevent the transmission of microorganisms from contaminated to aseptic areas. If moisture penetrates the gowns or drapes, it permits the passage of microorganisms from a contaminated surface to an aseptic surface; this is termed *strikethrough*. The need to prevent strikethrough is a critical factor in maintaining an aseptic field and is achieved by the use of waterproof drapes and gowns (or by the use of plastic aprons under gowns made of permeable material). However, if strikethrough occurs on either gown or drapes, they must be replaced. On completion of the surgical procedure and following the application of a wound dressing, the drapes are removed immediately using a 'contain and confine' approach, as described for the removal of gowns and gloves.

SCENARIO 6.4: ASEPTIC TECHNIQUE (CONTINUED)

While circulating for a surgical procedure, RN Cohen notices Dr West contaminate her glove while repositioning the operating light.

Critical Thinking Question

- How should RN Cohen handle this situation? Provide rationales for your answer.

INSTRUMENT CLEANING, DECONTAMINATION, DISINFECTION AND STERILISATION

All reusable medical devices (RMDs) used on a patient during a surgical or investigative procedure must undergo terminal decontamination procedures between each use to reduce the potential for cross-infection. Spaulding first proposed a system of classifying infection risk and the appropriate processing methods in 1968 (NHMRC, 2019). A modified Spaulding table is shown in Table 6.8.

The standards necessary to enable the safe and reproducible reprocessing of RMDs are detailed in Australian and New Zealand standard AS/NZS 4187: *Reprocessing reusable medical devices in health service organizations* (Standards Australia, 2014) and its 2019 Amendment 2 (Standards Australia, 2019). This governance-based standard provides a detailed chronological description of the essential requirements underpinning the reprocessing of RMDs to assist staff in sterilising services departments (SSDs), endoscopy units, operating suites, primary care and other facilities where RMDs may be reprocessed and rendered safe for reuse.

In adopting a governance approach to the reprocessing discipline, this latest version of AS/ANZ 4187, which

---

TABLE 6.8
Modified Spaulding Table – General Criteria for Reprocessing and Storage of RMDs in Health Service Organisations

Level of Risk	Process	Storage
Critical (a medical device that comes into contact with the vascular system or sterile tissue and that must be sterile at the time of use)	• Clean as soon as possible after using • Sterilise by moist heat after cleaning • If the RMD is heat sensitive, sterilise using an alternative process (e.g. automated low-temperature chemical sterilising process, liquid chemical sterilising process or ethylene oxide sterilising process)	• Sterility should be maintained • Packaged RMD should be stored to prevent environmental contamination in a designated storage area to protect RMD • RMDs processed through a liquid chemical sterilising process should be used immediately
Semi-critical (a medical device that comes into contact with mucous membranes or non-intact skin, e.g. flexible endoscopes)	• Clean as soon as possible after using • Sterilise by moist heat after cleaning • If the RMD will not tolerate moist heat sterilisation, use a low-temperature sterilisation process or thermal disinfection, or disinfection using a high-level, instrument-grade chemical disinfectant	• Store to prevent environmental contamination in a designated storage area to protect RMD
Non-critical (a medical device that only comes into contact with intact skin and not mucous membranes, e.g. stethoscope, sphygmomanometer cuff)	• Clean as necessary with detergent solution • If further treatment is necessary, disinfect with compatible low-level or intermediate-level, instrument-grade disinfectant after cleaning	• RMD shall be stored in a clean dry place to minimise environmental contamination

(Sources: Adapted from Standards Australia. (2014). AS/NZS 4187. *Reprocessing of reusable medical devices in health service organizations*. Sydney: Author.)

was first published in April 1994, has adopted many significant European and international standards, all of which are sector and/or device-specific and underpinned by applied science and engineering. This suite of referenced standards are overarched by quality- and risk-based standards.

These quality- and risk-based standards are used globally in setting the basis for service excellence in risk-averse production and operating environments such as are required in the reprocessing of RMDs.

This section should be read in conjunction with the ACORN (2020g) standard *Reprocessing re-usable medical devices*.

Decontamination and Cleaning

Decontamination procedures may include, but are not limited to, the following:

- initial postprocedural cleaning at point of use by the instrument nurse
- transport to a centralised SSD
- inspection and content verification
- manual cleaning to remove any remaining visual organic contamination
- mechanical cleaning
- process verification
- checking, calibration, assembly packaging
- terminal sterilisation, thermal or chemical disinfection.

Point of use care

In the perioperative context, the decontamination process begins in the OR during the procedure with the instrument nurse wiping used instruments with a sponge dampened with sterile water to keep them free of blood and tissue debris (WHO, 2018). If organic material is allowed to dry, this will reduce the safety and the potential function of the RMD, thus hindering effective use by the surgeon. Particular attention should be given to the tips, jaws, joints, channels and any moving and concealed parts of instruments to prevent build-up of organic debris (NHMRC, 2019). This important and consistent action throughout the procedure also helps reduce the bioburden, making the subsequent cleaning process easier and effective. Instruments with lumens or channels should be flushed through with sterile water to prevent blockage and adhesion of biomatter. Heavily contaminated instruments maybe cleaned in a splash bowl containing sterile water within the aseptic field or rinsed immediately following the procedure prior to transporting to SSD (according to local policy). Normal saline must not be used for cleaning, as it is corrosive and can damage instruments (Nania, 2015; WHO, 2016b).

At the conclusion of the procedure, an instrument tray check is carried out to ensure that all used RMDs are accounted for and are returned to their correct trays according to the trays lists/count sheets. This is particularly important where multiple trays and/or loan trays have been used. Loan trays (e.g. for orthopaedic joint replacement) are often presented into the surgical field in customised 'graphic trays'. These trays are designed with specific locations designated for the placement of these specialised and often-complex RMDs (Fig. 6.14).

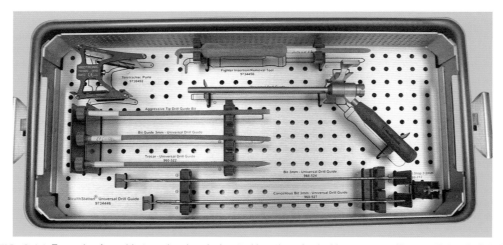

FIG. 6.14 Example of graphic tray showing designated location of spinal instruments. (Source: Tighe, S. (2016). Sterilization container system. In S. Tighe, *Instrumentation for the operating room* (9th ed., pp. 24–30). St Louis, MO: Mosby.)

PATIENT SCENARIOS

SCENARIO 6.5: CARE OF INSTRUMENTS

EN Noakes must ensure that all the instruments used in the procedure are cared for correctly.

Critical Thinking Question

- Describe four 'point of use care' actions that EN Noakes should take when managing her instruments during the surgical procedure. Give rationales for each answer.

Sterilising services department (SSD)

The SSD may be located adjacent to or some distance from the operating suite. Used RMDs must be transported to the SSD in covered or enclosed trolleys as an infection prevention measure (Standards Australia, 2014). In the SSD, the trays of RMDs are checked against the relevant tray list to verify that all contents are correct and to check on the degree of visibly remaining contamination on RMDs. Often, there may a time delay of greater than 30 minutes postprocedure, during which time organic debris will have begun to dry and adhere to the surfaces of inadequately rinsed RMDs. Such debris may affect the time it takes the SSD to effectively decontaminate the RMD and may also lead to the premature deterioration of an RMD, as organic debris is corrosive.

Before RMDs can be either sterilised or disinfected, they must be thoroughly cleaned of all residual organic material (bioburden). Failure to remove this material prevents the sterilising or disinfecting agent effectively coming into contact with all surfaces of the item and results in failure to achieve sterilisation or disinfection.

After inspection and verification, depending on the type of RMD being handled, RMDs will be processed by a manual-only method, a manual and partial mechanical cycle, or a manual and fully automated cycle. Ultimately, the process pathway selected will be dependent on the original equipment manufacturer's (OEM) instructions for use (IFU), sometimes also referred to as 'directions for use' (DFU) (NHMRC, 2019).

IFUs/DFUs are essential in establishing a safe and reproducible process pathway for any and all RMDs, particularly if the device is complex and may have several interconnected or related parts and/or may be heat sensitive. Such information is essential to guide SSD staff so as to ensure that the RMD is processed correctly.

Manual cleaning is often applied to RMDs if it is contraindicated that the particular device is non-submersible or heat sensitive. This category of equipment includes, for example, power drills and flexible gastroendoscopes.

Under such circumstances the correct detergent selection is essential to ensure the manual cleaning process will achieve a stated aim, which is to lower the bioburden. Where an RMD may be tolerant to mechanical reprocessing, the aim may achieved by using a combination of ultra-sonication, sometimes referred to as cavitation. The RMDs are then loaded into a large instrument washer, often called a indexing tunnel washer–disinfector (I-WD) or compact upright washer–disinfector (WD), which follows these stages:

- initial cold rinse ($<40°C$)
- thermal wash ($60°–70°C$)
- thermal rinse ($75°–85°C$)
- thermal disinfection ($70°–90°C$)
- drying ($100°–110°C$) (Standards Australia, 2014).

The success of these mechanical processes is dependent on the instruments such as scissors and clamps and other multisurfaced devices having their concealed and enclosed areas fully opened where possible, to allow all surfaces to be contacted by the circulating washing solutions.

The washers subject RMDs to a thermal disinfection and drying cycle, which serves two purposes:

- lowering the retained bioburden as temperatures attained during the disinfection stage deactivate vegetative organisms
- rendering the RMDs safer for technicians to handle in the assembly and checking stages.

The manual cleaning and rinsing of RMDs takes place in temperatures that do not exceed $44°C$, which can result in colonisation with microorganisms occurring. Therefore, the RMDs must be dried as soon as possible.

The testing of the success of the decontamination process can be achieved using protein test kits and digital technology, such a luminometer, to read a swab sample taken from an RMD. The latter technology can enable the SSD to focus on risk points on a difficult-to-clean RMD and, from the results, to design a device-specific reprocess protocol to ensure that the RMD is consistently reprocessed each time it is received for reprocessing (NHMRC, 2019; Standards Australia, 2014).

Inspection, Assembly and Packaging

Inspection

Following cleaning, manual/mechanical washing and drying, all instruments are visually inspected by the trained SSD technical staff to identify any obvious damage or defects and to ensure that the item is functioning correctly (i.e. scissors are sharp, the jaws of clamps are properly aligned, channels are unobstructed and optics are clear). Sterilising an item that is not functioning correctly could place the patient at risk should it fail during surgery. Material defects such as cracks within the instrument can harbour microorganisms, rendering the sterilisation process ineffective (NHMRC, 2019; Standards Australia, 2014).

Assembly

RMDs are assembled in trays or packaged individually. All operating suites have a range of instrument trays to cater for the procedures they commonly perform (e.g. laparotomy, hysterectomy), as well general trays of instruments to which individual items may be added, depending on the procedure. All trays are standardised and contain a specified number and type of instruments identified on a tray list or count sheet, which is packaged and sterilised with the tray. The tray list or count sheet is used by the instrument and circulating nurses to check the contents preoperatively and postoperatively to ensure that no items are inadvertently left inside the patient, discarded in the waste stream or misplaced within the OR (ACORN, 2020g; Standards Australia, 2014).

Packaging or sterile barrier system (SBS)

The aim of packaging RMDs is to protect the sterilised items against recontamination until they are opened ready for use in a subsequent surgical procedure. The term 'sterile barrier system' (SBS) is now commonly applied to packaging as it aligns with the principle of maintaining a barrier. Various materials are available and their selection depends on the item to be packaged and the sterilising process to be used. The product selected must comply with relevant international standards and provide a sustained and effective barrier against potential contamination (Standards Australia, 2014). Examples of packaging materials include:

- single-use wraps made from a combination of cellulose and/or synthetic polymer products for wrapping trays
- paper–synthetic-laminated pouches made of specialised paper and a flexible transparent multilayered plastic film-web. These can be used for individual items or for those items that require easy identification.

Trays, baskets or preformed containers in which instruments, endoscopes and specialised RMDs can be placed are made of a variety of durable materials such as moulded thermostable plastics, aluminium or stainless steel. They are designed with perforations to allow for circulation of cleaning agents during recommended cleaning stages, and to facilitate air removal and penetration by the sterilising agent.

Once assembled, the tray/container is wrapped in the selected packaging material (this may vary depending on the material and local policy) and folded in a manner that allows subsequent opening using aseptic technique. At a minimum, a piggyback easy-peel label identifying the tray is placed on the external surface. Once the item has been used, this label can be detached and placed on a tracking form, which remains in the patient's notes. This enables items to be traced back to the patient event should an investigation into a fault in the sterilisation process be required (WHO, 2016b).

Many hospitals now use an electronic tracking system which creates a barcode or QR code on the label with the RMD name, its model, size and the identity of the technician responsible for final reassembly/packaging. These codes are unique and are encrypted with the embedded information relating to the individual stages of reprocessing.

Depending on the sterilising agent to be used, the SBS will be sealed using a specialised chemically and pressure-sensitive indicator tape, which will change colour during the sterilising process. This also becomes a distinct visual check that the item has undergone the sterilisation process and is checked by the circulating nurse prior to opening the item. It must be noted that a change in colour of the external indicator tape alone does not guarantee sterility of the item. Other sterilising parameters must be met before sterility is assured and these are discussed below. However, if the indicator tape is found **not** to have changed colour, the item must be considered unsterile and not used.

Commercially packaged single-use items contain information from the manufacturer in the form of symbols on the package. These indicate the serial number, sterilisation method, that the item is for single use, whether it is latex free (if appropriate) and whether it requires specific storage conditions. This information should be checked to ensure that all the manufacturer's instructions are adhered to. Fig. 6.15 illustrates examples of commonly used symbols and their meanings.

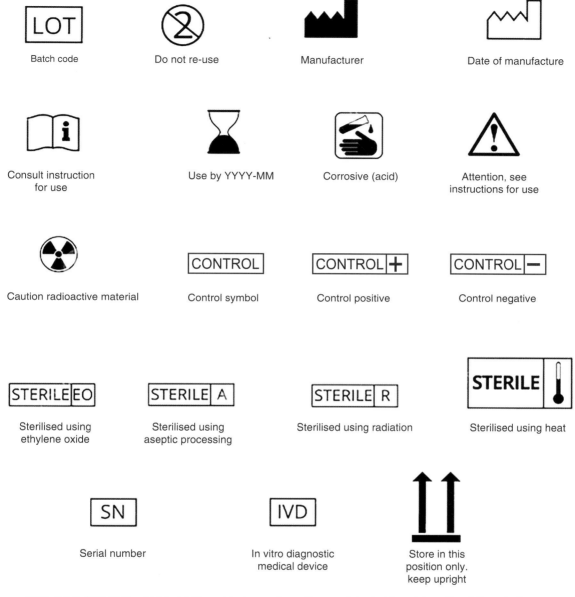

FIG. 6.15 Commonly used symbols and their meanings. (Source: Adapted from International Organization for Standardization. (2016). *ISO 15223-1. Medical devices: Symbols to be used with medical device labels, labelling and information to be supplied.* https://www.iso.org/obp/ui/#iso:std:iso:15223:-1:ed-3:v2:en.)

STERILISATION

Sterilisation is defined as 'the complete elimination or destruction of all forms of microbial life' (King & Spry, 2019). All items introduced into the aseptic field must be sterile in order to minimise the risk of surgical site (or other) infection and to promote an uneventful recovery. A number of different methods are employed to sterilise items used during surgical procedures. Their use is based on the physical properties of the item to be sterilised. For example, metal instruments, plastic disposable items, cotton swabs and linen drapes all require a different sterilisation method. Table 6.9

TABLE 6.9
Methods of Sterilisation

Method	Process	Action	Example of Items	Wrapping Material	Biological Indicator
High-temperature steam Temperature range 121°C–134°C	Saturated steam under pressure	Destroys cellular protein by coagulation	Stainless steel Alloy-based metals Textiles Moulded thermo-stable plastics	Textiles Cotton/polyester Paper Cellulose/synthetic wrap Heat-stable pouches	*Geobacillus stearothermophilus*
Dry heat (rarely used in hospital settings; used commercially) Temperature range 160°C–180°C	Non-pressurised sealed hot air chamber	Oxidises cellular protein	Powders Oils Paraffin gauze Carbon steel RMDs	Metal canisters Aluminium foil Glass tubes, bottles	*Bacillus subtilis niger*
Low-temperature ethylene oxide (EO)	100% ethylene oxide gas Temperature range 37°C–55°C	Alkylation: chemical interference, which inactivates reproductive process	Heat-sensitive RMDs (e.g. laparoscopes, cameras)	Paper pouches Perforated rigid containers Cellulose/synthetic wrap	*B. subtilis niger*
Low temperature steam and formaldehyde (LTSF)	2%–40% formaldehyde Temperature range 60°C–80°C	Alkylation: chemical interference, which inactivates reproductive process	Heat-sensitive RMDs (e.g. laparoscopes, cameras)	Paper pouches Perforated rigid containers Synthetic wrap	*G. stearothermophilus*
Low-temperature hydrogen peroxide (H$_2$O$_2$)	Low-temperature hydrogen peroxide vapour/plasma Temperature 50°C	Disrupts cellular activity	Heat-sensitive RMDs (e.g. laparoscopes, rigid cameras)	Synthetic wrap Synthetic pouches	*B. subtilis niger*
Wet processing	Low-temperature liquid peracetic acid 35%	Disrupts cellular activity	Flexible endoscopes (e.g. gastroscopes)	Unwrapped in specialised rigid tray within automated endoscope reprocessor (AER)	*G. stearothermophilus*
Gamma irradiation (commercial applications)	Cobalt-60 isotope	Destroys cellular DNA	Sponges Surgical gloves Petroleum gauze	Paper Plastic Cellulose	*Bacillus pumilus*

(Sources: Adapted from King, C., & Spry, C. (2019). Infection prevention and control. In J. Rothrock (Ed.), *Alexander's care of the patient in surgery* (16th ed., pp. 54–106). St Louis, MO: Elsevier; Standards Australia. (2014). AS/NZS 4187. *Reprocessing of reusable medical devices in health service organizations*. Sydney: Author.)

outlines methods of sterilisation; the 'biological indicator' is the challenge organism used to test the microbial destruction capabilities of the specific sterilising process. *Geobacillus stearothermophilus* is the common resistant organism used in commercial biological indicators (King & Spry, 2019).

Methods of Sterilisation
Steam
Saturated steam under pressure is one of the most effective and commonly used methods of sterilisation. It is an inexpensive method on a per-cycle basis and can be used on items capable of withstanding high temperatures (121°C–134°C), such as metal instruments and bowls. The steam sterilising process is designed to sterilise large loads of instruments within an SSD, the end result of which is a wrapped, sterile item with a shelf life ranging from 1 month to 1 year, depending on local policy.

Steam sterilisation takes place in specially designed sterilisers, often referred to as autoclaves, into which trays and individual items are carefully arranged to allow all surfaces to come into contact with the saturated steam. Fig. 6.16 shows an example of a steam steriliser loaded with RMDs for sterilisation. The sterilisers are preprogrammed to reach and maintain a specific temperature, pressure and time ratio depending on the type of load being sterilised (i.e. settings differ for metal ware, moulded plastic, linen or mixed loads). These are categorised as 'product families' and cycle parameters are designed around 'challenge' loads on the assumption that the most difficult to sterilise item determines the cycle program selected for the load (Standards Australia, 2014).

The steriliser chamber is sealed and the sterilisation process begins with the creation of a vacuum inside the chamber while steam is simultaneously injected into the chamber. This is known as fractionation and assists in chasing the air out of the chamber more quickly, while enabling the RMD to absorb latent heat more rapidly. It is during these presterilisation vacuum stages that there may be differences in the design of the cycle's parameters. These differences take into account the time it takes for the most dense or heaviest item(s) to attain the desired sterilisation temperature. Irrespective of the size or complexity of the RMD, this physical process occurs as the steam makes contact with the load contents and the heat of the steam is absorbed by the RMD; this heat is known as *latent heat* or *hidden heat*.

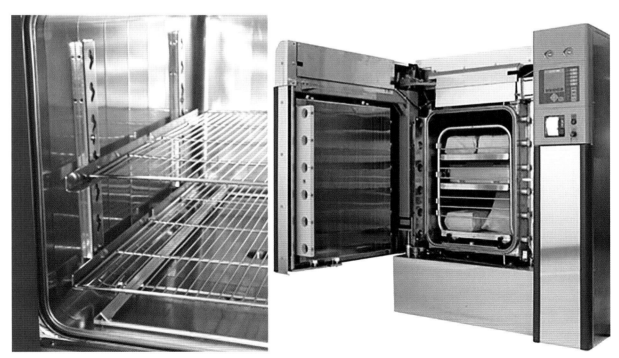

FIG. 6.16 Steam steriliser. (Source: King, C., & Spry, C. (2019). Infection prevention and control. In J. Rothrock (Ed.), *Alexander's care of the patient in surgery* (16th ed., pp. 54–106). St Louis, MO: Elsevier.)

Following removal of all the air and based on the onboard detection equipment, the chamber is now at the optimal temperature band for the holding or plateau stage, which is set at 134°C at 206 kPA (30–32 psi) for 3–4 minutes (or longer if a cycle program requires an elongated exposure as recommended by an OEM IFU). This is when sterilisation takes place as the chamber has reached a state of equilibrium.

When the sterilising cycle is completed, the steam is rapidly withdrawn by deep vacuum and the load is left to dry, using the residual radiant heat in the load contents and chamber walls. In the final stage of the process, HEPA-filtered air is introduced, which returns the chamber to normal atmospheric pressure, enabling the hitherto pressurised chamber to reach atmospheric pressure. It can now be opened and the load released for inspection. However, the load cannot be released for reuse until it has attained an ambient temperature in the range of 18°C–24°C.

Dry heat

Dry-heat sterilisation using the traditional hot air oven is rarely seen in healthcare facilities, but may be available commercially for sterilising paraffin gauze or petroleum jelly. It operates using fans to force hot air to circulate inside a sealed unpressurised chamber. It is reliant on heat being absorbed gradually to destroy microorganisms. The cycle times are long and impractical for rapid turnaround of RMDs and unsuitable for RMDs that may have a bonded component, such as adhesives (Centers for Disease Control and Prevention [CDC], 2008).

Ethylene oxide gas

Ethylene oxide (EO) gas is a low-temperature (37°C–55°C) chemical method of sterilisation that is suitable for items that cannot be exposed to the high temperatures associated with steam or to dry heat (e.g. RMDs with narrow lumens, and telescopes and drills). EO is a highly toxic and carcinogenic agent, and exposure can cause severe toxic reactions such as nausea, vomiting and respiratory difficulties in healthcare workers. Therefore, strict WH&S controls exist to protect operators of EO sterilisers. Few EO sterilisers remain in Australian hospitals, as many facilities have transitioned their older heat-sensitive inventory to steam-compatible RMDs and adopted hydrogen-peroxide-based low-temperature technologies as their means of low-temperature sterilisation.

EO is used by many commercial suppliers of disposable items (e.g. surgical sponges, custom packs). These commercial EO sterilisers are large machines with a capacity measured in cubic metres (pallets) rather than trays, baskets or packages.

While EO is becoming less used across Australia, it is a very effective means of sterilisation and can process items composed of materials such as elastomers, polymers and fabric. Items for sterilising are wrapped in single-use packaging or pouches and placed in the EO steriliser, where the temperature and humidity are controlled before the EO gas is introduced. The time taken to sterilise items can be up to 3–6 hours and, as EO is absorbed into the items, there must be a further 8 or more hours aeration or desorption time to ensure that the EO has been reduced to less than 1 part per million (ppm) from the items before they can be released for reuse. These limiting factors, combined with availability of more steam-tolerant RMDs, have contributed to the technology becoming almost obsolete in hospital-based reprocessing (King & Spry 2019; Standards Australia, 2014).

Hydrogen-peroxide-based low-temperature sterilisation

These sterilisers are very common across Australian hospitals as they offer a quick cycle time of 1–1.5 hours depending on the load. They operate using hydrogen peroxide as the sterilant, which is delivered to the chamber in a vapour and either is charged using a radiofrequency to produce a plasma/gaseous state or pressure is applied and a vapour or gas created. Both methods rely on a deep vacuum to be drawn inside the chamber to achieve permeation of the hydrogen peroxide to the load. The by-products are oxygen and water, thus making it substantially more environmentally sound than EO, as well as faster.

The technology is suitable to process RMDs such as cameras, telescopes and batteries. This method has, in many instances, superseded EO because it is a less toxic and more rapid form of sterilisation (King & Spry, 2019). There are limitations to the technology, however, as RMDs with long lumens or channels are difficult for hydrogen peroxide to penetrate effectively.

Low-temperature steam and formaldehyde (LTSF)

Low-temperature steam and formaldehyde (LTSF) sterilisation technique uses a 2%–40% concentration of formaldehyde to achieve sterilisation. The system operates using multiple vacuum stages to remove air and to prehumidify the chamber and load under pressure. This primes a humidified load for the injection of the pressurised gaseous formaldehyde, which rapidly permeates the load to achieve sterilisation. Following sterilisation of the load, formaldehyde is flushed out using steam and air.

The cycle times are approximately 3–4 hours duration and the penetration rate of RMD channels is similar to EO. Toxicity is high and it is only in recent years that the technology has been re-engineered to enable faster desorption, and therefore make it safer and a more viable low-temperature technology for daily use in hospitals (CDC, 2008).

Peracetic acid (PAA) and endoscope reprocessing

Peracetic acid is a low-temperature, liquid chemical sterilant that is suitable for the processing of flexible gastroendoscopes, which cannot be exposed to high temperatures. This category of reprocessing, while using the active chemical sterilant (PAA), is nonetheless not a guarantee that the endoscope is sterile. This is due to the variable that exists for all flexible-channelled endoscopes: the rigor to which the endoscope was subjected in its previous clinical usage. Flexible endoscopes are one of the most challenging and complex RMDs in circulation in contemporary healthcare. Their internal components are complex in design and construction, and the internal channels are not able to be examined for cleanliness prior to their exposure to a chemical reprocessing cycle. This is what is considered in the field of reprocessing as the 'limiting value'. As such, there is necessary caution in attributing the term 'sterile' to flexible-channelled endoscopes, which have undergone an exposure to a wet processing cycle in a liquid chemical sterilant-reprocessing system or automated endoscope reprocessor (AER). Most breaches of infection control in endoscope usage occur as a result of inadequate cleaning of flexible endoscopes and accessories (Gastroenterological Society of Australia [GESA], 2010).

Commercially produced liquid chemical sterilant-reprocessing systems are used to deliver the PAA in enclosed chambers (Figs 6.17, 6.18). AERs are used within ORs and endoscopy suites where flexible endoscopes (e.g. gastroscopes) are used frequently and require reprocessing close to the point of use or just-in-time (JIT) processing. Many newer-generation AER technologies also use a detergent and rinse sequence prior to the injection of the PAA. This has the added benefit of introducing deactivating chemicals to the channels of endoscopes and aids in the removal of biofilms and other potential organic debris. Following the cleaning and flushing stages, if the system is so equipped, PAA, at a concentration of 35%, is circulated through the channels and around the external surfaces of the endoscope. PAA is highly corrosive and is therefore used in combination with an anticorrosive

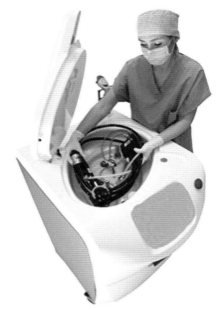

FIG. 6.17 Loading an endoscope into an automated endoscopic reprocessor (AER) (Source: Ecolab https://en-pl.ecolab.com/solutions/endoscope-reprocessing.)

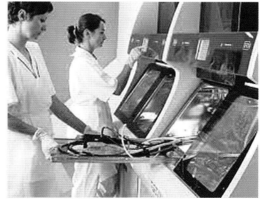

FIG. 6.18 ED-FLOW AER - allows for a physical barrier between soiled and clean sides with each chamber having two doors, one side for loading and the other side for unloading the endoscopes. (Source: Getinge Group https://www.getinge.com/siteassets/products-a-z/ed-flow-sd/getinge-aer-range-1922-en.pdf.)

buffering agent to reduce the potential harm to the delicate internal mechanisms of flexible endoscopes. These AER units are fully computerised and vary in design, with some featuring an interchangeable internal tray that accommodates a variety of equipment or a specially configured tray to fit a flexible endoscope, whereas others feature a universal chamber than can accommodate all conventional submersible endoscopes. A connection kit or hook-up fits onto the exposed ends of the internal lumen/channel system of the endoscope to ensure that the cleaning chemicals and PAA pass through each lumen/channel. Once the lid is closed and the processor activated, the endoscope is subjected to washing and flushing with deactivating chemistries and/or PAA. These chemicals mix with water and are flushed over and through the endoscope and its channels for preset periods of time – which are usually calibrated according to the type of endoscope being processed. Longer-channelled endoscopes may have longer cycles than shorter-channelled or non-channelled endoscopes. Following exposure to the PAA, there is a rinse cycle, which uses ultra-filtered or purified water to flush the PAA away, leaving an environmentally safe end product of acetic acid and water. The whole cycle takes approximately 20–30 minutes and the result is a wet endoscope ready for immediate use (King & Spry, 2019).

As with all RMDs intended to be reprocessed, thorough cleaning of an endoscope must occur prior to processing to ensure, as practicably possible, that all lumens are free of debris and bioburden (King & Spry, 2019; Standards Australia, 2014).

It is beyond the scope of this text to provide detailed description of the cleaning processes that must be undertaken for the safe reprocessing of endoscopes. Although much of the cleaning and reprocessing is automated, the need to oversee the process cannot be relinquished. Nursing staff working in endoscopic procedure areas, or in ORs where endoscopy may be performed as part of a surgical procedure, are still required to undertake some activities prior to endoscope reprocessing. This involves, for example, passing a brush down the channel after cleaning to check for patency or to ascertain the subtle nuances associated with minor damage/kinking of the endoscope. Failure to complete this activity has been identified by the Gastroenterological Nurses College of Australia (GENCA) as a matter of significant concern, with reports of haemostatic clips being retained within the endoscope channel; Feature box 6.6 details two incidents. Such incidents highlight that the staff engaged in the reprocessing task must be educated, trained and have demonstrable competency. GENCA and the Gastroenterological Society of Australia, Australian Gastrointestinal Endoscopy Association (AGEA) and NZ Society of Gastroenterology are key professional bodies involved in education, standard development and credentialling of staff involved in reprocessing endoscopes.

FEATURE BOX 6.6
TGA Medical Device Safety Alert

Two incidents reported to the Therapeutic Goods Administration (TGA) in 2014 highlighted issues with items being left behind in endoscopes despite multiple instances of cleaning and sterilisation.

In one incident, a small metal clip was flushed out of a colonoscope during cleaning. However, the type of clip involved had been used with the colonoscope 5 days earlier. It is thought that the clip had sucked into the device's internal biopsy channel during surgery and became lodged inside. The manufacturer could not rule out that the facility performed insufficient reprocessing or did not perform a biopsy channel inspection before or after use.

In the second incident, a 3 cm pancreatic stent was removed from a patient using a duodenoscope, but was noted not to have exited the device. Despite undergoing normal cleaning, brushing and leak testing, the stent remained inside. Over the next five days, four patients underwent procedures using this duodenoscope after it was cleaned and sterilised in the usual manner. The stent came out of the scope during the fourth procedure.

To help avoid incidents such as these, the TGA advises health facilities to ensure that appropriate education is in place for staff cleaning and sterilising endoscopes. These incidents also highlight the importance of following manufacturers' instructions carefully (American Society for Gastrointestinal Endoscopy [ASGE], 2011; AORN, 2015; the Gastroenterological Society of Australia [GESA], 2010).

Gamma radiation

Many commercially packaged products that are unsuitable for sterilisation by chemical or heat processes are sterilised by irradiation using the isotope cobalt-60, which produces gamma rays. Gamma rays can penetrate large cartons of items, making this an economical method for medical companies to sterilise items such as ointments, sponges, plastic drapes and surgical gloves. This method is suitable for commercial application only (CDC, 2008).

Sterilisation and Creutzfeldt–Jakob Disease

The causative prions of Creutzfeldt–Jakob disease (CJD) are highly resistant to conventional decontamination and sterilisation methods. Special protocols are required to manage instruments if they have been used on patients known to carry, or thought to be at risk of carrying, this disease. Ideally, single-use instruments should be used, but this may not prove to be practical. Many institutions quarantine reusable instruments used on suspected CJD patients until test results from the patient have been obtained. Negative results will mean that routine decontamination and sterilisation processes can be followed. Positive results will require instruments to be destroyed (King & Spry, 2019). The management of equipment exposed to CJD prions is still evolving as further research is carried out on this highly infective, but fortunately rare, disease (Australian Government Department of Health, 2013).

Monitoring Sterilisation Processes

All sterilising methods must undergo validation processes to ensure that items are sterile and may be safely used on patients. The validation process refers to documented procedures for obtaining, recording and interpreting results needing to show that a process will consistently produce a sterile item. This commences with the commissioning of new sterilising equipment and ongoing regular performance requalifications comprising microbiological and physical parameters (Standards Australia, 2014).

Physical

Regular maintenance, monitoring and testing of all sterilisers take place to ensure that they are functioning correctly in accordance with standard AS/NZS 4187 (Standards Australia, 2014). All sterilisers have external gauges, thermometers, timers and computer printouts to monitor their functions. Internal sensors can provide information about temperature, pressure and, where applicable, humidity for every load. Documentation of these parameters is captured both in analogue and more commonly in digital format to provide permanent records so as to provide proof that all loads have passed through the sterilisation process satisfactorily. This may be required in the event of a look-back following an infection or during a routine quality audit (Standards Australia, 2014).

Chemical

Chemical indicators and integrators (CIs) are calibrated chemical compounds, usually mounted on a paper or synthetic carrier. CIs are formulated to react incrementally when exposed to the physical and chemical agents active inside a sterilising chamber – a steam or low-temperature chemical steriliser or disinfector. The indicators may be attached to the outside of each package in the form of an adhesive tape, incorporated into the wrapping material, in the seam of paper-laminated pouches/rolls, or as independent strips/spots to be attached to the outside or inside, if preferred, of the wrapped RMD. CIs do not guarantee that the RMD is sterile, but they do provide an important visual indicator that the RMD has undergone a sterilisation or chemical disinfection process.

If the sterilisation parameters have been met, the CI should change colour. External CIs are verified at point of processing in the CSD and, subject to their satisfactory colour change, the RMDs are then released to the end user, who must check for CI colour change prior to opening the item. Internal indicators are verified at the point of use by the instrument nurse prior to using the instruments. If the integrator strip has not changed colour, the item must not be used, as sterilisation may not have occurred (Standards Australia, 2014).

Biological

Biological indicators (BIs) are standardised preparations of resistant bacterial spores that are included as part of the routine testing processes of sterilisers to demonstrate whether sterilisation conditions have been met. BIs are inoculated with a known concentration of resistant spores, usually retained on a carrier strip within a self-contained capsule or carrier in which there is a liquid growth media housed in a sealed vial. The spore population may vary depending on the sterilisation process that is being challenged. For example, the organism used to test steam sterilisation conditions is G. *stearothermophilis.*

While it is acknowledged that no one testing parameter alone will verify that sterilisation conditions have been met, the contemporary reprocessing of RMDs follows a measurable sequence of reduction stages using handling techniques and technologies which are performance verified in each cycle. Checking, assembly and wrapping processes are also undertaken against work procedures based on RMD manufacturers' IFUs. These sequenced components of RMD reprocessing culminate in the terminal processing in a steriliser or disinfector for which the cycle details enable careful analysis of the cycle stages, aiding in process verification (Standards Australia, 2014).

Tracking and Traceability

The ability to track instruments and trace their use for individual patients is an integral component of safety and risk management processes. Written and computerised records are maintained within the sterilising department to provide retrospective proof that an item has satisfactorily passed through a sterilisation or disinfection process. These records are important should an outbreak of infection occur and where investigations demonstrate that there may have been a breakdown in the sterilisation or disinfection process. Patients who have undergone procedures during the period in question and who may have been infected need to be traced and their infectious status investigated. Tracking systems rely on the accurate capture of all details relating to the contents of procedure trays and separate instruments.

The use of barcodes or QR codes attached to trays enables scanning during the various handling stages: collection, decontamination, checking, testing and terminal sterilisation or disinfection. Each time an RMD tray or single items is received for reprocessing, a new barcode or QR code number is generated. This facilitates the recording of the reprocess cycle, which is stored on a computer server for future reference. Optimally, a tracking system ought to be capable of tracking each individual RMD. However, this is not only labour intensive, but also restrictive for the turnaround of RMDs, which are often in short supply (Standards Australia, 2014).

It is, however, recognised that in some procedures, such as those associated with patients known or thought to be at risk of carrying CJD, RMDs should be individually tracked. This would quarantine those RMDs, separating them for more intensive reprocessing than conventionally practised (Standards Australia, 2014).

Disinfection

Disinfection is described as a process of destroying all pathogenic organisms except spores from inanimate objects (King & Spry, 2019). The process can be used on items identified as semi-critical or non-critical (see Table 6.8). Disinfection may be achieved by either thermal or chemical means. In the hierarchy of controls, thermal disinfection or pasteurisation is preferred to chemicals, which may leave a residue and may lead to gradual deterioration of the RMD.

Thermal disinfection has the benefit of being able to be supported through an SSD, as most contemporary instrument washers have a thermal disinfection stage as a default in their cycle programs.

Thermal disinfection can be achieved at different temperatures, classified as high, intermediate or low level depending on their killing capabilities. As with items for sterilisation, effective decontamination of the items or surfaces using enzymatic cleaners, detergents and water must occur prior to disinfection (King & Spry, 2019). Staff should wear PPE when using disinfecting agents, as contact can produce adverse skin or respiratory effects. Material safety data sheets (MSDSs) containing information on each chemical, its use, possible adverse effects and first aid and spill management should be available within the operating suite and SSD.

Storage of Sterile Equipment

Following sterilisation, RMDs and single-use items from external medical companies are stored in a stockroom within the restricted area of the operating suite. Sterility of RMDs and single-use items is event rather than time related and relies on the environment being controlled at a temperature of 18°C–22°C and a humidity range of 35%–70%. The storage area must be regularly cleaned and free of dust, insects and vermin. Open storage racks are recommended to reduce collection of dust and storage bins must be kept free of dust. Other 'events' which may compromise sterility include stacking too many instrument trays on top of one another and storing packages too tightly – both these events could lead to damage to the wrapping and render the item unsterile (WHO, 2016b). Any departure from the optimum conditions may compromise the sterility of the sterile items. Stock should be regularly rotated to ensure economical use of items, with attention paid to the date of manufacture (i.e. older items used first) (Standards Australia, 2014). (See Chapter 5 for further information.)

CONCLUSION

Understanding the modes of transmission of infection and applying the principles of infection prevention and control are a critical part of perioperative nurses' role in keeping themselves and patients safe during the perioperative period. The focus of this chapter has been on assisting perioperative nurses to implement a range of strategies aimed at preventing or minimising the risk of infection in the surgical patient. Perioperative nurses must work in collaboration with other members of the healthcare team to monitor infection control practices constantly to ensure quality care for patients.

RESOURCES

Australian College of Perioperative Nurses (ACORN)
https://www.acorn.org.au
Australian Commission on Safety and Quality in Health Care. Infection prevention and control learning modules
https://infectionprevention.kineoportal.com.au (registration) or information
https://www.safetyandquality.gov.au/our-work/infection-prevention-and-control/infection-prevention-and-control-elearning-modules
Centers for Disease Control and Prevention (CDC)
https://www.cdc.gov
Creutzfeldt–Jakob Disease (CJD) Support Group Network
https://www.cjdsupport.org.au
Department of Health (Australia)
https://www.health.gov.au
Department of Health (NZ)
https://www.health.govt.nz
National Hand Hygiene Initiative (through ACSQHC)
https://www.safetyandquality.gov.au/our-work/infection-prevention-and-control/national-hand-hygiene-initiative-nhhi/national-hand-hygiene-initiative-manual

National Health and Medical Research Council
https://www.nhmrc.gov.au
Perioperative Nurses College of New Zealand Nurses Organisation
https://www.pnc.org
Society for Healthcare and Epidemiology of America (SHEA)
https://www.shea-online.org
The Cochrane Collaboration
https://www.Cochrane.org/index.htm
World Health Organization (WHO) 5 Moments of Hand Hygiene
https://www.who.int/gpsc/tools/Five_moments/en/

Video Resources

Closed gloving method
https://www.youtube.com/watch?v=XizEHAc_jjY
Self-gowning and gloving
https://www.youtube.com/watch?v=jwcSdJlx17E

REFERENCES

Agency for Clinical Innovation (ACI). (2020). Personal protective equipment in the operating theatre during the COVID-19 pandemic. Retrieved from <https://aci.health.nsw.gov.au>.

American Society for Gastrointestinal Endoscopy (ASGE). (2011). Multisociety guideline on reprocessing flexible gastrointestinal endoscopes. *Gastrointestinal Endoscopy, 73*(6), 1075–1084. https://dx.doi.org/10.1016/j.gie.2011.03.1183

Association of periOperative Registered Nurses (AORN). (2015). *Guidelines for perioperative practice: Guideline for cleaning and processing flexible endoscopes and endoscope accessories*. Denver, CO: Author.

Association of periOperative Registered Nurses (AORN). (2019). *Perioperative standards and recommended practices*. Denver, CO: Author.

Australian and New Zealand College of Anaesthetics (ANZCA). (2015). *PS28 Guidelines on infection control in anaesthesia*. Melbourne: Author. Retrieved from <https://www.anzca.edu.au/getattachment/e4e601e6-d344-42ce-9849-7ae9bfa19f15/PS28-Guideline-on-infection-control-in-anaesthesia>.

Australian College of Perioperative Nurses (ACORN). (2020a). Perioperative attire. In *ACORN standards for perioperative nursing in Australia* (16th ed., Vol. 1). Adelaide: Author.

Australian College of Perioperative Nurses (ACORN). (2020b). Infection prevention. In *ACORN standards for perioperative nursing in Australia* (16th ed., Vol. 1). Adelaide: Author.

Australian College of Perioperative Nurses (ACORN). (2020c). Surgical hand antisepsis, gowning and gloving. In *ACORN standards for perioperative nursing in Australia* (16th ed., Vol. 1). Adelaide: Author.

Australian College of Perioperative Nurses (ACORN). (2020d). Cleaning and maintaining the perioperative environment. In *ACORN standards for perioperative nursing in Australia* (16th ed., Vol. 1). Adelaide: Author.

Australian College of Perioperative Nurses (ACORN). (2020e). Asepsis. In *ACORN standards for perioperative nursing in Australia* (16th ed., Vol. 1). Adelaide: Author.

Australian College of Perioperative Nurses (ACORN). (2020f). Preoperative patient skin antisepsis. In *ACORN standards for perioperative nursing in Australia* (16th ed., Vol. 1). Adelaide: Author.

Australian College of Perioperative Nurses (ACORN). (2020g). Reprocessing reusable medical devices. In *ACORN standards for perioperative nursing in Australia* (16th ed., Vol. 1). Adelaide: Author.

Australian Commission on Safety and Quality in Health Care (ACSQHC/the Commission). (2017). *Recommendations for the control of carbapenemase-producing Enterobacteriaceae (CPE): a guide for acute care health facilities*. Retrieved from <https://www.safetyandquality.gov.au/sites/default/files/migrated/Recommendations-for-the-control-of-Carbapenemase-producing-Enterobacteriaceae.pdf>.

Australian Commission on Safety and Quality in Health Care (ACSQHC/the Commission). (2018a). *Antimicrobial stewardship clinical care standard*. Sydney: Author.

Australian Commission on Safety and Quality in Health Care (ACSQHC/the Commission). (2018b). Hospital-acquired complications information kit: fact sheets to support safety and quality in Australian health services. Retrieved from <https://www.safetyandquality.gov.au/sites/default/files/migrated/SAQ7730_HAC_InfomationKit_V2.pdf>.

Australian Commission on Safety and Quality in Health Care (ACSQHC/the Commission). (2020). National Hand Hygiene Initiative (NHHI). 5 moments of hand hygiene. Retrieved from <https://www.safetyandquality.gov.au/our-work/infection-prevention-and-control/national-hand-hygiene-initiative-nhhi/national-hand-hygiene-initiative-manual>.

Australian Government Department of Health (2013). CJD Infection control guidelines. Retrieved from <https://www.health.gov.au/internet/main/publishing.nsf/content/icg-guidelines-index.htm>.

Australian Institute of Health and Welfare (2017). Staphylococcus aureus *bacteraemia in Australian public hospitals 2016–17: Australian hospital statistics.* Health services series no. 83. Cat. No HSE 198. Canberra: Author.

Australian Society for HIV Medicine (ASHM). (2020). Hepatitis B training, information and resources [webpage]. Retrieved from <https://www.ashm.org.au/HBV/>.

Ball, K. (2019). Surgical modalities. In J. Rothrock (Ed.), *Alexander's care of the patient in surgery* (16th ed., pp. 201–243). St. Louis, MO: Elsevier.

Ban, K. A., Minei, J. P., Laronga, C., Harbrecht, B. G., Jensen, E. H., Fry, D. E. … Duane, T. M. (2017). American College of Surgeons and Surgical Infection Society surgical site infection guidelines, 2016 update. *Journal of the American College of Surgeons, 224*(1), 59–74. https://dx.doi.org/10.1016/j.jamcollsurg.2016.10.029

Berrios-Torres, S. I., Umscheid, C. A., Bratzler, D. W., Leas, B., Stone, E. C., Kelz, R. R., … Healthcare Infection Control Practices Advisory Committee. (2017). Centers for Disease Control and Prevention guideline for the prevention of surgical site infection. *Journal of the American Medical Association – Surgery, 152*(8), 784–791.

Best, M., & Neuhauser, D. (2004). Ignaz Semmelweis and the birth of infection control. *Quality Safety Health Care, 13,* 233–234. http://dx.doi.org/10.1136/qshc.2004.010918

Bowden, S., & Locarnini, S. (2018). *Virology: viral replication, current therapy and progress to a cure.* Retrieved from <https://www.hepatitisb.org.au/virology-viral-replication-current-therapy-and-progress-to-a-cure/>.

Boyce, J. (2016). Modern technologies for improving cleaning and disinfection of environmental surfaces in hospitals. *Antimicrobial Resistance and Infection Control, 5,* 10. https://dx.doi.org/10.1186/s13756-016-0111

Centers for Disease Control and Prevention (CDC). (2008, updated 2019). *Guideline for disinfection and sterilization in healthcare facilities.* Retrieved from <https://www.cdc.gov/infectioncontrol/pdf/guidelines/disinfection-guidelines-H.pdf v>.

Centers for Disease Control and Prevention (CDC). (2021). Summary for healthcare facilities: strategies for optimizing the supply of N95 respirators during shortages. Retrieved from <https://www.cdc.gov/coronavirus/2019-ncov/hcp/checklist-n95-strategy.html>.

Clinical Excellence Commission (CEC). (2020a). Infection prevention and control practice handbook. Retrieved from <http://www.cec.health.nsw.gov.au/__data/assets/pdf_file/0010/383239/IPC-Practice-Handbook-2020.PDF>.

Clinical Excellence Commission (CEC). (2020b). Antimicrobial stewardship [webpage]. Retrieved from <http://www.cec.health.nsw.gov.au/patient-safety-programs/medication-safety/antimicrobial-stewardship/quah>.

Engelkirk, P., Fader, R., & Duben-Engelkirk, J. (2019). *Burton's microbiology for the health sciences* (11th ed.). Philadelphia, PA: Wolters Kluwer.

European Committee for Standardization (CEN). (2011). EN 13795. *Surgical drapes, gowns and clean air suits, used as medical devices for patients, clinical staff and equipment. General requirements for manufacturers, processors and products, test methods, performance requirements and performance levels.* Brussels: Author.

Gastroenterological Society of Australia (GESA), Gastroenterological Nurses College of Australia (GENCA), Australian Gastrointestinal Endoscopy Association (AGEA) (GESA/GENCA/AGEA). (2010). *Infection control in endoscopy.* Melbourne: GESA.

Gillespie, B., Bull, C., Walker, R., Lin, F., Roberts, S., & Chaboyer, W. (2018). Quality appraisal of clinical guidelines for surgical site infection prevention: a systemic review. *PLoS One.* 13(9), e0203354.

Guo, Y. P., Wong, P. M., Li, Y., & Or, P. P. L. (2012). Is double-gloving really protective? A comparison between the glove perforation rate among perioperative nurses with single and double gloves during surgery. *American Journal of Surgery, 204*(2), 210–215. https://dx.doi.org/10.1016/j.amjsurg.2011.08.017

Harkavy, L., & Novak, D. (2014). Clearing the air: surgical smoke and workplace safety practices. *OR Nurse, 8*(6), 1–7. https://dx.doi.org/10.1097/01.ORN.0000453446.85448.2f

Health Quality and Safety Commission New Zealand. (2014). Surgical skin antisepsis [webpage]. Retrieved from <https://www.hqsc.govt.nz/our-programmes/infection-prevention-and-control/news-and-events/news/1372/>.

Health Quality and Safety Commission New Zealand. (2018a). Surgical site infection improvement [webpage]. Retrieved from <https://www.hqsc.govt.nz/our-programmes/infection-prevention-and-control/projects/surgical-site-infection-improvement/>.

Health Quality and Safety Commission New Zealand. (2018b). Hand hygiene [webpage]. Retrieved from <https://www.hqsc.govt.nz/our-programmes/infection-prevention-and-control/projects/hand-hygiene>.

Hill, D. S., O'Neill, J. K., Powell, R. J., & Oliver, D. W. (2012). Surgical smoke: a health hazard in the operating theatre. A study to quantify exposure and a survey of the use of smoke extractor systems in UK plastic surgery units. *Journal of Plastic and Reconstructive Aesthetic Surgery, 65*(7), 911–916. https://dx.doi.org/10.1016/j.bjps.2012.02.012.23

International Organization for Standardization (ISO). (2016). ISO 15223-1. Medical devices: Symbols to be used with medical device labels, labelling and information to be supplied. Retrieved from <https://www.iso.org/obp/ui/#iso:std:iso:15223:-1:ed-3:v2:en>.

International Organization for Standardization (ISO). (2018). ISO 22610:2018. ISO/TC 94/SC13 Protective clothing. Retrieved from <https://www.iso.org/standard/63671.html>.

Jain, S., Clezy, K., & McLaws, M. (2018). Safe removal of gloves from contact precautions: the role of hand hygiene. *American Journal of Infection Control, 46*(7), 764–767. https://dx.doi.org/10.1016/j.ajic.2018.01.013

Kelkar, U., Gogate, B., Kurpad, S., Gogate, P., & Deshpande, M. (2013). How effective are face masks in operation theatre? A time frame analysis and recommendations. *International Journal of Infection Control, 9*(1). https://dx.doi.org/10.3396/ijic.v9i1.003.13

Khatoon, Z., McTiernan, C., Suuronen, E., Mah, T., & Alarcon, E. (2018). Bacterial biofilm formation on implantable devices and approaches to its treatment and prevention. *Heliyon, 4*(12). Retrieved from <https://www.cell.com/action/showPdf?pii=S2405-8440%2818%2936901-9>.

Kieser, D., Wyatt, M., Beswick, B., Kunutsor, S., & Hoopera, G. (2018). Does the type of surgical drape (disposable versus non-disposable) affect the risk of subsequent surgical site infection? *Journal of Orthopaedics, 15*(2), 566–570. https://dx.doi.org/10.1016/j.jor.2018.05.015

King, C., & Spry, C. (2019). Infection prevention and control. In J. Rothrock (Ed.), *Alexander's care of the patient in surgery* (16th ed., pp. 54–106). St. Louis, MO: Elsevier.

Lee, G., & Bishop, P. (2016). *Microbiology and infection control for health professionals* (5th ed.). Sydney: Pearson Australia.

Loveday, H., Wilson, J., Pratt, R., Golsorkhi, M., Tingle, A., Bak, A., ... UK Department of Health. (2014). National evidenced-based guidelines for preventing healthcare-associated infections in NHS hospitals in England. *Journal of Hospital Infection, 86,* S1–S70.

Makama, J. G., Okeme, I. M., Makama, E. J., & Ameh, E. A. (2016). Glove perforation rate in surgery: a randomized, controlled study to evaluate the efficacy of double gloving. *Surgical Infections, 17*(4), 436–442. https://dx.doi.org/10.1016/j.ajic.2018.01.013

Markel, T., Gormley, T., Greely, D., Ostojic, J., Wise, A., Rajala, J., Bharadwaj, R., & Wagner, J. (2017). Hats off: a study of different operating room headgear assessed by environmental quality indicators. *Journal of the American College of Surgeons, 225*(5), 57–581. https://dx.doi.org/10.1016/j.jamcollsurg.2017.08.014

Mischke, C., Verbeek, J., Saarto, A., Lavoie, M.-C., Pahwa, M., & Sharea Ijaz, S. (2014). Gloves, extra gloves or special types of gloves for preventing percutaneous exposure injuries in healthcare personnel. *Cochrane Database of Systematic Reviews, 3*, CD009573. https://dx.doi.org/ 10.1002/ 14651858.CD009573.pub2

Murphy, C. (2018). Surgical glove changing practices. ACORN Webinar series. Retrieved from <https://www.acorn.org.au/webinars>.

Murphy, C., Di Ruscio, F., Lynskey, M., Collins, J., McCullough, E., Cosgrave, R., … Fennel, J. (2017). Identification badge lanyards as infection control risk: a cross-sectional observation study with epidemiologic analysis. *Journal of Hospital Infection, 96*, 63–66. https://dx.doi.org/10.1016/j.jhin.2017.01.008

Murrell, L., Hamilton, E., Johnson, H., & Spencer, M. (2018). Influence of a visible-light continuous environmental disinfection system on microbial contamination and surgical site infection in an orthopedic operating room. *American Journal of Infection Control, 47*(7), 804–810. https://dx.doi.org/10.1016/j.ajic.2018.12.002

Nania, P. (2015). New guidance for reprocessing medical devices. *AORN Journal, 102*(4), 13–14. https://dx.doi.org/ 10.1016/s0001-2092(15)00824-8

National Health and Medical Research Council (NHMRC). (2019). Australian guidelines for the prevention and control of infection in healthcare. Retrieved from <https://www.nhmrc.gov.au/about-us/publications/australian-guidelines-prevention-and-control-infection-healthcare-2019>.

National Health Service (NHS). (2015). *Patient safety agency. Risk of death or severe harm due to inadvertent injection of skin preparation solution.* Patient safety alert (Stage One: Warning). London, UK: Author.

Neely, A., & Maley, M. (2000). Survival of enterococci and staphylococci on hospital fabrics and plastic. *Journal of Clinical Microbiology, 38*(2), 724–726. https://dx.doi.org/10.1128/JCM.38.2.724-726.2000

New Zealand (NZ) Ministry of Health. (2017). New Zealand antimicrobial action plan. Retrieved from <https://www.health.govt.nz/publication/new-zealand-antimicrobial-resistance-action-plan>.

New Zealand (NZ) Ministry of Health. (2018). Infection prevention and control and management of carbapenemase-producing Enterobacteriaceae (CPE). Retrieved from <https://www.health.govt.nz/publication/infection-prevention-control-and-management-carbapenemase-producing-enterobacteriaceae-cpe>.

NSW Health. (2011). *Safe use of alcohol-based skin preparations for surgical and anaesthetic procedures.* Safety Information Sheet 001/11. Sydney: Author.

NSW Health. (2019). Communicable diseases factsheet: Creutzfeld–Jakob disease (CJD). Retrieved from <https:// www.health.nsw.gov.au/Infectious/factsheets/Pages/creutzfeldt-jakob-disease.aspx>.

Patterson, T. (2019). *Aspergillus* species. In J. Mandell, R. Dolin & M. Blaser (Eds.), *Mandell, Douglas and Bennett's principles and practice of infectious diseases* (9th ed., Ch. 257). Philadelphia, PA: Elsevier Saunders.

Phillips, N. (2017). Surgical microbiology and antimicrobial therapy. In *Berry & Kohn's operating theatre technique* (13th ed., Ch. 14). St. Louis, MO: Mosby.

Royal Australasian College of Surgeons (RACS). (2015). Position paper: jewellery in the operating theatre. Ref. No. FES-PST-027. Retrieved from <https://umbraco.surgeons.org/media/1649/2015-06-24_pos_fes-pst-027_jewellery_in_the_operating_theatre.pdf>.

Schrank, G., & Branch-Elliman, W. (2017). Breaking the chain of infection in older adults. *Infectious Disease Clinics of North America, 31*(4), 649–671. https://dx.doi.org/10.1016/j.idc.2017.07.004

Schultz, L. (2015). Can efficient smoke evacuation limit aerosolization of bacteria? *AORN Journal, 102*(1), 7–14. https://dx.doi.org/10.1016/j.aorn.2015.04.023

Shaban, R., Macbeth, D., Russo, P., Mitchell, B., & Potter, J. (2019). Healthcare-associated infections and infectious diseases. In K. Curtis, C. Ramsden, R. Shaban, M. Fry & J. Considine (Eds.), *Emergency and trauma care* (3rd ed., pp. 717–738). Sydney: Elsevier.

Society for Healthcare Epidemiology of America (SHEA). (2014). Strategies to prevent surgical site infections in acute care hospitals. *Infection Control and Hospital Epidemiology, 35*(6), 605–627. https://dx.doi.org/10.1086/676022

South Australia Health. (2020). *Candida auris.* Adelaide: Author. Retrieved from <https://www.sahealth.sa.gov.au/wps/wcm/connect/public+content/sa+health+internet/clinical+resources/clinical+programs+and+practice+guidelines/infection+and+injury+management/healthcare+associated+infections/multidrug-resistant+organisms+mro/candida+auris>.

Spruce, L. (2017). Surgical head coverings: a literature review. *AORN Journal, 106*(4), 306–316.

Standards Australia. (2014). AS/NZS 4187. *Reprocessing of reusable medical devices in health service organizations.* Sydney: Author.

Standards Australia. (2019). AS/NZS 4187:2014/Amdt 2:2019. *Reprocessing of reusable medical devices in health service organizations.* Sydney: Author.

Stuart, R. A., Marshall, B. C., Harrington, G., Sasko, E. F., McLaws, M. A., & Ferguson, J. (2019). ASID/ACIPC position statement. Infection control for patients with *Clostridium difficile* infection in healthcare facilities. *Infection, Disease and Health, 24*(1), 32–43.

Tighe, S. (2016). Sterilization container system. In S. Tighe (Ed.), *Instrumentation for the operating room* (9th ed., pp. 24–30). St. Louis, MO: Mosby.

VanMeter, K., & Hubert, R. (2016). *Microbiology for the health professional* (2nd ed.). Sydney: Elsevier.

Vassello, A. (2016). Preventing surgical site infections with the SHEA bundle. Retrieved from <http://sdapic.org/

wp-content/uploads/2016/09/Vassallo-Prev-SSI-w-the-SHEA-Bundle-Sept-2016.pdf>.

Webster, J., Croger, S., Lister, C., Doidge, M., Terry, M., & Jones, I. (2010). Use of face masks by non-scrubbed operating room staff: a randomized controlled trial. *ANZ Journal of Surgery, 80*(3), 169–173. https://dx.doi.org/10.1111/j.1445-2197.2009.05200.x

Wilson, M., McNab, R., & Henderson, B. (2019). *Bacterial disease mechanisms: an introduction to cellular microbiology.* London: Cambridge University Press.

World Health Organization (WHO). (2009). WHO guidelines on hand hygiene in healthcare. Retrieved from <http://apps.who.int/iris/bitstream/10665/44102/1/9789241597906_eng.pdf>.

World Health Organization (WHO). (2016a). Global guidelines for the prevention of surgical site infection. Retrieved from <https://www.who.int/gpsc/ssi-prevention-guidelines/en/>.

World Health Organization (WHO). (2016b). Decontamination and reprocessing of medical devices for health-care facilities. Retrieved from <https://apps.who.int/iris/bitstream/handle/10665/250232/9789241549851-eng.pdf;jsessionid=F9B3E732E9DAE4BE8E57EB733CB8E735?sequence=>.

World Health Organization (WHO). (2018). *Global guidelines on the prevention of surgical site infection* (2nd ed.). Geneva: Author.

FURTHER READING

Australian Commission on Safety and Quality in Health Care (ACSQHC/the Commission). (2018). *Antimicrobial prescribing practice in Australian hospitals: results of the 2017 National Antimicrobial Prescribing Survey.* Sydney: Author.

Chobin, N. (2019). Surgical instrument decontamination: a multistep approach. *AORN Journal, 110*(3), 253–262. https://dx.doi.org/10.1002/aorn.12784

Link, T. (2019). Guideline implementation: sterile technique. *AORN Journal, 110*(4), 416–422. https://dx.doi.org/10.1002/aorn.12867

McKenna, E. (2019). Cloth hats: (w)hat's the issue. *Journal of Perioperative Practice, 32*(4), 21–25. https://dx.doi.org/10.26550/2209-1092.1069

Palmore, T. (2019). Infection prevention and control in the health care setting. In J. Bennett, R. Dolin & M. Blaser (Eds.), In *Mandell, Douglas and Bennett's principles and practice of infectious diseases* (9th ed., Ch. 298). Philadelphia, PA: Elsevier.

Rutala, W., & Weber, D. (2019). Best practices for disinfection of non critical environmental surfaces and equipment in health care facilities: a bundle approach. *American Journal of Infection Control, 47*, A96–A105.

Wilson, J. (2019). *Infection control in clinical practice* (3rd ed.). London: Elsevier.

CHAPTER 7

Patient Assessment and Preparation for Surgery

TRACEY LEE • KRISTEL ALKEN • SALLY SUTHERLAND-FRASER

EDITOR: SALLY SUTHERLAND-FRASER

LEARNING OUTCOMES

- Identify the functions of preoperative patient assessment and preparation for elective surgery
- Describe the pre-admission assessment processes, including patient selection, risk assessment, investigations and patient education
- Discuss the need for cultural safety during patient assessment and the use of interpreter services
- Identify the additional needs of special populations, including those at extremes of age and pregnant patients, as well as patients with conditions such as diabetes, obesity and a history of smoking
- Describe the patient's transfer to the perioperative department, including completion of the preoperative checklist and the patient's clinical handover in the preoperative holding room

KEY TERMS

cultural safety

interpreter services

patient education

pre-admission clinic

preoperative assessment

preoperative health questionnaire

preoperative (pre-op) holding area

recommendation for admission (RFA)

INTRODUCTION

This chapter explores the preoperative phase of the elective patient's perioperative journey, encompassing preoperative assessment and preparation for surgery. It discusses the important role of pre-admission clinics in the provision of preoperative assessment, which supports the process of patient selection and triage. The chapter also highlights the contribution of nurses in pre-admission clinics to the effectiveness of preoperative preparation and patient education.

This chapter acknowledges the increasing cultural diversity within the population and identifies the specialist knowledge and skills needed by perioperative nurses to provide culturally appropriate care during the preoperative period. Some elective surgical patients will present with common comorbidities such as diabetes, cardiac and vascular disease or cognitive impairment, while patients at extremes of age will require different assessments and preparation from the pregnant surgical patient or the patient presenting for emergency surgery. Other surgical patients may present with behaviours affecting their preoperative health, such as tobacco smoking or obesity.

The chapter outlines key features of the patient's admission to the healthcare facility and highlights the routine risk assessments required for elective patients. It describes the role of the preoperative ward nurse in preparation of the patient for transfer to the operating suite, as well as the clinical handover process performed in the preoperative holding area. The chapter concludes with an overview of the perioperative patient journey in ambulatory care settings such as a stand-alone day procedure unit (DPU).

Full-page examples of assessment pathways, screening tools and checklists have been sourced from healthcare facilities across Australia and New Zealand to exemplify the principles explored in the chapter. The reader is encouraged to refer to these examples at different stages throughout the chapter. The full-page examples appear at the end of the chapter (Figs 7.1 to 7.10.) while smaller figures appear within the chapter (Figs 7.8, 7.11 and 7.12).

PREOPERATIVE PATIENT CARE

Preoperative patient care aims to provide the unique holistic preparation of the patient's physical, psychological, emotional and spiritual needs prior to their surgery (He et al., 2018; Malley, Kenner, Kim, & Blakeney, 2015). The preoperative stage of the surgical journey is critical not only in the patient's preparation for surgery, but also prepares the family or carer and enables a process of planning for the patient's prompt and safe discharge (Agency for Clinical Innovation [ACI], 2018). For the patient undergoing an elective procedure, preoperative care encompasses the period of initial consultation with the surgeon or proceduralist (hereafter referred to collectively as the surgeon) followed by patient selection, assessment and investigation (Turunen, Miettinen, Setälä, & Vehviläinen-Julkunen, 2017). This preoperative stage may extend many weeks ahead of the scheduled admission date and may include a telephone interview with a preoperative nurse, or may require in-person attendance at a pre-admission clinic for more complex assessment and investigations by a perioperative team including nurses, anaesthetists, physiotherapists and dietitians.

The elective patient's preoperative preparation continues along a planned, standardised pathway through to the day of the surgery when they will be admitted to the preoperative area and prepared for surgery before being transferred to the preoperative holding area of the operating suite. Table 7.1 lists nine elements of perioperative care. These elements were identified by a multidisciplinary team which produced *The perioperative toolkit* (ACI, 2018). This resource describes the nine elements in detail and also contains model health questionnaires, preoperative assessment forms, pathways and checklists as well as resources to guide the development of patient information tools (ACI, 2018).

In practical terms, preoperative care starts when the patient and the surgeon discuss the patient's presenting problem. An example of a preoperative pathway is provided at the end of the chapter (see Fig. 7.1 from South Australia Health, 2019). The initial surgical consultation will explore the potential preoperative investigations that

TABLE 7.1 Elements of Perioperative Care	
1	The perioperative process prepares the patient, family and carer for the whole surgical/procedural journey
2	All patients require pre-admission review using a triage process
3	Preprocedure preparation optimises and supports management of the patient's perioperative risks associated with their planned surgery/procedure and anaesthesia
4	The multidisciplinary team collects, analyses, integrates and communicates information to optimise patient-centred care
5	Each patient's individual journey should follow a planned standardised perioperative pathway
6	Measurement for quality improvement, benchmarking and reporting should be embedded in the perioperative process
7	Integration with primary care optimises the patient's perioperative well-being
8	Partnering with patients, families and carers optimises shared decision making for the whole perioperative journey
9	Effective clinical and corporate governance underpins the perioperative process

(Source: Adapted from Agency for Clinical Innovation (ACI). (2018). The perioperative toolkit. GL2018_004. Anaesthesia Perioperative Care Network Surgical Services Taskforce.)

the patient may need to undergo, and the surgeon will propose a treatment plan. This process lays the foundations for an informed consent and, in many instances, the patient may be asked to sign the consent form at this early stage (Australian Commission on Safety and Quality in Health Care [ACSQHC/the Commission], 2020a).

As part of this consultation process, the surgeon will also identify the relevant clinical urgency category for the patient. These nationally agreed categories have been developed by the Royal Australasian College of Surgeons (RACS), the Royal Australian and New Zealand College of Ophthalmologists (RANZCO) and the Royal Australian and New Zealand College of Obstetricians and Gynaecologists (RANZCOG), and are:
- Category 1: procedures that are clinically indicated within 30 days
- Category 2: procedures that are clinically indicated within 90 days

- Category 3: procedures that are clinically indicated within 365 days (Australian Health Ministers' Advisory Council [AHMAC], 2015).

The surgeon will also discuss the patient's preference for admission to a public or private healthcare facility and will initiate any administrative processes such as a **recommendation for admission (RFA)**, sometimes known as a request for admission or an elective booking form.

DAY SURGERY

The practice of day surgery (or ambulatory surgery) has been evident in Australasia for several decades and, while it has grown continuously throughout this time, the pace of change has escalated. For example, 61% of hospitalisations in Australia for the year 2018–19 were for day surgery patients (Australian Institute of Health and Welfare [AIHW], 2020a). This figure represents an increase in presentations of almost 2% every year since 2014–15. Improvements in pharmacology as well as anaesthetic and surgical techniques have led to an increasing range of elective surgical procedures which may be performed safely in short-stay services, including stand-alone day only surgery (DOS) facilities or as a day of surgery admission (DOSA) (Bailey et al., 2019). Table 7.2 is a glossary of the more commonly used names and acronyms in this sector.

A shortened hospital stay is advantageous as it means reduced exposure to risks such as hospital-acquired infections and may also have a positive impact on the factors which can contribute to patient anxiety, such as the loss of control, a fear of pain, inadequate analgesia or surgical complications. There has been growth in the range of short-stay services in the healthcare sector extending beyond 12- to 23-hour wards to those providing stays of up to 72 hours.

Day surgery services may be provided in a range of settings including:

- units within a hospital setting but completely independent, with all services incorporated within an ambulatory care area
- units within a hospital setting but all perioperative services making use of the main theatre complex, whether day only, inpatient or DOSA patients
- a satellite unit where some services (e.g. sterilising) are carried out by another department, perhaps away from the main hospital campus.

The Australian Day Surgery Nurses Association (ADSNA) produces consensus guidelines to inform the practice of nurses working within day surgery settings (ADSNA, 2018). These guidelines may also be used to inform the development of local policies relating to patient selection and risk assessment for day surgery admission, as well as discharge planning and preoperative education and health promotion. Fig. 7.2 (see end of chapter) is an example of a clinical pathway for a day surgery patient.

TABLE 7.2
Glossary of Terms Used in Short-stay and Ambulatory Care Services

DOS	Day only surgery or ambulatory surgery	Planned surgery/procedures which allow patients to be admitted and discharged on the same day
DOSA	Day of surgery admission	Patients admitted on the same day as their surgery with an expected length of stay more than 23 hours
DPU	Day procedure unit or short-stay unit	A unit designed and staffed to provide complete care for DOS patients, sometimes as a stand-alone facility
EDO	Extended day only	Planned surgery/procedures requiring admission up to 23 hours
HVSSS	High-volume short-stay surgery	Planned surgery/procedures requiring admission up to 72 hours. It includes both day only surgery (DOS) and extended day only (EDO) surgery (23-hour surgery)
PAC	Pre-admission clinic	A multidisciplinary clinic where preoperative interviews, investigations and assessments can be conducted in the weeks prior to scheduled surgery/procedures
RFA	Recommendation for admission	A document used to initiate the admission of a patient to hospital. May also be called a request for admission or an elective booking form

(Sources: Agency for Clinical Innovation (ACI). (2012). High volume short stay surgical model toolkit. GL2012_001; ACI. (2018). The perioperative toolkit. GL2018_004. Anaesthesia Perioperative Care Network Surgical Services Taskforce; Australian and New Zealand College of Anaesthetists. (2018a). *PS15 Guidelines for the perioperative care of patients selected for day stay procedures*. Australian and New Zealand College of Anaesthetists and Faculty of Pain Medicine; State of Queensland (Queensland Health). (2014). *Statewide Anaesthesia and Perioperative Care Clinical Network (SWAPNET) guideline – 23 hour ward admission criteria*.)

PATIENT SELECTION AND ASSESSMENT FOR SURGERY

Patient selection processes determine whether the patient is a suitable candidate for a day surgery admission or will require overnight admission as an inpatient (ACI, 2018). This selection will be informed by the patient's clinical urgency category as well as the complexity of the intended surgery. It will also require evaluation of the patient's medical history and their social circumstances, which will be self-reported in a **preoperative health questionnaire**. Fig. 7.3 (see end of chapter) is an example of comprehensive health questionnaire for the preoperative screening of adult patients, and Fig. 7.4 (see end of chapter) is an example for paediatric patients (State of Queensland [Queensland Health], 2017).

Preoperative assessment is a collective term referring to the process of clinical investigation which provides data for the selection of an appropriate anaesthetic strategy (ANZCA, 2017). The ADSNA (2018) recognises preoperative assessment as a process which determines the patient's fitness and readiness for the impending admission, anaesthetic and surgical procedure. ACORN (2020a) sees further benefits in preoperative assessment and the opportunity it provides for the preoperative nurse to identify any gaps in the patient's knowledge, which will inform preoperative patient education.

Clear selection criteria, protocols and pathways guide the preoperative nurse's evaluation of preoperative health questionnaires and help identify which patients will require preoperative assessment and further investigation (Bailey et al., 2019). The preoperative nurse will also use this information to determine which patients are suitable candidates for telephone assessment and which patients will require in-person attendance at a pre-admission clinic. The preoperative health questionnaire will also identify the specific assessments and preparation needs of the patients. For example, a completed questionnaire will identify whether the patient needs an interpreter and, if so, for which language (see Fig. 7.3 and 7.4 at end of chapter). It will also identify whether the patient is in a special population such as Jehovah Witnesses, patients who may be pregnant, patients with diabetes or bleeding disorders, and patients with disabilities. For children, the health questionnaire will also identify in advance who will accompany the child to hospital and whether they are the legal guardian (see Fig. 7.4 (see end of chapter)).

Each of these patients will have differing needs and preoperative assessment can forecast any issues related to the patient's preoperative condition and medical history, biochemistry and current medications, which need to be addressed or altered before surgery can be safely scheduled (Joanna Briggs Institute, 2016a, 2016b). Clinicians can order appropriate tests and receive results during the preoperative period, which may reduce the likelihood of delays or cancellations in the patient's planned surgery, which, in turn, can increase patient well-being and improve patient satisfaction (Turunen et al., 2017, 2018).

There are many models and examples of preoperative assessment pathways, such as assessment conducted by telephone or requiring in-person attendance at a pre-admission clinic (Research boxes 7.1 and 7.2). The contribution of nurse-led telephone assessment can be seen in the preoperative pathway depicted in Fig. 7.1 (see end-of-chapter charts) (South Australia Health, 2019). The use of telephone assessments for low-risk patients is shown on the left side of the pathway. It also suggests that telephone assessment may be a useful triage tool for some moderate- to high-risk patients, shown on the right side of the pathway. Telephone assessment also plays an important role where distance is a problem because it can provide patients more promptly with information and access to services which may not be available locally.

Regardless of the patient's location or the patient's risk, preoperative assessment conducted by telephone requires patient consent and should be supported by a process of correct patient identification using approved patient identifiers, such as patient identity, site, procedure and consent (ACSQHC/the Commission, 2020a). A written summary of the telephone assessment should be included in the patient's health record so that it is available to other members of the perioperative team. Documentation and good lines of communication within the perioperative team ensure that the patient's preoperative requirements (including physical, cultural and psychological) and their specific education needs are identified and addressed in a timely manner (ACORN, 2020b). They also ensure that advanced bookings can be made for interpreter services, referrals can be made to other services (such as tobacco counselling, drug and alcohol services, dietitians, physiotherapists, etc.) and appointments scheduled at a pre-admission clinic for selected patients (ACORN, 2020a).

RESEARCH BOX 7.1
Evolving Models of Preoperative Assessment

The benefits of virtual models of preoperative care and telemedicine have been studied widely in recent decades. A retrospective review conducted by Mullen-Fortino and colleagues (2019) compared preoperative patients assessed by telemedicine ($n = 361$ patients) with those who attended pre-admission clinics ($n = 7442$ patients) on three telehealth outcome measures: access (time spent in evaluation), experience (patient satisfaction) and effectiveness (case cancellation rate). The study found improvements in all three telehealth quality measures, with telemedicine patients spending less time in evaluation (by 24 minutes), experiencing high levels of satisfaction and with no case cancellations reported during the study period. The authors concluded that the use of telemedicine for preoperative assessment was beneficial for patients and healthcare facilities (Mullen-Fortino et al., 2019).

Kamdar and colleagues (2020) conducted a descriptive study of preoperative anaesthesia assessment services of a large metropolitan medical centre in the US. The evaluated services were provided by a multidisciplinary team including surgeons and anaesthetists as well as nurse navigators, nurse practitioners and nurse anaesthetists. The study evaluated aspects of virtual assessment by telemedicine ($n = 419$ patients) and assessment by in-person presentation at a preoperative clinic ($n = 1785$ patients) over a 2-year period. The authors concluded that telemedicine assessments were associated with higher levels of patient satisfaction and lower rates of cancellation, and reduced the burden of time and costs both for patients and services (Kamdar et al., 2020).

One of the unexpected outcomes of the COVID-19 global pandemic was an increased uptake of telemedicine for preoperative assessment (Mihalj et al., 2020). Given the positive outcomes described above, it seems likely that such virtual models of care will continue to evolve.

RESEARCH BOX 7.2
Nurse-led Preoperative Assessment for Elective Surgery

Hines and colleagues' (2015) systematic review of the effectiveness of nurse-led preoperative assessment services reported on a total of 23 studies published since their earlier review in 2009. A number of outcome measures from the randomised controlled trials and before–after studies were selected, including patient no-shows on the day of surgery, cancellations, length of stay, adverse events, participant satisfaction and patient anxiety. Earlier reviews on similar practices by other authors have found little evidence to assess the effectiveness of a nurse-led service on similar outcome measures (Nicholson, Coldwell, Lewis, & Smith, 2013). Although Hines and colleagues (2015) found little evidence of a positive effect on some of these measures

(rates of surgical patient adverse events, morbidity and mortality), the authors did find a positive effect from nurse-led preadmission services on the following outcome measures, although the evidence was low level:

- Nurse-led pre-admission services may reduce the frequency of procedural cancellations, patient no-shows on the day of surgery and patient anxiety.
- Nurse-led pre-admission services may also improve patient preparation, and increase recognition of patients' postoperative needs and levels of patient satisfaction with the surgical process (Hines et al., 2015).

PATIENT SCENARIOS

Four patient scenarios and a brief description of the healthcare setting are provided at the front of the book for readers to review when answering the questions in these unfolding scenarios:

1. Mr James Collins is a 78-year-old man scheduled for a right total knee replacement – TKR.
2. Mrs Patricia Peterson is a 42-year-old Indigenous woman who requires an emergency laparoscopic cholecystectomy – lap chole.
3. Mrs Janine Clark is a 35-year-old woman scheduled for an elective lower segment caesarean section – LSCS.
4. Master Thanh Nguyen is a 3-year-old boy admitted as a day surgery patient for a left orchidopexy.

SCENARIO 7.1

Notice some of the differences in our four patients, in terms of their age, medical history and comorbidities, which may influence their selection and subsequent surgical care pathway.

Critical Thinking Questions

- Referring to Fig 7.2 at the end of the chapter, select one of our four patients who may be suitable for the Day Surgery Clinical Pathway.
- Referring to Figs 7.3 and 7.4 at the end of the chapter, select all patients who may be suitable for pre-procedure screening.
- Provide reasons to explain all of your selections.

INTERPRETER SERVICES

Healthcare facilities will need access to interpreter services for patients from non-English-speaking backgrounds and those with a significant hearing disability. **Interpreter services** include multi-language translation and sign-language interpretation, which ensure all patients have equitable access to information and social support in a method that works for their needs (NSW Ministry of Health, 2017a).

Each facility will have its own means of accessing interpreter services, with government departments commonly providing a wide range of public sector services including telephone- and video-supported translation and interpreter services for many language groups. For example, the services provided in Queensland include interpreter cards and graphic posters for waiting rooms translated into Mandarin and Cantonese, as well as Vietnamese, Korean, Japanese, Italian and Arabic (State of Queensland, Queensland Government, 2020). Interpreter services in New Zealand provide services for English and Te Reo Māori, as well as Samoan and Hindi (Health Navigator, 2019), reflecting the major language groups of the population.

Once the need for an interpreter has been confirmed during preoperative screening, for example, an alert should be entered in the patient's medical record. This should specify the patient's preferred language and dialect if relevant. Interpreter services are highly specialised and often in high demand, so advanced bookings are recommended and should be confirmed (NSW Ministry of Health, 2017a). It is also important to be aware of the distinction between the informal bilingual communication that staff may find helpful when they are providing direct patient care and the authorised, formal role provided by healthcare interpreter services when essential medical information must be communicated (NSW Ministry of Health, 2017a).

In the context of preoperative patient assessment and preparation for surgery, the most likely time that interpreter services will be needed is during discussions about the surgical patient's consent for treatment. This includes access to interpreter services initially when gaining consent and once again when the patient is admitted on the day of surgery. The presence of a health interpreter with the required language translation skills is important not only for identification of the patient but also for verification of the consent and reassurance for the patient that their wishes have been understood. This may include the presence of an interpreter in the admissions area as well as the preoperative holding area of the operating suite. Chapter 3 provides more detail on the medico-legal aspects of the consent processes.

PRE-ADMISSION CLINICS

The increasing use of the **pre-admission clinic** (PAC) has provided the opportunity to identify and manage patient comorbidities in advance of their admission date for surgery. Such clinics have played an important role in changing models of care towards shorter lengths of stay in hospital and the growth of ambulatory surgery, DPUs and DOSAs. These and other common terms used to describe these models of care are listed in Table 7.2.

Assessment involves a two-way pre-admission interview between the patient and the health practitioner so that the patient is assessed physically, psychologically and socially for surgery (Turunen et al., 2017). The consultation needs to occur at an appropriate time and place. Ideally, the patient should attend the pre-admission clinic several weeks before surgery. This is particularly important if there are significant comorbidities requiring management, special laboratory tests or procedures to be ordered, or planning/management of any anaesthetic concerns required, and to allow time for patient education (ACORN, 2020a; Turunen et al., 2017). Preoperative assessment at a pre-admission clinic has a clear advantage over telephone assessment: as a face-to-face meeting between the nurse and the patient (and parent or carer), it provides the additional opportunity for observation and physical assessments, which may not be possible over the telephone. It also facilitates a range of preoperative diagnostic tests, which can enable staff to provide perioperative care that has been tailored to individual patient needs. Patient assessment at a pre-admission clinic also enables more DOSA (see Table 7.2) patients to arrive on their day of surgery even for complex surgical procedures (Nelson et al., 2016).

Patient preparation in the weeks leading up to hospital admission is just as important for the healthcare service, improving the overall efficiency and theatre utilisation (Leite, Hobgood, Hill, & Muckler, 2019). Efficiency is also improved with the use of protocol-driven guidelines which standardise the processes for pre-admission and assessment and reduces the number of unnecessary preoperative tests (Bailey et al., 2019). A number of different healthcare professionals may be involved in the care and preparation of the patient prior to surgery; for example, the pre-admission nurse, dietitian, physiotherapist, pharmacist, social worker and occupational therapist, as well as the anaesthetist.

Anaesthesia Assessment

Anaesthetic evaluation is particularly important in patients identified as having previous or family problems with anaesthesia and includes patients who have a known (or possible) difficult airway, a history of malignant hyperthermia, a history of postoperative nausea and vomiting (PONV), obstructive sleep apnoea or drug/egg allergies. Recommendations provided by ANZCA (2017) on the preanaesthesia consultation indicate that all patients must be seen by an anaesthetist prior to anaesthesia and surgery to ensure that they are in an optimal state of health and to facilitate the planning of anaesthesia along with appropriate discussion and consent for the anaesthesia and related procedures.

The American Society of Anesthesiologists (ASA) classification is presented in Table 7.3. This is an internationally recognised system to classify the patient's health prior to surgery by a general assessment of illness severity (ASA, 2019). The patient's ASA score is used with other assessment information to triage patients and select the best pathway for their surgery (ACI, 2018). Box 7.1 outlines the conditions that determine the suitability of patients for ambulatory care procedures. The

TABLE 7.3
ASA Physical Status Classification System

ASA PS Classification	Definition	Adult Examples, Including, but not Limited to:	Pediatric Examples, Including but not Limited to:	Obstetric Examples, Including but not Limited to:
ASA I	A normal healthy patient	Healthy, non-smoking, no or minimal alcohol use	Healthy (no acute or chronic disease), normal BMI percentile for age	
ASA II	A patient with mild systemic disease	Mild diseases only without substantive functional limitations. Current smoker, social alcohol drinker, pregnancy, obesity (30<BMI<40), well-controlled DM/HTN, mild lung disease	Asymptomatic congenital cardiac disease, well controlled dysrhythmias, asthma without exacerbation, well controlled epilepsy, non-insulin dependent diabetes mellitus, abnormal BMI percentile for age, mild/moderate OSA, oncologic state in remission, autism with mild limitations	Normal pregnancy*, well controlled gestational HTN, controlled preeclampsia without severe features, diet-controlled gestational DM.
ASA III	A patient with severe systemic disease	Substantive functional limitations; One or more moderate to severe diseases. Poorly controlled DM or HTN, COPD, morbid obesity (BMI ≥40), active hepatitis, alcohol dependence or abuse, implanted pacemaker, moderate reduction of ejection fraction, ESRD undergoing regularly scheduled dialysis, history (>3 months) of MI, CVA, TIA, or CAD/stents.	Uncorrected stable congenital cardiac abnormality, asthma with exacerbation, poorly controlled epilepsy, insulin dependent diabetes mellitus, morbid obesity, malnutrition, severe OSA, oncologic state, renal failure, muscular dystrophy, cystic fibrosis, history of organ transplantation, brain/spinal cord malformation, symptomatic hydrocephalus, premature infant PCA <60 weeks, autism with severe limitations, metabolic disease, difficult airway, long term parenteral nutrition. Full term infants <6 weeks of age.	Preeclampsia with severe features, gestational DM with complications or high insulin requirements, a thrombophilic disease requiring anticoagulation.

Continued

TABLE 7.3
ASA Physical Status Classification System—cont'd

ASA PS Classification	Definition	Adult Examples, Including, but not Limited to:	Pediatric Examples, Including but not Limited to:	Obstetric Examples, Including but not Limited to:
ASA IV	A patient with severe systemic disease that is a constant threat to life	Recent (<3 months) MI, CVA, TIA or CAD/stents, ongoing cardiac ischemia or severe valve dysfunction, severe reduction of ejection fraction, shock, sepsis, DIC, ARD or ESRD not undergoing regularly scheduled dialysis	Symptomatic congenital cardiac abnormality, congestive heart failure, active sequelae of prematurity, acute hypoxic-ischemic encephalopathy, shock, sepsis, disseminated intravascular coagulation, automatic implantable cardioverter-defibrillator, ventilator dependence, endocrinopathy, severe trauma, severe respiratory distress, advanced oncologic state.	Preeclampsia with severe features complicated by HELLP or other adverse event, peripartum cardiomyopathy with EF <40, uncorrected/decompensated heart disease, acquired or congenital.
ASA V	A moribund patient who is not expected to survive without the operation	Ruptured abdominal/thoracic aneurysm, massive trauma, intracranial bleed with mass effect, ischemic bowel in the face of significant cardiac pathology or multiple organ/system dysfunction	Massive trauma, intracranial hemorrhage with mass effect, patient requiring ECMO, respiratory failure or arrest, malignant hypertension, decompensated congestive heart failure, hepatic encephalopathy, ischemic bowel or multiple organ/system dysfunction.	Uterine rupture.
ASA VI	A declared brain-dead patient whose organs are being removed for donor purposes			

ARD = acid reflux disease; BMI = body mass index; CAD = coronary artery disease; CVA = cerebrovascular accident; DIC = disseminated intravascular coagulation; DM = diabetes mellitus; ESRD = end-stage renal disease; HTN = hypertension; MI = myocardial infarction; PCA = post conceptual age; TIA = transient ischaemic attack.
*Although pregnancy is not a disease, the parturient's physiologic state is significantly altered from when the woman is not pregnant, hence the assignment of ASA 2 for a woman with uncomplicated pregnancy.**The addition of "E" denotes Emergency surgery: (An emergency is defined as existing when delay in treatment of the patient would lead to a significant increase in the threat to life or body part)
(Source: American Society of Anesthesiologists, 2019. ASA Physical Status Classification System.)

final decision is made by the anaesthetist (ANZCA, 2017, 2018a) and, at a minimum, will be based on the following information
• *Medical history* includes details of past surgical history, family medical history and current intake of medication. Many patients have comorbidities such as cardiac disease, liver disease, pulmonary disease, hypertension, type 2 diabetes (T2D) or latex allergy, thus requiring complex medication regimens – for example, patients with insulin-dependent type 1 diabetes (T1D) and

taking anticoagulants. In these cases, a specific clinical pathway should be initiated, indicating the necessary preoperative tests and patient management throughout the surgical experience. Those patients with an artificial heart valve or other prosthesis may also require prophylactic antibiotic therapy. New guidelines suggest many patients undergoing joint replacement surgery no longer require antibiotic prophylaxis, and associated risk factors should be identified instead (DeFroda, Lamin, Gil, Sindhu, & Ritterman, 2016).

BOX 7.1
Conditions that Determine the Suitability of Patients for Ambulatory Care Procedures

The procedure/surgery to be performed should:
- have a minimal risk of postoperative haemorrhage
- have a minimal risk of postoperative airway compromise
- be amenable to postoperative pain controllable by outpatient management techniques
- permit postoperative care to be managed by the patient and/or a responsible adult and any special postoperative nursing requirements met by day surgery, home or district nursing facilities
- be associated with a rapid return to normal fluid and food intake
- be scheduled, taking into account the anticipated recovery period. Where a prolonged recovery is anticipated, the procedure should be scheduled first on the list or as close to first as feasible.

(Source: Adapted from Australian and New Zealand College of Anaesthetists, 2018. *PS15 Guidelines for the perioperative care of patients selected for day stay procedures*.)

- *The patient's current medications* should be identified. Some prescribed medications have potential interactions with drugs used throughout the surgical procedure (Dagli, Kocaoglu, Bayir, Hakki, & Doylan, 2016). Herbal and complementary medicines can cause adverse effects in patients undergoing anaesthesia and surgery. There is the potential for drug interactions, and the side effects of herbal medicines can result in unanticipated perioperative anaesthetic or surgical problems. The anaesthetist will use this history to advise which medications the patient needs to take the day before and on the day of their surgery, as well as which medications should be ceased (see more in 'Preoperative instructions' below).

Fig. 7.5 (see end of chapter) is an example of a checklist used during anaesthetic assessment. It provides a record of the following factors:
- ASA status
- airway with Mallampati diagram
- anaesthetic discussed
- pain relief discussed
- anaesthetic history
- drug allergies.

The following body systems may also require assessment:

- respiratory
- circulatory
- endocrine
- gastrointestinal tract (GIT)
- hepatic/renal
- central nervous system (CNS).

The preanaesthetic assessment may also identify confused older patients with potential to develop postoperative delirium. This should inform the anaesthetic plan and trigger referral to other services prior to the patient's admission to hospital (ACI, 2019; Guenther, Riedel, & Radtke, 2016).

Nursing Assessment

Nurse-led pre-admission clinics have been found to be effective in preoperative patient screening, reducing inappropriate admission of unfit patients and reducing late cancellations (He et al., 2018; Hines et al., 2015). While the nurse's role in the pre-admission clinic may vary between healthcare agencies, the central responsibility should be to ensure that patients are prepared effectively for their intended surgery (ACORN, 2020a). Commonly, the pre-admission nurse would record baseline information about the patient, using a standardised pre-admission checklist (similar to Fig. 7.6, at end of chapter):

- *Demographic details* should be recorded, including confirming the patient's name, home address and other relevant details.
- *The patient's age* should be confirmed, as some healthcare facilities may have upper and/or lower age limits for admission.
- *Baseline vital signs* should be recorded, including the patient's height and weight; their body mass index (BMI) should also be calculated in the preoperative period. The information will be used for comparison throughout the patient's admission, so it is important to record these details in the patient's medical record on a pre-admission chart.
- *Hygiene, elimination and nutrition* may also be part of the pre-admission assessment. These factors may further inform assessment of the patient's skin condition or indicate additional risk factors for pressure injury. The nurse may also identify the need for referral to a dietitian in the lead-up to surgery.
- *Social history* is an important body of information for the perioperative journey. Preoperative assessment allows time for appropriate referral to other services and planning. For example, the patients may have special needs, such as the presence of a carer or significant other during the perioperative

period. Supporting patients' unique needs protects their dignity and allows them to maintain control over what is happening to them. Patients who are scheduled for day surgery and who are unable to make satisfactory arrangements for travel, or who do not have a responsible carer to take them home and provide care postoperatively, may be deemed unsuitable for day surgery. Alternative arrangements must also be considered when a patient is the sole carer of another person – for example, those patients with a spouse who has dementia. It is important that these patients are given additional assistance to enable them to attend hospital and then be supported while resuming their own role once they return home.

- *Risk assessment* for pressure injury (PI) and venous thromboembolism (VTE) will be required for all surgical patients (discussed in the following section). Additional screening and assessment will depend on the individual patient and may need to comply with national safety and quality standards. For example, preventing falls or delirium and managing cognitive impairment and delirium may be indicated for older surgical patients (Eamer et al., 2018) (discussed in a later section). There is also a requirement to screen patients for nutrition and hydration, aggression and violence (ACI, 2019; ACSQHC/the Commission, 2020b).

If any of these preoperative nursing assessments are not conducted preoperatively, they should be completed during the nursing admission processes on the patient's day of surgery. Fig. 7.3 (see end of the chapter) includes a section titled 'Planning for your care' where these potential risk factors are recorded.

Risk Assessments

Risk assessments may be mandated by local facility policy, state-based initiatives and safety and quality programs such as the national standards (ACSQHC/the Commission, 2017a, 2020b). The local facility policy should identify which tools are approved for local use (these should be validated assessment tools) and should specify the points of care, the required frequency of patient assessment, documentation and reporting requirements. Chapter 4 contains more information about the role of risk assessment and governance. Chapters 8–12 describe the specific nursing activities of the perioperative patient's journey that are designed to manage any risks of harm that may be identified during preoperative patient assessment and preparation.

Pressure injury

A number of PI risk assessment tools are used in Australasia, including the Norton Scale, Braden Scale and Waterlow Score, and these provide validated and reliable PI risk scores for adult patients. Other tools have been developed for patients with specific risk – for example, paediatric patients and patients with spinal cord injuries. These tools assess multiple risk factors considered as either intrinsic or extrinsic.

Risk assessment prior to admission facilitates the earliest possible identification of alterations in the patient's skin and also provides an opportunity for the preoperative nurse to plan and instigate preventative measures in a timely and efficient manner. Such measures may include access to lifting and patient transfer devices as well as PI support surfaces and mattresses on the operating table or postoperative ward, which may need to be ordered in advance from a supplier. Just as baseline vital signs are important for later comparison and indications of changes in the patient's condition, so too preoperative PI risk assessment ensures that pre-existing injuries are not misidentified later as hospital-acquired injuries. A further benefit is that patients can receive wound care advice and preoperative treatment.

The patient's PI score and preoperative nurse's recommendations for any preventative care should be included in the pre-admission history and in all subsequent clinical handovers of the patient's care during the perioperative journey (ACSQHC/the Commission, 2020c). Chapter 9 contains information on the intra-operative nursing considerations for prevention and management of PI.

Venous thromboembolism (VTE)

Adult surgical patients may be at risk of forming a life-threatening clot and/or bleeding and must be assessed for their risk as close as possible to the date of admission (ACSQHC/the Commission, 2018; Tran et al., 2019). It is important that the VTE risk assessment tool accurately identifies patients at risk (Figure 9.22 in Chapter 9 is an example of a VTE risk assessment tool) and enables the assessor to allocate the patient into a VTE risk category. This category will depend on the patient's risk factors including:

- age >60 years
- obesity (BMI >30 kg/m^2)
- moderate to major surgery (i.e. operating time >45 minutes and/or involves abdomen)
- prior history of VTE (NSW Health Clinical Excellence Commission [NSW CEC], 2018).

The results of the risk assessment will be used to inform the patient's VTE prevention strategies. These strategies may need to be implemented before the patient's admission or they may be required only from the admission day. For example, the patient may be measured for graduated compression stockings (GCSs) and instructed to wear these prior to their admission, while mechanical devices may not be recommended for use until the patient has been admitted to hospital (see later section). Chapter 9 contains information about the VTE preventative measures which are important during the intraoperative period.

PATIENT SCENARIOS

SCENARIO 7.2: FACTORS AFFECTING SELECTION FOR SURGERY – SOCIAL AND CULTURAL CONSIDERATIONS

Sometimes, patients present to the pre-admission clinic with social issues that may need to be resolved before the day of surgery. Mr James Collins arrives at his pre-admission clinic appointment with his daughter, Rebecca. He lives alone, but Rebecca says she will be staying with her father during his immediate recovery until he becomes more mobile.

Not all patients will have a support person at home and, for those patients, the preoperative nurse may need to consider the need for referral to appropriate social services. Fig. 7.3 (see end of the chapter) includes a section titled 'Planning for your care' where these social considerations are recorded.

Another common issue that the preoperative nurse will need to consider is communication, with many different language groups requiring the support of an interpreter service.

Critical Thinking Questions

- Does your facility have access to interpreter services? If so, what languages are included and does access include a telephone service?
- Explain why the interpreter service should be used during the admissions process instead of asking a family member to translate.

Preoperative Investigations

Not all of the preoperative information can be collected during nursing and anaesthetic assessments. Some patients may require further preoperative investigations in the preoperative period. Evidence-based guidelines now rationalise the use of preoperative investigations and pathology tests, reducing the volume of investigations ordered without compromising patient safety and reducing costs for both patients and healthcare systems (O'Neill, Carter, Pink, & Smith, 2016). Although some authors suggest that routine testing can be eliminated completely (Rusk, 2016), others propose that testing should be based on the patient's medical condition or comorbidities (Bock, Fritsch, & Hepner, 2016).

Blood investigations that may be required preoperatively include the following:

- Routine blood testing (including a full blood count [FBC], urea, electrolytes and glucose) should be undertaken for patients with severe systemic disease undergoing major surgery only (Martin & Cifu, 2017). For these patients, a blood group test and screen will also be required to ensure the availability of blood should a transfusion be required. Informed consent should be obtained prior to a surgical procedure for patients who may require a blood transfusion (NSW Ministry of Health, 2020).

- Investigation of the patient's international normalised ratio (INR) (clotting time) should be carried out for all patients on anticoagulant therapy.
- Patients with unstable diabetes may need a glycated haemoglobin (HbA_{1c}) test to determine their average blood glucose level (BGL) before admission. In stable patients with diabetes, HbA_{1c} may also be required if this has not been tested in the past 6 months.

Other patient groups who may require specific perioperative investigations are listed briefly below (O'Neill et al., 2016; State of Queensland, Queensland Health, 2018):

- Patients with cardiopulmonary conditions may require a chest X-ray and a resting electro-cardiograph (ECG).
- Patients with kidney disease or signs of infection may need kidney function tests (estimated glomerular filtration rate, electrolytes, creatinine and sometimes urea levels) and urine tests.
- Patient groups including overweight and obese patients with obstructed airways and sleep apnoea may benefit from polysomnography sleep studies.
- Patients undergoing thoracic or respiratory surgery may be candidates for lung function tests (spirometry, including peak expiratory flow rate, forced vital capacity and forced expiratory volume).

- Women of child-bearing age who are uncertain whether they may be pregnant should have a pregnancy test. If any doubt exists, the woman should be offered a pregnancy test on the day of surgery. This is particularly important in high-risk surgeries which may risk the viability of the fetus or if a pregnancy result is likely to affect the plan of care for the patient (Bock et al., 2016). The woman must give consent to be tested (NSW Ministry of Health, 2020).

As many of these investigations will have been conducted prior to admission, it is important to remind the patient to bring any test results with them on their admission day to ensure the results can be reviewed prior to anaesthesia and surgery.

ADDITIONAL CONSIDERATIONS FOR PATIENT ASSESSMENT AND PREPARATION

In addition to these routine preoperative investigations and assessments, it may be necessary to consider the needs of patients from special populations such as:
- culturally and linguistically diverse (CALD) patients
- paediatric patients
- older patients
- pregnant patients
- patients with diabetes.

Other considerations relate to the health behaviours and risk factors for some patients, such as the intake of tobacco smoking, as well as overweight and obesity. These considerations are explored in the following sections.

Special Populations
Culturally and linguistically diverse (CALD) patients

Australian and New Zealand populations are becoming increasingly multicultural and linguistically diverse (Waitemata District Health Board [WDHB], 2018a). The different needs of CALD patients have been known for some time (Crawford, Candlin, & Roger, 2017). It is important for healthcare facilities to provide support and resources for their workforce to develop **cultural safety** and facilitate the delivery of culturally safe and appropriate care to CALD patients (WDHB, 2018a; 2018b), as well as Indigenous peoples and their families (AHMAC, 2016).

Perioperative nurses must have the knowledge and skills to practise effectively in multicultural teams; furthermore, they have a duty of care to provide culturally safe and appropriate care to their patients (ACORN, 2020c; Nursing and Midwifery Board of Australia [NMBA], 2018). It is important for perioperative nurses not only to be aware of the cultural and linguistic

---

BOX 7.2
Release of Human Tissue

Although not commonplace in Australia, it is routine in New Zealand that, in every case where hair, specimen or tissue is removed, patients are offered the opportunity to have this returned to them on completion of the histology or other required testing. In Māori culture, body parts are revered; if a Māori patient's body part is to be removed, the nurse needs to establish whether the patient requires it to be disposed of according to practice or returned to them (New Zealand Health and Disability Commissioner, 2020). Patient information resources should be provided to patients and families outlining the public health and safety risks and how these must be managed, especially during transportation of such tissues, and when returned tissues have been preserved in formalin (Canterbury District Health Board [CDHB], 2016).

Furthermore, written consent is routinely required before such tissues can be authorised for release back to the patient or the next of kin (Department of Health, Government of Western Australia, 2020). This should be included in clinical handover and may also be recorded on the preoperative checklist (see Figure 7.10 at end of chapter). In the case of emergency surgery where no wishes have been noted, any body part/tissue removed may need to be retained for subsequent return to the patient (CDHB, 2016).

Patients may also consent to the removed tissue being used for other purposes such as bone banking and research (Australian Tissue Donation Network, 2019). This requires a separate consent and needs to comply with the Australian Human Tissue Act 1983. For example, patients who are undergoing total hip replacement may be asked whether they consent to donate their femoral head for bone banking. In 2018, over 10,000 Australians benefited from eye and tissue donation (Organ and Tissue Authority, 2019).

---

needs of their patients, but they must also be able to demonstrate this awareness so that their patients feel that their beliefs and culture are valued and recognised. The range of beliefs for patients from CALD backgrounds may include specific dietary requirements, as well as different beliefs about blood products, medical interventions, return of body parts (Box 7.2) and care of the body after death (ACORN, 2020d; Swihart, Yarrarapu, & Martin, 2020).

The pre-admission nurse should consider whether the care that can be provided to patients during their perioperative journey is appropriate to their beliefs. The nurse may need to modify the patient's care plan to reflect the needs of a CALD patient. For example, women of certain cultures, such as Muslim women, may have a preference to be cared for by female nurses only. In some cultures, the head area of the body is deemed sacred and must not be touched. Sharing such cultural information with other members of the preoperative team can assist them to make to adjustments to assessment processes, where required.

Health services for Aboriginal and Torres Strait Islander peoples must also be accessible and culturally appropriate (AHMAC, 2016). Coordinated, culturally appropriate services across the health system will improve the patient journey and health outcomes for Indigenous populations. Aboriginal and Torres Strait Islander people are fearful of the dislocation from family and Country when accessing health services, particularly for treatment as inpatients (Commonwealth of Australia, Department of Health, 2017). Health professionals need to practise with cultural respect and have cultural competency to be more effective in their care of Indigenous people, and an increasing range of education initiatives is available to support health professionals to do so. Cultural safety is discussed in more detail in Chapter 1.

Paediatric patients

Collectively, paediatric patients may include the following age ranges (ANZCA, 2019; NSW Ministry of Health, 2010):

- neonate: 1–28 days
- infant: 1–12 months
- toddler: 1–3 years
- child: 4–11 years
- adolescent: 12–19 years.

Preparation and assessment of the paediatric patient must be tailored to the relevant age and will need to include the parent, a member of the child's family or a carer in most instances (referred to simply as parent and child) (Sydney Children's Hospitals Network [SCHN], 2018a). Parents who are calm and supportive with their child when presenting at a healthcare facility may be able to allay the child's fears and assist with physical examinations, history taking and measurement of baseline observations. Medical play is a strategy that may help the child relax as they become familiar with healthcare equipment in their own time before the actual day of surgery. Research suggests that medical play in a non-threatening environment provides an opportunity for the child to express any emotions and fear related to their contact with healthcare professionals (SCHN, 2019) (see also

> ### RESEARCH BOX 7.3
> ### Paediatric Patient Education
>
> For preoperative education to be effective for the paediatric surgical patient, it must first be age appropriate.
>
> Research has been undertaken to evaluate whether preoperative anaesthetic education delivered to children on the day of surgery reduces anxiety behaviour during induction of anaesthesia. The results showed that, for children 6 years and older, preoperative education delivered up to a week prior to surgery reduced anxiety during induction of anaesthesia, while anxiety was not reduced in children under 6 years and, in fact, increased in children less than 3 years old (Kassai et al., 2016). In this younger age group, interventions such as riding to the operating theatre in a toy car have been found to reduce anxiety on day of surgery (Liu et al., 2018). Educational programs for children that have been effective in reducing preoperative anxiety include play therapy, interactive books and videos, and orientation tours. Multimedia with interactive and educational elements is one effective method of providing age-related education (Dai & Livesley, 2018; Stålberg, Sandberg, Coyne, Larsson, & Söderbäck, 2019). Medical play is another approach to education which allows the paediatric surgical patient to express any emotions and fear related to their contact with healthcare professionals (SCHN, 2019).

Research box 7.3). Preoperative education in all its forms should be central in the planning for the admission of the child and may also serve to inform the parent and allay their fears.

Being able to keep a favourite toy with them is another strategy that can allay the child's fears; so too is the parent's presence for as long as possible on the perioperative journey. It may be possible for one parent to be present at the induction of their child's anaesthetic. No guarantees should be made in advance, however, as the child's clinical care and safety are the priorities at all times. The anaesthetic team will make the final decision about this on the day of surgery; however, the option can be part of the preoperative assessment and discussion (SCHN, 2018a).

Irrespective of their age, paediatric surgical patients can cause stress for their parents and other family members. The stress burden is often worsened by the realisation that the parent will be responsible for the child's care postoperatively. Thus, it is extremely important that the child's parents are well prepared and understand their role throughout the perioperative experience.

PATIENT SCENARIOS

SCENARIO 7.3: PAEDIATRIC PATIENT

Master Thanh Nguyen has arrived from the admissions area with his parents. Thanh is looking around a lot and is holding tightly onto his mother. Mrs Nguyen is very nervous and has been crying. Her husband explains to EN Marcus Macedo that his wife does not speak English and that she had a very bad experience in hospital herself as a child when she had her tonsils removed.

Critical Thinking Questions

- What actions could EN Macedo take to provide comfort and assurance to Thanh and his parents while they are in the waiting area?
- Only one of Thanh's parents will be able to come with him into the anaesthetic room when the team is ready. Which of Thanh's parents would you anticipate accompanying him into the anaesthetic room? Include your rationales and consider how this decision is made in your facility.

Older patients

The perioperative nurse must also be skilled in the assessment of older persons being admitted for surgery. Preoperative planning should also include the older patient's family, whenever possible, to ensure the surgical treatment and postoperative goals are realistic (Kim, Brooks, & Groban, 2015).

The AIHW (2020b) classifies older persons as those aged 65 years and older. Indigenous Australians, by contrast, are considered to be older persons when aged 50 years and older, because of their nationally higher mortality rates and lower life expectancy (AIHW, 2020c). In 2016–17, older persons accounted for more than 40% of hospitalisations in Australia, including same-day admissions and overnight stays. Of this group, nearly a quarter of patients were aged 85 years or older (AIHW, 2020b). The older person is likely to experience many changes in their preoperative health, which may be triggered by the normal age-related decline in the body's metabolic processes. These changes include:

- decreased muscle strength and aerobic capacity
- decreased bone density and joint flexibility
- vasomotor instability
- skin thinning and loss of elasticity
- changes in nutritional requirements and loss of appetite
- changes in bladder and bowel function
- decreased glucose tolerance
- reduction in sensory perception
- memory loss and reduced cognitive awareness
- changes in mental health and well-being
- altered sexual functioning (State of Victoria, 2020).

When caring for the older person as a surgical patient, it is important to recognise these normal changes and their potential association with postoperative complications and negative effect on the patient's capacity to recover (Mistry, Gaunay, & Hoenig, 2017).

Cognition and delirium screening. Cognitive impairment should be considered in older patients such as Mr Collins undergoing elective orthopaedic procedures, as it may lead to an extended length of stay due to postoperative delirium (Culley et al., 2017; Daiello et al., 2019). Delirium is an acute change in mental status that is common among older patients in hospital. Each year, patients in Australian public hospitals experience more than 22,700 recognised episodes of delirium. It is a serious condition associated with increased mortality and significant morbidity that may precipitate long-term cognitive decline and premature entry to residential care (ACSQHC/the Commission, 2016). Key risk factors for postoperative delirium in the older patients include:

- pre-existing cognitive impairment and/or dementia
- age ≥65 years (≥45 years for Aboriginal and Torres Strait Islander peoples)
- severe medical illness
- hip fracture.

Falls screening. Hearing loss and a decline in visual acuity and mobility are common conditions which increase the older patient's risk of falls. All patients should be screened for the risk of falls and harm from falls, with older patient populations at higher risk while in hospital (ACSQHC/the Commission, 2017a). Falls risk is associated with the following patient characteristics and health conditions:

- aged ≥65 years
- vision impairments including cataracts and disorders of the retina
- postural hypotension, syncope and balance disorders
- recent history of falls.

Pregnant patients

Many factors need to be considered during the assessment of the pregnant patient presenting for surgery. This is not only because of the presence of the fetus and gestational age, but also because of the physiological changes in the woman during her pregnancy. The woman may be admitted for obstetric surgery related to the pregnancy itself (such as cerclage of the cervix, ovarian cysts and lower segment caesarean section [LSCS]) or she may need non-obstetric surgery which is unrelated to her pregnancy. Examples of non-obstetric surgery include:

- diagnostic procedures
- abdominal surgery for appendicitis, cholecystitis, etc.
- orthopaedic surgery for laceration, tendon repair and bone fractures, etc. (Rasmussen, Christiansen, Uldbjerg, & Nørgaard, 2019).

The incidence of non-obstetric surgery during pregnancy is low, reportedly between 1% and 2% (Vujic et al., 2019; Yu et al., 2018). However, some maternal characteristics are associated with a higher prevalence of surgery performed during pregnancy, such as increasing age and higher BMI. Smoking and multiple pregnancies are two other maternal characteristics found to be more prevalent in the pregnant surgical patient (Rasmussen et al., 2019).

The pregnant surgical patient may be considered 'two patients in one' (Webb et al., 2018). During preoperative consultations, the surgeon and the anaesthetist should inform the woman of the potential risks to herself and her fetus. Anaesthetic assessment should consider the woman's weight and access to her airway (which may be difficult depending on the stage of pregnancy), has well as her cardiovascular health and lower back mobility, particularly if neuraxial anaesthesia is a possibility (Webb et al., 2018). The potential for hypertension needs to be assessed, as well as insulin resistance and development of gestational diabetes, coagulation issues and thromboembolism (Rasmussen et al., 2019; Upadya & Saneesh, 2016). Thus, preoperative screening for VTE is essential, while both mechanical and pharmacological VTE prophylaxis are recommended preventative practices throughout the perioperative period (American College of Obstetricians and Gynecologists [ACOG] (2019).

PATIENT SCENARIOS

SCENARIO 7.4: PLANNING FOR SOCIAL AND CULTURAL CONSIDERATIONS

Mrs Janine Clark is a 35-year-old woman scheduled for an elective lower segment caesarean section (LSCS). Her partner Ari would like to be with her during the delivery of their baby. Ari explains that he and Janine would like the placenta returned to them after the delivery, which is an important part of his Māori culture.

Critical Thinking Question

- What are the processes for the return of tissue such as a placenta?
  Box 7.2 will help you to prepare your answer.

Patients with diabetes

The patient with diabetes is vulnerable to the effects of both the anaesthetic and the surgery, with postoperative complications including infection, hypoglycaemia and hyperglycaemia (Kuzulugil, Papeix, Luu, & Kerridge, 2019). The type of diabetes and control of blood glucose levels will determine the plan created by the surgeon or anaesthetist. Consequently, regular monitoring of blood glucose level (BGL) in the diabetic fasted patient is necessary in the preoperative period (Auckland District Health Board, 2017; Australian Diabetes Society, 2012). The preoperative nurses should report any BGL measurements outside the normal range to the anaesthetist and seek advice about potential treatment. Box 7.3 summarises recent advances in diabetes treatments and their perioperative implications.

Leading up to the day of admission, patients with diabetes should be assessed to determine their glycaemic control, and this should be optimised by establishing an individualised management plan prior to surgery (O'Neill et al., 2016). If the diabetes is uncontrolled, this should be weighed up against the urgency for surgery. This also provides the opportunity for support from the diabetes specialist team where necessary. Complications from uncontrolled diabetes require consideration and planning, such as patients with neuropathy or peripheral vascular disease with regards to VTE assessment and prevention interventions. The role and engagement of the patient in planning are essential.

Organisational policy should guide diabetes management in surgical patients pre-/intra- and postoperatively (AIHW, 2020d; Kuzulugil et al., 2019). Assessment and planning should be completed and documented at the time of surgical booking or the point of admission. This should include all relevant preoperative testing such as electrocardiograms,

---

BOX 7.3
Recent Advances in Diabetes Treatments and Their Perioperative Implications

- Adhere to standardised clinical pathways and reduce variation in practice to improve perioperative outcomes.
- Arrange preoperative assessment as soon as possible after the decision is taken to proceed with surgery to optimise care.
- Identify and manage patients with suboptimal diabetes control, especially hyperglycaemia, to improve postoperative outcomes.
- Review haemoglobin A1c (HbA1c) preoperatively for all patients with diabetes. The optimal blood glucose level (BGL) is approximately 106–180 mg/dL (6–10 mmol/L) for hospitalised patients.
- Ensure that comorbidities are recognised, documented and optimised prior to admission:
  - Patients with peripheral vascular disease or neuropathy may not be suitable for VTE antiembolism stockings.
  - Patients with 'at risk' diabetic feet may need referral for specialist assessment.
  - All diabetic patients should be managed to prevent pressure injuries.

- Recommendations for the management of antihyperglycaemic medications vary among national guidelines.
  - It may not be necessary to cease all antihyperglycaemic agents prior to surgery.
  - Cease sulfonylureas and sodium-glucose co-transporter 2 inhibitors (SGLT2i) before moderate or major surgery. SGLT2i may provoke euglycaemic diabetic ketoacidosis in the perioperative period and should be withheld until the patient is well and eating normally. SGLT2i are associated with higher rates of ketoacidosis, especially in acutely unwell and postsurgical patients.
- Day of surgery admission (DOSA) should be the 'default' position.
- Prioritise surgical patients to ensure that patients with diabetes are scheduled for morning lists to minimise duration of fasting.
- Anaesthetic technique should minimise fasting time and the risk of postoperative nausea and vomiting.

(Sources: Adapted from Joint British Diabetes Societies for Inpatient Care. (2016). *Management of adults with diabetes undergoing surgery and elective procedures: improving standards*; Kuzulugil, D., Papeix, G., Luu, J., & Kerridge, R. K. (2019). Recent advances in diabetes treatments and their perioperative implications. *Current Opinion in Anaesthesiology, 32*(3), 398–404.)

---

blood potassium levels and renal tests. Ideally, patients with diabetes should be placed first on an elective list to prevent longer than necessary fasting (Australian Diabetes Society, 2012). In an emergency situation where planning is not possible, BGL should be monitored regularly, and an insulin or glucose infusion may be necessary depending upon the result (Auckland District Health Board, 2017).

PATIENT SCENARIOS

SCENARIO 7.5: PATIENTS WITH DIABETES

Consider the target blood glucose range for Mrs Peterson, an Indigenous woman with T2D admitted for an emergency laparoscopic cholecystectomy.

Critical Thinking Questions

- What actions would be necessary before surgery commenced if Mrs Peterson's BGL was found to be higher than 12 mmol/L?

- Outline the preoperative pathway for an elective surgical patient with T2D in your facility, including instructions for preoperative fasting and day of surgery medications. Identify any differences in this pathway for a patient with T1D.
- What is the required frequency of BGL measurements by the nursing staff during the perioperative journeys of patients with diabetes?

HEALTH BEHAVIOURS AND RISK FACTORS
Tobacco Smoking

The Australian Medical Association (AMA) states there is no safe level for tobacco smoking (AMA, 2015) and yet it remains the leading cause of cancer, preventable illnesses, disease and deaths in Australia (AIHW, 2020e). The New Zealand and Australian governments have introduced strategies to reduce tobacco smoking in the general population (Commonwealth of Australia, Department of Health, 2019; Ministry of Health – Manatū

Hauora, 2019a). While the level of tobacco smoking is decreasing in our populations, the use of electronic cigarettes and vaping has been increasing for current smokers, with reported rates climbing from 31% in 2016 to 39% in 2019 (AIHW, 2020e). The Royal Australasian College of Surgeons (RACS) identifies the need for additional research not only on the long-term health effects of vaping and e-cigarettes but also on the effectiveness of these products as part of an overarching smoking cessation strategy (RACS, 2018).

All healthcare organisations have smoke-free policies, making it all the more important for healthcare professionals to understand the nature of nicotine dependence in their patients (Ministry of Health – Manatū Hauora, 2019a). Patients who report smoking within 30 minutes of waking or those who typically smoke more than 10 cigarettes in a day may be considered to be nicotine dependent (NSW Ministry of Health, 2016), making them candidates for nicotine replacement therapy (NRT). Options for patients coming into the smoke-free hospital environment range from medicinal NRT lozenges and patches, e-cigarettes, bupropion, nortriptyline and varenicline to other strategies such as behavioural support (Ministry of Health, 2014). Brief counselling preoperatively, along with referral information, has been shown to increase the likelihood of patients quitting preoperatively when compared with no advice at all (Carrick, Robson, & Thomas, 2019; Young-Wolff, Adams, Fogelberg, Goldstein, & Preston, 2019).

The length of time a smoker should be advised to cease smoking prior to surgery remains unclear; times ranging from 12 hours to 8 weeks have been suggested (Carrick et al., 2019). Refraining from smoking for as little as 24 hours before surgery, however, is likely to be beneficial (RACS, 2018). Cessation advice and support should be provided during the patient's first preoperative interview. ANZCA (2014) recommends that the smoking habits of all preoperative patients are assessed by the primary person making the surgical referral well before surgery. Tables 7.4 and 7.5 outline some simple questions to identify nicotine-dependent patients during preoperative assessment and provide them with the support they need.

The importance of smoking cessation should be provided, with an explanation of the possible consequences of not stopping smoking (ANZCA, 2014; RACS, 2018). Tobacco smoking is a risk factor for surgical patients, being associated with impaired bone healing, postoperative wound dehiscence, wound infections and delayed wound healing (Carrick et al., 2019). Smoking also increases liver enzyme numbers used to break down many medications, resulting in reduced blood concentrations of the medications

TABLE 7.4
Assessing Nicotine Dependence

Question to Ask	Response Indicating Nicotine Dependence
'How soon after waking do you smoke your first cigarette?'	Within 30 minutes of waking
'How many cigarettes do you smoke on a typical day?'	More than 10 cigarettes per day
'If you have previously attempted to quit, did you experience withdrawals or cravings?'	A history of withdrawal symptoms in previous quit attempts
Client is considered to be nicotine dependent if a positive response is given to one or more of the above questions.	

(Source: Adapted from NSW Ministry of Health, 2016. Tool 3. Assessing nicotine dependence. Tools for health professionals.)

TABLE 7.5
Smoking Cessation Before Surgery

In Australia, the Practice is to Use AAR: Ask – Advise – Refer

A	Ask patients about their smoking status. This reinforces the message that tobacco use is a significant issue
A	Advise patients of specific perioperative risks and the risks of cancer and cardiorespiratory disease
R	Refer the patient to counselling and evidence-based cessation treatment

In New Zealand, the Practice is to Use ABC: Ask – Brief – Cessation

A	Ask about and document every person's smoking status
B	Give brief advice to stop to every person who smokes
C	Strongly encourage every person who smokes to use cessation support (a combination of behavioural support and stop-smoking medicine works best) and offer to help them access it. Refer to, or provide, cessation support to everyone who accepts your offer

(Sources: Adapted from Ministry of Health – Manatū Hauora, 2019a. *The New Zealand guidelines for helping people to stop smoking*; RACS, 2018. News, media releases and advocacy. Cessation of smoking.)

(Ministry of Health, 2014). Furthermore, smokers have a higher incidence of perioperative respiratory and cardiovascular complications compared with non-smokers (Carrick et al., 2019).

PATIENT SCENARIOS

SCENARIO 7.6: HEALTH BEHAVIOURS AND RISK

Mr James Collins arrives at his pre-admission clinic appointment with his daughter, Rebecca. During the nursing interview, Rebecca corrects her father when he describes himself as a non-smoker. She explains that her father has been a heavy smoker most of his life and, while he says he gave them up years ago, she knows that he still smokes a few cigarettes a day. He also enjoys one or two drinks in the evening. Mr Collins says to her 'They help me relax. What can a couple of ciggies and a few tots of rum do to me now, eh Bec?'

Rebecca asks RN George Markham to explain the risks of her father's continued smoking. She also asks whether e-cigarettes or nicotine gum might be better alternatives for him prior to his admission for surgery the following month.

Locate any information provided by your facility for patients to help them to give up smoking and use this to formulate your answers to the following questions.

Critical Thinking Questions

- What are the main risks of smoking for patients such as Mr Collins?
- Outline the benefits for Mr Collins in ceasing smoking completely before his surgery and explain how he can access a smoking cessation program that uses nicotine replacements such as gum or patches.

Obesity

Obesity is a recognised risk factor for surgical patients, owing to its association with sleep apnoea, T2D and cardiovascular disease, any of which will increase the complexity of risk for the patient (Australian Diabetes Society, 2016) (Box 7.4). The World Health Organization (WHO) defines overweight and obesity as having an abnormal or excessive accumulation of fat that can affect a person's health (WHO, 2020a). Body mass index (BMI) is a measure commonly used to classify weight with a simple calculation, expressed as kg/m^2. A person with a BMI of 30 or more is classified as obese (WHO, 2020a). Table 7.6 describes BMI and waist circumference, which are the accepted units of measurement to assess a person's risk for developing chronic disease associated with obesity (AIHW, 2020f). Common health consequences for overweight and obese people include cardiovascular disease, diabetes, musculoskeletal disorders and endometrial, breast and colon cancers (WHO, 2020b). Effects on cardiac

---

BOX 7.4
Overweight and Obesity

Obesity is a global health issue. Large-scale, longitudinal studies have shown obesity in 'never-smokers' to be associated with increased mortality in nearly all regions of the world (Global BMI Mortality Collaboration et al., 2016), while the World Health Organization (WHO) estimates nearly 3 million people die each year from issues related to obesity and being overweight (WHO, 2020b).

According to 2017–18 national data in Australia, two-thirds of the adult population (over 18 years of age) were classified as either overweight or obese, with similar rates for men and women in general (AIHW, 2020f). Obesity was more common in older populations than in younger populations, with one-quarter of the population of children and adolescents (aged under 18 years) classified as overweight or obese. These rates also appear to be related to living conditions, with higher rates of overweight and obesity in remote areas away from major cities, as well as areas with a lower socioeconomic status (AIHW, 2020f). The equivalent national data for the period 2018–19 in Australia reported three-quarters of the Indigenous adult population as being overweight or obese (AIHW, 2020f).

In New Zealand, nearly one-third of all adults are considered as obese, which is the third highest rate among Organisation for Economic Co-operation and Development (OECD) countries (Gray et al., 2018). According to 2018–19 national data, Māori adults were almost twice as likely to be obese as non-Māori adults, while Pacific adults were 2.5 times more likely than non-Pacific adults to be obese (Ministry of Health – Manatū Hauora, 2019b). The rates of overweight or obesity for Māori children and Pacific children were also higher compared with children in non-Māori, non-Pacific populations. As with the Australian population, the rates of overweight and obesity were higher in socioeconomically deprived areas.

TABLE 7.6
Measuring Overweight and Obesity

BODY MASS INDEX

The international standard for classifying weight in adults is the body mass index (BMI). It is calculated by dividing a person's weight in kilograms by their height in metres squared, as follows:

$$\text{Body mass index} = \frac{\text{weight (kg)}}{\text{height (m)}^2}$$

The table below depicts the classification of weight according to a person's BMI score.

BMI (kg/m²)	Classification
Less than 18.5	Underweight
18.5 to less than 25	Normal weight range
25 to less than 30	Overweight
30 or more	Obese

WAIST CIRCUMFERENCE

Waist circumference is another common measure of weight in adults. A high waist circumference is associated with an increased risk of chronic disease. The table below depicts the categories of risk for people of Caucasian ethnicity.

	Increased Risk	Substantially Increased Risk
Men	94 cm	102 cm
Women	80 cm	88 cm

(Source: Adapted from Australian Institute of Health and Welfare, 2020f. Overweight and obesity. Snapshot.)

function include increased cardiac output, increased sympathetic responses and increased circulating blood volume. Respiratory problems associated with obesity have further implications for anaesthesia, such as obstructive sleep apnoea, hypoxaemia, restrictive lung disease, chronic obstructive pulmonary disease and hypercapnia (Tsai & Schumann, 2016).

For obese surgical patients, extra preparations required for securing airway access and providing respiratory support should be identified and organised during preoperative assessment by the anaesthetic and surgical teams (Chung et al., 2016; Nightingale et al., 2015). Consideration and planning are also required for these patients with regard to theatre bed weight capacity, transfer equipment, extensions for bed sides, and positioning equipment and its weight capabilities, as well as extra staffing requirements for transfer and

considerations for emergency management of the patient (ACORN, 2020e). Ideally, this information should be communicated at the time of surgical scheduling and following pre-admission assessment (Chung et al., 2016). Assessment of risk for the obese surgical patient also requires appropriate education for all perioperative staff and the development of policies and guidelines (ACORN, 2020f).

Additional considerations will be required when the obese surgical patient is being assessed for bariatric surgery (when weight loss is the primary intention) or for metabolic surgery to control diabetes and hyperglycaemia (Rubino et al., 2014). For a patient with a BMI higher than 35, such surgical techniques may also be successful in decreasing comorbidities and can improve the patient's quality of life (Lee & Almalki, 2017). It is common for patients undergoing bariatric or metabolic surgery to be put on very-low-energy diets (VLEDs) in an attempt to lose weight preoperatively (Lee & Dixon, 2017). While this can reduce the risk of surgical complications, many patients will be nutritionally compromised, so a thorough nutritional assessment is required to ensure correction of any deficiencies before admission. In addition to physical assessment and preparation, the patient's understanding and expectations of the surgery as well as their commitment and motivation need to be assessed. If depression or anxiety is part of the patient's medical history, a referral to a psychologist or similar service may be needed as part of the patient's preoperative preparation. More information about the care and management of the obese surgical patient is provided in Chapters 8 and 9.

PREOPERATIVE INSTRUCTIONS
Medications

The anaesthetist will provide instructions for the patient about their regular medications and whether any should be ceased prior to their surgery. While most medications can continue to be taken preoperatively, there are exceptions including blood-thinning medications such as aspirin, antiplatelets (e.g. clopidogrel) and anticoagulants (e.g. warfarin). Due to the risk of periprocedural diabetic ketoacidosis (DKA), the Australian Diabetes Society (ADS) recommends cessation of sodium-glucose co-transporter-2 inhibitor (SGLT2i) oral medications for some patients in the days prior to admission for surgery (ADS, 2020). Clinicians should refer to the detailed recommendations in the ADS alert update (2020) to ensure patients with diabetes are given the correct preoperative advice about these medications. Other medications may need to be adjusted prior to surgery. The patient may also need to seek advice from their endocrinologist, cardiologist, oncologist or general practitioner (GP), who may have prescribed some of the patient's regular medications.

Some herbal products may also need to be avoided in the preoperative period, owing to their potential association with unanticipated excessive bleeding. These products include garlic, *Ginkgo biloba* and ginger. Common herbal drinks such as green tea can interact with vitamin K, thereby reducing the blood-thinning effects of warfarin, while ginger has the opposite effect and may increase bleeding (Dagli et al., 2016). The ASA suggests that surgical patients should cease using herbal products at least 1 week prior to their planned date of admission (Donoghue, 2018). An awareness of these over-the-counter 'natural' products and the risks they pose to patients during their perioperative journey requires understanding, assessment and patient education by all members of the multidisciplinary team.

Procedural Fasting

Procedural fasting is an essential component of preoperative preparation, which should be explained in simple written instructions for the patient (ACI, 2016a). These instructions should be based on the expected timing of anaesthesia (or sedation) to reduce the potential for extended periods of fasting, which may result in fluid depletion (ANZCA, 2017). The ANZCA fasting guidelines are:

    i. *For adults having an elective procedure, limited solid food may be taken up to six (6) hours prior to anaesthesia and clear fluids may be taken up to two (2) hours prior to anaesthesia.*

    ii. *For children over six (6) months of age having an elective procedure, breast milk or formula and limited solid food may be given up to six (6) hours and clear fluids (no more than 3 mL/kg/h) up to one hour prior to anaesthesia.*

    iii. *For infants under six (6) months of age having an elective procedure, formula may be given up to four (4) hours, breast milk up to three (3) hours and clear fluids (no more than 3 mL/kg/h) up to one hour prior to anaesthesia.*

    iv. *Prescribed medications may be taken with a sip of water less than two (2) hours prior to anaesthesia unless otherwise directed (for example oral hypoglycaemics and anticoagulants).*

(ANZCA (2017), PS07 Appendix 1, p. 5)

Additional considerations may be required for patients at risk of regurgitation or vomiting, such as patients with hiatus hernia or abdominal disorder and patients who have had bariatric surgery or are suspected to have delayed gastric emptying, as well as emergency surgical patients and labouring women (ANZCA, 2017).

The preoperative nurse should identify any patients who require further explanation about the small but important differences in fluid descriptions and times in their fasting instruction, such as:

- *clear fluids* – fluids or foods that liquefy at room temperature. All liquids containing fat are excluded, sugar, sweeteners and salt are allowed (e.g. clear soup, pulp-free fruit juice, cordial, soft drink, black tea or coffee and water)
- *full fluids* – liquid foods that require no chewing (e.g. pureed soups, milk, drinking yoghurt or smooth yoghurt without fruit pieces, etc.) (ACI, 2016b).

It is most likely that the elective surgical patient will need to fast the night before they are admitted to hospital, so if the patient has not attended a pre-admission clinic the preoperative team will need to provide this information in the admission information pack or preoperative telephone call.

Preoperative Bathing

Patients being admitted for elective procedures may be instructed to bathe or shower with an antimicrobial solution once or twice on the day prior to their procedure. The Association of periOperative Registered Nurses (AORN) recommends this practice to reduce the microbial colony count on the patient's skin, which is thought to lower the incidence of surgical site infection (SSI) (Cowperthwaite & Holm, 2015). Preoperative bathing has been the subject of systematic reviews (Dumville, McFarlane, Edwards, Lipp, & Holmes, 2013; Kamel, McGahan, Polisena, Mierzwinski-Urban, & Embil, 2012; Webster & Osborne, 2015) and interest remains in whether one antimicrobial product is more effective than another or plain soap and water. Edmiston and Leaper (2017) reviewed the evidence and recommend 4% aqueous chlorhexidine gluconate (CHG) for preoperative bathing or showering to reduce the risk of SSI, ideally as part of a care bundle (see also Box 7.5).

Bowel Preparation

Many surgical patients will require bowel preparation before their admission to hospital. Patient education is important for these patients as it can provide them with the opportunity to clarify the instructions for the specifically timed regimen for taking their bowel preparation and ask questions about modifications to their diet (Hassan et al., 2019). The preoperative nurse will need to allow adequate time to explain these instructions and may need to provide supporting educational materials such as videos and brochures. It is also recommended that the preoperative nurse attend to the diverse linguistic and cultural needs of their patients by including patients'

BOX 7.5

Steps to Implement Preoperative Bathing With Chlorhexidine Gluconate (CHG)

1. Patient education, emphasising the benefit of the pre-admission antiseptic shower as an element of the presurgical checklist
2. Oral and written showering instructions to the patient
3. Use of a standard 118 mL amount of 4% aqueous CHG for each shower
4. The taking of a minimum of two showers
5. 1-minute pause per shower to be observed prior to the rinsing of CHG from the skin surface
6. Instruction to patients not to apply lotions, creams or emollients following CHG showering as they may mask or adversely (pharmacologically) affect antimicrobial activity
7. Avoidance of CHG contact with eyes or ears and, if exposed, advice to rinse immediately
8. Advice to undertake immediate and copious rinsing if significant burning or itching occurs after application of CHG with reporting of the occurrence to the healthcare provider
9. Provision of appropriate CHG showering materials to the patient by the healthcare institution or provider
10. Enhancement of patient compliance to completing the showering using SMS texting, email or voice-mail alert system (all commercial vendors of 4% aqueous CHG support a computer-based alert system)

(Source: Edmiston, C. E., Jr, & Leaper, D. (2017). Should preoperative showering or cleansing with chlorhexidine gluconate (CHG) be part of the surgical care bundle to prevent surgical site infection? *Journal of Infection Prevention, 18*(6), Table 1, p. 313.)

BOX 7.6

Guidelines for Bowel Preparation Before Colonoscopy

The latest evidence-based guidelines from the European Society for Gastrointestinal Endoscopy (ESGE) include strong recommendations for preoperative patients instructed to take bowel preparation before colonoscopy.

ESGE recommends:

- a low-fibre diet on the day preceding colonoscopy
- the use of enhanced instructions for bowel preparation
- split-dose bowel preparation for elective colonoscopy
- a same-day bowel preparation for patients undergoing afternoon colonoscopy, as an acceptable alternative to split dosing
- starting the last dose of bowel preparation within 5 hours of colonoscopy and completing it at least 2 hours before the beginning of the procedure
- the use of high-volume or low-volume polyethylene glycol (PEG)-based regimens as well as that of non-PEG-based agents that have been clinically validated for routine bowel preparation. In patients at risk for hydroelectrolyte disturbances, the choice of laxative should be individualised.

ESGE suggests:

- adding oral simethicone to bowel preparation (*weak recommendation*).

(Source: Adapted from Hassan, C., East, J., Radaelli, F., Spada, C., Benamouzig, R., Bisschops, R., . . . Dumonceau, J.-M. (2019). Bowel preparation for colonoscopy: ESGE Guideline – update 2019. *Endoscopy, 51*(08), 775–794.)

guardians, carers or interpreter services during preoperative education to ensure their patients understand these instructions (ACORN, 2020a).

It is important that preoperative nurses maintain their knowledge of current practice guidelines relating to the preparation and care of patients undergoing such procedures, particularly the information relating to any modifications to preoperative diets and the correct regimen for bowel preparation. Box 7.6 outlines the latest evidence-based guidelines from the European Society for Gastrointestinal Endoscopy (ESGE). A national clinical care standard has been developed in Australia to ensure that colonoscopy patients not only receive timely assessment and evidence-based information, but also that they are instructed in effective preoperative bowel preparation (ACSQHC/the Commission,

2020d). Additional patient information is provided by relevant health ministries as well as organisations such as Bowel Cancer Australia and the Gastroenterological Society of Australia (GESA), which also provides information in other languages.

PATIENT EDUCATION

Preoperative instructions may need the additional support of **patient education** to help patients prepare for their time in hospital, as well as their recovery period and follow-up appointments. Furthermore, timely preoperative patient education aims to assist the surgical patient to make informed decisions about their care options and provide them with adequate time to reflect on information delivered by the multidisciplinary team (ACORN, 2020a).

Providing information in advance of the admission date has also been shown to decrease patient anxiety,

BOX 7.7
Preoperative Visiting

This practice developed at a time when the prevailing model of care for elective surgical patients required an advanced admission to hospital the day before surgery. This was a system-centred model of care in which clinicians used the extended preoperative time to complete preoperative assessments and investigations, pathology tests and to attend to the general physical preparation of the surgical patient (Malley et al., 2015). Nurses' preoperative visits were expected to reduce preoperative anxiety for surgical patients and, as such, it was considered an important aspect of the perioperative nurse's role and a way of articulating the patient-centred focus. It was thought to be particularly helpful strategy in preparing children for surgery (Dai & Livesley, 2018) (see also Research box 7.3).

Changes in models of surgical patient care mean that today's elective surgical patient is likely to meet perioperative nurses well before their arrival in the perioperative department and instead will have time to ask questions during the comprehensive assessment processes at a pre-admission clinic (ADSNA, 2018).

which can reduce postoperative pain and length of stay in hospital and may increase overall levels of patient satisfaction (Mitchell, 2017). Fear of the unknown and anxiety are common feelings for many surgical patients. Health professionals have a duty to care to identify and manage the effects of preoperative anxiety on a patient's psychological status (ACORN, 2020a). This anxiety may be attributed to the forthcoming surgical procedure, loss of autonomy or fear of the unknown (pain or death), and these responses may be seen in abnormal haemodynamic readings such as hypertension or tachycardia (Wilson et al., 2016). Personality characteristics and underlying psychological comorbidities are also important factors to be considered when assessing anxious patients (Tong, Dannaway, Enke, & Eslick, 2020). Preoperative visiting is an example of patient education that was once considered an effective strategy to manage preoperative patient anxiety (Shetler, 1972) (Box 7.7). This once common daily activity for perioperative nurses is less suited to present models of care such as day surgery and DOSA where patients are no longer admitted the afternoon prior to their scheduled surgery.

Nursing staff play a central role in the provision of patient education (ACORN, 2020a). Fig. 7.3 (see end of chapter) includes a section titled 'Patient education', where potential topics can be recorded. The preoperative nurse should try to assess the patient's understanding about their impending surgical procedure. It is equally important, following the provision of any education, that the nurse assesses whether the patient has understood that information. This can be done by asking patients to summarise the information in their own words. Individual patient factors which may influence the amount of information provided in the preoperative period include the patient's education level, gender and cultural background (Koivisto et al., 2019). Fig. 7.7 (see end of chapter) is a checklist of information that may be helpful when provided to patients and their carers during the preoperative preparation. When written patient information is provided, it should be available in a variety of languages, to meet the diverse cultural and linguistic needs of the local population.

Additional patient follow-up by telephone in the days prior to admission can also ensure that the patient has understood all of the preparation requirements including:

- cessation of medications
- preoperative fasting
- specific bowel preparations for gastrointestinal procedures
- planned admission times
- paperwork or X-rays the patient needs to provide
- advice about staying comfortably warm before surgery
- advice about discharge home with a support person for day surgery patients.

These phone calls may also require the support of interpreter services.

ADMISSION TO HOSPITAL

The next phase in the perioperative journey for the elective surgical patient is their admission to hospital. While the local facility policy will designate the exact procedure to be followed, the perioperative nurse should take a systematic and planned approach (ACORN, 2020a). Admission processes rely on coordinated teamwork, with the admissions clerical staff providing essential support to the clinical team of nurses, anaesthetists and surgeons, dietitians, pharmacists, porters and interpreters.

On the day of the procedure or surgery (referred to collectively as the procedure from here onwards), the admissions team ensures each patient detail is checked and confirmed according to the National Safety and Quality Health Service (NSQHS) Standards (ACSQHC/the Commission, 2017a). Professional standards and best-practice guidelines such as the ACORN Standards, ADSNA best practice guidelines, ANZCA professional documents and RACS position papers may also guide these admission processes, but, most importantly, admissions processes will need to follow the specific local facility policies.

If any of the admission processes are left incomplete, or if any patient details are found to be incorrect, the patient's procedure might be delayed and, in some cases, it may need to be cancelled. Cancellation of a planned procedure has a major impact on theatre utilisation and efficiency of the system, but, more importantly, it can have a huge negative impact on the patient and their family. All members of the admissions team should therefore work together to avoid cancellations on the day and aim to have all patients prepared and ready for their specific procedure. The surgical patient's admission to hospital can be divided broadly into administrative processes, which ensure that all information is available and correct, and clinical preparations, which ensure that the patient is physically ready for transfer to the operating suite.

Administrative processes ensure the following information has been checked, assembled and recorded in the patient's health record:

- preoperative health questionnaire and pre-admission assessments
- results of preoperative investigations and risk assessments
- old notes, imaging and other patient records
- surgical patient care plan with relevant clinical pathway, including baseline observation charts, anaesthetic record and preoperative checklist
- patient identification including printed labels and identification bands with or without allergies (see details in section below)
- consent forms (see details in section below).

Clinical preparation of the patient by the admitting nurse needs to be tailored to each patient's specific needs, with the following minimum requirements:

- *measurement of baseline observations* such as vital signs including temperature, height and weight, BGL
- *risk assessments* not completed at pre-admission such as pressure injury, VTE, falls, delirium, etc.
- *surgical site verification and marking* (see details in section below)
- *physical preparation* such as removal of jewellery and other personal belongings, skin assessment, preoperative warming, VTE prophylaxis, hydration and voiding, and premedication (see details in section below)
- *completion of the preoperative checklist* and clinical handover (see details below)

Patient Identification

To comply with the NSQHS Standards, healthcare facilities in Australia are required to use information systems which ensure consistent, reliable and correct **patient identification** (ACSQHC/the Commission, 2017b, 2017c). The administrative systems in place should confirm the hospital admission is for:

- the correct patient, who is correctly prepared
- for the correct surgery
- at the correct time.

A minimum of three approved patient identifiers should be used throughout the patient journey, starting at patient admission (ACSQHC/the Commission, 2017c). These identifiers will be used on the patient's charts to confirm patient identity during all clinical handovers. These will also be used to confirm correct patient identity whenever care is provided, such as medication administration. The three identifiers may include any of the following patient details:

- full name including family name and given names
- date of birth
- gender
- address with postcode (note that patients may have moved address since previous admissions and any address appearing in old notes or electronic health record [EHR] or electronic medical record [EMR] must be verified by the patient as their current address)
- Individual Healthcare Identifier (IHI)
- healthcare record number.

As part of this identification process, adult patients should be asked to state their full name and their date of birth. When the patient is unable to communicate because of age, physical condition or mental capacity, a parent, guardian or carer may be asked to confirm the patient's details. Once confirmed, the patient's personal details should be matched to any preprinted patient identification labels, as well as the scheduled admission records and any earlier documentation from the preadmission period. These records are likely to include a combination of EHR, printed charts and care pathways as well as patient identification bands. The attention and diligence of admitting staff are important when confirming these details at this initial stage of the patient's journey and can reduce the potential for wrong patient, wrong site, wrong surgeries to occur (see more detail in Chapter 4). The confirmed patient identification bands should then be placed on the patient's wrist and ankle according to local facility policy. The following principles apply to patient identification bands:

- A transparent or white-coloured patient identification band must be used to record the mandatory patient identifiers with black text on a white background (ACSQHC/the Commission, 2017c).
- Patients with allergies or sensitivities should instead wear two red identification bands with the confirmed patient details (ACSQHC/the Commission, 2017c). Red bands are an alert and indication to all staff throughout the patient's perioperative journey to check the patient's EHR where the full details of the allergy, sensitivity risk or adverse drug reaction should be recorded.
- Two or more patient identification bands are required for patients undergoing procedures where it is likely that a band may be removed or become inaccessible to staff during the procedure.
- One patient identification band should be easily accessible to staff throughout the procedure (e.g. details can be read by staff without the need to move procedural drapes, adjust equipment or disrupt the procedural flow) (NSW Ministry of Health, 2014).

Allergies and Sensitivities

The admitting nurse must take a thorough history of patient allergies or sensitivities and record the details in the patient's health record, with the type of reaction noted. These patient details will be referred to at each clinical handover so it is important to obtain as much detail as possible during the admission process before the patient has received any premedication.

The National Inpatient Medication Charts (NIMC) for Adults include a section on allergies and adverse drug reactions (ADR). The admitting nurse should record whether the patient has 'nil known, unknown or known' reactions. Where known, the admitting nurse should record the name of the medicine (or other substance), the type of reaction the patient experienced and, where possible, the date of adverse reaction.

This history should include food allergies and sensitivities as well as previous reactions and sensitivities to drugs. Examples include any previous unfavourable reactions to anaesthesia, blood transfusions, iodine, adhesive tapes or dressings and the risk of latex allergy. The Australian and New Zealand Anaesthetic Allergy Group (ANZAAG) and ANZCA recognise that the number of patients who are allergic to chlorhexidine is increasing (ANZCA/ANZAAG, 2016a). All care should be taken to avoid the patient's exposure to these common allergens, and special consideration is required before

the patient is transferred to locations where these products may be present (ANZCA/ANZAAG, 2016b). This will allow time to prepare an environment free of potential allergens. Chapter 5 contains more information about these patient risks.

The likelihood of an allergic reaction to anaesthetic agents is estimated at 1 in every 1250 to 10,000 anaesthetics, and at least 60% of all hypersensitivity reactions observed occur within the perioperative period (World Allergy Organization, 2019). Anaphylaxis is a life-threatening emergency that requires prompt recognition of signs and symptoms, and should be considered if the patient demonstrates skin signs with bronchospasm or hypotension (ANZCA/ANZAAG, 2016b).

Consent

Healthcare facilities must ensure their processes for gaining informed consent comply with legislation and national standards (NSW Ministry of Health, 2020). These requirements are described in more detail in Chapter 3, including situations involving guardianship and substitute consents. The administrative systems in place should ensure that the patient's consent form is included in the admission papers. The consent form is one of the most important documents in the surgical patient's health record and both its availability and its completion must be prioritised. Legislation in some states requires that written consent is obtained from patients undergoing significant treatment and procedures (NSW Ministry of Health, 2020) (see also Box 7.8).

A missing consent form should trigger immediate administrative follow-up, with phone calls to the consultant's rooms and pre-admission clinics. If the original consent form cannot be located, then the surgeon (or a senior member of the surgical team) will need to see the patient as soon as possible and together they will complete a new consent form. This must be resolved before the admission can progress any further and before administration of any strong analgesia or premedications, which may render the consent invalid. Local policies commonly mandate that patients should not be transferred to the preoperative holding area without their consent form. This is to reduce the risk of wrong site, wrong patient surgeries (NSW Ministry of Health, 2020).

The next step is for the admitting nurse to check and confirm the following:

- the consent form has been completed correctly, including all patient details, signatures and dates
- the planned procedure is written legibly without abbreviations (i.e. sites, sides or levels must be clearly written in full)

- patients who used an interpreter during the con-senting process should have the interpreter's decla-ration on their consent form
- patients who may need a blood transfusion should have this section completed.

A further confirmation of the patient's consent is achieved by the admitting nurse asking the patient to describe, in their own words, the operation or proce-dure they have consented to as part of their admis-sion. The admitting nurse should seek clarification as soon as practical from the surgical team or nurse manager if there is uncertainty about any aspect of the patient's written consent. A brief clarification of con-sent details before the patient's scheduled surgery may avert a subsequent delay, cancellation, or a wrong site surgery.

Surgical Site Verification and Marking

If the patient is to undergo surgery on a limb or any other body part where the potential for operating on an incorrect site exists (such as digit, kidney, breast, etc.), the patient should not proceed to the operating room unless the surgical site is clearly marked (NSW Ministry of Health, 2017b). The surgeon should mark

the site with a single-use indelible pen. The marking should use an arrow pointing to the site or level of the planned incision (positioned close to the site but not directly on top of the site). This arrow must remain visible to the perioperative team for the conduct of the Surgical Safety Checklist (SSC) and remain visible af-ter the patient has been draped (NSW Ministry of Health, 2017b).

Some surgical sites cannot be marked owing to their location, such as perineal areas, teeth and other areas of the body that are unable to be seen (Phillips & Hornacky, 2020). If the details of the intended proce-dure differ between the operating list and the consent/agreement to treatment form, or the patient's opinion, the surgeon should be informed immediately. The surgical site marking on the patient will need to be postponed until there is confirmation of the correct procedure and correct site. The patient should not be transferred to the preoperative holding area until this process has been completed.

Physical Preparation
Jewellery and body piercings

In preparation for admission, the patient may have been given preoperative instructions to come to the hospital without any jewellery or body piercings. Patients with genital piercings may be at increased risk of injury during positioning or thermal injuries from electrosurgery (Smith, 2016). The Association of peri-Operative Registered Nurses (AORN) recommends that the nurse explains these risks during the preoperative assessment phase and advises relevant patients to re-move genital piercings before admission (Smith, 2016). Hence, the presence of such items will require some decisions by the admitting nurse. Depending upon the location of the surgery, the patient may be asked to remove the item. This is not only for the purpose of security, but also to minimise the risk of infection, traumatic removal, or thermal injury risk (as conductive metal may provide an alternative pathway for the elec-trosurgical current during surgery) (ACORN, 2020g). All mouth, tongue, nasal and facial jewellery must be removed, as the risk of dislodgement creates a risk to patients undergoing anaesthetic and operative proce-dures. Removed jewellery may be given to a family member, or labelled and secured safely in the patient's locker or ward safe.

If any jewellery does remain in place, such as a wedding band, this needs to be taped to prevent its loss (ACORN, 2020g; Smith, 2016). If there are any doubts about jewellery or piercings, these should be discussed with the anaesthetist and the surgeon and the patient should be advised of the potential risks (Smith, 2016).

Implants

Patient implants include joint replacement prostheses, breast implants, permanent pacemakers (PPMs), automatic internal cardiac defibrillators (AICDs), cochlear implants and port-a-caths. The admitting nurse should record the location of these implants on the preoperative checklist and ensure that this information is included in clinical handover with the perioperative nurse in the preoperative holding area. This information will assist the perioperative team with patient positioning (e.g. taking care with joint replacements) as well as placement of the return electrode (diathermy plate) when electrosurgery is required. Some implants are large in size and these may have scar tissue encircling them, such as internal defibrillators or chest ports. Scar tissue has a high resistance to the electrosurgical current and the perioperative team will need to avoid placing a return electrode (diathermy plate) over scarred tissue (Ball, 2018).

Skin integrity

Guidelines recommend that initial skin assessments should be completed as soon as possible, within 8 hours of the patient's admission (ACSQHC/the Commission,

2020b; National Pressure Ulcer Advisory Panel, European Pressure Ulcer Advisory Panel and Pan Pacific Pressure Injury Alliance [NPUAP/EPUAP/PPPIA], 2019). While this simple top-to-toe visual inspection is separate from the patient's PI risk assessment (described in previous sections), it does contribute to PI prevention, because the condition of the patient's skin and underlying tissues are early indicators of the patient's PI risk. Local policies may require comprehensive skin assessments for some patients using a validated tool where skin changes can be recorded on body diagrams.

The admitting nurse is ideally placed to inspect the preoperative patient's skin and tissue condition efficiently when the patient has removed their street clothes and changed into the hospital gown. The nurse can use this time to confirm whether the patient has followed preoperative instructions to bathe or shower with an antimicrobial solution and can ensure that the patient's skin and tissue at the procedural site are clean and free from visible debris prior to transfer to the procedure rooms or operating suite (Cowperthwaite & Holm, 2015) (Fig. 7.8) (see below).

The WHO strongly recommends that hair should not be removed preoperatively unless absolutely necessary – for example, if it will obscure the incision site. If the surgical team subsequently decides that hair

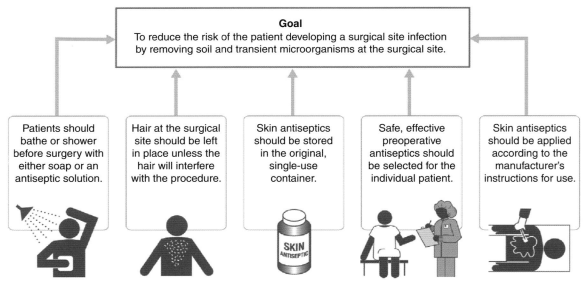

FIG. 7.8 Elements of preoperative patient skin antisepsis. (Source: Cowperthwaite, L., & Holm, R. L., 2015. Guideline implementation: preoperative patient skin antisepsis, *AORN Journal, 101*(1), p. 73, Figure 1.)

removal is warranted, the WHO recommends clippers only and strongly discourages shaving at any time owing to resulting skin trauma (Health Quality and Safety Commission New Zealand [HSQCNZ], 2014; WHO, 2019).

For the paediatric patient, the parent's presence during skin inspection may be helpful. For example, the child may be able to remain in their pyjamas or loose clothing (SCHN, 2018b) so the skin inspection cannot be done quite as easily as when the adult patient is in a hospital gown. An infant's nappy should always be changed before transfer to the preoperative holding area and this is another opportunity to inspect the skin. If any of this is difficult, or distressing, to complete while the child is awake, it may need to be handed over to the perioperative staff, who can complete this assessment during patient positioning. The handover principle applies to all preoperative patients with incomplete patient assessments; the admitting nurse should include this advice at clinical handover so that the required assessments and any subsequent care are not missed.

Patient warming

The admitting nurse should aim to keep the preoperative patient comfortably warm, which can be difficult in the cold hospital environment during physical assessments (ACORN, 2020h). Maintenance of normothermia is the aim for all patients throughout the perioperative period, with 36°C the target temperature (ANZCA, 2018b; National Institute for Health and Care Excellence [NICE], 2016). If the patient's temperature falls below 36°C, the admitting nurse should take action to bring the patient's temperature back to acceptable levels (Australian College of Perianaesthesia Nurses [ACPAN], (2020). The patient may request additional bed coverings or warmed blankets and, while these passive warming methods may provide quick comfort, they are less effective than active warming methods to manage inadvertent perioperative hypothermia (IPH) (Watson, 2018). For example, forced-air warming blankets are commonly used to manage the patient's temperature in the operating room and this active warming method can be used preoperatively with good effect and patient comfort.

The paediatric patient is more at risk of IPH than the adult patient because of a greater surface area-to-volume ratio, higher metabolic rate and poorer insulation due to lower levels of subcutaneous adipose tissue. Consequently, a preoperative temperature of 36.5°C may be recommended for child patients (Riley & Andrzejowski, 2018). More information about the risks of IPH and strategies for intraoperative management can found in Chapters 8 and 9.

VTE prophylaxis

Patients who have been assessed preoperatively and identified at risk of VTE should be placed on a care pathway with a range of prevention measures prescribed by a medical professional (NSW CEC, 2018). These measures include mechanical prophylaxis, such as the wearing of GCSs to encourage venous return in the patient's legs, the application of mechanical sequential compression devices (SCDs), which compress the veins in the patient's legs intermittently, venous foot pumps (VFPs) as well as pharmacological prophylaxis. The choice of prophylaxis will vary depending on the patient's risk factors and those associated with the planned procedure. The admitting nurse must be knowledgeable and skilled in the application of these mechanical devices to ensure that they are applied safely and without injury to the patient's skin. This is usually done as part of the admitting nurse's final preparation of the patient for surgery and should be guided by the documentation requirements of the facility-approved preoperative checklist (ACORN, 2020b). More information about the risks of VTE and intraoperative prophylaxis is provided in Chapter 9.

Hydration and voiding

The elective surgical patient should be given an opportunity to go to the toilet and empty their bowel and bladder before they are transferred to the preoperative holding area. This situation can be made easier for the paediatric patient by the presence and supervision of a parent. Infants should have a clean nappy. The admitting nurse should ensure that any drainage bags (urinary, stomal, etc.) are emptied and the volume charted where relevant in the patient's health record. This should occur before any premedication is due to be administered, so that the premedicated patient can remain comfortably in bed until transfer to the preoperative holding area.

Premedication

Administration of medications should always follow standard protocols for medication safety, including correct patient identification and confirmation of any allergies (ACSQHC/the Commission, 2017c). This is important in all healthcare settings, and especially so in a busy admissions ward when the preoperative nurses are working in an open-practice environment with many patients arriving and departing from the same area.

While the practice of premedication is less common than it once was, special consideration needs to be given to those patients who have been administered opioids, sedatives and anxiolytic premedications (Conway, Rolley, & Sutherland, 2016). These patients need close observation of vital signs for any significant changes, such as a slowing respiratory rate or change in level of responsiveness. Regular oral medications may be taken preoperatively with a sip of water at prescribed times unless documented otherwise by the anaesthetist. If the patient is due other medications while they are going to be in the operating suite, the escorting nurse needs to include this information in the patient's clinical handover and may need to transfer some prescribed medications with the patient to ensure timely intraoperative administration.

PREPARING THE PATIENT FOR TRANSFER TO THE OPERATING SUITE

The following section describes the final checks in preparation of an adult patient for transfer to the preoperative holding area in the operating suite. This process should be guided by the preoperative checklist, which records the most important patient details collected during admission. Preparing the paediatric patient for transfer may require additional considerations, including the presence of a parent who may be able to stay with the child in the preoperative holding area and also during anaesthetic induction (SCHN, 2018a). An interpreter may also be required for these final checks and for the subsequent transfer and clinical handover.

Preoperative Checklist

The preoperative checklist is often used as the front sheet in the preoperative patient's health record, which guides the escorting nurse's clinical handover in the preoperative holding area. It also serves as a quick reference tool for the perioperative team during the subsequent surgical safety checks. Therefore, it is vital for the preoperative nurses to check that all details are completed and verified with the patient.

The patient's escort nurse may not have participated in the patient's admission and may be unfamiliar with the patient's history. Preoperative conversations with the admitting nurse may be significant or require follow-up, so when a team of preoperative nurses is involved any remaining admission processes, assessments or documentation must be handed over to the escort nurse for their attention prior to the patient's transfer. For example, the patient may have raised questions during admission for the anaesthetic or surgical

teams, or they may have expressed concern about the safety of their belongings during their surgery (i.e. spectacles, dentures and hearing aids), or they have requested a postoperative call to a family member. Not all of these processes are prompted by a review of the preoperative checklist; however, they may be a source of anxiety and priorities for the preoperative patient. Figs 7.9 and 7.10 (see end of chapter) are examples of preoperative checklists being used in Australia and New Zealand respectively. While there will be variations in the preoperative checklist content and layout between different healthcare facilities, the common features are likely to include:

- confirmation of completed consent, patient site marking
- patient alerts including allergies, infections, skin integrity issues
- a record of recent vital signs, including temperature, blood pressure, weight
- fasting status
- medications, infusions, continence
- personal items with patient, including spectacles, dentures and hearing aids
- names, signatures, designations and times.

CLINICAL HANDOVER IN THE PREOPERATIVE HOLDING AREA

The **preoperative (pre-op) holding area** is an area specifically allocated for receiving patients into the operating suite. Characteristically, the environment is quiet, provides privacy and is staffed by an appropriately qualified nurse (or registered anaesthetic technician [AT] in New Zealand) with skills in patient assessment and decision making, and an understanding of perioperative processes and procedures. Some pre-op holding areas use calming, quiet music to minimise the patient's anxiety, while those admitting the paediatric patient may have wall murals, busy fish tanks and play areas to create a colourful and welcoming environment for the child and parents.

Together with the patient (and the interpreter, parent or guardian when required), the escorting nurse and perioperative nurse work through the items on the preoperative checklist (Figs 7.9 and 7.10 at end of chapter) and the patient's health record to ensure that the patient is ready for surgery with all documentation required. Figs 7.11 and 7.12 depict two preoperative holding areas. (Note the participation of the escorting nurse and perioperative nurse, as well as the patient [and parent].) This is a process of clinical handover and should allow for a temporary transfer of the patient's

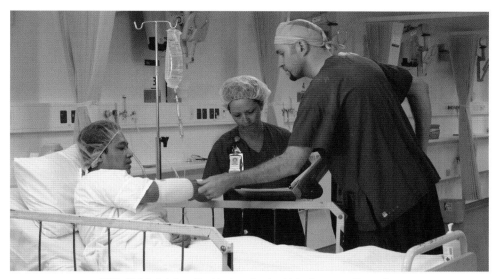

FIG. 7.11 Adult patient being checked into the operating suite.

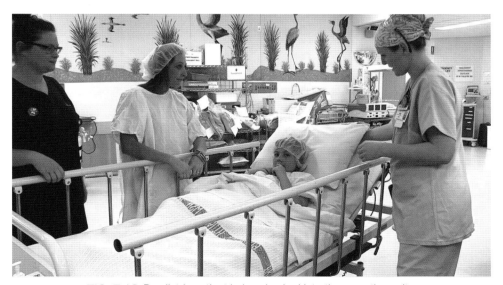

FIG. 7.12 Paediatric patient being checked into the operating suite.

care to the perioperative team and a safe continuation of the elective surgical patient's perioperative journey.

EMERGENCY SURGERY

While this chapter has described the routine preoperative patient care that is delivered during the elective patient's perioperative journey, it is important to acknowledge the differences in the preoperative period for the patient requiring an emergency procedure and the impact on patient preparation and assessment processes.

An emergency procedure is one being performed on a patient whose clinical acuity is assessed by the clinician as requiring the surgery within 24 hours or in less than

72 hours where the patient is not physiologically stable enough to be discharged from hospital prior to the required surgery . . . These patients whether undergoing surgery or not, are also described in various ways including emergency, unplanned, unbooked, acute or urgent surgery patients.

(NSW Ministry of Health, 2009, p. 24)

Emergency surgery definitions will include two main components:

- *An unplanned nature of identification of the need for surgery; and*
- *A relative urgency for surgical intervention, without which the patient's health may deteriorate and risk poor clinical outcomes (including loss of life, limb, or function, or reduced quality of life)*

(ACI, 2011, p. 6)

The patient requiring emergency surgery may be admitted via the emergency department or a specialist outpatient service, or they may be an inpatient who has a sudden deterioration (State of Queensland [Queensland Health], 2017). Just as there are categories of urgency for elective surgery (described earlier), the patient requiring emergency surgery will also need to be categorised according to the degree of urgency. These categories are described in Table 7.7.

Occasionally, there is such urgency that some preoperative investigations and assessments need to be prioritised or omitted. For example, patient consent is generally not required when the treatment is potentially life, sight or limb saving or where the patient lacks capacity and immediate treatment is needed to prevent further serious injury to their health (NSW Ministry of Health, 2020). Perioperative nurses need to consider the additional risks for such patients as there will be less time available for the routine checks, administrative processes and patient preparation to be completed before the emergency surgical patient is transferred to the operating suite.

TABLE 7.7
Emergency Surgery Urgency Categorisation System

Priority Level	Timeframe for Surgery (Time From Booking to Arrival in Operating Theatre)	Obstetric Cases	Definition
1	<15 minutes; immediate life threatening	Category 0 and 1 (includes code green)	Immediate life threatening The patient is in immediate risk of loss of life, shocked or moribund, resuscitation not providing positive physiological response
2	<1 hour; life threatening	Category 2	Life threatening The patient has a life-threatening condition, but is responding to resuscitative measures
3	<4 hours; organ/limb-threatening obstetric morbidity	Category 3	Organ/limb-threatening obstetric morbidity The patient is physiologically stable, but there is immediate risk of organ survival or systemic decompensation
4	<8 hours; non-critical, emergent	Includes Category 4	Non-critical, emergent The patient is physiologically stable but the surgical problem may undergo significant deterioration if left untreated
5	<24 hours; non-critical, non-emergent, urgent		Non-critical, non-emergent, urgent The patient's condition is stable No deterioration is expected
6	<48 hours; semi-urgent, not stable for discharge	Category 5	Semi-urgent, not stable for discharge The patient's condition is stable No deterioration is expected but the patient is not suitable to be discharged

(Source: State of Victoria, 2012. A framework for emergency surgery in Victorian public health services. Department of Health and Human Services, State Government of Victoria. Appendix 2, p. 26, Table 1.)

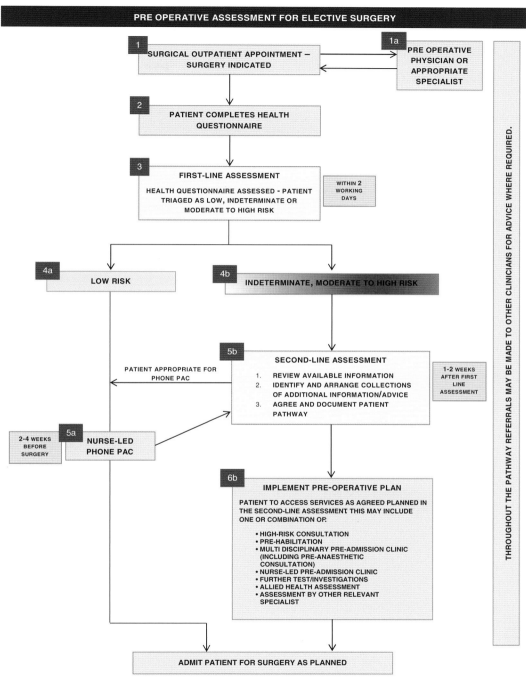

FIG. 7.1 Preoperative assessment pathway for elective surgery. (Source: South Australia Health, 2019. Preoperative pathway for adult elective surgery. SA Health Government of South Australia. Adelaide: Author.)

Queensland Government

Day Surgery Clinical Pathway

Extended day surgery / Day only

Facility: ....

(Affix identification label here)	
URN:	
Family name:	
Given name(s):	
Address:	
Date of birth:	Sex: ☐ M ☐ F ☐ I

» Clinical pathways **never replace clinical judgement.**
» Care outlined in this pathway **must be varied if it is not clinically appropriate** for the individual patient.

Procedure:

Consultant: | Admission date: / / | Time: :

Documentation instructions

- **Initial** - Indicates action / care has been ordered / administered.
- **N/A** - Indicates preceding care / order / recovery phase is not applicable.
- **Crossing out** - Indicates that there is a change in the care outlined. A neat line is to be drawn through the change and initialed.
- **V** - Indicates a variation from the pathway on that day, in that section. When applicable **flag it** in the "Variance column", then document in the free text area as instructed. If this variance occurs more than once daily, document the additional times of the variance in the variance free text area and in the patient's progress notes as applicable.

1		**Admission** ☐ Day case ☐ Overnight stay	Initial	N/A	V
Admissions	1.1	• Pre-admission screen completed and reviewed with patient (refer to MO if required): ☐ Pre-procedure Screening Tool (e.g. SW269) ☐ Day Surgery Agreement - Patient and Carer Responsibilities (e.g. SW331)			
	1.2	• Discharge destination: ☐ Home ☐ Community Care ☐ Residential Care ☐ Other:			
	1.3	• Planned transport home with responsible adult by: ☐ Private Car ☐ Taxi ☐ Public Transport ☐ Community Transport Booked: ☐ Hospital Transport Booked: ☐ Ambulance Booked: ☐ Other: Booked:			
	1.4	• Patient requires: ☐ Medical certificate ☐ Centrelink certificate ☐ Work cover certificate ☐ Travel documentation ☐ Other:			

Signature Log (Every person documenting in this Care Plan **must** supply a sample of their initials and signature below)

Initials	Signature	Print name	Role	Initials	Signature	Print name	Role

DO NOT WRITE IN THIS BINDING MARGIN

DAY SURGERY CLINICAL PATHWAY

FIG. 7.2 Day surgery clinical pathway (excerpt). (Source: Queensland Health. © The State of Queensland (Queensland Health), 2017.)

Queensland Government

Perioperative Patient Record

Facility:

(Affix identification label here)

URN:

Family name:

Given name(s):

Address:

Date of birth: Sex: ☐ M ☐ F ☐ I

Preoperative checklist Patient must not be transferred to operating suite unless Procedural Consent is completed

Date / /	Temp °C	Pulse	Resps	Blood pressure /	BGL mmol/L Time :	O₂ sats

Beta HCG	Weight kg	Height cm	BMI	Pressure injury risk score ☐ Adult ☐ Paediatric	Ward from	Ward to

Check 1 – Preoperative preparation area — Checked / N/A / Variance
Check 2 – Patient handover/transfer — Checked / N/A / Variance
Check 3 – Patient handover/transfer — Checked / N/A / Variance

1 Patient/parent/legal guardian to state full name and DOB; full name DOB and URN match ID band and medical record Patient's preferred name:

2 Procedural Consent Form completed

3 Patient/parent/legal guardian to state procedure in own words, procedure stated corresponds with signed consent form Response:

4 Intended surgical site marked by surgeon

5 X-rays/Medical Imaging/PACS ☐ Queensland Health ☐ Private Number of packets:

ALERTS

6 Allergy status documented ☐ Yes (note on page 2) ☐ Nil known

7 Infection alert ☐ Contact ☐ Droplet ☐ Airborne ☐ MRO Contact operating theatre

8 Cytotoxic medication administered in the last 7 days ☐ Yes (note on page 2) ☐ No

9 Anticoagulant / antiplatelet agent / fish oil administered within the last 7 days ☐ Yes (note on page 2) ☐ No

10 Pregnant ☐ Yes ☐ Suspected/Unknown (document as variance) ☐ No

11 Diabetic status ☐ NIDDM ☐ IDDM

12 Other alerts (e.g. falls, interpreter, aggression) (if yes, document as variance)

13 Fasted Last food intake: / / : hrs Last fluid intake: / / : hrs

14 Pre-medication administered ☐ Yes ☐ No
  Other medication taken ☐ Yes (note on page 2) ☐ No
  Other medication withheld ☐ Yes (note on page 2) ☐ No

15 Haematology documented ☐ Group and hold ☐ INR ☐ Blood cross-match ☐ Blood product refusal

16 Existing implants/prostheses ☐ Yes (note on page 2)

17 Caps/crowns/loose teeth or dentures documented
  ☐ Caps ☐ Crowns ☐ Loose teeth Specify site(s):
  ☐ Dentures: ➔ ☐ Upper ☐ Lower ☐ Partial ☐ Full ☐ Insitu ☐ Remain on ward

18 Preparation ☐ Pre-op shower ☐ Surgical attire
  ☐ Removed/taped: jewellery, body jewellery, hair pins, make-up, nail polish
  - Operation site prepared: ☐ Clip ☐ Bowel prep and return:
  - Anti-embolic devices applied ☐ TEDs™ ☐ SCDs/IPCs ☐ Other:

19 Skin integrity assessed ☐ Rash ☐ Bruise ☐ Tears ☐ Pimples ☐ Pressure injury ☐ Other
  Site:

20 Personal aides/items documented Specify:
  Glasses: ☐ Insitu ☐ Remain on ward Contact lenses: ☐ Removed
  Hearing aid: ☐ Insitu ☐ Remain on ward

21 Passed urine: hrs ☐ IDC insitu ☐ Nappy/Pad

22 Relevant documentation
  ☐ Medical record ☐ Fluid order sheet ☐ Medication chart ☐ Fluid balance chart
  ☐ Diabetic chart ☐ 3 sheets of patient labels ☐ Observation sheet ☐ ECG

23 Patient/parent/legal guardian agrees to clinicians discussing the procedure with the nominated support person ☐ Yes ☐ No
  Support person Name: Phone number:

Ck1	Print name:	Designation:	Signature:	Time: :
Ck2	Print name:	Designation:	Signature:	Time: :
Ck3	Print name:	Designation:	Signature:	Time: :

DO NOT WRITE IN THIS BINDING MARGIN

PERIOPERATIVE PATIENT RECORD

Page 1 of 3

FIG. 7.9 Australian checklist for admission into the OR (excerpt). (Source: Queensland Health. © The State of Queensland (Queensland Health), 2014.)

AUCKLAND
DISTRICT HEALTH BOARD
Te Toka Tumai

Pre-operative Checklist

MUST ATTACH PATIENT LABEL HERE

SURNAME: .... NHI: ....

FIRST NAMES: .... DOB: ....

Please ensure you attach the correct visit patient label

Attach patient label after checking that information matches the Visit Record Front Sheet (CR2685).

Important: Complete the checklist with either a ✓ Yes or ✗ No or N/A and circle as appropriate

Parent or legal guardian present for consent			
Escort person / overnight support			
Currently nursed in isolation? Yes / No		MRSA+ VRE+ ESBL+ TB+ Other	

PATIENT PREPARATION

Ward	Preop	OR	
			Name verbally communicated by patient, if non verbal, identification verified by caregiver / power of attorney
			Identification band cross checked against Front Sheet / Consent
			Surgical / Procedural Agreement to Treatment Form signed and dated
			Anaesthetic Agreement to Treatment Form signed and dated
			Operation site marked
			Patient / Family requests return of body part tissue - CR2547 completed Yes ☐ No ☐
			Interpreter required Language:
			Interpreter: Phone number:
			Patient is oriented / disoriented GCS: E M V
			Impairments: vision / hearing / speech / mobility Aids location: with patient / ward / support person
			Last food (time and date): **Last clear fluid (time and date):**
			Allergies / Adverse Reactions / Alerts Details:
			Medic Alert Bracelet Details:
			Regular medication administered ☐ Withheld for valid medical reason
			Pre-medication given
			Diabetic / metabolic disorder Blood sugar level: Time:
			Medication infusions / Meds due
			Fluid Balance Chart ☐ Medication Chart ☐ 20 patient labels checked against front sheet ☐
			Old notes with patient / electronic Xrays with patient / electronic
			Pre-operative investigations ECG ☐ CT ☐ MRI ☐ US ☐ Other:
			Group and Screen / Cross Match **Date:** **Valid Until:**
			Haematology Results electronic / paper Date:
			Biochemistry Results electronic / paper Date:
			Urine voided (time): Catheter insitu ☐ Bowel prep:
			Possibility of Pregnancy (Y / N) Last Menstrual Period: Pregnancy test: Pos / Neg / Refused
			Skin Integrity intact / broken / bruised / rashes Site:
			Pressure Area Assessment completed (DD3087 or CR3987) Details:
			Teeth natural / chipped / crowns / caps / loose / dentures / full / partial Details:
			Jewellery / Taonga : removed / taped (details):
			Metalware / Implants / Pacemaker
			Clean appropriate pyjamas / gown VTE Risk assessment ☐ Plan Implemented ☐
			Removed: hair clips / nail polish / make up / contact lenses
			Patient property:

Additional Information:		Weight	Temp
		Height	BP
			HR
			Sats
			Resp Rate

	WARD STAFF	PRE-OPERATIVE STAFF	INTRA-OPERATIVE STAFF
Name			
Signature			
Designation			
Date / Time			

P R E O P E R A T I V E   C H E C K L I S T

CR4048

FIG. 7.10 New Zealand checklist for admission into the OR. (Source: Auckland District Health Board © Crown Copyright, 2017.)

CONCLUSION

This chapter has explored the elective surgical patient's journey before they arrive in the operating suite. It has also explored the day surgery model and emergency surgery. The focus has been on patient assessment. Some patients have few comorbidities, whereas others will need to be seen in a pre-admission clinic where thorough investigations will take place to ensure the patient is fit for surgery. Each patient is an individual with their own needs, which need to be valued. Their care needs be a collaborative journey between the patient and the healthcare team. Cultural issues will need to be acknowledged and included in care planning. The preoperative phase becomes crucial in the provision of effective and efficient patient-centred care. Despite the increase in the complexity of surgery, hospital stays and recovery times are getting shorter. This makes the role of the preoperative nurse even more important, because they will need the knowledge and skills to provide the most appropriate care for each patient in a shortened preoperative period.

RESOURCES

Agency for Clinical Innovation
https://www.aci.health.nsw.gov.au
Australian and New Zealand College of Anaesthetists & Faculty of Pain Medicine
https://www.anzca.edu.au
Australian Day Surgery Nurses Association
http://adsna.info
Australian Diabetes Society
https://www.diabetessociety.com.au/position-statements.asp
Australian Institute of Health and Welfare
https://www.aihw.gov.au
British Association of Day Surgery
https://www.bads.co.uk
International Association for Ambulatory Surgery
https://iaas-med.com
New Zealand Health Statistics
https://www.health.govt.nz/nz-health-statistics
Queensland Health Clinical Excellence Division Pre-anaesthetic Evaluation Framework
https://www.clinicalexcellence.qld.gov.au/resources/pre-anaesthetic-evaluation-framework

Interpreter Services

New South Wales https://www.health.nsw.gov.au/multicultural/Pages/default.aspx
New Zealand https://www.healthnavigator.org.nz/languages/i/interpreter-services/
Queensland https://www.forgov.qld.gov.au/find-translator-or-interpreter

REFERENCES

Agency for Clinical Innovation (ACI). (2011). *NSW health emergency surgery implementation project final report October 2011.* PricewaterhouseCoopers. Retrieved from <https://www.aci.health.nsw.gov.au/resources/surgical-services/delivery/predictable-surgery/8>.

Agency for Clinical Innovation (ACI). (2012). High volume short stay surgical model toolkit. GL2012_001. Retrieved from <https://www1.health.nsw.gov.au/pds/Pages/doc.aspx?dn=GL2018_004>.

Agency for Clinical Innovation (ACI). (2016a). Key principles for preoperative fasting: nutrition, anaesthesia perioperative care and endocrine networks. Retrieved from <https://aci.health.nsw.gov.au/__data/assets/pdf_file/0006/299301/ACI_Key_Principles_Preoperative_fasting_in_NSW_public_hospitals.pdf>.

Agency for Clinical Innovation (ACI). (2016b). *FAQs: preoperative oral fluid.* Nutrition, Anaesthesia Perioperative Care and Endocrine Networks. Retrieved from <https://www1.health.nsw.gov.au/pds/Pages/doc.aspx?dn=GL2018_004>.

Agency for Clinical Innovation (ACI). (2018). *The perioperative toolkit.* GL2018_004. Anaesthesia Perioperative Care Network Surgical Services Taskforce. Retrieved from <https://www1.health.nsw.gov.au/pds/Pages/doc.aspx?dn=GL2018_004>.

Agency for Clinical Innovation (ACI). (2019). Care of confused hospitalised older persons (CHOPS). Delirium risk factors [webpage]. Retrieved from <https://aci.health.nsw.gov.au/chops/chops-key-principles/delirium-risk-identification-and-preventive-measures/delirium-risk-factors>.

American College of Obstetricians and Gynecologists (ACOG). (2019). Nonobstetric surgery during pregnancy. ACOG Committee Opinion mo. 775. *Obstetrics and Gynecology, 133,* e285–e286. Retrieved from <https://www.acog.org/clinical/clinical-guidance/committee-opinion/articles/2019/04/nonobstetric-surgery-during-pregnancy>.

American Society of Anesthesiologists (ASA). (2019). ASA Physical Status Classification System. Retrieved from <https://www.asahq.org/standards-and-guidelines/asa-physical-status-classification-system>.

Auckland District Health Board. (2017). Diabetes care for an adult. Retrieved from <https://misur.com/Diabetes_care_of_an_adult.pdf>.

Australian Diabetes Society (ADA) and New Zealand Society for the study of Diabetes. (2020). Periprocedural diabetic ketoacidosis (DKA) with SGLT2 inhibitor use. Retrieved from <https://diabetessociety.com.au/documents/ADS_DKA_SGLT2i_Alert_update_2020.pdf>.

Australian and New Zealand College of Anaesthetists (ANZCA). (2014). Guidelines on smoking as related to the perioperative period. Retrieved from <https://www.anzca.edu.au/safety-advocacy/standards-of-practice/policies,-statements,-and-guidelines>.

Australian and New Zealand College of Anaesthetists (ANZCA). (2017). *PS07. Guidelines on pre-anaesthesia consultation and patient preparation.* Australian and New Zealand College of Anaesthetists and Faculty of Pain Medicine. Retrieved from

<https://www.anzca.edu.au/safety-advocacy/standards-of-practice/policies,-statements,-and-guidelines>.

Australian and New Zealand College of Anaesthetists (ANZCA). (2018a). *PS15 Guidelines for the perioperative care of patients selected for day stay procedures*. Australian and New Zealand College of Anaesthetists and Faculty of Pain Medicine. Retrieved from <https://www.anzca.edu.au/safety-advocacy/standards-of-practice/policies,-statements,-and-guidelines>.

Australian and New Zealand College of Anaesthetists (ANZCA). (2018b). Clinical audit guide for perioperative normothermia. Retrieved from <https://www.anzca.edu.au/safety-advocacy/standards-of-practice/policies,-statements,-and-guidelines>.

Australian and New Zealand College of Anaesthetists (ANZCA). (2019). *PS29 Guidelines for the provision of anaesthesia care to children*. Australian and New Zealand College of Anaesthetists and Faculty of Pain Medicine. Retrieved from <https://www.anzca.edu.au/safety-advocacy/standards-of-practice/policies,-statements,-and-guidelines>.

Australian and New Zealand College of Anaesthetists, Australian and New Zealand Anaesthetic Allergy Group (ANZCA/ANZAAG). (2016a). Perioperative anaphylaxis management guidelines background paper. Retrieved from <http://www.anzaag.com/Mgmt%20Resources.aspx>.

Australian and New Zealand College of Anaesthetists, Australian and New Zealand Anaesthetic Allergy Group (ANZCA/ANZAAG). (2016b). Perioperative anaphylaxis management guidelines. Retrieved from <http://www.anzaag.com/Mgmt%20Resources.aspx>.

Australian College of Perianaesthesia Nurses (ACPAN). (2020). PG01 Perioperative hypothermia prevention and management guideline. Retrieved from <https://acpan.edu.au/pdfs/acpan-guideline-pg01-perioperative-hypothermia-prevention-and-management-guideline.pdf>.

Australian College of Perioperative Nurses (ACORN). (2020a). Preoperative patient assessment and education nurse. In *ACORN standards for perioperative nursing* (16th ed., Vol. 2). Adelaide: Author.

Australian College of Perioperative Nurses (ACORN). (2020b). Documentation and patient information management. In *ACORN standards for perioperative nursing* (16th ed., Vol. 1). Adelaide: Author.

Australian College of Perioperative Nurses (ACORN). (2020c). Cultural diversity. In *ACORN standards for perioperative nursing* (16th ed., Vol. 2). Adelaide: Author.

Australian College of Perioperative Nurses (ACORN). (2020d). Disposal of human tissue and explanted items. In *ACORN standards for perioperative nursing* (16th ed., Vol. 1). Adelaide: Author.

Australian College of Perioperative Nurses (ACORN). (2020e). Manual handling. In *ACORN standards for perioperative nursing* (16th ed., Vol. 1). Adelaide: Author.

Australian College of Perioperative Nurses (ACORN). (2020f). Patient positioning. In *ACORN standards for perioperative nursing* (16th ed., Vol. 1). Adelaide: Author.

Australian College of Perioperative Nurses (ACORN). (2020g). Preoperative patient skin antisepsis. In *ACORN standards for perioperative nursing* (16th ed., Vol. 1). Adelaide: Author.

Australian College of Perioperative Nurses (ACORN). (2020h). Hypothermia. In *ACORN standards for perioperative nursing* (16th ed., Vol. 1). Adelaide: Author.

Australian Commission on Safety and Quality in Health Care (ACSQHC/the Commission). (2016). *Delirium clinical care standard*. Sydney: Author. Retrieved from <https://www.safetyandquality.gov.au/our-work/clinical-care-standards/delirium-clinical-care-standard>.

Australian Commission on Safety and Quality in Health Care (ACSQHC/the Commission). (2017a). *Comprehensive care standard*. Sydney: Author. Retrieved from <https://www.safetyandquality.gov.au/standards/nsqhs-standards/comprehensive-care-standard>.

Australian Commission on Safety and Quality in Health Care (ACSQHC/the Commission). (2017b). *Communicating for safety standard*. Sydney: Author. Retrieved from <https://www.safetyandquality.gov.au/standards/nsqhs-standards/communicating-safety-standard>.

Australian Commission on Safety and Quality in Health Care (ACSQHC/the Commission). (2017c). *Specifications for a standard patient identification band*. FAQs. Sydney: Author. Retrieved from <https://www.safetyandquality.gov.au/our-work/communicating-safety/patient-identification/specification-standard-patient-identification-band>.

Australian Commission on Safety and Quality in Health Care (ACSQHC/the Commission). (2018). *Venous thromboembolism prevention clinical care standard*. Sydney: Author. Retrieved from <https://www.safetyandquality.gov.au/our-work/clinical-care-standards/venous-thromboembolism-prevention-clinical-care-standard>.

Australian Commission on Safety and Quality in Health Care (ACSQHC/the Commission). (2020a). *Informed consent in health care: fact sheet for clinicians*. September 2020. Sydney: ACSQHC. Retrieved from <https://www.safetyandquality.gov.au/publications-and-resources/resource-library/informed-consent-fact-sheet-clinicians>.

Australian Commission on Safety and Quality in Health Care (ACSQHC/the Commission). (2020b). *Comprehensive care standard: screening and assessment for risk of harm*. AS18/14 version 3.0, October 2020. Sydney: Author. Retrieved from <https://www.safetyandquality.gov.au/publications-and-resources/resource-library/as1814-comprehensive-care-standard-screening-and-assessment-risk-harm>.

Australian Commission on Safety and Quality in Health Care (ACSQHC/the Commission). (2020c). *Fact sheet: NSQHS standards – preventing pressure injuries and wound management*. Sydney: Author. Retrieved from <https://www.safetyandquality.gov.au/publications-and-resources/resource-library/nsqhs-standards-preventing-pressure-injuries-and-wound-management>.

Australian Commission on Safety and Quality in Health Care (ACSQHC/the Commission). (2020d). *Colonoscopy clinical care standard*. Sydney: Author. First released 2018. Updated (minor revisions) January 2020. Retrieved from <https://www.safetyandquality.gov.au/standards/clinical-care-standards/colonoscopy-clinical-care-standard>.

Australian Day Surgery Nurses Association (ADSNA). (2018). *Best practice guidelines for ambulatory surgery and procedures.* Osborne Park: Cambridge Publishing.

Australian Diabetes Society. (2012). Peri-operative diabetes management guidelines July 2012. Retrieved from <https://diabetessociety.com.au/documents/PerioperativeDiabetesManagementGuidelinesFINALCleanJuly2012.pdf>.

Australian Diabetes Society. (2016). The Australian Obesity Management Algorithm. Statement developed with the Australian and New Zealand Obesity Society and the Obesity Surgery Society of Australian and New Zealand. Retrieved from <http://diabetessociety.com.au/position-statements.asp>.

Australian Diabetes Society (ADS). (2020). Periprocedural diabetic ketoacidosis (DKA) with SGLT2 inhibitor use. Alert Update January 2020. Australian Diabetes Society and New Zealand Society for the study of Diabetes. Retrieved from <https://diabetessociety.com.au/documents/ADS_DKA_SGLT2i_Alert_update_2020.pdf>.

Australian Health Ministers' Advisory Council (AHMAC). (2015). National elective surgery urgency guideline – April 2015. Retrieved from <http://www.coaghealthcouncil.gov.au/Portals/0/National%20Elective%20Surgery%20Categorisation%20-%20Guideline%20-%20April%202015.pdf>.

Australian Health Ministers' Advisory Council (AHMAC). (2016). Cultural respect framework 2016–2026. Retrieved from <https://www1.health.gov.au/internet/main/publishing.nsf/Content/indigenous-crf>.

Australian Institute of Health and Welfare (AIHW). (2020a). *Australia's hospitals at a glance 2018–19.* Cat. no. HSE 247. Canberra: Author. Retrieved from <https://www.aihw.gov.au/reports/hospitals/australias-hospitals-at-a-glance-2018-19/contents/summary>.

Australian Institute of Health and Welfare (AIHW). (2020b). *Older Australians at a glance.* Cat. no. AGE 87. Canberra: Author. Retrieved from <https://www.aihw.gov.au/reports/older-people/older-australia-at-a-glance>.

Australian Institute of Health and Welfare (AIHW). (2020c). Health risk factors among Indigenous Australians. Snapshot. [webpage]. Retrieved from <https://www.aihw.gov.au/reports/australias-health/health-risk-factors-among-indigenous-australians>.

Australian Institute of Health and Welfare (AIHW). (2020d). *Diabetes.* Cat. no. CVD 82. Canberra: AIHW. Retrieved from <https://www.aihw.gov.au/reports/diabetes/diabetes>.

Australian Institute of Health and Welfare (AIHW). (2020e). Tobacco smoking. Snapshot [webpage]. Retrieved from <https://www.aihw.gov.au/reports/australias-health/tobacco-smoking>.

Australian Institute of Health and Welfare (AIHW). (2020f). Overweight and obesity. Snapshot [webpage]. Retrieved from <https://www.aihw.gov.au/reports/australias-health/overweight-and-obesity>.

Australian Medical Association (AMA). (2015). Tobacco smoking and E-cigarettes – 2015. The AMA position. Retrieved from <https://ama.com.au/position-statement/tobacco-smoking-and-e-cigarettes-2015>.

Australian Tissue Donation Network. (2019). About us [webpage]. Retrieved from <https://tissuedonationnetwork.org.au/about/>.

Bailey, C. R., Ahuja, M., Bartholomew, K., Bew, S., Forbes, L., Lipp, A., . . . Stocker, M. (2019). Guidelines for day-case surgery 2019. *Anaesthesia, 74,* 778–792. https://dx.doi.org/10.1111/anae.14639

Ball, K. A. (2018). Surgical modalities. In J. C. Rothrock (Ed.), *Alexander's care of the patient in surgery* (16th ed., pp. 201–243). St. Louis, MO: Elsevier Mosby.

Bock, M., Fritsch, G., & Hepner, D. L. (2016). Preoperative laboratory testing. *Anesthesiology Clinics, 34*(1), 43–58.

Canterbury District Health Board (CDHB). (2016). Volume 11: Clinical return of tissue/body parts to patients. Retrieved from <http://edu.cdhb.health.nz/Hospitals-Services/Health-Professionals/CDHB-Policies/Clinical-Manual/Documents/4632-Return-body-tissue-parts.pdf>.

Carrick, M., Robson, J., & Thomas, C. (2019). Smoking and anaesthesia. *British Journal of Anaesthesia Education, 19*(1), 1–6.

Chung, F., Memtsoudis, S. G., Ramachandran, S. K., Nagappa, M., Opperer, M., Cozowicz, C. . . . Auckley, D. (2016). Society of anesthesia and sleep medicine guidelines on preoperative screening and assessment of adult patients with obstructive sleep apnea. *Anesthesia and Analgesia, 123,* 452–473.

Commonwealth of Australia, Department of Health. (2017). My life my lead – opportunities for strengthening approaches to the social determinants and cultural determinants of Indigenous health: report on the national consultations December 2017. Retrieved from <https://www1.health.gov.au/internet/main/publishing.nsf/Content/indigenous-ipag-consultation>.

Commonwealth of Australia, Department of Health. (2019). *National framework for alcohol, tobacco and other drug treatment 2019–2029.* Department of Health. Retrieved from <https://www.health.gov.au/health-topics/smoking-and-tobacco>.

Conway, A., Rolley, J., & Sutherland, J. R. (2016). Cochrane review. Midazolam for sedation before procedures. Retrieved from <https://www.cochrane.org/CD009491/EMERG_midazolam-sedation-procedures>.

Cowperthwaite, L., & Holm, R.L. (2015). Guideline implementation: preoperative patient skin antisepsis. *AORN Journal, 101*(1), 72–77. https://dx.doi.org/10.1016/j.aorn.2014.11.009

Crawford, T., Candlin, S., & Roger, P. (2017). New perspectives on understanding cultural diversity. *Collegian, 24*(1), 63–69. https://dx.doi.org/10.1016/j.colegn.2015.09.001

Culley, D. J., Flaherty, D., Fahey, M. C., Rudolph, J. L., Javedan, H., Huang, C. C., ... Crosby, G. (2017). Poor performance on a preoperative cognitive screening test predicts postoperative complications in older orthopedic surgical patients. *Anesthesiology, 127*(5), 765–774.

Dagli, R., Kocaoglu, N., Bayir, H., Hakki, M., & Doylan, M. R. (2016). Evaluation of medical drug and herbal product use before anesthesia. *International Journal of Clinical and Experimental Medicine, 9*(2), 4670–4674.

Dai, Y., & Livesley, J. (2018). A mixed-method systematic review of the effectiveness and acceptability of preoperative psychological preparation programmes to reduce paediatric preoperative anxiety in elective surgery. *Journal of Advanced Nursing, 74*, 2022–2037. https://dx.doi.org/10.1111/jan.13713

Daiello, L. A., Racine, A. M., Yun Gou, R., Marcantonio, E. R., Xie, Z., Kunze, L. J., . . . Jones, R. N. (2019). Postoperative delirium and postoperative cognitive dysfunction: overlap and divergence. *Anesthesiology, 131*(3), 477–491.

DeFroda, S. F., Lamin, E., Gil, J. A., Sindhu, K., & Ritterman, S. (2016). Antibiotic prophylaxis for patients with a history of total joint replacement. *Journal of the American Board of Family Medicine, 29*, 500–507.

Department of Health, Government of Western Australia. (2020). Release of human tissue and explanted medical devices policy. MP 0129/20. Retrieved from <https://ww2.health.wa.gov.au/About-us/Policy-frameworks/Public-Health/Mandatory-requirements/Regulatory/Release-of-Human-Tissue-and-Explanted-Medical-Devices-Policy>.

Donoghue, T. J. (2018). Herbal medications and anesthesia case management. *Journal of American Association of Nurse Anesthetists, 86*(3), 142–248.

Dumville, J. C., McFarlane, E., Edwards, P., Lipp, A., & Holmes, A. (2013). Preoperative skin antiseptics for preventing surgical wound infections after clean surgery. *Cochrane Database of Systematic Reviews, 28*(3), CD003949. https://dx.doi.org/10.1002/14651858.CD003949.pub3

Eamer, G., Al-Amoodi, M. J. H., Holroyd-Leduc, J., Rolfson, D. B., Warkentin, L. M., & Khadaroo, R.G. (2018). Review of risk assessment tools to predict morbidity and mortality in elderly surgical patients. *American Journal of Surgery, 216*(3), 585–594. https://dx.doi.org/10.1016/j.amjsurg.2018.04.006. Epub 2018 Apr 18.PMID: 29776643.

Edmiston, C. E., Jr., & Leaper, D. (2017). Should preoperative showering or cleansing with chlorhexidine gluconate (CHG) be part of the surgical care bundle to prevent surgical site infection? *Journal of Infection Prevention, 18*(6), 311–314. https://dx.doi.org/10.1177/1757177417714873

Global BMI Mortality Collaboration, di Angelantonio, E., Bhupathiraju, S. N., Wormser, D., Gao P., Kaptoge, S., . . . Hu, F. (2016). Body-mass index and all-cause mortality: individual-participant-data meta-analysis of 239 prospective studies in four continents. *The Lancet, 388*, 776–786.

Gray, L., Stubbe, M., Macdonald, L., Tester, R., Hilder, J., & Dowell, A. C. (2018). A taboo topic? How general practitioners talk about overweight and obesity in New Zealand. *Journal of Primary Health Care, 10*(2), 150–158.

Guenther, U., Riedel, L., & Radtke, F. M. (2016). Patients prone for postoperative delirium: preoperative assessment, perioperative prophylaxis, postoperative treatment. *Current Opinion in Anaesthesiology, 29*(3), 384–390.

Hassan, C., East, J., Radaelli, F., Spada, C., Benamouzig, R., Bisschops, R., . . . Dumonceau, J.-M. (2019). Bowel preparation for colonoscopy: ESGE guideline – update 2019. *Endoscopy, 51*(08), 775–794. https://dx.doi.org/10.1055/a-0959-0505. Retrieved from <https://www.thieme-connect.de/products/ejournals/abstract/10.1055/a-0959-0505>.

He, J., llego, B., Stubbs, C., Scott, A., Dawson, S., Forrest, K., & Kennedy, C. (2018). Improving patient flow and satisfaction: an evidence-based pre-admission clinic and transfer of care pathway for elective surgery patients. *Collegian, 25*(2), 149–156. https://dx.doi.org/10.1016/j.colegn.2017.04.006

Health Navigator. (2019). Interpreter services [webpage]. Retrieved from <https://www.healthnavigator.org.nz/languages/i/interpreter-services/#Overview>.

Health Quality and Safety Commission New Zealand (HQSCNZ). (2014). Guidelines: clipping not shaving intervention guidelines. Retrieved from <https://www.hqsc.govt.nz/our-programmes/infection-prevention-and-control/publications-and-resources/publication/1392/>.

Hines, S., Munday, J., & Kynoch, K. (2015). Effectiveness of nurse-led preoperative assessment services for elective surgery: a systematic review update. *JBI Database of Systematic Reviews and Implementation Reports, 13*(6), 279–317. https://dx.doi.org/10.11124/jbisrir-2015-1996

Joanna Briggs Institute. (2016a). JBI evidence summary. Hospital: patient pre-admission. Joanna Briggs Institute EBP Database, JBI@Ovid. JBI820.

Joanna Briggs Institute. (2016b). Recommended practice. Pre-operative nursing care. Joanna Briggs Institute EBP Database, JBI@Ovid. JBI820.

Joint British Diabetes Societies for Inpatient Care. (2016). Management of adults with diabetes undergoing surgery and elective procedures: improving standards [Internet]. Retrieved from <https://abcd.care/sites/abcd.care/files/resources/Surgical_guidelines_2015_full_FINAL_amended_Mar_2016.pdf>.

Kamdar, N. V., Huverserian, A., Jalilian, L., Thi, W., Duval, V., Beck, L., ... Cannesson, M. (2020). Development, implementation, and evaluation of a telemedicine preoperative evaluation initiative at a major academic medical center. *Anesthesia and Analgesia, 31*(6), 1647–1656. https://dx.doi.org/10.1213/ANE.0000000000005208

Kamel, C., McGahan, L., Polisena, J., Mierzwinski-Urban, M., & Embil, J. M. (2012). Preoperative skin antiseptic preparations for preventing surgical site infections: a systematic review. *Infection Control and Hospital Epidemiology, 33*(6), 608–617. https://dx.doi.org/10.1086/665723

Kassai, B., Rabilloud, M., Dantony, E., Grousson, S., Revol, O., Malik, S., ... Pereira de Souza Neto, E. (2016). Introduction of a paediatric anaesthesia comic information leaflet reduced preoperative anxiety in children. *British Journal of Anaesthesia, 117*(1), 95–102.

Kim, S., Brooks, A. K., & Groban, L. (2015). Preoperative assessment of the older surgical patient: honing in on geriatric syndromes. *Clinical Interventions in Aging, 10*, 13.

Koivisto, J. M., Saarinen, I., Kaipia, A., Puukka, P., Kivinen, K., Laine, K. M., & Haavisto, E. (2019). Patient education in relation to informational needs and postoperative complications in surgical patients. *International Journal for Quality in Health Care, 32*(1), 35–40. https://dx.doi.org/10.1093/intqhc/mzz032

Kuzulugil, D., Papeix, G., Luu, J., & Kerridge, R. K. (2019). Recent advances in diabetes treatments and their perioperative implications. *Current Opinion in Anaesthesiology, 32*(3), 398–404. https://dx.doi.org/10.1097/ACO.0000000000000735

Lee, P. C., & Dixon, J. (2017). Bariatric–metabolic surgery: a guide for the primary care physician. *Australian Family Physician, 46*(7), 465–447.

Lee, W.-J., & Almalki, O. (2017). Recent advancements in bariatric/metabolic surgery. *Annals of Gastroenterological Surgery, 1,* 171–179.

Leite, K. A., Hobgood, T., Hill, B., & Muckler, V. C. (2019). Reducing preventable surgical cancellations: improving the preoperative anesthesia interview process. *Journal of PeriAnesthesia Nursing, 34*(5),929–937. https://dx.doi.org/10.1016/j.jopan.2019.02.001

Liu, P. P., Sun, Y., Wu, C., Xu, W. H., Zhang, R. D., Zheng, J. J., . . . Wu, J. Z. (2018). The effectiveness of transport in a toy car for reducing preoperative anxiety in preschool children: a randomised controlled prospective trial. *British Journal of Anaesthesia, 121*(2), 438–444.

Malley, A., Kenner, C., Kim, T., & Blakeney, B. (2015). The role of the nurse and the preoperative assessment in patient transitions. *AORN Journal, 102*(2), 181.e1–181.e1819. https://dx.doi.org/10.1016/j.aorn.2015.06.004

Martin, S. K., & Cifu, A. S. (2017). Routine preoperative laboratory tests for elective surgery. *Journal of the American Medical Association, 318*(6), 567–568.

Mihalj, M., Carrel, T., Gregoric, I. D., Andereggen, L., Zinn, P. O., Doll, D., ... Luedi, M. M. (2020). Telemedicine for preoperative assessment during a COVID-19 pandemic: recommendations for clinical care. *Best practice & research. Clinical Anaesthesiology, 34*(2), 345–351. https://dx.doi.org/10.1016/j.bpa.2020.05.001

Ministry of Health. (2014). Background and recommendations of the New Zealand guidelines for helping people to stop smoking. Retrieved from <https://www.health.govt.nz/system/files/documents/publications/background-recommendations-new-zealand-guidelines-for-helping-stop-smoking-mar15-v2.pdf>.

Ministry of Health – Manatū Hauora. (2019a). The New Zealand guidelines for helping people to stop smoking. Retrieved from <https://www.health.govt.nz/publication/new-zealand-guidelines-helping-people-stop-smoking>.

Ministry of Health – Manatū Hauora. (2019b). Annual data explorer 2018/19: New Zealand Health Survey [data file]. Retrieved from <https://minhealthnz.shinyapps.io/nz-health-survey-2018-19-annual-data-explorer>.

Mistry, P. K., Gaunay, G. S., & Hoenig, D. M. (2017). Prediction of surgical complications in the elderly: can we improve outcomes? *Asian Journal of Urology, 4*(1), 44–49.

Mitchell, M. (2017). Day surgery nurses' selection of patient preoperative information. *Journal of Clinical Nursing, 26*(1–2), 225–237

Mullen-Fortino, M., Rising, K. L., Duckworth, J., Gwynn, V., Sites, F. D., & Hollander, J. E. (2019). Presurgical assessment using telemedicine technology: impact on efficiency, effectiveness, and patient experience of care. *Telemedicine Journal and e-Health, 25*(2), 137–142. https://dx.doi.org/10.1089/tmj.2017.0133

National Institute for Health and Care Excellence (NICE). (2016). *Hypothermia: prevention and management in adults having surgery: clinical guideline [CG65].* UK: Author.

National Pressure Ulcer Advisory Panel, European Pressure Ulcer Advisory Panel and Pan Pacific Pressure Injury Alliance (NPUAP/EPUAP/PPPIA). (2019). *Prevention and treatment of pressure ulcers/injuries. Quick reference guide* [e-book]. Retrieved from: <https://pppia.org/guideline/>.

Nelson, O., Quinn, T. D., Arriaga, A. F., Hepner, D. L., Lipsitz, S. R., Cooper, Z., . . . Bader, A. M. (2016). A model for better leveraging the point of preoperative assessment: patients and providers look beyond operative indications when making decisions. *A & A Case Reports, 6*(8), 241–248.

New Zealand Health and Disability Commissioner. (2020). The Code of Health and Disability Services Consumers' Rights (The Code) Regulations 1996. Retrieved from <https://www.hdc.org.nz/your-rights/about-the-code/code-of-health-and-disability-services-consumers-rights/>.

Nicholson, A., Coldwell, C. M., Lewis, S. R., & Smith, A. F. (2013). Nurse-led versus doctor-led preoperative assessment for elective surgical patients requiring regional or general anaesthesia. *Cochrane Database of Systematic Reviews, 11,* CD010160. https://dx.doi.org/10.1002/14651858.CD010160.pub2

Nightingale, C. E., Margarson, M. P., Shearer, E., Redman, J. W., Lucas, D. N., Cousins, J. M., . . . Ireland Society for Obesity and Bariatric Anaesthesia. (2015). Peri-operative management of the obese surgical patient 2015: Association of Anaesthetists of Great Britain and Ireland Society for Obesity and Bariatric Anaesthesia. *Anaesthesia, 70*(7), 859–876.

NSW Health Clinical Excellence Commission (NSW CEC). (2018). Patient safety programs, VTE risk assessment tool. Retrieved from <http://www.cec.health.nsw.gov.au/__data/assets/pdf_file/0010/458821/Venous-Thromboembolism-VTE-Risk-Assessment-Tool.pdf>.

NSW Ministry of Health. (2009). GL 2009_009 New South Wales health emergency surgery guideline. Retrieved from <https://www1.health.nsw.gov.au/pds/Pages/doc.aspx?dn=GL2009_009>.

NSW Ministry of Health. (2010). Guidelines for the care of children and adolescents in acute care settings – PD2010_034. Retrieved from <https://hospitals.sydney/kidsfamilies/paediatric/Pages/policies-and-guidelines.aspx>.

NSW Ministry of Health. (2014). *PD2014_024 Patient identification bands.* Sydney: Author. Retrieved from <https://www1.health.nsw.gov.au/pds/Pages/doc.aspx?dn=PD2014_024>.

NSW Ministry of Health. (2016). Tool 3. Assessing nicotine dependence. Tools for health professionals [webpage]. Retrieved from <https://www.health.nsw.gov.au/tobacco/Pages/tools-for-health-professionals.aspx>.

NSW Ministry of Health. (2017a). PD2017_044 Interpreters – standard procedures for working with health care interpreters. Retrieved from <https://www1.health.nsw.gov.au/pds/ActivePDSDocuments/PD2017_044.pdf>.

NSW Ministry of Health. (2017b). Policy directive: clinical procedure safety PD2017_032. Retrieved from <https://www1.health.nsw.gov.au/pds/Pages/doc.aspx?dn=PD2017_032>.

NSW Ministry of Health. (2020). Consent to medical and healthcare treatment manual. Retrieved from <https://www.health.nsw.gov.au/policies/manuals/Pages/consent-manual.aspx>.

Nursing and Midwifery Board of Australia. (2018). Fact sheet: Code of conduct for nurses and Code of conduct for midwives. Retrieved from <https://www.nursingmidwiferyboard.gov.au/Codes-Guidelines-Statements/FAQ/Fact-sheet-Code-of-conduct-for-nurses-and-Code-of-conduct-for-midwives.aspx>.

O'Neill, F., Carter, E., Pink, N., & Smith, I. (2016). Routine preoperative tests for elective surgery: summary of updated NICE guidance. *British Medical Journal (Clinical research ed.)*, 354, i3292. https://dx.doi.org/10.1136/bmj.i3292

Organ and Tissue Authority. (2019). *Australian donation and transplantation activity report 2019*. Australian Government. Retrieved from <https://donatelife.gov.au/about-donation/frequently-asked-questions/facts-and-statistics>.

Phillips, N., & Hornacky, A. (2020). *Berry & Kohn's operating room technique* (14th ed.). St. Louis, MO: Elsevier.

Rasmussen, A. S., Christiansen, C. F., Uldbjerg, N., & Nørgaard, M. (2019). Obstetric and non-obstetric surgery during pregnancy: a 20-year Danish population-based prevalence study. *British Medical Journal Open*, 9, e028136. https://dx.doi.org/10.1136/bmjopen-2018-028136

Riley, C., & Andrzejowski, J. (2018). Inadvertent perioperative hypothermia. *British Journal of Anaesthesia*, 18, 227–233. https://dx.doi.org/10.1016/j.bjae.2018.05.003

Royal Australasian College of Surgeons (RACS). (2018). News, media releases and advocacy. Cessation of smoking [webpage]. Retrieved from <https://www.surgeons.org/News/Advocacy/2015-06-12-cessation-of-smoking>.

Rubino, F., Shukla, A., Pomp, A., Moreira, M., Ahn, S. M., & Dakin, G. (2014). Bariatric, metabolic, and diabetes surgery: what's in a name? *Annals of Surgery, 259*(1), 117–122. https://dx.doi.org/10.1097/SLA.0b013e3182759656

Rusk, M. H. (2016). Avoiding unnecessary preoperative testing. *Medical Clinics of North America*, 100(5), 1003–1008. https://dx.doi.org/10.1016/j.mcna.2016.04.011. PMID: 27542420.

Shetler, M. (1972). Operating room nurses go visiting. *American Journal of Nursing*, 72(7), 1266–1269. https://dx.doi.org/10.2307/3422454

Smith, F.D. (2016). Caring for surgical patients with piercings. AORN Journal, 103(6), 583-596. Retrieved from <https://doi.org/10.1016/j.aorn.2016.04.005>.

South Australia Health. (2019). *Pathway for pre-operative assessment for booked adult elective surgery*. Adelaide: Author. Retrieved from <https://www.sahealth.sa.gov.au/wps/wcm/connect/public+content/sa+health+internet/clinical+resources/clinical+programs+and+practice+guidelines/elective+surgery/pre-operative+assessment+for+booked+adult+elective+surgery>.

Stålberg, A., Sandberg, A., Coyne, I., Larsson, T., & Söderbäck, M. (2019). Using an interactive communication tool in healthcare situations: patterns in young children's use of participation cues. *Journal of Child Health Care, 23*(4), 613–625. https://dx.doi.org/10.1177/1367493518814928

State of Queensland (Queensland Government). (2020). Find a translator or interpreter [webpage]. Retrieved from <https://www.forgov.qld.gov.au/find-translator-or-interpreter>.

State of Queensland (Queensland Health). (2014). Statewide Anaesthesia and Perioperative Care Clinical Network (SWAPNET) guideline – 23 hour ward admission criteria. Retrieved from <https://clinicalexcellence.qld.gov.au/resources/service-delivery-models/23-hour-ward>.

State of Queensland (Queensland Health). (2017). *Emergency surgery access guideline*. Clinical Excellence Division Healthcare Improvement Unit. Retrieved from <https://www.health.qld.gov.au/__data/assets/pdf_file/0033/635784/qh-gdl-440.pdf>.

State of Queensland (Queensland Health). (2018). *Queensland hospital admission guidelines*. Queensland Hospital Admitted Patient Data Collection (QHAPDC) manual appendix F 2018–2019 v2.0. Retrieved from <https://www.health.qld.gov.au/hsu/collections/qhapdc>.

State of Victoria. (2012). *A framework for emergency surgery in Victorian public health services*. Department of Health and Human Services, State Government of Victoria. Retrieved from <https://www2.health.vic.gov.au/getfile/?sc_itemid=%7bF0CEB373-020C-4CB0-927E-FF7D911F6FAE%7d&title=A%20framework%20for%20emergency%20surgery%20in%20Victorian%20public%20health%20services>.

State of Victoria. (2020). *Assessment and ageing* [webpage]. Department of Health and Human Services, State Government of Victoria. Retrieved from <https://www2.health.vic.gov.au/hospitals-and-health-services/patient-care/older-people/comm-topics/assessment/assessment-ageing>.

Swihart, D. L., Yarrarapu, S. N. S., & Martin, R. L. (2020). Cultural religious competence in clinical practice. In *StatPearls* [online]. Treasure Island, FL: StatPearls Publishing. Retrieved from <https://pubmed.ncbi.nlm.nih.gov/29630268/>.

Sydney Children's Hospitals Network (SCHN). (2018a). *Anaesthesia: parents attending the induction of – CHW*. Policy no.: 2006-8179 v5. Retrieved from <https://www.schn.health.nsw.gov.au/_policies/pdf/2006-8179.pdf>.

Sydney Children's Hospitals Network (SCHN). (2018b). *Preparing a patient for surgery – CHW*. Guideline no.: 2006-8073 v4. Retrieved from <https://www.schn.health.nsw.gov.au/_policies/pdf/2006-8073.pdf>.

Sydney Children's Hospitals Network (SCHN). (2019). Fact sheet. Medical play. Retrieved from <https://www.schn.health.nsw.gov.au/fact-sheets/medical-play>.

Tong, F., Dannaway, J., Enke, O., & Eslick, G. (2020). Effect of preoperative psychological interventions on elective orthopaedic surgery outcomes: a systematic review and meta-analysis. *Australian and New Zealand Journal of Surgery, 90*(3), 230–236. https://dx.doi.org/10.1111/ans.15332.

Tran, H. A., Gibbs, H., Merriman, E., Curnow, J. L., Young, L., Bennett, A., . . . Nandurkar, H. (2019). New guidelines from the thrombosis and haemostasis society of Australia and New Zealand for the diagnosis and management of venous thromboembolism. *Medical Journal of Australia, 210*, 227–235. https://dx.doi.org/10.5694/mja2.50004

Tsai, A., & Schumann, R. (2016). Morbid obesity and perioperative complications. *Current Opinion in Anaesthesiology, 29*(1), 103–108.

Turunen, E., Miettinen, M., Setälä, L., & Vehviläinen-Julkunen, K. (2017). An integrative review of a preoperative nursing care structure. *Journal of Clinical Nursing, 26*(7–8), 915–930. https://dx.doi.org/10.1111/jocn.13448

Turunen, E., Miettinen, M., Setälä, L., & Vehviläinen-Julkunen, K. (2018). The impact of a structured preoperative protocol on day of surgery cancellations. *Journal of Clinical Nursing, 27*, 288–305. https://dx.doi.org/10.1111/jocn.13896

Upadya, M., & Saneesh P. J. (2016). Anaesthesia for non-obstetric surgery during pregnancy. *Indian Journal of Anaesthesia, 60*(4), 234–241. Retrieved from <https://www.wfsahq.org/components/com_virtual_library/media/778ea9709529109c62d9c62b9e339d92-Update-34-Anaes-Non-obs-Surgery-in-Pregnancy.pdf>.

Vujic, J., Marsoner, K., Lipp-Pump, A. H., Klaritsch, P., Mischinger, H. J., & Kornprat, P. (2019). Non-obstetric surgery during pregnancy – an eleven-year retrospective analysis. *BMC Pregnancy Childbirth, 19*, 382. https://dx.doi.org/10.1186/s12884-019-2554-6

Waitemata District Health Board (WDHB). (2018a). *Toolkit for working in a culturally diverse workplace.* Auckland: Author, eCALD® Services. Retrieved from <http://www.ecald.com/Resources/Cross-Cultural-Resources>.

Waitemata District Health Board (WDHB). (2018b). *Cross-cultural resource for health practitioners.* Auckland: Author, eCALD® Services. Retrieved from <http://www.ecald.com/Resources/Cross-Cultural-Resources>.

Watson, J. (2018). Inadvertent postoperative hypothermia prevention: passive versus active warming methods. *Journal of Perioperative Nursing, 31*(1), 43–43. https://dx.doi.org/10.26550/2209-1092.1025

Webb, M. P., Helander, E. M., Meyn, A. R., Flynn, T., Urman, R. D., & Kaye, A. D. (2018). Preoperative assessment of the pregnant patient undergoing nonobstetric surgery. *Anesthesiology Clinics, 36*(4), 627–637. https://dx.doi.org/10.1016/j.anclin.2018.07.010

Webster, J., & Osborne, S. (2015). Preoperative bathing or showering with skin antiseptics to prevent surgical site infection. *Cochrane Database of Systematic Reviews, 2*, CD004985. https://dx.doi.org/10.1002/14651858.CD004985.pub5

Wilson, C. J., Mitchelson, A. J., Tzeng, T. H., El-Othmani, M. M., Saleh, J., Vasdev, S., . . . Saleh, K. J. (2016). Caring for the surgically anxious patient: a review of the interventions and a guide to optimizing surgical outcomes. *American Journal of Surgery, 212*(1), 151–159.

World Allergy Organization. (2019) Perioperative allergic reactions. Retrieved from <https://www.worldallergy.org/education-and-programs/education/allergic-disease-resource-center/professionals/allergy-to-anesthetic-agents>.

World Health Organization (WHO). (2020a). Body mass index (BMI) [webpage]. Retrieved from <https://www.who.int/data/gho/data/themes/theme-details/GHO/body-mass-index-(bmi)?introPage=intro_3.html>.

World Health Organization (WHO). (2020b). Obesity and overweight [fact sheet]. Retrieved from <https://www.who.int/news-room/fact-sheets/detail/obesity-and-overweight>.

Young-Wolff, K. C., Adams, S. R., Fogelberg, R., Goldstein, A. A., & Preston, P. G. (2019). Evaluation of a pilot perioperative smoking cessation program: a pre-post study. *Journal of Surgical Research, 237*, 30–40.

Yu, C., Weng, S., Ho, C., Chen, Y. C., Chen, J. Y., Chang, Y. J., . . . Chu C., C. (2018). Pregnancy outcomes following nonobstetric surgery during gestation: a nationwide population-based case-control study in Taiwan. *BMC Pregnancy Childbirth, 18*, 460. https://dx.doi.org/10.1186/s12884-018-2079-4

FURTHER READING

Agency for Clinical Innovation (ACI). (2011). Extended day only admission policy. PD2011_045. Retrieved from <https://www1.health.nsw.gov.au/PDS/pages/doc.aspx?dn=PD2011_045>.

Agency for Clinical Innovation Aged Health Network. (2015). Key principles for the care of confused hospitalised older persons (CHOPS). Version 1.2 March 2015. Retrieved from <https://aci.health.nsw.gov.au/__data/assets/pdf_file/0006/249171/CHOPS-key-principles1-2-web.pdf>.

Allen + Clarke Consulting. (2020). *Baseline data capture: cultural safety, partnership and health equity initiatives.* Wellington: Medical Council of New Zealand and Te Ohu Rata o Aotearoa. Retrieved from <https://www.mcnz.org.nz/assets/Publications/Reports/f5c692d6b0/Cultural-Safety-Baseline-Data-Report-FINAL-September-2020.pdf>.

Australian Diabetes Society. (2020). Australian blood glucose treatment algorithm for type 2 diabetes. Retrieved from <http://t2d.diabetessociety.com.au/plan/>.

Australian Institute of Health and Welfare (AIHW). (2017). *Impact of overweight and obesity as a risk factor for chronic conditions.* Cat. no: BOD 12. Canberra: Author. Retrieved from <https://www.aihw.gov.au/reports/burden-of-disease/impact-of-overweight-and-obesity-as-a-risk-factor-for-chronic-conditions/contents/table-of-contents>.

Barker, P., Creasey, P. E., Dhatariya, K., Levy, N., Lipp, A., . . . Woodcock, T. (2015). Peri-operative management of the surgical patient with diabetes 2015: Association of Anaesthetists of Great Britain and Ireland. *Anaesthesia, 70*(12), 1427–1440.

Canterbury District Health Board. CDHB (2019). Stop for your op: become smokefree before your surgery. Retrieved from <http://edu.cdhb.health.nz/Hospitals-Services/Health-Professionals/CDHB-Policies/Clinical-Manual/Documents/Stop-For-Your-Op-Smokefree-Fact-Sheet.pdf#search5Stop%20for%20your%20op%20become%20smokefree%20before%20your%20surgery>.

Cosson, E., Catargi, B., Cheisson, G., Jacqueminet, S., Ichai, C., Leguerrier, A. M., . . . Valensi, P. (2018). Practical management of diabetes patients before, during and after surgery: a joint French diabetology and anaesthesiology position statement. *Diabetes & Metabolism, 44*(3), 200–216. doi.org/10.1016/j.diabet.2018.01.014

Dekkers, T., Melles, M., Groeneveld, B. S., & de Ridder, H. (2018). Web-based patient education in orthopedics: systematic review. *Journal of Medical Internet Research, 20*(4), e143.

Department of Health. (2018). *Clinical practice guidelines: pregnancy care.* Canberra: Australian Government Department of Health. Retrieved from <https://www.health.gov.au/resources/collections/pregnancy-care-guidelines-and-related-documents>.

Haas, D. M., Morgan, S., Contreras, K., & Kimball, S. (2020). Vaginal preparation with antiseptic solution before cesarean section for preventing postoperative infections. *Cochrane Database of Systematic Reviews, 4*, CD007892. https://dx.doi.org/10.1002/14651858.CD007892.pub7

Hadiati, D. R., Hakimi, M., Nurdiati, D. S., Masuzawa, Y., da Silva Lopes, K., & Ota, E. (2020). Skin preparation for preventing infection following caesarean section. *Cochrane Database of Systematic Reviews, 6*, CD007462. https://dx.doi.org/10.1002/14651858.CD007462.pub5

Lee, C. M., Rodgers, C., Oh, A. K., & Muckler, V. C. (2017). Reducing surgery cancellations at a pediatric ambulatory surgery center. *AORN Journal, 105*(4), 384–391. https://dx.doi.org/10.1016/j.aorn.2017.01.011.

Liu, Z., Dumville, J. C., Norman, G., Westby, M. J., Blazeby, J., McFarlane, E., . . . Cheng, H. (2018). Intraoperative interventions for preventing surgical site infection: an overview of Cochrane Reviews. *Cochrane Database of Systematic Reviews, 2*, CD012653. https://dx.doi.org/10.1002/14651858.CD012653.pub2

Madrid, E., Urrútia, G., Roqué i Figuls, M., Pardo-Hernandez, H., Campos, J., Paniagua, P., ... Alonso-Coello, P. (2016). Active body surface warming systems for preventing complications caused by inadvertent perioperative hypothermia in adults. *Cochrane Database of Systematic Reviews, 4*, CD009016. https://dx.doi.org/10.1002/14651858.CD009016.pub2

National Blood Authority. (2014). Preoperative anaemia identification, assessment and management case study. Retrieved from <https://www.blood.gov.au/case-studies>.

NSW Ministry of Health. (2017). Policy directive: clinical procedure safety PD2017_032. Retrieved from <https://www1.health.nsw.gov.au/pds/Pages/doc.aspx?dn=PD2017_032>.

Royal Australasian College of Surgeons (RACS). (2015). Position statement on emergency surgery. Retrieved from <https://www.surgeons.org/about-racs/position-papers/emergency-surgery-2015>.

Royal Australian College of General Practitioners (RACGP). (2016). *General practice management of type 2 diabetes: 2016–18.* East Melbourne: Author. Retrieved from <https://www.diabetesaustralia.com.au/wp-content/uploads/General-Practice-Management-of-Type-2-Diabetes-2016-18.pdf>.

Smaling, J. (2018). Health targets: improved access to elective surgery. Wellington: Ministry of Health. Retrieved from https://www.health.govt.nz/new-zealand-health-system/health-targets/about-health-targets/health-targetsimproved-access-elective-surgery.

Steliga, M. A. (2018). Smoking cessation in clinical practice: How to get patients to stop. *Seminars in Thoracic and Cardiovascular Surgery, 30*(1), 87–91.

Tariq, H., Ahmed, R., Kulkarni, S., Hanif, S., Toolsie, O., Abbas, H., & Chilimuri, S. (2016). Development, functioning, and effectiveness of a preoperative risk assessment clinic. *Health Services Insights, 9*(Suppl. 1), 1–7. https://dx.doi.org/10.4137/HSI.S40540. doi.org/10.4137/HSI.S40540

CHAPTER 8

Patient Care During Anaesthesia

JULIE WALTERS • FIONA NEWMAN
EDITOR: MENNA DAVIES

LEARNING OUTCOMES

- Examine the role of the anaesthestic nurse when caring for the patient during anaesthesia
- Explore the different modalities of anaesthesia
- Describe the physiological changes that occur during anaesthesia
- Identify the drugs commonly used in anaesthesia
- Describe equipment used for management of the patient during anaesthesia
- Explain airway management strategies
- Discuss the fluid and electrolyte requirements of a patient undergoing anaesthesia
- Highlight complications that may arise during anaesthesia and their management
- Explore the management of paediatric, older, obstetric and obese patients

KEY TERMS

airway management	general anaesthesia
anaesthetic emergencies	haemodynamic monitoring
central neural blockade	regional anaesthesia
epidural anaesthesia	special populations
fluid and electrolyte balance	spinal (subarachnoid) anaesthesia

INTRODUCTION

This chapter presents the concepts of perianaesthesia care of the patient, with an emphasis on the anaesthestic assistant's role, including the different types of anaesthesia commonly used, management of the patient's airway and the monitoring required during the perianaesthesia period. Anaesthesia has a physiological impact on all body systems and these are described, together with a discussion on anaesthetic complications and their management. The chapter also discusses fluid and electrolyte management, including blood replacement. Finally, it examines management of older, obstetric, obese and paediatric patients, although detailed information on paediatric anaesthesia is beyond the scope of this text.

The complexity of surgery and advances in surgery require the anaesthetist to be supported by an assistant, who may be a nurse (the term used in this chapter) or an anaesthetic technician (depending on the healthcare facility's protocol). The assistant must be educated and competent in the range of anaesthetic procedures carried out within the local healthcare facility in order to provide safe and effective support to both the anaesthetist and the patient. The anaesthestic nurse has a responsibility to act in accordance with a number of professional standards, policies and guidelines, all of which guide the anaesthetic team in the care of the patient during the perianaesthesia period:

- Australian College of Perioperative Nurses (ACORN, 2020) Standards (2020)
- New Zealand Nurses Organisation (NZNO) Knowledge and Skills Framework (2014)
- Australian and New Zealand College of Anaesthetists (ANZCA), in particular *PS08 Statement on the assistant for the anaesthetist* (ANZCA, 2016a)

- Australian College of PeriAnaesthesia Nurses (ACPAN) Professional Standards for Perianaesthesia Nursing (2019).

Consider the patient scenario of Mr James Collins, a 78-year-old man scheduled for a right total knee replacement, detailed in the Introduction to this book, as you read this chapter.

HISTORY OF ANAESTHESIA

General anaesthesia dates back to William T. Morton, an American dentist who was credited as being the first to use inhalational ether as a surgical anaesthetic in 1846. This discovery revolutionised surgery, making it possible for more complex procedures to be undertaken because patients could now be rendered unconscious with anaesthesia. Since then, anaesthesia practice has seen many advances incorporating new drugs, inhalational agents, techniques and sophisticated equipment to provide patients with safe and pain-free surgery.

MEDICAL PREANAESTHETIC ASSESSMENT OF THE PATIENT

The American Society of Anesthesiologists (ASA) grading system was introduced in the 1960s as a description of the physical state of the patient, along with an indication of whether the patient's surgery is elective or an emergency (see Chapter 7 for more information). This classification influences the anaesthetist's decisions about anaesthetic care and postoperative (PO) management. These decisions include whether the patient requires PO care in the day surgery unit, an inpatient bed, a high-dependency unit or an adult intensive care unit (ANZCA, 2018; Tibble, 2019).

Prior to the patient undergoing an anaesthetic, a full medical assessment must be carried out by a member of the anaesthetic team. This assessment, which often takes place in a pre-admission clinic, must take into consideration the patient's:

- baseline physiological state including BMI and VTE
- current and past medical and surgical history
- family history
- social history (e.g. smoking, alcohol, illicit drugs)
- planned procedure
- drug sensitivities or allergies
- current medications, including herbal dietary supplements
- previous anaesthetic experiences including a family history of previous anaesthestic experiences
- psychological make-up (Marley & Sheets, 2018).

See Chapter 7 for more information on preoperative patient assessment and preparation.

After the patient's history, examination and relevant investigations have been collated, the anaesthetist can plan the patient's care more accurately. The decisions being considered regarding anaesthetic care, pain management and possible blood transfusions should be discussed with the patient and opportunities should be made available for the patient to ask questions. Nurses in the pre-admission clinic or on the ward will inform patients about fasting times and whether regular medications should be taken or omitted on the day of surgery.

Assessment of the Airway

As part of the preanaesthetic assessment, it is essential that the anaesthetist predicts airway and intubation difficulties and plans **airway management** accordingly. Assessment criteria include the following:

- length of incisors – this may impede the introduction of a laryngoscope blade into the mouth
- mobility of cervical spine, and length and thickness of neck – to facilitate neck movement during intubation
- the ability to see the soft palate and uvula with the mouth open and tongue protruded, known as the Mallampati assessment
- the ability to sublux lift the mandible forwards and upwards at the temporomandibular joint (subluxation)
- the thyromental distance (less than three fingers) – this is measured from the thyroid notch to the inner border of the mandible when the patient's head is extended (Cook, 2019).

Mallampati assessment

The Mallampati assessment is used to examine and assess the patient's oral cavity and soft palate visually, in order to predict any possible difficulties with tracheal intubation. It is conducted during the preanaesthetic assessment. Fig. 8.1 shows the classification. Classes III and VI, which indicate that viewing of the soft palate is difficult or impossible, suggest a higher degree of difficulty with intubation in these patients (Kirkbride, 2019).

Nursing Assessment and Preparation of the Patient

It is important that the anaesthetic nurse, in consultation with the anaesthetic team, is familiar with the patient's history and assessment, in order to ascertain any special requirements for the patient's anaesthetic management. This will help the anaesthetic nurse to plan nursing care and prepare equipment to ensure safe patient outcomes.

Mallampati Classification

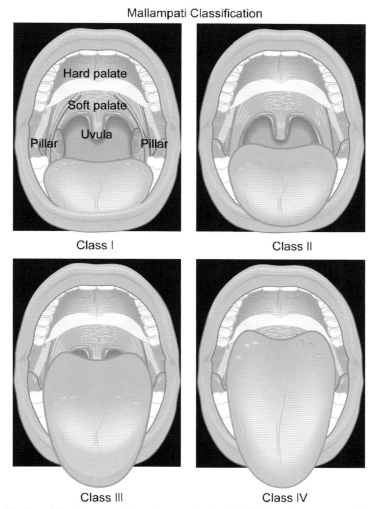

Class I

Class II

Class III

Class IV

FIG. 8.1 Classification of the pharyngeal view when performing the Mallampati assessment. (Source: Heiner, J. (2018). Airway management. In J. Nagelhout & E. Sass (Eds.), *Nurse anesthesia* (6th ed., Chapter 24, Fig. 24.9). St Louis, MO: Elsevier. Modified Mallampati classification.)

Verification of all patient details must comply with the National Safety and Quality Health Service (NSQHS) Standards (the National Standards) on patient identification and procedure matching (Australian Commission on Safety and Quality in Health Care [ACSQHC/the Commission], 2017). Correct patient identification continues throughout each stage of the patient's journey to reduce the risk of mismatch between the patient and the intended procedure (see Chapters 4 and 7 for further information). When the patient is accompanied to the operating suite by a nurse from the ward, a clinical handover is completed by both nurses and the patient using a preoperative patient checklist. When the patient arrives unaccompanied (i.e. from the day surgery ward), the perioperative nurse will use the checklist to verify details with the patient. This checklist may vary according to hospital policy, but will include asking the patient to confirm:

• their name
• date of birth
• fasting times – when the patient last ate or drank
• allergies
• their consent – the patient confirms the procedure, the site and the side of surgery; in most hospitals

the site of surgery should already be marked by the surgeon, although this may be carried out following admission to the operating suite

- any preoperative medications given.

This information is checked against the patient identification bracelet, marked operative site and consent form (ACSQHC/the Commission, 2017). (See Chapter 7 for further information on patient admission to the operating suite.)

In addition, the anaesthetic nurse should ensure that the anaesthetic assessment documentation is present and complete. Any discrepancies that the perioperative nurse notes on admission must be reported to the anaesthetic and surgical teams and rectified before commencement of anaesthesia (ACORN, 2020; ACPAN, 2018).

Prior to the induction of anaesthesia, the anaesthetic nurse should take and document the patient's pulse, temperature and blood pressure, oxygen saturation as baseline observations. The nurse should also attach electrocardiograph (ECG) leads and other monitoring devices as well as instituting active warming measures, if required (ANZCA, 2017a). In addition, the nurse may prepare for intravenous (IV) access or ensure that lines present are secured and labelled in compliance with the national recommendations for user-applied labelling of injectable medicines, fluids and lines (ACSQHC/the Commission, 2017) (Fig. 8.2).

The period just before induction of anaesthesia can be a highly anxious time for the patient, and the anaesthetic nurse plays an important role in reducing the patient's anxiety by demonstrating good communication skills to explain to the patient what is happening and providing quiet reassurance. Therapeutic touch and other anxiety-reduction measures (e.g. music) may

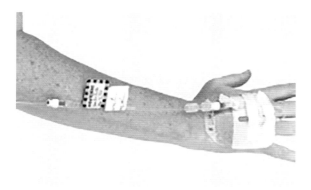

FIG. 8.2 IV line label placed on the patient side close to the injection port. (Source: Australian Commission on Safety and Quality in Health Care. (2015). *National recommendations for user-applied labelling of injectable medicines, fluids and lines*.)

be used, or an anxiolytic medication such as midazolam and an opioid may be given, depending on the surgery.

TYPES OF ANAESTHETICS

It is important that the anaesthetic nurse has an understanding of the different types of anaesthetics in order to provide support to the anaesthetist and the patient in the safe administration of anaesthesia, as well as effective assistance during critical anaesthetic situations (ACORN, 2020; ACPAN, 2018). Anaesthesia is defined as the 'loss of the sensations of pain, pressure, temperature and touch in a part or the whole of the body' (Bryant, Knights, Darroch, & Rowland, 2019). The main categories of anaesthesia are:

- general
- local infiltration
- regional – spinal and epidural – these can be continued in the immediate PO period, to provide the patient with pain relief
- sedation/analgesia.

General Anaesthesia

General anaesthesia is a reversible, unconscious state characterised by amnesia, analgesia and suppression of reflexes (Campbell, 2019). The drugs and inhalational agents used to induce and maintain anaesthesia have a profound physiological effect on body systems, notably the central nervous system (CNS). The area in the CNS that is most affected is the sensory pathway from the thalamus to the cortex, thus depressing conscious thought, motor control, perception, memory and sensation. The medullary centres are the final cerebral area to be affected by anaesthesia and unconsciousness then occurs, with both respiratory and cardiovascular centres temporarily depressed. The stages of anaesthesia were first described by the American anaesthetist Arthur Guedel and are outlined in Table 8.1. These stages can be observed by the anaesthetic team – for example, checking eyelash reflex, altered pupil size – signs that assist in assessing when anaesthesia has been achieved. Measures of these signs indicate the depth of anaesthesia; however, advances in techniques and monitoring have enabled accompanying methods of assessing that anaesthesia has been achieved.

Agents used to induce general anaesthesia

Intravenous (IV) induction agents. IV induction agents, such as short-acting propofol, are commonly used to induce **general anaesthesia** because they provide a smoother and more rapid induction than most

TABLE 8.1
Stages of Anaesthesia

Stage	Respiration	Pupils	Eye Reflexes	Upper Respiratory Tract and Respiratory Reflexes
1. Analgesia	Regular, small volume			
2. Excitement	Irregular		Eyelash absent	
3. Anaesthesia				
Plane I	Regular, large volume		Eyelid absent, conjunctival reflex depressed	Pharyngeal and vomiting reflexes depressed
Plane II	Regular, large volume		Corneal reflex depressed	
Plane III	Regular, becoming diaphragmatic, small volume			Laryngeal reflex depressed
Plane IV	Irregular, diaphragmatic, small volume			Carinal reflex depressed
4. Overdose	Apnoea			

(Source: Kirkbride, D. (2019). The practical conduct of anaesthesia. In J. Thompson, I. Moppett, & M. Wiles (Eds.), *Smith and Aitkenhead's textbook of anaesthesia* (7th ed., pp. 441–455). Edinburgh: Churchill Livingstone.) (Modified from Guedel.)

inhalational agents. Anaesthesia is maintained for the duration of the surgical procedure by using a combination of gases such as oxygen, nitrous oxide and inhalational agents (e.g. sevoflurane). Some anaesthetists may use an IV induction agent as a continuous infusion to maintain anaesthesia, eliminating the need for inhalational agents (Kirkbride, 2019). This is known as total intravenous anaesthesia (TIVA), and the use of target-controlled infusion (TCI) devices enables the theoretical concentration of propofol in the plasma to be continuously controlled, as well as administered (Kirkbride, 2019).

Propofol is known to cause allergic reactions in patients who are allergic to eggs, so an alternative induction agent, such as thiopental sodium (pentothal), can be used. As well as being used for induction of general anaesthesia, thiopental sodium has several other clinical uses:
- as supplementation to other drugs
- in conjunction with regional anaesthesia
- to treat status epilepticus
- as a sedative
- for cerebral protection with raised intracranial pressure (Kirkbride, 2019).

Inhalational agents. Inhalational agents remain popular for the maintenance of anaesthesia and may be used to induce anaesthesia in paediatrics to avoid the need to insert IV cannulae, which can be traumatic for a child. Inhalational agents include nitrous oxide, which is colourless, essentially odourless and the only inorganic anaesthetic gas in clinical use (Nagelhout, 2018c). Although it possesses some analgesic properties, it will not maintain narcosis; however, it does reduce the amount of other opioid medications needed. The addition of an inhalational agent or 'volatile' inhalational agent (e.g. sevoflurane) is required to maintain the patient in an unconscious state.

Volatile inhalational agents are liquid at room temperature and administered through a specialised vaporiser attached to the anaesthetic machine. Oxygen, which must be used in all general anaesthesia, passes through the vaporiser and mixes with the liquid agent, changing the volatile agent into a gas. The mixture is administered to the patient via the airway and delivery equipment attached to the anaesthetic machine. The percentage of inhalational agents delivered to the patient is adjusted by the anaesthetist, depending on the depth of anaesthesia required (Kossick, 2018).

Table 8.2 provides a summary of the IV and inhalational agents used in general anaesthesia.

Adjuncts to general anaesthesia
There are a variety of drugs that are used as adjuncts to anaesthesia and they include analgesics, sedatives,

TABLE 8.2
Intravenous and Inhalational Anaesthetic Agents

Drugs	Advantages	Disadvantages	Nursing Interventions
IV AGENTS			
Barbiturates			
Thiopentone	Rapid induction, duration of action less than 5 minutes	Adverse cardiac effects, hypotension, tachycardia, respiratory depression	Usually have minimal PO effects owing to extremely short duration. Repeated doses may lead to 'hangover effect'
Non-barbiturate hypnotics			
Propofol	Ideal for short outpatient procedures because of rapid onset of action, rapid distribution and high metabolic clearance; may be used for maintenance of anaesthesia as well as induction	May cause bradycardia and other dysrhythmias, hypotension, apnoea, phlebitis, nausea and vomiting, hiccups. May cause hypertriglyceridaemia	Short action leads to minimal PO effects; monitor injection site for phlebitis; cardiac monitoring if unstable. Monitor serum triglycerides every 24 h for sedation greater than 24 h
INHALATIONAL AGENTS			
Volatile liquids			
Isoflurane Desflurane Sevoflurane	All volatile liquids: muscle relaxation, low incidence of nausea and vomiting. Isoflurane: less cardiac depression, devoid of toxicity to body organs. Desflurane: rapid induction and emergence, widely used volatile agent. Sevoflurane: predictable effects on cardiovascular and respiratory systems, rapid acting, non-irritating to respiratory system	All volatile liquids: myocardial depression, early onset of pain because of rapid elimination. Sevoflurane: may be associated with emergence delirium	Assess and treat pain during early anaesthesia recovery; assess for adverse reactions such as cardiopulmonary depression with hypotension and prolonged respiratory depression; monitor for nausea and vomiting
Gaseous agents			
Nitrous oxide	Potentiates volatile agents, allowing a reduction in their dosage and their negative side effects and increases the rate of induction; has high analgesic potency	Weak anaesthetic, rarely used alone; must be administered with oxygen to prevent hypoxaemia; nausea and vomiting more common than with other inhaled anaesthetics	Produces little or no toxicity at therapeutic concentrations; monitor for effects of volatile liquids when nitrous oxide used as an adjunct
Dissociative anaesthetics			
Ketamine	Can be administered intravenously or intramuscularly; potent analgesic and amnesic	May cause hallucinations and nightmares, increased intracranial and intraocular pressure, increased heart rate, hypertension	Anticipate administration of a benzodiazepine if agitation and hallucinations occur; calm quiet environment is essential in PO care

(Source: Tizani, A. (2017). *Harvard's nursing guide to drugs* (10th ed.). Sydney: Elsevier.)

TABLE 8.3
Adjuncts to General Anaesthesia

Agents	Uses During Anaesthesia	Adverse Effects	Nursing Interventions
OPIOIDS			
Fentanyl Sufentanil Morphine sulfate Alfentanil Remifentanil Methadone	Induce and maintain anaesthesia, reduce stimuli from sensory nerve endings, provide analgesia during surgery and anaesthetic recovery	Respiratory depression, stimulation of vomiting centre, possible bradycardia and peripheral vasodilation (when combined with anaesthetics), high incidence of pruritus with both regional and intravenous administration	Assess respiratory status, monitor pulse oximetry (for a late sign of hypoxaemia), protect airway in anticipation of vomiting, use standing orders for antipruritics, such as diphenhydramine
BENZODIAZEPINES			
Midazolam Diazepam Lorazepam	Induce and maintain anaesthesia	Potentiation of the effects of opioids, increasing the potential for respiratory depression, hypotension and tachycardia	Monitor cardiopulmonary status, level of consciousness
NEUROMUSCULAR BLOCKING AGENTS			
Depolarising agent: Suxamethonium **Non-depolarising agents:** Vecuronium Atracurium Pancuronium Rocuronium Mivacurium	Facilitate endotracheal intubation, promote skeletal muscle relaxation (paralysis) to enhance access to surgical sites; effects of non-depolarising agents are usually reversed towards the end of surgery by the administration of anticholinesterase agents (e.g. neostigmine, pyridostigmine, edrophonium)	Apnoea related to paralysis of respiratory muscles, prolonged muscle relaxation due to longer action of non-depolarising agents than reversal agents, cardiac alterations; recurrence of muscle weakness with correction of hypothermia	Monitor respiratory rate and pattern until the patient is able to cough and return to previous levels of muscle strength; maintain patent airway; ensure availability of non-depolarising reversal agents and respiratory support equipment, monitor temperature and levels of muscle strength with temperature changes
ANTIEMETICS			
Droperidol Ondansetron Dolasetron Metoclopramide Prochlorperazine Promethazine	Prevention of vomiting with aspiration during surgery, counteract the emetic effects of inhalation agents and opioids; droperidol often used during surgery; others more often used postoperatively	Droperidol: dysrhythmias, laryngospasm, bronchospasm, tachycardia, hypotension, central nervous system alterations, extrapyramidal reactions; contraindicated in patients with Parkinson's disease or hypomagnesaemia Other antiemetics: headache, dizziness, sedation, malaise, fatigue, musculoskeletal pain, shivers, diarrhoea, acute dystonic reactions, cardiovascular alterations; contraindicated in patients with hypomagnesaemia	Monitor cardiopulmonary status, level of consciousness and ability to move limbs Droperidol: administer with caution in patients with heart disease

(Source: Tizani, A. (2017). *Harvard's nursing guide to drugs* (10th ed.). Sydney: Elsevier.)

antiemetics and neuromuscular blocking agents (muscle relaxants). Table 8.3 provides a summary of the adjuncts most commonly used in general anaesthesia. As can be seen from Tables 8.2 and 8.3, many of the agents used to induce anaesthesia and as adjuncts have a powerful effect on the patient's cardiovascular and respiratory systems. This requires the anaesthetist and the anaesthetic nurse to monitor the patient closely using their observational skills and a variety of invasive and non-invasive haemodynamic monitoring techniques described later in the chapter.

Analgesia

In addition to the drugs designed to keep the patient under general anaesthesia, it is important to provide pain relief during the procedure. Opioid analgesic drugs (e.g. fentanyl) are given intraoperatively and in the immediate PO period when further pain protocols are initiated in the postanaesthesia care unit (PACU). *Opioid* is a term used to refer to a group of drugs, both naturally occurring and synthetically produced, that possess the properties of opium or morphine. The anaesthetic nurse can monitor the patient's pain response by observing for physiological changes or reactions to surgical interventions and alerting the anaesthetist.

Muscle relaxation

The discovery of curare, a naturally occurring muscle relaxant, by Harold Griffith and Enid Johnson in 1942 was a milestone in anaesthesia. Curare greatly facilitated endotracheal intubation and provided excellent relaxation for abdominal surgery. For the first time, surgery could be performed on patients without having to administer large doses of anaesthetic agents, which was necessary to produce the muscle relaxation or paralysis required to incise through muscles and enter the abdominal cavity. A wide range of muscle relaxant or neuromuscular blocking agents have been developed since then, giving today's anaesthetist a variety of drugs for use in clinical practice (Hunter & Shields, 2019).

Muscle relaxation or paralysis is achieved by blocking neuromuscular activity at the motor end plate of skeletal muscles, where the receptors for acetylcholine are located. Acetylcholine, a naturally occurring neurotransmitter, plays an important role in facilitating the transmission of nerve impulses. Interference with the transmission of nerve impulses results in paralysis of skeletal muscle, which includes the muscles of respiration. There are two types of neuromuscular blocking agents: depolarising and non-depolarising (Naguib, Lien, & Mistelman, 2015).

Depolarising neuromuscular blockers.

Suxamethonium is a short-acting *depolarising* muscle relaxant that acts in 30–60 seconds and lasts 3–5 minutes before it is metabolised by plasma cholinesterase, a naturally occurring enzyme. It is the only agent that creates good conditions for tracheal intubation in emergency airway management situations or when rapid sequence induction is required. Its onset of action is characterised by facial twitching or fasciculations. However, the effect wears off rapidly owing to the build-up of plasma cholinesterase (Naguib et al., 2015). It is the only example of a depolarising muscle relaxant (Bryant et al., 2019).

Non-depolarising neuromuscular blocking agents.

To maintain muscle paralysis for the duration of the vast majority surgical procedures, a longer acting neuromuscular blocking agent is required. These agents are known as *non-depolarising* agents (e.g. rocuronium) and they have a different mode of action to that of depolarising blocking agents. Non-depolarising blocking agents compete with naturally occurring acetylcholine for receptors at the motor end plate of skeletal muscles, causing paralysis.

To terminate the action of non-depolarising blocking agents, a reversal drug (i.e. neostigmine, glycopyrrolate or sugammadex) is administered towards the end of the procedure. This allows acetylcholine to build up to normal levels and enables normal muscle contraction to return. This results in the patient commencing unassisted respiration once all other anaesthetic agents have been stopped. A side effect of neostigmine is bradycardia, which is counteracted by the simultaneous administration of an antimuscarinic drug (e.g. atropine, glycopyrrolate), which blocks parasympathetic stimuli and increases pulse rate (Bryant et al., 2019).

Anaesthetists may select an alternative muscle relaxant for patients with renal impairment – for example, cisatracurium, which is metabolised in a manner that does not compromise renal function (Nagelhout, 2018b).

The anaesthetic team must be alert to the possibility of administering insufficient inhalation agents or TIVA, which can lead to the patient suffering awareness of the procedure. Feature box 8.1 provides information about this distressing condition and how it can be avoided.

Antiemetics

Nausea and vomiting can be an unpleasant side effect of general anaesthesia and cause patients distress and discomfort. In order to minimise nausea, vomiting and possible aspiration of stomach contents into the lungs, which can cause serious complications of pneumonitis, the anaesthetist may administer an antiemetic drug intraoperatively. The effects of antiemetic drugs should continue into the immediate PO period, providing the patient with a more comfortable recovery period. Examples of antiemetic drugs can be seen in Table 8.3.

PROCEDURE FOR GENERAL ANAESTHESIA
Preparation and Equipment

Anaesthetic machines deliver gases and volatile agents to the patient via delivery tubing that attaches to the patient's airway management equipment (e.g. endotracheal tube [ETT], supraglottic airway, also known as a laryngeal mask airway [LMA]). Oxygen, nitrous oxide and medical

FEATURE BOX 8.1
Awareness Under General Anaesthesia

Awareness occurs when the patient is paralysed with muscle relaxants but has been given insufficient doses of anaesthetic agents to maintain an unconscious state. Paralysed patients have no way of indicating their awareness to the anaesthetic team. The possibility of patients remaining aware during general anaesthesia is a concern for both the anaesthetic team and patients. Accounts in the media of patients experiencing awareness during anaesthesia have heightened patient fears. A 2014 report published by the Royal College of Anaesthetists in the UK found that awareness under anaesthesia occurs in approximately 1 in 19,000 cases of general anaesthesia. Sensations reported by patients who remain aware included tugging, stitching, pain, paralysis, choking, feelings of dissociation, panic, extreme fear, suffocation and even feeling that they may be dying. Longer-term psychological harm often includes features of post-traumatic stress disorder (Royal College of

Anaesthetists and the Association of Anaesthetists of Great Britain and Ireland, 2014). Although rare, awareness under general anaesthesia is distressing for those who experience it.

To reduce the possibility of patients remaining aware during general anaesthesia, constant observation is required and this can be achieved using bispectral index (BIS) monitoring or entropy. A sensor strip attached externally to the patient's forehead monitors the patient's brain waves relative to the depth of anaesthesia and relays this information to a monitor, which can alert the anaesthetic team if the patient's level of awareness is increasing (Fig. 8.3). The numerical reading is shown on the monitor: a BIS value of 0 indicates electroencephalograph (EEG) silence, whereas a value near 100 is the expected value in a fully awake adult; between 40 and 60 is the recommended reading for general anaesthesia (Pandit & Cook, 2014).

(Source: Pandit, J., & Cook, T. (Eds). (2014). *Accidental awareness during general anaesthesia in the United Kingdom and Ireland. NAPP5 report and findings*. Royal College of Anaesthetists and the Association of Anaesthetists of Britain and Ireland.)

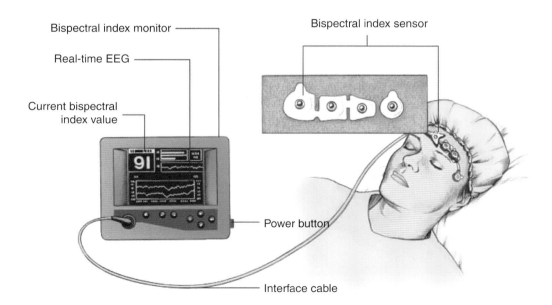

FIG. 8.3 Bispectral index (BIS) monitoring electrodes. (Source: https://nursekey.com/wp-content/uploads/2016/07/DA2CBISPECTRAL_INDEX_MONITORINGFFU28.jpg.)

air are delivered into the operating room (OR) via a network of pipes from a central bulk store of gases within the hospital. A pendant attached to the ceiling delivers the gases to the anaesthetic machine through colour-coded tubes, which are standardised and internationally recognised (white for oxygen, blue for nitrous oxide). The fixtures for each gas outlet are gas specific and pin indexed – an important safety feature ensuring that oxygen tubing cannot be attached to the nitrous oxide outlet, and vice versa. Similarly, the gas cylinders attached to the anaesthetic machines are pin-index yoked, to ensure that cylinders cannot be interchanged (Campbell, 2019). These cylinders provide back-up gases if the pipeline supplies fail, although in smaller facilities they may be the main source of gas supply. Another safety feature of anaesthetic machines is that they are fitted with gas analysers to monitor gas outflow from the pipeline system.

The anaesthetic machine is more than a gas delivery unit. It also contains a range of sophisticated equipment necessary to monitor the patient's condition throughout the perianaesthesia period (e.g. ECG, pulse oximetry and capnography) and the means to provide various types of ventilation inclusive of paediatrics and neonates. Prior to the commencement of the operating list, it is important that the anaesthetist and the anaesthetic nurse check the anaesthetic machine in accordance with ANZCA and the manufacturer's guidelines (ANZCA, 2014a). Fig. 8.4 is an example of an anaesthetic machine and its components.

Other preoperative equipment checks include suction, airway equipment, drugs and additional equipment such as infusion pumps, warming devices and monitoring equipment. These must be available and in working order prior to the patient's arrival in order to ensure a smooth and safe anaesthesia process for the patient.

Airway Management Equipment and Techniques

To understand how artificial airways are used, it is important to review the anatomy of the airway. The airway is

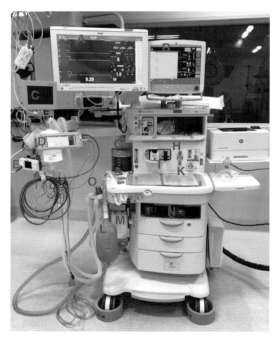

FIG. 8.4 Anaesthetic machine and monitoring devices.
A Vital sign monitoring
B Ventilator and anaesthetic agent monitor
C BIS monitor
D Transport vital sign monitor
E Neuromuscular monitor
F Carbon dioxide monitor
G Ventilator bellows
H On/off suction switch

I Sevoflurane inhalational cartridge
J Ventilator bellows
K Anaesthetic machine on/off switch
L Anaesthetic circuit
M Carbon dioxide absorber
N Spare inhalational agent storage (desflurane and isoflurane)

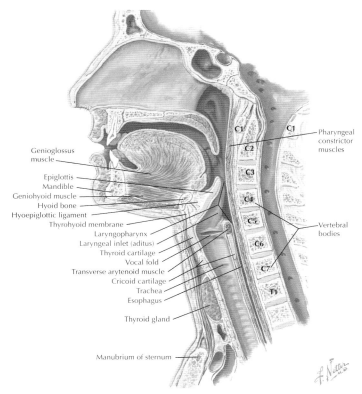

Genioglossus muscle
Epiglottis
Mandible
Geniohyoid muscle
Hyoid bone
Hyoepiglottic ligament
Thyrohyoid membrane
Laryngopharynx
Laryngeal inlet (aditus)
Thyroid cartilage
Vocal fold
Transverse arytenoid muscle
Cricoid cartilage
Trachea
Esophagus
Thyroid gland
Manubrium of sternum

C1
C2
C3
C4
C5
C6
C7
T1

Pharyngeal constrictor muscles
Vertebral bodies

FIG. 8.5 Anatomy of the upper airway. (Source: netterimages.com)

divided into two sections, upper and lower, which are separated at the level of the cricoid cartilage (Heiner, 2018). Fig. 8.5 illustrates the anatomy of the upper airway.

Artificial airways

When the patient loses consciousness, muscle tone of the upper airway is also lost, causing the tongue and epiglottis to fall back against the posterior wall of the pharynx, obstructing the airway. An artificial airway (e.g. Guedel's airway) is inserted into the patient's mouth to prevent airway obstruction. Manoeuvres such as chin lift and jaw thrust may also be required in conjunction with Guedel's airway to maintain a clear airway. Nasopharyngeal airways are also available to prevent PO trauma to the mouth following oral or dental surgery. Nasopharyngeal airways require lubrication before insertion via the patient's nose; they are well tolerated during light anaesthesia or during emergence from anaesthesia (Cook, 2019).

Face masks

Face masks used in anaesthesia are made of silicone or polyvinyl chloride (PVC) and are designed to fit firmly over the nose and mouth, following the contours of the face, as this will assist in providing effective ventilation of an unconscious patient. Several types of transparent face masks are available, which allow observation of exhaled gas and immediate recognition of vomiting, and cushioned masks, which allow for contouring to facial bone structures (Cook, 2019).

Holding face masks in situ requires correct technique to maintain a patent airway. The technique involves holding the mask with a downward pressure using the thumb and index finger, while the middle and ring fingers grasp the mandible to extend the atlanto-maxillary joint. The little finger slides under the angle of the jaw and pulls it anteriorly (Fig. 8.6). Poor technique when applying a face mask can result in pressure on the soft tissues of the face and neck, which can lead to obstruction and excessive bag pressure, causing inflation of the stomach.

Difficulties in obtaining an effective seal with face masks may be experienced in edentulous patients (without teeth) and those patients with congenital abnormalities, facial and eye trauma, tumours, infections or limited neck extension.

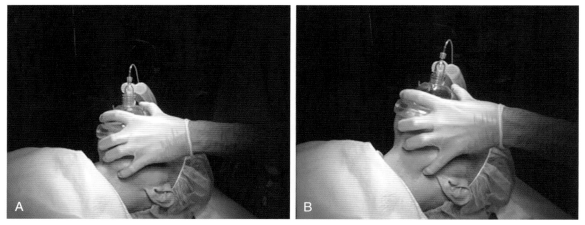

FIG. 8.6 (**A**, **B**) Techniques for holding a face mask with one hand. (Source: Heiner, J. (2018). Airway management. In J. Nagelhout & E. Sass (Eds.), *Nurse anesthesia* (6th ed., Chapter 24, Fig. 24.5). St Louis, MO: Elsevier. Modified Mallampati classification.)

High-flow nasal oxygen

Many anaesthetists use high-flow nasal oxygen (HFNO) via cannulae to preoxygenate the patient prior to airway management and also during sedation. HFNO therapy consists of a warmed, humidified oxygen/air mixture delivered at flow rates of up to 70 L/min by purpose-built nasal cannulae. The use of HFNO has increased considerably in recent years as it provides effective apnoeic oxygenation and administration of high FiO_2 without the need for a tight-fitting face mask or endotracheal intubation.

HFNO can be used to improve preoxygenation prior to intubation and also to maximise apnoea time prior to desaturation, which may occur during certain ear, nose and throat procedures. A major advantage of HFNO is that it can be continued while airway instrumentation takes place, while face-mask oxygen must be removed following induction of general anaesthesia (Millette, Athanassoglou, & Patel, 2018) (Fig. 8.7).

Supraglottic airway device

A supraglottic airway device (SAD), also known as a laryngeal mask airway (LMA), provides an alternative to face masks or ETTs (see next section). It consists of a silicone or PVC tube that is slightly shorter than an ETT, with an inflatable elliptical cuff at the distal end which resembles a miniature face mask. When this cuff is inflated the LMA is designed to provide a relatively airtight seal around the perimeter of the larynx, above the glottis – hence its name supraglottic – but it does so without passing through the vocal cords. LMAs are inserted by hand without the aid of a laryngoscope (Figs 8.8 and 8.9). LMAs are available in sizes for both paediatric and adult patients. Indications for their use include:

- patients who do not require tracheal intubation to facilitate their surgical procedure and are breathing spontaneously
- providing a clear airway without the need for the anaesthetist's hands to support a mask.

As the LMA does not pass through the vocal cords and thus provides the same security from aspiration as ETTs, it is not suitable for all patients, especially those who are at high risk of aspiration. Contraindications to use of the LMA include:

- a full stomach – or unknown fasting status
- pregnancy
- hiatus hernia
- high airway resistance
- pharyngeal abscess
- low pulmonary compliance, such as obesity (Campbell, 2019).

Endotracheal tubes

ETTs are designed to deliver gases directly into the trachea and onwards into the lungs. They are disposable and made of PVC or silicone, with

OPTIFLOW THRIVE

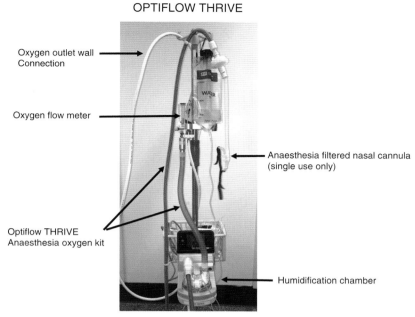

Oxygen outlet wall Connection

Oxygen flow meter

Anaesthesia filtered nasal cannula (single use only)

Optiflow THRIVE Anaesthesia oxygen kit

Humidification chamber

FIG. 8.7 Optiflow for delivery of high-flow nasal oxygen. (Courtesy: Fisher-Paykel. Source: author.)

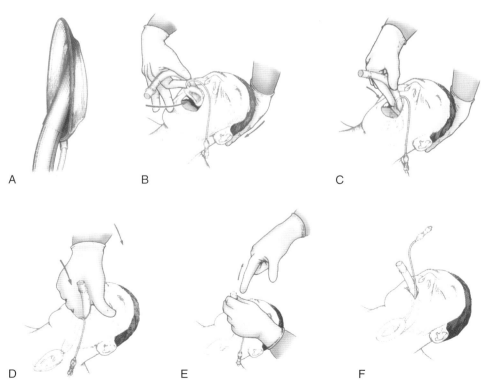

A   B   C

D   E   F

FIG. 8.8 Insertion of laryngeal mask airway. (Source: Campbell, B. (2019). Anesthesia. In J. Rothrock (Ed.), *Alexander's care of the patient in surgery* (16th ed., Fig 5.5). St Louis, MO: Elsevier.)

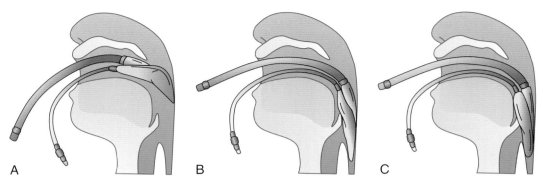

A   B   C

FIG. 8.9 A–C Laryngeal mask airway in situ. (Source: Adapted from Campbell, B. (2019). Anesthesia. In J. Rothrock (Ed.), *Alexander's care of the patient in surgery* (16th ed., Fig 5.6). St Louis, MO: Elsevier.)

the distal end bevelled to aid visualisation and insertion through the vocal cords. The Murphy eye is an additional hole at the distal end and is designed to lessen the risk of obstruction by secretions, blood or other matter. Resistance to air flow depends primarily on the tube diameter, but is also affected by tube length and curvature. ETTs may have an inflatable cuff at the distal end that, when inflated with air, provides a seal, permitting positive pressure ventilation and decreasing the risk of aspiration.

ETTs have been modified for a variety of specialised applications. Reinforced ETTs have been designed to reduce obstruction when the patient is in the prone position. Ring–Adair–Elwyn (RAE) tubes are used in orofacial surgery as they are angled to avoid encroaching on the surgical site (e.g. during ear, nose and throat surgery, plastic surgery and ophthalmology). Nasal RAE tubes are also used for oral and faciomaxillary surgery. Indications for intubation include:
- patients who are at risk of aspiration and require the airway to be protected, as discussed later in the section on rapid sequence induction
- patient positioning, where the airway is at a greater risk of being compromised (e.g. when it must be protected from blood loss at the operative site during ear, nose and throat, facial, plastic or dental surgery) and to facilitate access to the surgical site
- abdominal surgery requiring muscle relaxation and mechanical ventilation

- thoracic surgery that requires specific control of ventilation and sometimes one-lung ventilation
- patients with a Mallampati score of class III or IV, where a difficult airway is anticipated
- patients with significant comorbidities (Kirkbride, 2019).

Intubation equipment
The anaesthetic nurse must be aware of the requirements for intubation in order to provide effective assistance to the anaesthetist and a safe outcome for the patient (ACORN, 2020). The equipment required includes the following (Fig. 8.10):
- laryngoscope handle and blades in working order (the anaesthetic nurse should ensure that the blade fits and locks onto the handle, confirm the light-source strength by opening the blade and viewing the light, and be aware that brands are generally not interchangeable)
- appropriately sized tubes, plus lubricant
- 10 mL syringe for cuff inflation
- tape to secure tube in place (this may depend on anaesthetist preference, e.g. linen tape, adhesive plaster)
- suction equipment, including Yankauer and Y-suction catheters.

Additional requirements that should be available include:
- a malleable introducer
- Magill forceps
- intubating bougie (for difficult or awkward airways).

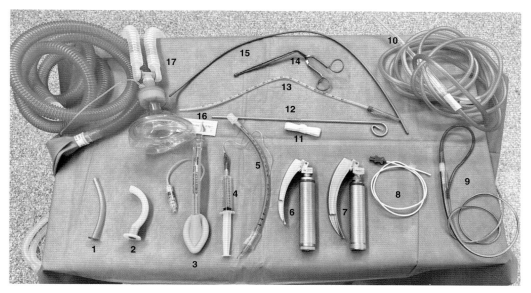

FIG. 8.10 Anaesthetic equipment:
1. Nasopharyngeal airway
2. Oropharyngeal airway (Guedel)
3. Supraglottic device (SAD)
4. Air syringe for inflating cuff on endotracheal tube
5. Endotracheal tube (ETT)
6. Mackintosh (MAC) laryngoscope blade size 3
7. Mackintosh (MAC) laryngoscope blade size 4
8. Temperature probe
9. Nasogastric tube
10. Yankauer sucker and suction tubing
11. Linen tape for securing ETT
12. Malleable introducer (stylet)
13. Y-suction catheter
14. Magill forceps
15. Intubating bougie
16. Lubricant gel
17. Anaesthetic circuit including mask and heat and moisture exchanger filter
(Source: Courtesy Zoe Kumar.)

PATIENT SCENARIOS

Mr James Collins is a 78-year-old man who has been admitted for an elective right total knee replacement (TKR). Mr Collins' full history and a brief description of the healthcare setting is provided in the Introduction at the front of the book for readers to review when answering the questions in this unfolding scenario.

SCENARIO 8.1: PREPARATION FOR ANAESTHESIA

Mr Collins is to undergo his TKR procedure under a spinal anaesthetic and sedation. However, it is a requirement that equipment is prepared to administer a general anaesthetic in the event that the spinal anaesthetic fails to be effective or an emergency arises requiring Mr Collins to be anaesthetised.

The anaesthetic team caring for Mr Collins comprises Dr Marion Thomas and Dr Vince De Silva, consultant anaesthetist and registrar, and RN Margaret McCormack, an experienced anaesthetic nurse.

> ### Critical Thinking Question
>
> - Considering Mr Collins has a history as a smoker, is being treated for hypertension and has polypharmacy, identify the equipment the anaesthetic team will prepare should Mr Collins require a general anaesthetic. Provide rationales for your answer.

Complications of Intubation

The anaesthetic nurse must be aware of and alert to complications that may arise during intubation in order to provide effective and prompt assistance to the anaesthetist, such as obtaining additional equipment. Complications include:

- oesophageal intubation or endobronchial intubation, as neither will provide effective ventilation and could be fatal as the patient will receive little or no oxygen
- complications when in situ, such as malposition due to changes in patient position, unintentional extubation or ignition of anaesthetic gases resulting in fire during use of lasers
- obstruction of the Murphy eye with secretions, which could compromise the ability to ventilate the patient
- airway trauma, such as damage to the teeth, lip and mucosal laceration, sore throat or dislocation of the mandible
- tube malfunction or cuff perforation
- laryngospasm (Heiner, 2018; Hewson & Hardman, 2019b).

Rapid Sequence Induction

On occasions, it is necessary to secure the airway rapidly in order to reduce the risk of pulmonary aspiration of the acid stomach contents. The technique to achieve this is called a rapid sequence induction. Aspiration can result in severe pneumonitis, which is known as Mendelson's syndrome and is often fatal (Rieker, 2018). The indications for rapid sequence induction include patients who are at risk of aspiration due to:

- unknown fasting time
- pregnancy
- hiatus hernia
- bowel obstruction
- gastrointestinal bleeding
- gastric reflux
- trauma sustained after eating.

The technique involves the anaesthetic nurse using their fingers to apply pressure on the cricoid cartilage, pressing it firmly backwards onto the cervical vertebral bodies behind it and occluding the upper end of the oesophagus, thus preventing aspiration of gastric contents. This is known as a Sellick's manoeuvre and was first described in 1961 (Heiner, 2018). The sequence of the technique is as follows:

- locate appropriate equipment (e.g. ETT, laryngoscope and suction)
- secure IV access
- apply haemodynamic monitoring
- preoxygenate the patient using a face mask
- locate the cricoid cartilage and apply pressure using two fingers when instructed to do so by the anaesthetist, usually as the induction agent is being administered (Fig. 8.11)

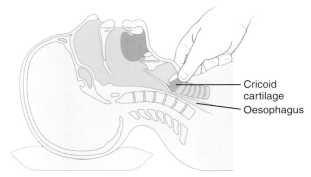

FIG. 8.11 Applying cricoid pressure. (Source: Heiner, J. (2018). Airway management. In J. Nagelhout & E. Sass (Eds.), *Nurse anesthesia* (6th ed., Chapter 24, Fig. 24.26). St Louis, MO: Elsevier. Modified Mallampati classification.)

Labels: Cricoid cartilage; Oesophagus

- administer IV induction agent and short-acting muscle relaxant (e.g. suxamethonium)
- observe for muscle twitching or fasciculations, which indicate the muscle relaxant is taking effect
- intubate, inflate cuff and ventilate patient
- confirm correct position of ETT (i.e. equal chest inflation and end-tidal carbon dioxide displayed waveform)
- release cricoid pressure *only* on the advice of the anaesthetist once the position of the ETT has been confirmed (Heiner, 2018).

It is important that patients are warned that they will feel pressure on their neck as their anaesthetic is being induced.

Note that Sellicks' manoeuvre is different from the application of external laryngeal manipulation, which the anaesthetist may ask the anaesthetic nurse to perform in order to facilitate a view of the larynx for routine intubation. This is sometimes referred to as BURP, an acronym for 'backward, upward, rightward pressure'.

Sequence of General Anaesthesia

Once the anaesthetic equipment has been assembled and checked, the anaesthetic team is ready and the patient has been prepared, the sequence of general anaesthesia can commence.

The anaesthetic team must follow standard precautions, undertake hand hygiene and don PPE (mask, eye protection and gloves) to reduce the risks from contamination from aerosolised sputum or vomit during intubation. If additional precautions are required, local facility policies should be followed. Feature box 8.2 provides information about the precautions put in place during the COVID-19 pandemic.

FEATURE BOX 8.2
Anaesthetic Management of Patients With COVID-19

COVID-19 is a virus thought to be spread primarily via droplets, but also via contact with contaminated surfaces. In the perioperative environment, these patients are treated with *airborne and contact* precautions owing to the potential aerosolisation of this pathogen.

During the anaesthetic care of the patient, particularly at intubation and extubating, additional practices and precautions must be followed to minimise the risk to healthcare involved in these procedures.

A team 'huddle' prior to the arrival of the patient is important to ensure all staff involved in the care of the patient are fully briefed and all equipment is available and checked.

Practices include:

PREANAESTHETIC

- PPE (including P2/N95[a] mask and visor) should be donned in the designated areas and checked by a 'buddy'
- PPE should remain in situ for duration of case
- The number of staff working in the OR should be kept to a minimum
- During intubation and extubation, only the intubating anaesthetist, second anaesthetist and anaesthetic nurse should be present in the room. All other staff must leave
- All staff should be positioned behind the patient to minimise risk of patient coughing/aerosolisation
- One anaesthetist (most senior) manages the airway, while a second anaesthetist monitors the patient, administers drugs and participates in other patient care activities to avoid contamination. The anaesthetic nurse will be assigned to assist with airway management.

INTUBATION

- Preoxygenation for all patients is essential (be aware that high gas flows may increase aerosolisation)
- A viral filter must be inserted between face mask and anaesthetic circuit
- Two hands are used to ensure tight face-mask seal – to reduce leakage around mask

- Use of positive pressure ventilation should be minimised to reduce risk of aerosolisation
- The head of bed is elevated for staff protection and to improve gas exchange
- Rapid sequence induction is used with a high-dose neuromuscular blocking agent
- Fresh gas flows are ceased before face mask is removed
- Use of disposable video laryngoscope is recommended
- Once the patient is intubated and the cuff inflated, a pressure monitor is used to check the seal is adequate and there are no air leaks around the ETT. The usual practice of listening for air leak close to the patient's mouth should not occur to reduce risk of contamination by aerosolisation
- The laryngoscope/blade is placed in a sealed bag for reprocessing
- Consider use of peripheral nerve stimulator to ensure adequate relaxation

EXTUBATION

- Administer antiemetic prophylaxis prior to extubation to reduce risk of vomiting
- Use suction while patient is deeply anaesthetised
- Elevate the head of the bed, if appropriate, prior to extubation to direct any coughing away from staff
- The patient is extubated while still deeply anaesthetised, but breathing spontaneously
- The patient may be recovered in the operating theatre with a PACU or anaesthetic nurse and anaesthetist in attendance
- When transferring the patient to the ward or ICU, they will be accompanied by the anaesthetic team. A 'clean' runner (anaesthetic nurse runner or scout nurse runner in existing PPE) will be required to clear the way and open door/lifts during transfer

Following transfer of the patient, cleaning protocols as per local policy should be undertaken to restore the environment ready for subsequent patients.

[a]Fit testing uses specialised equipment to provide quantitative data on how well a P2/N95 mask/respirator seals against the wearer's face, thus ensuring maximum protection. Records must be kept of the staff member's details, overall fit factor; make, model, style and size of respirator used; and date tested. The staff member must ensure they don the mask/respirator of the correct fit factor and must be fit checked following donning to ensure the mask/respirator is properly applied (Clinical Excellence Commission, 2020).
ETT = endotracheal tube; OR = operating room; PACU = postanaesthesia care unit ; PPE = personal protective equipment.
(Sources: Adapted from Randwick Campus Operating Suite Procedures (2020) (Dr A Duggan & CNC, P Bhusal) from sources: Australian Government, Department of Health (2020). *Environmental cleaning and disinfection principles for COVID-19*; Clinical Excellence Commission. (2020). *CEC guidelines – COVID-19 infection prevention and control*; NSW Health (2017). *PD2017_01. Infection prevention and control policy*. Wong, J. et al., (2020). Preparing for a COVID-19 pandemic: a review of operating room outbreak response measures in a large tertiary hospital in Singapore. *Canadian Journal of Anesthesia/Journal Canadien d'Anesthésie, 67*, 732–745; World Health Organization. (2020). *Infection prevention and control during health when COVID-19 is suspected*; Brewster, D., Chrimes, N., Do, T., Fraser, K., Groombridge, C., Higgs, A., … Gatward, J. (2020). Consensus statement: Safe Airway Society principles of airway management and tracheal intubation specific to the COVID-19 adult patient group. *MJA, 212* (10), 472–481.)

Table 8.4 illustrates this sequence and the rationale for each step and the anaesthetic nurse considerations during general anaesthesia.

In addition to the information contained in Table 8.4, the anaesthetic nurse must be aware of other considerations during the patient's anaesthesia.

Induction of anaesthesia

Induction of anaesthesia is a critical time during the patient's perioperative care and the anaesthetic nurse must ensure that all equipment is prepared prior to induction. Any delay due to lack of equipment can compromise patient safety. As mentioned earlier, this is an

TABLE 8.4
Sequence of General Anaesthesia

Sequence	Rationale
INDUCTION	
Preoxygenation	Provides a reserve supply of oxygen in the patient's lungs during induction and prior to intubation; can be delivered using HFNO
Administration of midazolam and opioid	Provides sedation and commences pain management
Administration of anaesthetic drug, i.e. propofol	Induces anaesthesia
Ventilation with bag/mask and oxygen	Manages apnoea caused by the anaesthetic induction agent and muscle relaxant drug
Administration of neuromuscular blocking agent	Provides paralysis to facilitate intubation and the surgical procedure; it takes 1–2 minutes to act, hence bag/mask ventilation, which provides airway support
Intubation with ETT	Facilitates ventilation for surgical procedure as patient's muscles are paralysed
Inflation of ETT cuff	Seals airway and facilitates positive pressure ventilation
ETT secured using tape of anaesthetist's choice	Prevents ETT being dislodged and resultant airway compromise
Confirmation of correct location of ETT using stethoscope and monitoring of CO_2	Ensures equal inflation of each lung and that the ETT is not located in the right main bronchus or in the oesophagus
Attachment of ETT to ventilator on anaesthetic machine and delivery of appropriate levels of oxygen, nitrous oxide and volatile agent	As the patient is paralysed and unable to breathe unassisted, they must be attached to the mechanical ventilator; and anaesthesia must be maintained using a combination of agents
MAINTENANCE	
Delivery of oxygen, nitrous oxide and volatile agent (e.g. sevoflurane) or continuous TIVA	Provides continuing anaesthesia
Further neuromuscular blocking agents may required	Provides continuing paralysis for surgical procedure
Haemodynamic monitoring, including temperature monitoring; continued IV access maintained	Provides data on the patient's physiological status, alerting the anaesthetic team to potential problems. Provides access to circulation for administration of drugs (e.g. analgesia) and IV fluids, if required
Depth of anaesthesia monitoring such as BIS, train of four, MAC and TCI	Provides adequate data on the patient's depth of anaesthesia throughout surgery or procedure
Ongoing analgesia will be administered	Provides continuing pain relief
EMERGENCE	
Reversal of neuromuscular blocking agents using appropriate reversal agents (i.e. neostigmine, glycopyrrolate or sugammadex)	Non-depolarising neuromuscular blocking agents require reversing to allow return of spontaneous respiration

TABLE 8.4
Sequence of General Anaesthesia—cont'd

Sequence	Rationale
Switching off of inhalation agents and administration of 100% oxygen; cessation of TIVA and TCI if in use	Cessation of inhalation agents assists the patient to emerge from general anaesthesia; delivery of 100% oxygen 'washes out' residual anaesthetic agents
Suction of oropharynx	Removes secretions and prevents aspiration and laryngospasm
Removal of ETT when the patient is breathing spontaneously, responding to verbal commands and is haemodynamically stable	Demonstrates successful emergence from general anaesthesia and maintenance of airway with minimal support
Continual monitoring until transfer to PACU; suction and oxygen must be available for transfer	Monitoring facilitates management of potential relapse in the patient's condition Availability of suction ensures the patient's airway can be kept clear Oxygen administration maintains optimal oxygen saturation of the patient's blood during transfer

BIS = bispectral index; ETT = endotracheal tube; HFNT = high-flow nasal oxygen; PACU = postanaesthesia care unit; TCI = target-controlled infusion; TIVA = total intravenous anaesthesia.
(Sources: Campbell, B. (2019). Anesthesia. In J. Rothrock (Ed.), *Alexander's care of the patient in surgery* (16th ed., pp. 107–141). St Louis, MO: Elsevier; Kirkbride, D. (2019). The practical conduct of anaesthesia. In J. Thompson, I. Moppett, & M. Wiles (Eds.), *Smith and Aitkenhead's textbook of anaesthesia* (7th ed., pp. 441–455). Edinburgh: Churchill Livingstone.)

anxious time for the patient and the nurse should seek assistance from the other members of the surgical team to provide an environment that is as quiet as possible to facilitate a smooth induction. Noise from music, people talking or the instrument and circulating nurses setting up equipment should be reduced (Kirkbride, 2019). The anaesthetic nurse must have knowledge of the indications for intubation (as discussed earlier) in order to ensure that the appropriate equipment is prepared.

Establishment of the airway

Once anaesthesia is induced, the patient will proceed through the stages of anaesthesia shown in Table 8.1. The establishment of an airway now becomes a priority. As well as ensuring that the intubation equipment is readily available, the anaesthetic team will ensure:

- correct patient positioning, head extension and flexion (the patient appears to be 'sniffing the morning air') (Fig. 8.12)
- the height of the patient trolley or the operating table should be adjusted to facilitate access by the anaesthetist
- all members of the anaesthetic team should don PPE (mask, eye protection and gloves).

Direct laryngoscopy and intubation

It is important that the anaesthetic nurse has assembled and prepared all the equipment ready for intubation

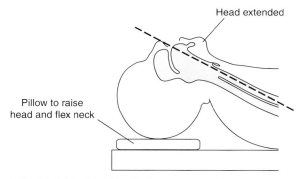

FIG. 8.12 Head position for laryngoscopy. (Source: Cook, T. (2019). Airway management. In J. Thompson, I. Moppett, & M. Wiles (Eds.), *Smith and Aitkenhead's textbook of anaesthesia* (7th ed., Fig. 23.9). Edinburgh: Churchill Livingstone.)

prior to induction of anaesthesia. Any delay in intubating the patient could compromise the patient's airway. The anaesthetic nurse should be positioned preferably to the right side of the patient's head. This allows for the intubation equipment to be handed to the anaesthetist without obstructing their view of the patient's airway. The procedure for intubation is as follows:

- the laryngoscope is designed to be used in the anaesthetist's left hand and is handed to them so

that the blade is inserted into the right side of the patient's mouth and the tongue is swept to the left, locating the epiglottis
- the blade is inserted into the vallecula (posterior oropharynx) and the patient's head is lifted perpendicular to the patient's mandible to expose the vocal cords
- the anaesthetic nurse holds the ETT so that it can be taken by the anaesthetist's right hand and inserted so that the cuff is just below the vocal cords, noting the level on the tube and at the lips
- the ETT is then connected to the anaesthetic delivery tubing (Figs 8.13 and 8.14).

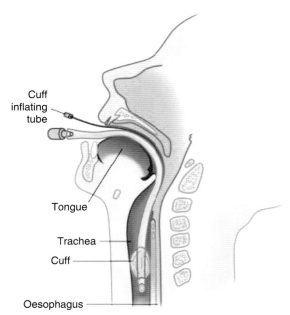

FIG. 8.14 Endotracheal tube in correct position. (Source: Campbell, B. (2019). Anesthesia. In J. Rothrock (Ed.), *Alexander's care of the patient in surgery* (16th ed., Fig 53.1). St Louis, MO: Elsevier.)

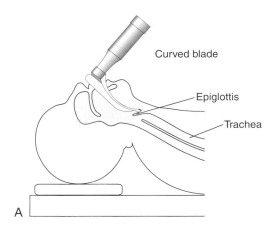

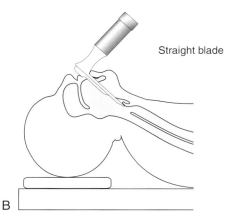

FIG. 8.13 Using a laryngoscope. (**A**) With curved blade. (**B**) With straight blade. (Source: Wright, S. (2018). Assessment and management of the airway. In J. Odom-Forren (Ed.), *Drain's perianaesthesia nursing: a critical approach* (7th ed., Ch. 30, Fig. 30.9). St Louis, MO: Saunders.)

Maintenance of anaesthesia

Once the airway is established, the patient will be positioned ready for surgery. The anaesthetic nurse may assist with positioning, ensuring that the patient remains covered with a sheet or blanket to maintain privacy and dignity and reduce the incidence of inadvertent perioperative hypothermia (IPH). The nurse will also assist with the placement of additional equipment, such as warming devices and further monitoring equipment. During maintenance of anaesthesia, when the operative procedure is taking place, there are a variety of activities the anaesthetic may undertake:
- monitoring the patient under anaesthesia in conjunction with the anaesthetist
- assisting and monitoring patient pressure area care
- managing IV fluids
- equipment management (i.e. decontaminating equipment, keeping areas clean and uncluttered)
- documenting fluid balance
- arranging postoperative care (e.g. liaising with the PACU or ICU)
- preparing equipment and the environment for the next patient

- collaborating with the anaesthetist for any additional patient requirements such as postoperative orders.

It is important that anaesthetic nurse demonstrates good situational awareness (as discussed in Chapter 2) by watching the progress of the surgery and listening to the conversations of the nursing and surgical team, so that they are aware of any possible changes in the patient's condition or in the progress of the procedure that may require action on the part of the anaesthetic team.

Emergence from general anaesthesia
Emergence from anaesthesia is a crucial time in the care of the patient and the anaesthetic team should don PPE prior to extubation and be prepared with the extubation equipment, including suction and oxygen delivery equipment, ready for post-intubation care of the patient and transfer to the PACU. Prior to transferring the patient to the bed/trolley, the nursing team, assisted by the anaesthetist and the surgical team, should carry out a check of the patient's skin integrity and record their observations on the perioperative nursing record (see Chapter 9 for further information). If any pressure injuries are evident, in addition to informing the PACU staff, these injuries must be treated as an adverse event and an incident form should be completed, in line with the National Standards (ACSQHC/the Commission, 2017). The patient's skin should be clean and dry – that is, any blood or skin preparation solution must be removed – and the patient should be dressed in a gown and placed on a clean sheet ready for transfer. The lateral position (recovery position) may be adopted to assist in maintaining an unobstructed airway, unless the anaesthetist is satisfied that this is unnecessary or the nature of the surgery prohibits it. The recovery position involves flexing the patient's upper leg and extending the lower leg, and positioning the patient's head on one side so that the tongue falls forwards under gravity, thus avoiding airway obstruction and/or inhalation of secretions (Kirkbride, 2019).

Clinical Handover
When the anaesthetist is satisfied that the patient's condition is stable, the patient will be transferred to the PACU accompanied by the anaesthetist and, depending on local policy, either the instrument nurse or the circulating nurse. An anaesthetic and nursing clinical handover to PACU nursing staff is important to ensure continuity of care.

On arrival in PACU, the anaesthetist will stay with the patient until a PACU nurse is available to care for the patient and carry out an initial assessment of airway, breathing and circulation, including noting the patient's skin colour. A pulse oximeter, non-invasive blood pressure cuff and, frequently, ECG electrodes will be attached to the patient and the readings noted. Often while this is occurring, the anaesthetist will commence the formal handover to the PACU nurse. This is followed by the nursing handover provided by the instrument or circulating nurse. The handover procedures are covered in detail in Chapter 12, PACU. Following both handovers, the PACU nurse should seek clarification of any postoperative management issues and be satisfied that the patient is in a stable condition before both the anaesthetist and the instrument or circulating nurse leave the PACU.

REPROCESSING USED ANAESTHETIC EQUIPMENT
Following the transfer of the patient to the PACU, the anaesthetic nurse will be required to dispose of or reprocess all the equipment used on the patient and undertake final preparations of equipment and the environment for the next patient. These are important steps to reduce the risk of cross-infection between patients, and the cleaning processes are dependent on local policies.

PPE should be worn while undertaking cleaning procedures, followed by hand hygiene prior to setting up equipment for the next patient. Cleaning procedures include the following:
- laryngoscope handles – in many facilities these are disposable or covered with a disposable cover. If the handles are reusable, they may be sent to the sterilising department for reprocessing or wiped with disinfectant solution (as per local policy)
- anaesthetic circuits – generally used all day (may depend on local policy) and then disposed of in general waste. If the patient required additional precautions, the circuit would be disposed of and a new one attached for subsequent patients
- surfaces (e.g. drug trolley, IV poles, workbenches) are wiped over with disinfectant solution (as per local policy)
- BP cuffs and ECG leads (if not disposable) are also wiped with disinfectant
- care should be taken to ensure any sharps (e.g. syringes, needles, cannulas) are disposed of in sharps containers (ACORN, 2020; ANZCA, 2015).

AIRWAY EMERGENCIES AND MANAGEMENT
Airway Complications
Management of the patient's airway usually occurs without incident but occasionally, due to unanticipated

circumstances, the anaesthetic team may be faced with a patient whose airway is difficult to secure. This requires urgent management and the whole team acting quickly and decisively to secure the patient's airway.

Difficulties with airway management contribute to a large number of situations that are collectively known as 'can't intubate, can't oxygenate' (CICO). Some patients will experience difficulties with tracheal intubation due to congenital abnormalities or acquired conditions, such as trauma to the head, neck and cervical spine, or tumours in the mouth (among many). Several options are available for the anaesthetic team to achieve control of the airway, depending on the patient's presenting condition. These include different sizes and designs of laryngoscopes, supraglottic devices (e.g. an AuroGain laryngeal mask, which has integrated gastric access and intubating capabilities), video laryngoscopes, such as the C-MAC and Glidescope, and fibreoptic intubating bronchoscopes (Figs 8.15–8.17). This equipment will be located in a difficult intubation/ algorithm trolley, and the anaesthetic nurse must be familiar with its location and contents.

Managing the difficult airway can be complex and often occurs in a time-pressured situation; therefore, it is essential to follow a systematic approach to ensuring all reasonable techniques are considered and attempted to resolve the underlying obstruction. Cognitive aids have been adapted and developed to assist the anaesthetics team in the management of a difficult airway. These are prominently displayed in anaesthetic areas for easy reference during an emergency. A team approach to decision making using technical and non-technical skills is essential to successfully manage the emergency and ensure a good patient outcome. Most cognitive aids refer to having a planned approach to managing the airway, and attempts at recommended techniques should be considered in the context of the individual patient situation (ANZCA, 2016b). There are many cognitive aids to manage airway emergencies, with different practice settings developing their own version. It is

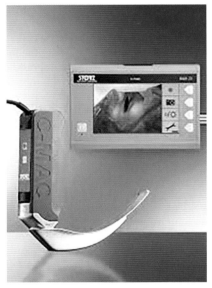

FIG. 8.16 C-MAC video laryngoscope. (Source: © Karl Storz Endoscopy.)

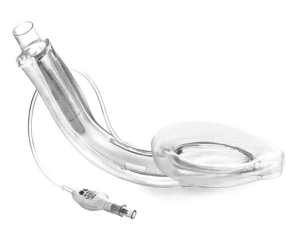

FIG. 8.15 AuraGain laryngeal mask. (Courtesy Ambu Australia.)

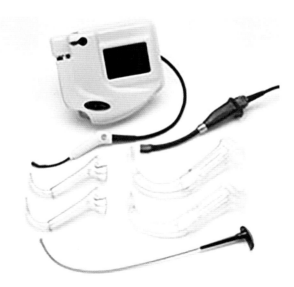

FIG. 8.17 Glidescope. (Source: Courtesy: Zoe Kumar.)

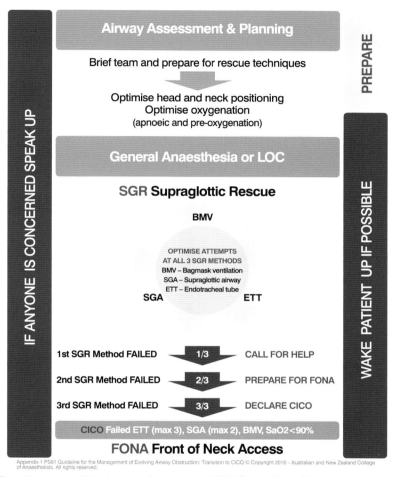

Appendix 1 PS61 Guideline for the Management of Evolving Airway Obstruction: Transition to Can't Intubate Can't Oxygenate (CICO)

ANZCA FPM

Cognitive Aid

Airway Assessment & Planning

Brief team and prepare for rescue techniques

Optimise head and neck positioning
Optimise oxygenation
(apnoeic and pre-oxygenation)

General Anaesthesia or LOC

SGR Supraglottic Rescue

BMV

OPTIMISE ATTEMPTS
AT ALL 3 SGR METHODS
BMV – Bagmask ventilation
SGA – Supraglottic airway
ETT – Endotracheal tube

SGA ETT

PREPARE

IF ANYONE IS CONCERNED SPEAK UP

WAKE PATIENT UP IF POSSIBLE

1st SGR Method FAILED	1/3	CALL FOR HELP
2nd SGR Method FAILED	2/3	PREPARE FOR FONA
3rd SGR Method FAILED	3/3	DECLARE CICO

CICO Failed ETT (max 3), SGA (max 2), BMV, SaO2<90%

FONA Front of Neck Access

FIG. 8.18 Transition to 'can't intubate can't oxygenate' (CICO) cognitive aid. (Source: Australian and New Zealand College of Anaesthetists. (2016b). *PS61. Guidelines for the management of evolving airway obstruction: transition to the can't intubate can't oxygenate airway emergency*. Melbourne: Author.)

important that the anaesthetic nurse identifies and becomes proficient with the system available in their workplace to manage difficult airway situations.

ANZCA (2016b) has based the cognitive aid (Fig. 8.18) on the Vortex model developed by Australian anaesthetist, Nicholas Chrimes. The Vortex is based around a 'high-acuity implementation tool', specifically designed for use during the high-stakes, time-critical situation of an evolving airway emergency. It is intended to help clinical teams perform under pressure by providing a simple, consistent approach that can be taught to all involved in advanced airway management, irrespective of critical care discipline. It is also able to be used in any context in which an airway management takes place.

Key factors behind this and other cognitive aids emphasise a limit of three best-effort attempts at techniques, or 'lifelines', such as bag mask ventilation (BMV), supraglottic airway device (SGA) and ETT. If alveolar oxygen delivery is not restored after these attempts, a spiral to airway crisis represents the need to declare a CICO situation. This will result in proceeding to immediate infraglottic rescue or front of neck access (FONA) technique and performing an emergency cricothyroidotomy using a needle/scalpel or cannula/bougie to puncture the trachea. A fine-bore tracheostomy tube is inserted to ventilate the patient (ANZCA, 2016b; Chrimes, 2016).

Laryngospasm

Laryngospasm is irritation of the vocal cords leading to an involuntary spasm of the superior laryngeal nerve, which can result in complete or partial obstruction of the vocal cords. This can occur during a light plane of anaesthesia (e.g. stage 3, plane I) and can be caused by: the presence of secretions, vomitus, blood or inhalation agents; placement of oropharyngeal or nasopharyngeal airways or the laryngoscope blade; or painful stimuli. The larynx can become completely closed by a reflex closure of the cords and the anaesthetist will not be able to ventilate the patient. A less-severe reaction that occurs when the cords only partially close is characterised by a 'crowing' sound or stridor and by a 'rocking' obstructed pattern of breathing. If left untreated,

hypoxia, hypercarbia and acidosis will result, leading to hypertension and tachycardia and, finally, to cardiac arrest (Heiner, 2018).

Management

Initially, deepening the anaesthetic and removing the stimulus (e.g. suctioning any blood or mucus from the airway) will remove the irritant and relieve the laryngospasm. Positive end-expiratory pressure (PEEP) is used to force 100% oxygen into the lungs. If this is ineffective, suxamethonium may be given, which will relax the vocal cords so that intubation can take place. The anaesthetic nurse must be alert to this condition and have drugs and intubation equipment immediately available. Fig. 8.19 shows a flowchart for the management of laryngospasm.

Bronchospasm

General anaesthesia can alter airway resistance and cause reactions within the bronchial tree, which may result in bronchospasm. This is characterised by an expiratory wheeze, which, if the patient is intubated, can make ventilation difficult. Bronchospasm can be caused by local airway irritation due to the presence of secretions, airway equipment, pulmonary aspiration or drug hypersensitivity. Bronchospasm can also be

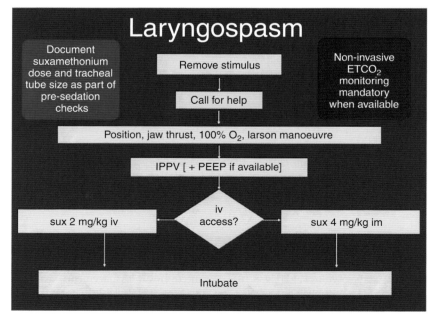

FIG. 8.19 Flowchart for the management of laryngospasm. (Source: Department of Anesthesiology, Division of Pediatric Anesthesia, Tufts Medical Center, Boston, Massachusetts, USA.)

precipitated by the rapid introduction of volatile anaesthetic agents. Patients who smoke, have a history of asthma or have suffered a recent respiratory tract infection are more susceptible to bronchospasm.

Management

If the patient is intubated, repositioning the ETT may reduce the physical irritation to the bronchial tree. Deepening the anaesthetic by increasing the level of inhalational agent will frequently overcome bronchospasm. Bronchodilators such as salbutamol can be administered intravenously and other drugs – such as steroids, ketamine and adrenaline – can also be used.

Aspiration

Patients who are at risk of aspiration are most likely to undergo a rapid sequence induction, as noted earlier. A patient's airway reflexes are depressed by general anaesthesia, which increases the risk of aspiration of gastric contents into the lungs. The occurrence of vomiting and regurgitation when the airway is unprotected can lead to bronchospasm, hypoxaemia, atelectasis, tachypnoea, tachycardia and hypotension. The severity of the symptoms depends on the volume and pH of the gastric contents. Patients who have aspirated may require ventilatory support in the intensive care unit for a period of time, depending on the severity of the condition (Heiner, 2018).

With at-risk patients, local and regional anaesthetic modalities may be an option, negating the need for a general anaesthetic and airway management. Thorough preoperative assessment is essential to prepare a care plan for such patients and ensure that all necessary equipment is available. Many operating suites have a difficult intubation/algorithm trolley that contains a range of anaesthetic equipment that the anaesthetist may require when managing a patient with a difficult airway (see 'Airway complications').

The role of the anaesthetic nurse during emergency situations is vital to ensure safe patient outcomes and they must have a good understanding of the equipment and proposed procedures (ANZCA, 2014b).

OTHER TYPES OF ANAESTHESIA

Sedation/Analgesia

Sedation/analgesia refers to the administration of sedatives (e.g. midazolam) and analgesia (e.g. fentanyl) to produce a depressed level of consciousness, but patient retains the ability to maintain their own airway. ANZCA (2014b) guidelines on sedation/analgesia note that 'the patient is in a state of drug-induced tolerance of uncomfortable or painful diagnostic or interventional medical, dental or surgical procedures'; however, they should be rousable. Patients may also be able to respond to commands or physical stimuli. Sometimes, patients may receive sedation in a non-OR environment for diagnostic or therapeutic procedures and must be managed to strict protocols and guidelines (ANZCA, 2014b; Sobey & Tracy, 2018).

Sedation/anaesthesia can range from a pleasant, relaxed feeling to deepening levels of unconsciousness, depending on the drug and amount administered. With increasing dosage, the areas of the brain controlling cardiac and respiratory function will be depressed to the point where breathing and blood pressure are adversely affected (Agency for Clinical Innovation [ACI], 2013). It is therefore a minimum requirement that all patients are assessed for suitability for sedation, that a trained clinician is present to monitor and manage the patient's airway and that the person is trained in bag/mask ventilation (ACI, 2013).

This method is often used for endoscopy procedures such as colonoscopy because it facilitates a rapid recovery and return to normal activities, although patients must be warned not to drive or operate machinery for 24 hours post-sedation. These procedures often take place outside the perioperative environment in dedicated endoscopy units. In countries such as the UK and the US, sedation anaesthesia is often administered by non-medical clinicians such as nurses who have undergone specialised training for the role (Jones, Long, & Zeitz, 2011). Such a role is being trialled in Australia. (See Chapter 1 for further information about the role of the nurse sedationist.)

Local Anaesthetic Techniques

Local anaesthesia refers to a group of anaesthetic techniques that involve the use of local anaesthetic drugs (e.g. lignocaine, bupivacaine, ropivacaine) to block sensory nerve pathways, thus allowing surgery to proceed without pain and without loss of consciousness (Nagelhout, 2018b; Whitman & Thompson, 2019). These techniques include peripheral nerve blocks, eye blocks, local infiltration at the site of surgery, local anaesthetic sprays to the vocal cords prior to intubation and topical anaesthetic gels, which are often used prior to cannulation in paediatric patients. They are particularly useful for patients who may have comorbidities that may contraindicate the use of general anaesthesia. In many cases, they may be used in combination with general anaesthesia, providing a degree of PO pain relief for the patient. Other advantages for the patient include:

- minimal respiratory impairment
- less nausea and vomiting
- being able to eat and drink sooner
- more rapid mobilisation and discharge
- simplicity of administration
- sympathetic blockade (Hewson & Hardman, 2019a).

Central neural blockade

Central neural blockade refers to the administration of local anaesthetic drugs into the spinal (subarachnoid) or epidural space, thus blocking nerve impulses as they exit the spinal cord and causing large areas of the lower body to lose sensation (hence the term 'block'). These techniques are particularly useful for surgery of the abdomen and lower limbs.

Spinal (subarachnoid) anaesthesia refers to a single administration of local anaesthetic directly into the subarachnoid space at the level of lumbar vertebrae L3–4 or L5–6, thus blocking the spinal nerve roots and producing a loss of sensation to the areas supplied by the nerves from this level of the spinal cord. The anaesthetist advances a hollow spinal needle through the intervertebral space into the subarachnoid space until drops of cerebrospinal fluid (CSF) appear. The local anaesthetic, which can be combined with opioids such as fentanyl, can be injected into the subarachnoid space and the needle is then removed (Pellegrini, 2018).

The patient must be closely observed by the anaesthetic nurse in the immediate post-injection period as local anaesthesia injected into the CSF can cause complications such as hypotension. This occurs as a result of blocking the sympathetic nerves that control vasomotor tone, thus producing vasodilation. This effect can be managed by rapid infusion of IV fluids and the administration of adrenaline. If the local anaesthetic agent inadvertently reaches the nerves controlling respiration, the patient may require ventilator support and the nurse must be alert to any changes in the patient's respiratory function.

Postoperatively, some patients may complain of a severe headache, which is caused by the hole in the dura and the leakage of CSF. The patient may have to remain supine for 24 hours and receive additional IV fluids until the headache subsides. Occasionally, the anaesthetist may perform a 'blood patch', which involves injecting 5–20 mL of blood into the epidural space at the puncture site to seal up the hole in the dura (Pellegrini, 2018).

Epidural anaesthesia involves the intermittent or continuous injection of local anaesthesia through a catheter that is inserted between the vertebrae at the L3–4 or L5–6 level into the epidural space. The epidural space is not really a space but rather an area of loose adipose tissue, lymphatic and blood vessels that lies between the dura mater and the ligamentum flavum (Bryant et al., 2019). The anaesthetist uses a hollow Tuohy needle attached to an empty syringe, which is marked at 1 cm intervals and has a Huber point that allows the fine catheter to be directed along the axis of the epidural space. When the needle penetrates the ligamentum flavum, there is a sudden loss of resistance to pressure on the plunger of the syringe, indicating to the anaesthetist that the correct location has been reached. Advancing the needle further would result in the dura being penetrated. A fine catheter is then inserted via the needle into the epidural space and local anaesthetic is injected (Hewson & Hardman, 2019a). The catheter is secured to the patient and is available to provide 'top-up' doses of local anaesthetic drugs at intervals to maintain effectiveness of the block. This may continue during the PO period as part of the patient's pain management.

As with spinal anaesthesia, epidural anaesthesia can also cause hypotension, although onset is usually slower. However, if a blood vessel in the epidural space is inadvertently punctured and the local anaesthetic agent is released into the bloodstream, sudden and profound hypotension, convulsions and respiratory compromise can occur. Postoperative backache and urinary retention have also been reported as a complication of epidural anaesthesia (Pellegrini, 2018).

Fig. 8.20 shows the location of the spinal cord and epidural space. Table 8.5 outlines the differences between spinal and epidural anaesthesia.

It may not be possible for some patients to receive either spinal or epidural anaesthesia. Patients for whom these are contraindicated include patients with:

- no consent given
- hypovolaemia – increased risk of hypotension
- local sepsis – danger of septicaemia and meningitis
- raised intracranial pressure – both blocks can dangerously alter intracranial pressure
- previous spinal surgery – anatomy may be altered
- coagulopathies – if a blood vessel is accidentally punctured, there is a risk of haemorrhage (Hewson & Hardman, 2019a).

Management of the patient undergoing spinal or epidural anaesthesia. With both spinal and epidural anaesthesia, patients are positioned with their back arched into the shape of a C in order to maximise the space between the spinous processes and to facilitate access for positioning the spinal/epidural needles

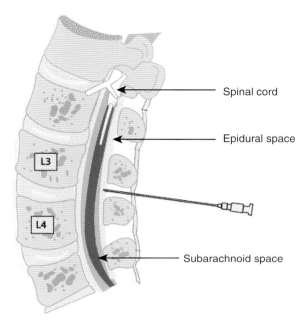

Spinal cord

Epidural space

L3

L4

Subarachnoid space

FIG. 8.20 Location of the spinal cord and epidural space. (Source: Gurch, https://commons.wikimedia.org/wiki/File:Epidural_blood_patch.svg.)

(Fig. 8.21). The position is similar to that used for a lumbar puncture. For those patients with physical disabilities this position is difficult and they can be sat upright, a position that some anaesthetists also favour (Hewson & Hardman, 2019a). Prior to administration of either block, the routine checks of the anaesthetic machine and equipment must be carried out because, if the block should fail or resuscitation is required, all resuscitation equipment must be available and in working order. Monitoring, IV access and baseline observations are obtained to determine variations during the administration of the block (ANZCA, 2014c).

In many instances, patients receive a combination of a central block and general anaesthesia, particularly for complex abdominal surgery where the central block can provide PO pain relief, or it is used as an adjunct to reduce the other drugs required during anaesthesia. However, the administration of central neural blockade is not without risk, as can be seen in Feature box 8.3.

The procedure to insert both spinal and epidural anaesthesia must be undertaken using surgical aseptic non-touch technique to prevent microorganisms from entering the spinal canal or epidural space, which could lead to infection (ANZCA, 2014c). The anaesthetic nurse assists the anaesthetist by assembling the

TABLE 8.5
Differences in the Effect of Spinal and Epidural Anaesthetics

	Spinal Anaesthesia	Epidural Anaesthesia
Dose of drug used	Small: minimal risk of systemic toxicity	Large: possibility of systemic toxicity after (accidental) intravascular injection or total spinal blockade after subarachnoid injection
Rate of onset	Fast: 2 minutes for initial effect; 20 minutes for maximum effect	Slow: 5–15 minutes for initial effect; 30–45 minutes for maximum effect
Intensity of block	Usually complete anaesthesia	Often incomplete anaesthesia for some segments
Pattern of block	May be dermatomal for first few minutes but rapidly develops appearance of cord transection	Dermatomal
Addition of vasoconstrictor	Reliably prolongs block when used with tetracaine (amethocaine) but not with other drugs	Reliably prolongs block when used with lignocaine; may prolong block with bupivacaine but not in all patients

(Sources: Hewson, D. & Hardman, J. (2019a). Regional anaesthetic techniques. In J. Thompson, I. Moppett, & M. Wiles (Eds.), *Smith and Aitkenhead's textbook of anaesthesia* (7th ed., pp. 527–557). Edinburgh: Churchill Livingstone; Pellegrini, J. E. (2018). Regional anesthesia: spinal and epidural anesthesia. In J. Nagelhout & E. Sass (Eds.), *Nurse anesthesia* (6th ed., pp. 1015–1041). St Louis, MO: Elsevier Saunders.)

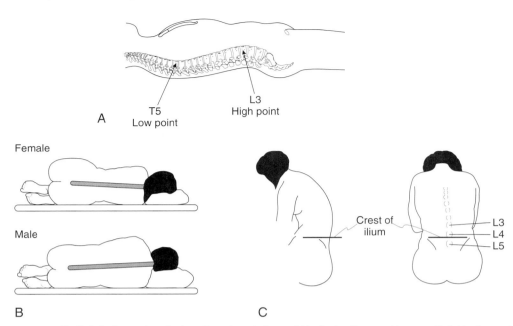

FIG. 8.21 **(A–C)** Spinal curvature for insertion of central neural blockade. (Source: Hewson, D. & Hardman, J. (2019a). Regional anaesthetic techniques. In J. Thompson, I. Moppett, & M. Wiles (Eds.), *Smith and Aitkenhead's textbook of anaesthesia* (7th ed., Ch, 25, Fig. 25.7). Edinburgh: Churchill Livingstone.)

FEATURE BOX 8.3
Epidural Error

In 2010 a patient in a large Sydney teaching hospital went into labour with her first child. During administration of an epidural anaesthetic, chlorhexidine (an antiseptic skin preparation) was mistakenly injected into the patient's epidural space instead of normal saline (used to check the position of the epidural needle). This had a catastrophic effect on the patient's nervous system, causing her excruciating pain and leaving her virtually paralysed. How did such a mistake occur? It appears from reports on the incident that both normal saline and the chlorhexidine 0.5% in alcohol solution were placed in separate unlabelled gallipots on the aseptic field. The anaesthetist drew up 8 mL chlorhexidine in a syringe by mistake and injected the substance via a Tuohy's needle into the patient's epidural space (Bogod, 2012).

In 2018, the ANZCA and the ACSQHC/the Commission issued a joint safety statement outlining steps to be taken to avoid a repeat of such an incident. These include:

- Skin preparation must precede preparation of any medication for the procedure.
- Receptacles containing skin preparation solutions must be removed from the aseptic field following preparation of the skin.
- Medications must be carefully checked by two people, one of whom is the proceduralist (ANZCA and ACSQHC/the Commission, 2018).

In addition, syringes containing medication must be labelled in accordance with national recommendations for user-applied labelling of injectable medicines, fluids and lines (ACSQHC/the Commission, 2015).

---

necessary equipment and by providing physical and emotional support to the patient, who is likely to be awake during the administration of the block. Once the block has been administered, the patient must be closely monitored for any of the complications discussed earlier. The effectiveness of the block must also be assessed prior to surgery taking place. This may be accomplished by using ice to test numbness in the required (specific dermatome) area and by asking the patient for feedback as to any sensations.

Local infiltration

Infiltration of local anaesthetic agent facilitates minor surgery (e.g. removal of skin cancer or suturing of lacerations) or the insertion of invasive monitoring devices and may be the only anaesthetic agent required for the procedure. This involves direct injection into tissues to block sensory nerve pathways, thus resulting in an absence of pain, which may continue post-procedure to provide the patient with pain relief for a period of time. Patients remain conscious and aware of their surroundings, although mild sedation may also be given, depending on the patient's condition (Bryant et al., 2019). Adrenaline may be added to local anaesthetic agents for vasoconstriction properties in the area to be injected. However, this combination should not be used when infiltrating digits (e.g. nail-bed repair or laceration) owing to possible necrosis of tissue caused by the effects of vasoconstriction (Campbell, 2019). Examples of drugs used in local infiltration are lignocaine, bupivacaine and ropivacaine.

Regional anaesthesia

Techniques of **regional anaesthesia** involve injecting local anaesthetics anywhere along a pathway of a nerve, resulting in anaesthesia to a region of the body. Regional anaesthesia may be used alone or in combination with a general anaesthetic (Hewson & Hardman, 2019a). Regional anaesthesia may be administered by:

- a single dose
- intermittent bolus – repeated injections or indwelling catheter for repeat administration
- continuous infusion via a catheter – can be used for PO pain management.

Regional blocks, which are available using local anaesthetics (e.g. bupivacaine, lignocaine, ropivacaine), include:

- upper limb – axillary nerve blocks for elbow, forearm and hand surgery
- lower limb – femoral nerve blocks for femoral fractures and knee and foot surgery (Hewson & Hardman, 2019a).

Prior to performing a regional anaesthesia technique, the procedure must be discussed with the patient and, prior to the block, the skin must be marked close enough to the block site to be visible while performing the block. These form part of the 'Sign In' section of the WHO Surgical Safety Checklist (SSC), which should be performed to ensure the correct side and site for insertion of the block (see Chapter 9 for more information on the SSC). Verification with another clinician (i.e. nurse, assistant or medical officer) is required and must be documented appropriately.

To assist with the safe and accurate placement of the block and administration of local anaesthetic, ANZCA recommends that ultrasound equipment is made available for visualising the nerve and surrounding vessels to be blocked. Alternatively, a peripheral nerve stimulator may be required to assist in the identification of the nerves to be blocked (ANZCA, 2014c).

The Awake Patient – Nursing Considerations

Prior to and during the administration of local, regional or central blocks, the anaesthetic nurse should provide the patient with explanations and reassurance at all times. While undergoing surgery, the patient will be awake and lightly sedated, and vigilance is required by the surgical team to ensure patient safety and provide reassurance. The anaesthetic nurse should sit at the patient's head during the procedure, using verbal and non-verbal communication to reduce the patient's anxiety. Patients must understand that, although this type of anaesthesia will block painful stimuli, they may still be aware of pressure in the area of the surgical procedure. To alleviate anxiety they will also receive drugs (e.g. midazolam). Haemodynamic monitoring by the anaesthetic team is important to detect any complications or unwanted effects of the local anaesthetic drugs. Oxygen may be applied by a Hudson mask or nasal prongs. It is important that the surgical and anaesthetic teams are aware that they should not make unnecessary noise, especially conversations, as the patient may still be semiconscious and able to hear.

PATIENT SCENARIOS

SCENARIO 8.2: PREPARATION FOR ANAESTHESIA (CONTINUED)

RN Margaret McCormack, anaesthetic nurse, is assisting Dr Marion Thomas to prepare Mr Collins for the insertion of the spinal anaesthetic. He appears quite anxious and asks RN McCormack about the insertion procedure, in particular if he will be awake for the surgery and if he will feel anything.

Critical Thinking Questions

- Identify the equipment RN McCormack will prepare for insertion of the spinal anaesthetic.
- Describe how RN McCormack should answer Mr Collins' questions and allay his anxiety.

FEATURE BOX 8.4
Local Anaesthetic Toxicity

A young woman undergoing cosmetic breast surgery in a Sydney clinic suffered a cardiac arrest, the cause of which was suspected to have been an overdose of a local anaesthetic. She was treated with Intralipid infusion and transferred to hospital where she made a full recovery (Patty, 2015).

(Source: Patty, A. (2015). Cardiac arrest during cosmetic surgery: overdose of local anaesthetic likely. *Sydney Morning Herald*, 28 July.)

Local Anaesthetic Toxicity

Toxicity can occur when an accidental overdose of local anaesthetic is administered during a regional or local anaesthetic block or is accidentally injected into the bloodstream. The result is life-threatening circulatory collapse, convulsions, agitation and loss of consciousness. This situation requires immediate cessation of the local anaesthetic injection and resuscitation measures to support circulation and breathing. The administration of lipid emulsion (Intralipid) is also recommended as a treatment for local toxicity (Association of Anaesthetists of Great Britain and Ireland [AAGBI], 2020; Australian and New Zealand Anaesthetic Allergy Group [ANZAAG], 2016). Feature box 8.4 provides an example of local anaesthetic toxicity.

HAEMODYNAMIC MONITORING DURING ANAESTHESIA

Regardless of the type of anaesthesia or sedation the patient receives, **haemodynamic monitoring** is a vital component of the patient's management and safety. Advances in haemodynamic monitoring have greatly decreased the mortality and morbidity of patients undergoing anaesthesia. Both the ANZCA *PS18 Guideline on monitoring during anaesthesia* (2017a) and ACORN (2020) stipulate the minimum standards for monitoring to be provided. The anaesthetic nurse should consult with the anaesthetist regarding the type of monitoring equipment appropriate for the patient and the procedure being undertaken (Fig. 8.22). Monitoring equipment available includes:

- oxygen supply failure alarm
- oxygen analyser
- pulse oximeter
- breathing system disconnection or ventilator failure alarm
- electrocardiograph
- intermittent non-invasive blood pressure monitor

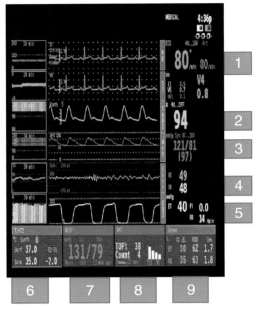

FIG. 8.22 Monitor showing vital signs.
1 ECG
2 Oxygen saturation
3 Arterial BP
4 BIS waveform
5 End tidal CO_2 (capnography)
6 Temperature
7 NIBP (non-invasive BP)
8 Train of 4 nerve stimulator
9 Gas analysis

- continuous invasive blood pressure monitor
- temperature monitor
- carbon dioxide monitor
- neuromuscular monitor – a peripheral nerve stimulator, also known as train of four monitor, can be used to assess the level of neuromuscular blockade (ANZCA, 2017a)
- volatile anaesthetic agent monitor
- bispectral index (BIS) monitoring (see Feature box 8.3)
- cardiac output, spirometry, central venous pressure (CVP) or transoesophageal echocardiogram (TOE) when clinically indicated (ANZCA, 2017a).

Circulation
Electrocardiograph
Monitoring of the patient's cardiovascular system involves observation of the patient's blood pressure and continuous ECG analysis. The ECG will detect arrhythmias, myocardial ischaemia, electrolyte imbalance and pacemaker dysfunction. The anaesthetic nurse must ensure that ECG

monitoring electrodes are not placed close to the proposed surgical site. Electrode placement requires a minimum of two sensing electrodes and a third reference (grounding) lead. The lead that displays the most prominent P waves on the ECG monitor is the preferred option because it follows the direction of the normal electrical impulse. Five-lead ECG monitoring provides more precise recording, with more accurate detection of myocardial ischaemia, and is used if the patient has a history of cardiac disease (Kossick, 2018). When using a three-lead ECG, the electrodes can be placed one on each shoulder and one on the left side of the rib cage.

Blood pressure

Indirect blood pressure monitoring is a minimum requirement for all patients. Changes in systolic blood pressure correlate with changes in myocardial oxygen requirements, and changes in diastolic blood pressure reflect coronary perfusion pressure. Care must be taken to ensure that the blood pressure cuff is the correct size. The cuff must be neither too tight nor too loose, as either will affect the readings, giving false results (Kossick, 2018).

Direct blood pressure monitoring involves cannulation of an artery to provide continuous measurement of arterial blood pressure. This invasive method is required when the patient is at risk of haemodynamic instability due to the nature of the surgery or has comorbidities that require close observation. Indicators for invasive blood pressure monitoring are listed in Feature box 8.5.

FEATURE BOX 8.5
Indicators for Invasive Blood Pressure Monitoring

- Patient-dependent factors
  - Haemodynamic instability (shock)
  - Cardiac disease
  - Respiratory insufficiency
  - Increased intracranial pressure
  - Polytrauma
- Type of surgery
  - Cardiac surgery
  - Craniotomy
  - Major thoracic surgery
  - Major abdominal surgery (Nagelhout, 2018a)

(Sources: Australian and New Zealand College of Anaesthetists. (2017a). *PS18 Guideline on monitoring during anaesthesia.* Melbourne: Author; Kossick, M. A. (2018). Clinical monitoring 1: Cardiovascular system. In J. Nagelhout & E. Sass (Eds.), *Nurse anesthesia* (6th ed., pp. 272–-289). St Louis, MO: Elsevier Saunders.)

Central venous pressure

A CVP catheter is often inserted prior to commencement of anaesthesia. The purpose of CVP monitoring is to:
- measure right heart filling pressure as a guide to intravascular volume
- administer drugs
- provide IV access in patients with poor peripheral veins.
  Additional reasons for CVP insertion include to:
- provide a route for long-term parenteral nutrition
- inject dye for diagnostic purposes
- remove air emboli.

Sites used for CVP catheter insertion include the internal jugular, subclavian, external jugular, cephalic, axillary and femoral veins. The anaesthetic nurse will provide assistance to the anaesthetist in preparing the required equipment using a surgical non-touch aseptic technique (ANZCA, 2015). The CVP catheter is inserted using the Seldinger technique, which involves insertion of a needle and use of a guide wire to thread the CVP catheter over the guide wire. Chest X-ray is carried out post-insertion to check the catheter position and to exclude pneumothorax. Documentation of insertion of the CVP must be completed by the anaesthetist and kept in the patient's medical record (NSW Health, 2011).

Complications of CVP catheter placement include:
- arrhythmias (atrial and ventricular)
- carotid or subclavian artery puncture (subclavian vein cannulation is contraindicated in patients on anticoagulants owing to the inability to compress the vessel)
- pneumothorax, hydrothorax, infection or air embolism (Scott, 2019).

Respiration

Monitoring the patient's respiratory function during anaesthesia involves the mandatory use of pulse oximetry and capnography.

Pulse oximetry

Pulse oximetry is a non-invasive measurement of haemoglobin oxygen saturation (S_pO_2) at the arteriole level that measures changes in the light absorbed by an extremity (Al-Shaikh & Stacey, 2018). It works by detecting the differences in absorption of oxygenated and deoxygenated blood. Normal values are 95% or above, and the anaesthetic nurse should monitor the patient's S_pO_2. If the patient's saturation level drops below 95%, the anaesthetic team should consider increasing the oxygen concentration in the patient's anaesthesia and/or check the equipment and placement of the probe. The pulse oximeter probe is usually placed on the fingers or toes and the reading is displayed on a monitor as a percentage. Cold or poorly perfused extremities can affect the accuracy of the pulse oximeter, and newer technologies using forehead oximetry may be more effective, providing more accurate readings (Welliver, 2018).

Capnography

Capnography is a graphical representation of expired carbon dioxide (CO_2) and is termed end-tidal CO_2 (Schick, 2018). Monitoring end-tidal CO_2 assists the anaesthetic team in the early detection of either technical catastrophes (e.g. inadvertent oesophageal intubation, breathing circuit leaks) or changes in the patient's respiratory, circulatory or metabolic condition. It is usually the initial indicator of malignant hyperthermia, which can be an anaesthetic emergency. The normal value of end-tidal CO_2 is 35–45 mmHg. CO_2 is collected by an adapter that is placed in the breathing circuit close to the airway so that the CO_2 collected will approximate the alveolar concentration. The expired CO_2 is then analysed using an infrared ray, which converts it to a waveform displayed on a monitor.

Temperature

Inadvertent perioperative hypothermia (IPH) is defined as a core temperature below 36°C (Duff et al., 2018). IPH is a preventable consequence of surgery and anaesthesia; during major surgery, a temperature probe placed orally, nasally or in the bladder (incorporated as part of a urinary catheter) is used to measure core temperature. If IPH is not addressed during the perioperative period, it can lead to a variety of complications, including:

- increased recovery time due to increased demand for oxygen consumption
- increased wound infections due to suppression of the immune system
- impaired cardiac function
- coagulopathy
- increased morbidity and mortality (ANZCA, 2017a; Duff et al., 2018).

In addition, maintaining normothermia (36°C) provides the patient with a feeling of well-being and comfort (Duff et al., 2018). Despite extensive evidence demonstrating the importance of providing intraoperative warming, a retrospective chart audit of 400 patients in four Australian hospitals revealed that almost one-third experienced IPH: this study highlights poor compliance by staff with established recommended evidence-based practice in relation to providing perioperative patient warming (Duff et al., 2018). See Chapter 9 for more information on the intraoperative management of IPH.

Neonates are more prone to hypothermia owing to their immature temperature regulation centres, as are older patients owing to their lower metabolic rates. Particular care should be taken to prevent IPH in these **special populations** and strategies are discussed later in the chapter.

Planned hypothermia may be required and deliberately induced to reduce oxygen requirements and create optimum operating conditions in specific surgery (e.g. neurosurgery and cardiac surgery).

Maintenance of normothermia should commence in the preoperative period, with nursing staff in the pre-admission area monitoring the patient's temperature and applying additional bed coverings or clothing or using forced-air warming devices if the patient's temperature drops below 36°C (ANZCA, 2017a) (see Chapter 7 for more information). Specialised gowns incorporating forced-air warming capabilities are commercially available, as are devices that use a disposable warming blanket connected to a hose and warming unit. The warm air inflates the blanket and the temperature can be regulated as required. The blankets are available in various configurations (e.g. full length or half length) to facilitate warming while allowing access to the surgical site for the surgeon. The anaesthetic nurse prepares the appropriately sized warming blanket and assists in positioning it on the patient as soon as practicable in the anaesthetic bay or immediately prior to the commencement of surgery.

Other methods of maintaining normothermia include:
- controlling the OR temperature
- warming IV fluids
- using overhead heating lamps for paediatric patients
- avoiding unnecessary exposure of the patient's body
- prewarming the patient.

PATIENT SCENARIOS

SCENARIO 8.3: THE ANAESTHETIC NURSE'S ROLE

Mr Collins' spinal anaesthetic has been successfully inserted and RN McCormack is applying monitoring equipment prior to commencement of his surgery.

Critical Thinking Questions

- Identify the monitoring equipment required for Mr Collins. Provide rationales for your answer.
- Describe the role of RN McCormack during Mr Collins' surgery. What are her priorities for patient care?

FLUID AND ELECTROLYTE BALANCE

The average adult requires water to replace gastrointestinal losses (100–200 mL/day), losses through respiration and perspiration (500–1000 mL/day) and excretion of urine (1000 mL/day). Adults need to consume about 2500 mL of fluids per day to ensure their renal function is adequate (Trinsoon & Patel, 2018).

Electrolyte Balance

When electrolyte values are abnormal, this affects the **fluid and electrolyte balance** and acid–base balance, resulting in renal, neuromuscular, endocrine or skeletal dysfunction. The levels of serum electrolytes affect the movement of fluid between the body compartments. The major extracellular electrolytes are sodium, calcium, chloride and bicarbonate (Table 8.6). Sodium is the most common cation and chloride the most common anion. Potassium, magnesium and phosphate are the major intracellular electrolytes, potassium being the most common cation and phosphate the most common anion. An imbalance in the serum electrolyte levels has ramifications for metabolic activity (Trinsoon & Patel, 2018).

Fluid and Blood Loss

When patients arrive in the OR, they have usually been fasting for some hours. Frequently, they also endure some loss of blood and other fluids during the surgical procedure. This can put them at risk of hypovolaemia, which can lead to other complications such as tachycardia, hypotension and reduced urine output.

The fluid requirements of a patient undergoing major surgery where considerable blood loss may occur can be difficult to estimate; patients may experience losses of up to 20 mL/kg per hour. The circulating nurse may be asked to provide the anaesthetist with an estimate of blood loss. In addition, the anaesthetist will monitor the suction canisters for blood that has been suctioned from the surgical site. The instrument nurse will be able to provide the amount of intraoperative irrigation fluid used. The anaesthetist may also use invasive monitoring such as CVP in a patient with potential blood loss to clinically manage the loss.

A patient who is adequately hydrated before, during and after surgery will have a better outcome. Therefore, all patients undergoing surgery or any procedure requiring an anaesthetic or sedation must have some form of venous access, not only to facilitate induction and maintenance of anaesthesia but also to enable provision of fluids during and after the procedure. There is increasing evidence that intraoperative fluid therapy may influence PO outcomes. Both too little and too much fluid can adversely affect patient outcomes, and fluid therapy guided by flow-based haemodynamic monitors improves perioperative outcomes (Trinsoon & Patel, 2018).

The anaesthetic nurse should ensure that a wide range of cannulae and IV administration sets, as well as a variety of IV fluids, are available. The usual practice for most general anaesthetic procedures is to prepare a litre of IV fluid on an administration set ready for the beginning of the surgery. The ability to warm the IV fluid is also required, as well as a rapid infuser if there is a risk of severe haemorrhage. The anaesthetist determines the site of placement of the IV cannulae after considering the type of surgery, the IV fluid requirements and the surgeon and patient's preferences, and the anaesthetic nurse assists with inserting, securing and labelling the IV lines. The anaesthetic nurse commences documentation of IV fluids, blood loss and urine output on a fluid balance chart. If irrigating fluids are being used during the procedure, this must be taken into account when calculating the patient's fluid status. Maintaining accurate documentation is particularly important with complex and trauma surgery, paediatric patients and patients with significant comorbidities, such as cardiac and renal disease.

IV solutions available include the following:

- *Crystalloid solutions* – these fluids (e.g. normal saline, Ringer's lactate solution, Plasmalyte) are isotonic and are equivalent to plasma in osmolarity. They are used to maintain normal fluid requirements and replace evaporative and third-space losses (Trinsoon & Patel, 2018).
- *Colloid solutions* – these fluids (e.g. albumin) are hypotonic and are greater in osmolarity than plasma. This causes the solutes to move from the bloodstream into the cells, so that the cells swell. They are used to replace blood loss or restore intravascular volume.

TABLE 8.6 Normal Electrolyte Values	
Sodium	134–145 mEq/L
Potassium	3.5–5.0 mmol/L
Chloride	96–106 mmol/L
Calcium	2.20–2.55 mmol/L
Bicarbonate	22–31 mmol/L
Magnesium	0.70–0.9 mmol/L

(Source: Adapted from AUSMED. (2018). Electrolyte imbalance 1 normal ranges and disturbances for common electrolytes. Retrieved from <https://ausmed.com/cpd/articles/normal-electrolytelevels>; Murphy, E. (2019). Patient safety and risk management. In J. Rothrock (Ed.), *Alexander's care of the patient in surgery* (16th ed., pp. 16–45). St Louis, MO: Elsevier Saunders.)

• *Blood transfusions* – these are used to replace lost blood volume or a specific component (e.g. red cells, platelets or coagulation factors) (Boer, Bossers, & Koning, 2018; Higgins Roche & Schwartz, 2018).

Blood Transfusions

If the patient's hypovolaemia is moderate and due to loss of blood, the anaesthetist may decide to administer a blood transfusion, which, in these patients, will improve oxygen-carrying capacity.

Fig. 8.23 shows templates published by National Blood Authority (2013) to guide the anaesthetist when managing patients with critical intra- or postoperative bleeding who require a massive transfusion.

In addition, the anaesthetist may have access to rotation thromboelastometry with a ROTEM machine – a device that is used for point-of-care blood analysis to streamline the management of blood requirements in a patient who is bleeding. It replaces standard laboratory tests of INR/APTT and fibrinogen in most scenarios and assists the anaesthetist to decide which blood products are best suited to the patient. The ability of the blood to clot is crucial in the management of bleeding and the ROTEM ensures that blood products are administered according to an individual's blood-clotting capacity. Fig. 8.24 shows the ROTEM machine (Haemoview Diagnostics, 2019).

There are numerous potential complications with critical bleeding/massive blood transfusion, including transfusion reactions, development of coagulopathies, hypothermia and sepsis. One of the most common causes of a transfusion reaction is the administration of the wrong blood type (Higgins Roche & Schwartz, 2018). Therefore, local protocols for the checking of blood, based on national guidelines (addressed later)

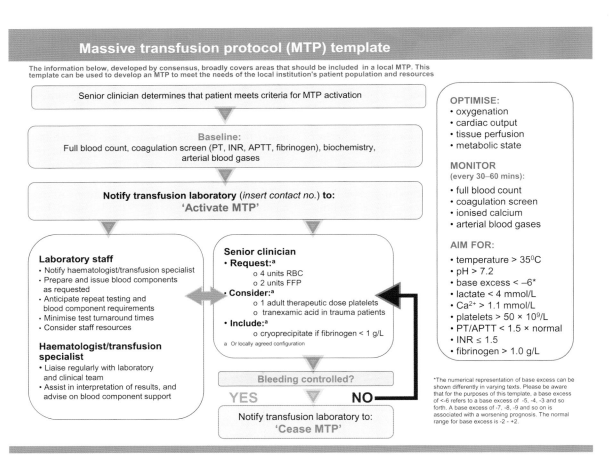

FIG. 8.23 (**A**) Massive transfusion protocol (MTP) template.

Suggested criteria for activation of MTP

- Actual or anticipated 4 units RBC in < 4 hrs, + haemodynamically unstable, +/– anticipated ongoing bleeding
- Severe thoracic, abdominal, pelvic or multiple long bone trauma
- Major obstetric, gastrointestinal or surgical bleeding

Initial management of bleeding

- Identify cause
- Initial measures:
  - compression
  - tourniquet
  - packing
- Surgical assessment:
  - early surgery or angiography to stop bleeding

Specific surgical considerations

- If significant physiological derangement, consider damage control surgery or angiography

Cell salvage

- Consider use of cell salvage where appropriate

Dosage

Platelet count < 50 x 10⁹/L	1 adult therapeutic dose
INR > 1.5	FFP 15 mL/kgᵃ
Fibrinogen < 1.0 g/L	cryoprecipitate 3–4 gᵃ
Tranexamic acid	loading dose 1 g over 10 min, then infusion of 1 g over 8 hrs

a Local transfusion laboratory to advise on number of units needed to provide this dose

Resuscitation

- Avoid hypothermia, institute active warming
- Avoid excessive crystalloid
- Tolerate permissive hypotension (BP 80–100 mmHg systolic) until active bleeding controlled
- Do not use haemoglobin alone as a transfusion trigger

Special clinical situations

- Warfarin:
  - add vitamin K, prothrombinex/FFP
- Obstetric haemorrhage:
  - early DIC often present; consider cryoprecipitate
- Head injury:
  - aim for platelet count > 100 × 10⁹/L
  - permissive hypotension contraindicated

Considerations for use of rFVIIaᵇ

The *routine* use of rFVIIa in trauma patients is not recommended due to its lack of effect on mortality (Grade B) and variable effect on morbidity (Grade C). Institutions may choose to develop a process for the use of rFVIIa where there is:
- uncontrolled haemorrhage in salvageable patient, and
- failed surgical or radiological measures to control bleeding, and
- adequate blood component replacement, and
- pH > 7.2, temperature > 34°C

Discuss dose with haematologist/transfusion specialist

ᵇ rFVIIa is not licensed for use in this situation; all use must be part of practice review.

ABG	arterial blood gas	FFP	fresh frozen plasma	APTT	activated partial thromboplastin time
INR	international normalised ratio	BP	blood pressure	MTP	massive transfusion protocol
DIC	disseminated intravascular coagulation	PT	prothrombin time	FBC	full blood count
RBC	red blood cell	rFVIIa	activated recombinant factor VII		

FIG. 8.23, cont'd (B) Suggested criteria for activation of MTP. (Source: National Blood Transfusion Authority (2013).)

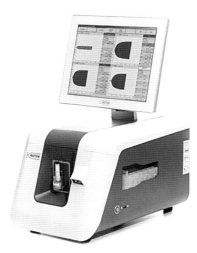

FIG. 8.24 ROTEM thromboelastometry. (Source: Instrumentation Laboratory, A Werfen Company. https://www.instrumentationlaboratory.com/en/rotem-sigma.)

must be followed. Signs and symptoms of an acute transfusion reaction include:

- mild allergic reaction – localised urticaria, pruritus and rash
- severe allergic reaction – flushing, wheezing, hypotension, anaphylaxis
- febrile reaction – unexpected fever (e.g. a temperature rise >1°C; may have accompanying chills and rigors).

Management of a suspected transfusion reaction includes the following:

- stop the transfusion immediately
- check vital signs
- maintain IV access
- check the right pack has been given to the right patient
- notify the medical officer and transfusion service provider
- send freshly collected blood and urine samples along with the blood pack and IV line as required by the transfusion service provider (National Blood Authority, 2011).

Australia and New Zealand have blood transfusion services that provide guidelines for the management of patients undergoing blood transfusions (National Blood Authority, 2011; New Zealand Blood Service, 2017).

ANAESTHETIC EMERGENCIES

Despite patients being closely monitored while under anaesthesia, emergencies still occur that require prompt and effective action. The anaesthetic nurse must have knowledge of the commonly occurring **anaesthetic emergencies** and their management in order to provide effective support to the anaesthetic and possibly the surgical teams.

Anaphylaxis

Anaphylaxis is an antibody-mediated reaction to an antigen that can cause a sudden life-threatening response involving the skin, respiratory and cardiovascular systems. Anaphylaxis is a rare occurrence during anaesthesia and depends on the antigen involved; for example, adverse reactions to muscle relaxants occur in 1 in 5000 to 1 in 10,000 cases (Hewson & Hardman, 2019b). Other causes are the administration of antibiotics, chlorhexidine, blood and blood products or contrast media (Cook & Harper, 2018). More than 90% of these reactions usually occur within 3 minutes of administration of the agent and it is vital for the anaesthetic nurse to remain with the anaesthetist at the beginning of the anaesthetic to assist in resuscitating the patient should a reaction occur.

Treatment of anaphylaxis includes:

- if the causative agent is known, stopping administration immediately
- administering 100% oxygen while maintaining the airway
- ceasing all anaesthetic drugs
- commencing fluid replacement with colloid or crystalloid
- treating bronchospasm with salbutamol
- administering adrenaline – bolus IV 0.001 mg/kg.

Adrenaline is the drug of choice for anaphylactic reactions. It is a direct-acting sympathomimetic agent that exerts its effect on alpha and beta adrenoreceptors. It is a powerful cardiac stimulant with vasopressor and antihistamine actions. It is also an excellent bronchodilator and has a rapid onset. Once the patient has been stabilised, an adrenaline infusion may be commenced and other drugs, such as hydrocortisone, administered. It is recommended that the patient be followed-up once this episode is resolved to determine the cause of the reaction (ANZAAG, 2016; ANZCA, 2016c; Cook & Harper, 2018).

Malignant Hyperthermia

Malignant hyperthermia (MH) is a rare, autosomal-dominant muscle disorder. It is a life-threatening disease that is regarded as one of the true emergencies within the perioperative environment. The condition can be triggered by any of the commonly used inhalational anaesthetic agents or muscle relaxants, particularly suxamethonium. If left untreated, MH can result in death. MH has very clear, discernible clinical manifestations. These include:

- a sudden unexplained increase in end-tidal CO_2 levels
- unexplained tachycardia, tachypnoea, labile blood pressure and arrhythmias
- hypercarbia in the spontaneously breathing patient
- acidosis, hypoxaemia, hyperkalaemia
- muscle rigidity, in particular of the masseter (jaw) muscle
- fever, which is described as a late sign and occurs in only 30% of MH cases
- myoglobinuria, with dark-coloured urine
- mottled cyanotic skin (Marley & Clapp, 2018).

Treatment

Prompt diagnosis and treatment of MH can reduce mortality and morbidity and, even though the condition is rare, knowledge of the condition and treatment is vital. Dantrolene sodium for injection is the only effective treatment for MH and functions by inhibiting calcium uptake. The anaesthetic nurse plays an important role in the management of an acute episode of MH by being aware of the location of the MH emergency equipment and the need for it to be checked daily to ensure the availability of at least 36 ampoules of dantrolene sodium for injection and drawing-up equipment (Gillerman, 2020).

PAEDIATRIC CONSIDERATIONS IN ANAESTHESIA

It is beyond the scope of this text to provide detailed content on paediatric anaesthesia as it is an anaesthetic specialty in its own right; however, a brief summary of some of the key paediatric anaesthesia considerations follow.

The physiological, pharmacological and psychological differences between children and adults must be understood in order to provide a safe outcome, and special considerations must be given to preterm infants and those with congenital malformations. Anaesthetic nurses must receive education in the anaesthetic management of paediatric patients, given the specialised equipment and pharmacology requirements.

Preoperative Assessment and Preparation

The preoperative assessment and preparation of the child for surgery are important considerations, as it is during this time that the anaesthetist will evaluate the child's medical condition, the needs of the planned surgical procedure and the psychological make-up of the child and family. The anaesthetist also formulates the approach to induction of anaesthesia, explains the possibilities regarding induction and, together with the anaesthetic nurse, helps soothe family concerns. In many operating suites, a parent or carer will accompany the child (usually under 6 years of age) and provide comfort to the child during induction of anaesthesia.

Fasting guidelines vary between healthcare facilities and anaesthetists, but Feature box 8.6 lists the ANZCA (2017b) guidelines.

FEATURE BOX 8.6
Guidelines for Fasting

For children over 6 months of age having an elective procedure, breast milk or formula and limited solid food may be given up to 6 hours and clear fluids up to 1 hour prior to anaesthesia.

For infants under 6 months of age having an elective procedure, formula may be given up to 4 hours, breast milk up to 3 hours and clear fluids up to 1 hour prior to anaesthesia.

Food and fluids are withheld prior to surgery as follows:

CHILDREN OVER 6 MONTHS OF AGE:
6 hours
- Limited solid foods
- Breast milk or formula

1 hour
- Clear fluids (no more than 3 mL/kg per hour)

INFANTS UNDER 6 MONTHS OF AGE
4 hours
- Formula

3 hours
- Breast milk

1 hour
- Clear fluids such as water/apple juice

(Source: ANZCA. (2017b). *PS07. Guideline on pre-anaesthesia consultation and patient preparation. Appendix 1 – Fasting guidelines.*)

Equipment

The equipment used for paediatric patients (e.g. face masks, ETTs, laryngoscopes and anaesthetic delivery systems) is scaled down to match the size and differing anatomy of paediatric patients. It is also modified to manage the different ventilator pressures required.

- *Laryngoscope* – curved or straight blades can be used, although the straight blade laryngoscope is recommended in young children, because it is designed to lift the epiglottis (which is comparatively large and floppy in children) under the tip of the blade, allowing a better view of the vocal cords (Figs 8.25 and 8.26).

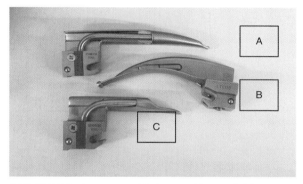

FIG. 8.25 Laryngoscope blades used in paediatrics.
A Seward blade
B Macintosh blade
C Miller blade

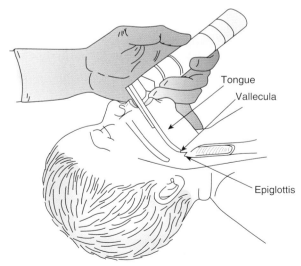

FIG. 8.26 Position of the laryngoscope blade for paediatric intubation. (Source: https://aneskey.com/wp-content/uploads/2016/06/B9781416037736100497_gr14.jpg.)

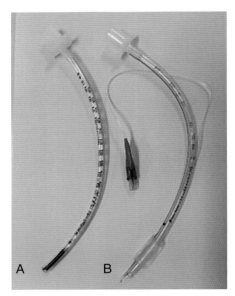

FIG. 8.27 Uncuffed and cuffed endotracheal tubes.
A Uncuffed
B Cuffed

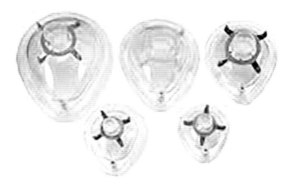

FIG. 8.28 Paediatric face masks.

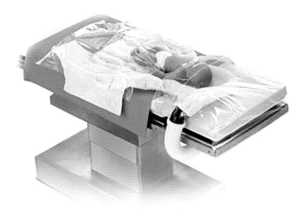

FIG. 8.29 Infant underbody body blanket. (Source: Reproduced with permission of 3M. Bair Hugger is a trademark of 3M.)

- *Endotracheal tubes* – traditionally, uncuffed endotracheal tubes have been preferred for use in children up to 8 years of age to reduce the risk of trauma and oedema to the trachea at the cricoid ring, which is the narrowest part of the airway (Fig. 8.27). However, it is becoming more common to use adjusted-size cuffed ETTs to ensure adequate tidal volume delivery (Rieker, 2018).
- *Supraglottic airway device (SAD)* – scaled-down versions of adult SADs are available for use in children under 5 kg in weight.

Anaesthetic Induction

Induction is usually carried out using inhalational agents via a face mask (Fig. 8.28) and with a parent present, supported by the anaesthetic nurse, to provide comfort to the child. Face masks are available with a pleasant fruity smell to provide further comfort to the child. IV access is usually secured following induction to reduce distress.

Temperature

Maintaining normothermia is extremely important in babies and neonates as their capacity to regulate temperature is not well developed. This is accomplished by the use of warming devices similar to those described earlier in the chapter. In addition, overhead heating devices can be used, providing radiant heating during the procedure when forced-air warming devices cannot be placed over the child. Alternatively, as can be seen in Fig. 8.29, a forced-air warming device can be placed underneath the child (Ip, Walker, & Thomas, 2019).

Drugs and IV Fluids

Drugs and IV fluids are titrated according to the child's weight and are delivered through micro IV burettes to prevent fluid overload. Careful checking and documentation of medications used is vital, as drug calculations are often complex in neonates (NSW Health, 2015).

PATIENT SCENARIOS

SCENARIO 8.4: TRANSFER OF CARE

Mr Collins' surgery has been successfully completed and he is ready for transfer to the PACU.

Critical Thinking Question

- Describe how RN Margaret McCormack will prepare Mr Collins for transfer from the operating table onto his bed/trolley.

ANAESTHETIC CONSIDERATIONS FOR THE OLDER PATIENT

While age is not synonymous with poor physiological function, the ageing process does bring with it physiological changes affecting all body systems that require consideration when planning anaesthetic management of the older surgical patient. The anaesthetic nurse must be cognisant of these changes in order to plan the care of the patient and their special needs; see Table 8.7, which summarises patient care considerations and actions which the anaesthetic team should consider. Of particular significance is the decrease in subcutaneous body fat in many older patients, which increases risks of pressure injury and hypothermia. Careful preoperative assessment of the patient and careful transfers to and from the table, avoiding shearing/friction and use of appropriate positioning devices, are vital to ensure the patient's skin remains intact. Monitoring the patient's temperature and the

---

TABLE 8.7
Patient Care Considerations and the Ageing Process

System	Physiological Changes	Significance	Action
Cardiovascular	Structural and functional changes to the heart; vascular system less compliant	Reduced capacity to increase heart rate in response to hypotension, hypovolaemia Delay with onset of IV drugs Severe bradycardia with potent opioids Comorbidities of hypertension and ischaemic heart disease	Monitor during surgery for any evidence of cardiovascular episodes; maintain normothermia to reduce workload on the heart; consider PO care in high-dependency unit Awareness of current medications and interactions with anaesthetic agents, especially anticoagulant therapy
Respiratory	Calcification in chest wall, intervertebral and intercostal joints, reduction in muscle strength, loss of elastic tissue recoil High incidence of pulmonary disease, e.g. chronic obstructive pulmonary disease Teeth may be missing	Decrease in chest wall compliance and reduction in functional alveolar surface area for gas exchange Increased risk of respiratory failure Opioids and other anaesthetic agents may cause respiratory depression Missing teeth or removed dentures may hinder ability to maintain bag/mask ventilation	Limit high inspired O_2, maintain P_aCO_2 near normal preoperative values Consider use of regional anaesthesia with sedation Close observation following administration of opioids in immediate pre- and postoperative period Maintaining bag/mask ventilation may need additional care or dentures to remain in situ until intubation
Musculoskeletal	Decrease in skeletal muscle mass, subcutaneous fat, loss of collagen and elastin Higher incidence of osteoarthritis	May affect mobility of joints and cervical spine, affecting airway management; patient positioning Increases risk of pressure injuries	Preassessment of cervical spine to plan appropriate airway management; assess and document skin integrity pre- and postoperatively Assemble additional equipment to facilitate positioning/transfer and prevent shearing forces

Continued

TABLE 8.7
Patient Care Considerations and the Ageing Process—cont'd

System	Physiological Changes	Significance	Action
Renal	Progressive atrophy of kidney tissue Deterioration of renal vascular structures Decreased renal blood flow	Decreased renal drug clearance leading to increased recovery time from anaesthesia Increased incidence of PO delirium	Careful fluid balance to avoid fluid overload Titration of drug dosage Monitor for respiratory depression in immediate PO period If renal impairment present, consider alternative anaesthetic agents Awareness of preoperative cognitive impairment Reassure patient to time and place to reduce effect of delirium/confusion Ensure bedrails are raised to prevent injury
Thermoregulation	Decrease in basal metabolic rate	Increased risk of hypothermia	Monitor core temperature and use active warming devices
Other	Hearing deficit Sight deficit Immune system not as effective and greater susceptibility to infection		Ensure hearing aid is present; remove mask when speaking to patient to allow lip reading Patient may wish to retain glasses until induction to allow for awareness of surroundings and aid in effective communication Strict adherence to aseptic practices; administration of antibiotics

PO = postoperative.
(Sources: Bordi, S. (2018). Geriatrics and anesthesia practice. In J. Nagelhout & E. Sass (Eds.), *Nurse anesthesia* (6th ed., pp. 1136–1145). St Louis, MO: Elsevier; Dhesi, J., Moppett, I., & Partridge, J. (2019). Surgery under anaesthesia for the older surgical patient. In J. Thompson, I. Moppett, & M. Wiles (Eds.), *Smith and Aitkenhead's textbook of anaesthesia* (7th ed., pp. 666–681). Edinburgh: Churchill Livingstone.)

use of warming devices to prevent hypothermia must also be a priority for the anaesthetic nurse. In addition, older patients may suffer hearing and visual impairment, requiring greater emphasis on clear communication (Bordi, 2018; Dehsi, Moppett, & Partridge, 2019).

ANAESTHETIC CONSIDERATIONS FOR THE OBESE PATIENT

Worldwide, obesity is one of the greatest health challenges facing Western medicine and yet it is preventable (WHO, 2018). According to the Australian Institute of Health and Welfare (AIHW), in 2014–15, 11.2 million Australian adults were overweight (BMI 25–29.9) or obese (BMI 30–34.9 Class 1), equivalent to a national rate of 63.4% (AIHW, 2018). Furthermore, 1 in 4 children are classified as obese or overweight (AIHW, 2018; WHO, 2018). Bariatric is a term

which is sometimes used interchangeably with obese. However, the term *bariatric* originates from the Greek words *baros* meaning weight and *iatrics* meaning medical treatment, and generally refers to surgery to treat obese patients, for example gastric banding (Cambridge University Press, 2020). Therefore, the term obese is used in this text.

Preoperative assessment

As the world's population increases and along with it the number of people who are obese, it is likely that increasing numbers of obese patients will present to hospitals for surgery. Chapter 7 discusses some of the general issues to be considered when managing obese patients in the perioperative environment, including the importance of preoperative assessment for possible underlying cardiac and pulmonary conditions that could lead to perioperative complications. In addition,

TABLE 8.8
Conditions Associated With the Pathophysiology of Obesity

System	Conditions
Airway	Increased incidence of difficulty in bag/valve mask ventilation due to increased adipose tissue in the pharyngeal wall
Respiratory	Decreased lung compliance due to increased pulmonary blood flow Decreased chest wall compliance due to presence of adipose tissue Decreased functional residual capacity (FRC), leading to possible hypoxia at rest, worse when supine Obstructive sleep apnoea Obesity hyperventilation syndrome
Cardiovascular	Increased blood volume Cardiomyopathy Hypertension Increased O_2 consumption and CO_2 production Ischaemic heart disease Pulmonary hypertension (secondary to obstructive sleep apnoea/obesity hyperventilation syndrome) Thromboembolic disease
Other	Increased risk of gastric aspiration secondary to reflux hiatus hernia Altered drug kinetics Diabetes Fatty liver disease Dyslipidaemia Metabolic syndrome Osteoarthritis

(Source: Bouch, C. (2019). Anaesthesia for the obese patient. In J. Thompson, I. Moppett, & M. Wiles (Eds.), *Smith and Aitkenhead's textbook of anaesthesia* (7th ed., pp. 656-665). Edinburgh: Churchill Livingstone.)

patients who are obese may face other complications in surgery and procedures. For example, there may difficulty with intubation due to increased adipose tissue around the face and pharynx, with secondary displacement of the larynx and enlarged tongue (Nightingale et al., 2015). Table 8.8 summarises the main conditions associated with obesity which require consideration when planning surgical and anaesthetic interventions.

Airway and Ventilation

Patients must be assessed preoperatively for the possibility of a difficult intubation. In the likelihood of a difficult intubation, it is important for the anaesthetic team to discuss the plan of action prior to any anaesthetic agents being administered so as to ensure that all appropriate difficult intubation equipment is available (see the discussion on difficult intubation earlier in the chapter).

Prior to the induction of anaesthesia, it is advisable to preoxygenate the patient with 100% oxygen via a Hudson mask and apply positive end-expiratory pressure (PEEP) (up to 10 cm H_2O), to reduce the incidence of dependent atelectasis (partial or complete collapse of the lung).

Symptoms of obstructive sleep apnoea and obesity hyperventilation syndrome can become worse in the supine position and induction of anaesthesia can be particularly problematic owing to patients being unable to lie flat. Neck flexion and movement can also be hindered in an obese patient, and correct positioning is vital to ensure visualisation of the vocal cords. This can be achieved by using extra pillows or blankets to 'ramp' the patient up, ensuring that their head, upper body and shoulders are substantially higher than the chest and that the ear canal is level with the sternal notch. This is typically referred to as 'sniffing the morning air' (see Chapter 9 for further information). An intubation wedge or pillow can be useful to ensure correct positioning. An example of this is an intubation wedge, which can be positioned deflated under the patient's head and shoulders and then inflated by the anaesthetist to the required height and position (Fig. 8.30).

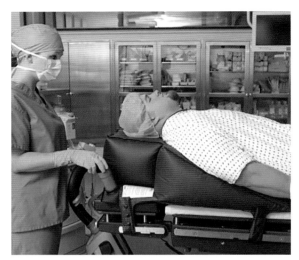

FIG. 8.30 HT-Wedge adjustable positioning device. (Source: https://marlinmedical.com.au/product/ht-wedge-adjustable-positioning-device/.)

Intraoperative Care

As with any unconscious patient, caution must be taken to ensure optimal patient positioning and protection of pressure areas. Nerve injuries can occur more frequently in obese patients (Fawcett, 2019). Patients placed in a steep Trendelenburg position are at greater risk of slipping down the table, so placement of safety straps (usually two) across the patient is advised. Operating tables can generally accommodate patients up to 250 kg, although some tables can take much greater weight. Side supports can also be fitted to accommodate patients too wide for regular operating tables. Other equipment to be considered includes extra-large calf compression stockings to prevent venous thromboembolism (VTE) and extra-long blood pressure cuffs to ensure accurate blood pressure monitoring. Transfer devices such as a Hovermatt should be positioned prior to the patient arriving in the operating suite to facilitate safe transfer and positioning during the perioperative period (Krogh, 2018).

ANAESTHETIC CONSIDERATIONS FOR THE OBSTETRIC PATIENT

Alterations in hormone levels (progesterone and oestrogen) that occur during pregnancy precipitate numerous physiological changes that have implications when an obstetric patient undergoes surgery and anaesthesia (Pillai, 2019) (Table 8.9). There are a number of risks to be considered, and anaesthetic nurses must have knowledge and skills to manage these risks to ensure a safe outcome for both mother and baby (Kasson, 2018).

Obstetric patients present the attending anaesthetist with a number of unique challenges. The most challenging aspect involves management of the airway, which, due to a number of anatomical and physiological changes that take place during pregnancy, places the pregnant patient into the difficult airway category.

Preparation for Surgery and Anaesthesia

Although this section will concentrate on the management of a patient undergoing a caesarean section, it is important to acknowledge that patients who are pregnant may undergo non-obstetric related surgery and many of the same risks exist.

Many patients undergoing elective or emergency caesarean section surgery will do so under regional anaesthesia, which may already be in situ if the patient has been transferred from the labour suite, or a spinal or epidural anaesthetic will be inserted on arrival in the OR. (See 'Central neural blockade'.)

Regional Anaesthesia

The use of effective regional anaesthesia is the preferred option for surgery as it negates the risks associated with securing the airway and administering a general anaesthetic. It also enables the patient to remain awake during the procedure, hear the first cry of the baby and experience skin-to-skin contact with the newborn baby, which has been found to be beneficial in promoting bonding (Moore, Bergman, Anderson, & Medley, 2016). The effectiveness of the regional anaesthesia will be assessed by the anaesthetist to ensure that all the nerves associated with innervating the layers between the skin and the uterus, peritoneum, vagina and perineum are anaesthetised. Therefore the block may extend up to at least T4 and T5 and also include the sacral roots (S1–5) (Kasson, 2018) (Fig. 8.31).

Managing the Airway

The anaesthetic team must ensure that equipment is prepared to administer a general anaesthetic using rapid sequence induction, should the regional anaesthesia fail or an emergency occur.

Rapid tracheal intubation, using the standard Macintosh laryngoscope, can be hindered in obstetric patients by the handle of the laryngoscope hitting the patient's engorged breasts and the hand of the assistant applying

TABLE 8.9
Patient Care Considerations and the Obstetric Patient

System	Physiological Changes	Significance	Action
Cardiovascular	Increased circulating volume resulting in an increase in cardiac output, stroke volume and heart rate Decreased systemic vascular resistance Peripheral venous engorgement and stasis Increased mucosal vascularity	Vital signs may remain stable despite large blood loss, but condition can deteriorate rapidly Haemodynamic instability Potential for aortocaval compression from ≈ 20 weeks gestation Venous stasis varicose veins, deep vein thrombosis May result in bleeding in nasal passages and gums, which can compromise airway	Close monitoring of haemodynamic status for signs of compromise Avoid nursing the woman flat on her back to reduce risk of aortocaval compression, e.g. tilt bed or use pillows/wedges under right side to obtain a lateral tilt of at least 15° to maintain placental flow (see Fig. 8.30) Thromboprophylaxis – compression devices Care to avoid any trauma during intubation, suction
Respiratory	Soft tissue oedema of the upper airway, weight gain Increased fat deposits around the neck, breast enlargement Elevation of diaphragm and flaring of rib cage	May cause pressure on neck when in supine and compromise airway and respiratory function Increased minute ventilation and oxygen consumption Decreased functional residual capacity	Preoxygenation Careful monitoring of oxygen saturation levels Rapid sequence induction
Gastrointestinal	Smooth muscle vasodilation Relaxation of cardiac sphincter Increased gastric acidity	Delayed gastric emptying High risk of aspiration pneumonitis	Rapid sequence induction Administration of sodium citrate solution immediately preoperatively to reduce acidity of gastric contents in the event of aspiration
Haematological	Dilution of plasma proteins, increase in plasma volume, decrease in red blood cell volume Increase in clotting factors, platelet consumption and increased platelet aggregation	Woman is in a hypercoagulable state with increased risk of bleeding	Ensure a current group and hold and blood has been cross-matched Accurate fluid balance
Renal	Increased renal blood flow as a result of increased cardiac output	Increased urine output with increased excretion of protein and glucose Dilated ureters, which can lead to urine stasis and increased risk of urinary tract infection Gravid uterus can cause mechanical obstruction	Check urine for proteinuria and blood sugar levels

(Source: Kasson, B. (2018). Obstetric anesthesia. In J. Nagelhout & E. Sass (Eds.), *Nurse anesthesia* (6th ed., pp. 1064–1091). St Louis, MO: Elsevier; Pillai, A. (2019). Obstetric anaesthesia and analgesia. In J. Thompson, I. Moppett, & M. Wiles (Eds.), *Smith and Aitkenhead's textbook of anaesthesia* (7th ed., pp. 800–830). Edinburgh: Churchill Livingstone.)

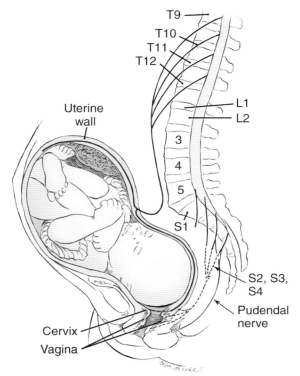

FIG. 8.31 Spinal cord, nerve roots and sensory innervation to uterus, cervix and vagina. (Source: Kasson, B. (2018). Obstetric anesthesia. In J. Nagelhout & E. Sass (Eds.), *Nurse anesthesia* (6th ed., Ch. 51, Fig. 51.3). St Louis, MO: Elsevier.)

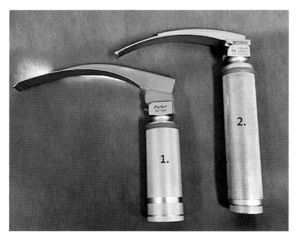

FIG. 8.32 Standard and short blades and handles.
1 Stubby handle and Kessel blade
2 Standard handle and Mackintosh blade

Positioning the patient is an important consideration. Fig. 8.33 shows how the patient should be positioned on the operating table. The anaesthetic nurse must ensure the wedge is placed under the right side of the patient to reduce the risk of aortocaval compression.

CONCLUSION

It is important that perianaesthesia anaesthetic nurses work in collaboration with the anaesthetist and other members of the surgical team to ensure patient safety during all phases of anaesthetic management. An in-depth knowledge of anaesthetic modalities and agents commonly used, together with haemodynamic monitoring and specialised anaesthetic equipment across different age groups and patients with comorbidities, will contribute to a smooth and safe anaesthetic for the patient.

cricoid pressure. To overcome these difficulties, a variation of the laryngoscope, a Kessel blade and a stubby (shorter) handle may be requested as well as a videolaryngoscope. The Kessel blade can be opened by a further 20 degrees to facilitate intubation (Fig. 8.32).

Supine   **Left uterine displacement**

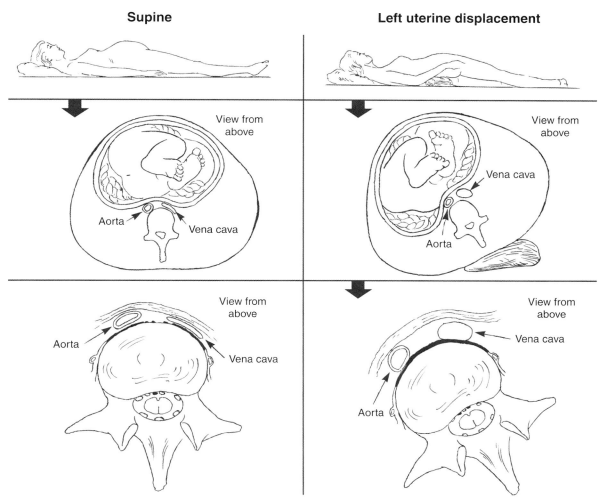

FIG. 8.33 Effects of uterine displacement on the diameter of the abdominal aorta and vena cava (Source: Kasson, B. (2018). Obstetric anesthesia. In J. Nagelhout & E. Sass (Eds.), *Nurse anesthesia* (6th ed., Ch. 51, Fig 51.1. St Louis, MO: Elsevier.)

RESOURCES

Association of Anaesthetists – Management of severe local anaesthetic toxicity
https://anaesthetists.org
Australian and New Zealand College of Anaesthetists
https://www.anzca.edu.au
Australian College of Critical Care Nurses
https://www.acccn.com.au
Australian College of Perianaesthesia Nurses
https://acpan.edu.au/about/

Difficult Airway Society
https://www.das.uk.com
Lipid Rescue Resuscitation
http://lipidrescue.squarespace.com
Malignant hyperthermia
https://malignanthyperthermia.org.au
National Blood Authority Australia
https://www.blood.gov.au
New Zealand Blood Service
https://www.nzblood.co.nz

REFERENCES

Agency for Clinical Innovation (ACI), Anaesthesia Perioperative Care Network. (2013). *Safe procedural sedation project phase 1: Diagnostic and solution design report.* Sydney: Author.

Al-Shaikh, B., & Stacey, S. (2018). *Essentials of anaesthetic equipment, critical care & peri-operative management* (5th ed.). London: Elsevier.

Association of Anaesthetists of Great Britain and Ireland (AAGBI). (2020). Management of severe local anaesthetic toxicity. Retrieved from <https://anaesthetists.org/Portals/0/PDFs/Guidelines%20PDFs/Guideline_management_severe_local_anaesthetic_toxicity_v2_2010_final.pdf?ver=2018-07-11-163755-240&ver=2018-07-11-163755-240>.

AUSMED. (2018). Electrolyte imbalance + normal ranges and disturbances for common electrolytes. Retrieved from <https://ausmed.com/cpd/articles/normal-electrolyte-levels.>

Australian and New Zealand Anaesthetic Allergy Group (ANZAAG). (2016). Anaphylaxis management guidelines. Retrieved from <http://www.anzaag.com/Mgmt%20Resources.aspx>.

Australian and New Zealand College of Anaesthetists (ANZCA). (2014a). *PS31 Guidelines on checking anaesthesia delivery systems.* Melbourne: Author. Retrieved from <https://www.anzca.edu.au/resources/professional-documents/guidelines/ps31-guidelines-on-checking-anaesthesia-delivery-s>.

Australian and New Zealand College of Anaesthetists (ANZCA). (2014b). *PS09 Guidelines on sedation and/or analgesia for diagnostic and interventional, medical, dental or surgical procedures.* Melbourne: Author. Retrieved from <https://www.anzca.edu.au/resources/professional-documents/guidelines/ps09-guidelines-sedation-analgesia-for-diagnostic>.

Australian and New Zealand College of Anaesthetists (ANZCA). (2014c). *PS03 Guideline for the management of major regional analgesia.* Melbourne: Author. Retrieved from <https://www.anzca.edu.au/getattachment/159a8905-b558-480b-82d7-79a653ff83a0/PS03-Guideline-for-the-management-of-major-regional-analgesia>.

Australian and New Zealand College of Anaesthetists (ANZCA). (2015). *PS28 Guidelines on infection control in anaesthesia.* Melbourne: Author. Retrieved from <https://www.anzca.edu.au/resources/professional-documents/guidelines/ps28-guidelines-on-infection-control-in-anaesthesi>.

Australian and New Zealand College of Anaesthetists (ANZCA). (2016a). *PS08 Statement on the assistant for the anaesthetist.* Melbourne: Author. Retrieved from <https://www.anzca.edu.au/resources/professional-documents/standards-(1)/ps08-statement-on-the-assistant-for-the-anaestheti>.

Australian and New Zealand College of Anaesthetists (ANZCA). (2016b). *PS61. Guidelines for the management of evolving airway obstruction: transition to the can't intubate can't oxygenate airway emergency.* Melbourne: Author. Retrieved from <https://www.anzca.edu.au/getattachment/71f54974-314a-4d96-bef2-c03f39c8a8e9/PS61-Guideline-for-the-management-of-evolving-airway-obstruction-transition-to-the-Can't-Intubate-Can't-Oxygenate-airway-emergency>.

Australian and New Zealand College of Anaesthetists (ANZCA). (2016c). *Perioperative anaphylaxis management guidelines.* Melbourne: Author. Retrieved from <http://anzaag.com/Docs/PDF/Management%20Guidelines/Guidelines-Anaphylaxis_2016.pdf>.

Australian and New Zealand College of Anaesthetists (ANZCA). (2017a). *PS18 Guideline on monitoring during anaesthesia.* Melbourne: Author. Retrieved from <https://www.anzca.edu.au/getattachment/0c2d9717-fa82-4507-a3d6-3533d8fa844d/PS18-Guideline-on-monitoring-during-anaesthesia>.

Australian and New Zealand College of Anaesthetists (ANZCA). (2017b). PS07. Guideline on pre-anaesthesia consultation and patient preparation. Appendix 1 – Fasting guidelines. Retrieved from <https://www.anzca.edu.au/resources/professional-documents/guidelines/ps07-guidelines-on-pre-anaesthesia-consultation-an>.

Australian and New Zealand College of Anaesthetists (ANZCA). (2018). PS15 Guideline for the perioperative care of patients selected for day stay procedures. Retrieved from <https://www.anzca.edu.au/getattachment/021e4205-af5a-415d-815d-b16be1fe8b62/PS15-Guideline-for-the-perioperative-care-of-patients-selected-for-day-stay-procedures>.

Australian and New Zealand College of Anaesthetists and Australian Commission on Safety and Quality in Health Care (ANZCA & ACSQHC/the Commission). (2018). Joint Safety Statement: topical application of chlorhexidine and the risks of accidental injection in regional anaesthesia and vascular access procedures. Retrieved from <https://www.safetyandquality.gov.au/sites/default/files/migrated/ANZCA-and-Commission-joint-statement-on-Chlorhexidine-second-edition-Nov-2018.pdf>.

Australian College of PeriAnaesthesia Nurses (ACPAN). (2018). Statement 3. Minimum training requirements for the anaesthetic nurse. Retrieved from <https://acpan.edu.au/pdfs/statement-competencies-and-education-anaesthetic-nurse-v1.pdf>.

Australian College of PeriAnaesthesia Nurses (ACPAN). (2019). Professional standards for perianaesthesia nursing. Retrieved from <https://acpan.edu.au/pdfs/standards/acpan-professional-standards-v1.pdf>.

Australian College of Perioperative Nurses (ACORN). (2020). Anaesthetic nurse. In *ACORN standards for perioperative nursing in Australia* (Vol. 2., 16th ed.). Adelaide: Author. Retrieved from <https://www.acorn.org.au/standards/>.

Australian Commission on Safety and Quality in Health Care (ACSQHC/the Commission). (2015). National recommendations for user-applied labelling of injectable medicines, fluids and lines. Retrieved from <https://www.safetyandquality.gov.au/wp-content/uploads/2015/09/National-Standard-for-User-Applied-Labelling-Aug-2015.pdf>.

Australian Commission on Safety and Quality in Health Care (ACSQHC/the Commission). (2017). Comprehensive care. National safety and quality health service standards (2nd ed.). Retrieved from <https://www.safetyandquality.gov.au/wp-content/uploads/2017/12/National-Safety-and-Quality-Health-Service-Standards-second-edition.pdf>.

Australian Government, Department of Health. (2020). Environmental cleaning and disinfection principles for COVID-19. Retrieved from <https://www.health.gov.au/sites/default/files/documents/2020/03/environmental-cleaning-and-disinfection-principles-for-covid-19.pdf>.

Australian Institute of Health and Welfare (AIHW). (2018). *Australia's health report: overweight and obesity rates across Australia 2014–2015*. Canberra: Author. Retrieved from <https://www.aihw.gov.au/getmedia/7c42913d-295f-4bc9-9c24-4e44eff4a04a/aihw-aus-221.pdf>.

Boer, C., Bossers, S. M., & Koning, N. J. (2018). Choice of fluid type: physiological concepts and perioperative indications. *British Journal of Anaesthesia, 120*(2), 384–396. https://dx.doi.org/10.1016/j.bja.2017.10.022

Bogod, D. (2012). Editorial. The sting in the tail: antiseptics and the neuraxis revisited. *Anaesthesia, 68* (2), 224. https://dx.doi.org/10.1111/anae.12060. Retrieved from <https://associationofanaesthetists-publications.onlinelibrary.wiley.com/doi/full/10.1111/anae.12060>.

Bordi, S. (2018). Geriatrics and anesthesia practice. In J. Nagelhout & E. Sass (Eds.), *Nurse anesthesia* (6th ed., pp. 1136–1145). St. Louis, MO: Elsevier.

Bouch, C. (2019). Anaesthesia for the obese patient. In J. Thompson, I. Moppett, & M. Wiles (Eds.), *Smith and Aitkenhead's textbook of anaesthesia* (7th ed., pp. 656–665). Edinburgh: Churchill Livingstone.

Brewster, D., Chrimes, N., Do, T., Fraser, K., Groombridge, C., Higgs, A., ... Gatward, J. (2020). Consensus statement: Safe Airway Society principles of airway management and tracheal intubation specific to the COVID-19 adult patient group. *Medical Journal of Australia, 212* (10), 472–481.

Bryant, B., Knights, K., Darroch, S., & Rowland, A. (2019). *Pharmacology for health professions* (5th ed.). Sydney: Elsevier.

Cambridge University Press. (2020). Bariatric. In *Cambridge dictionary*. Retrieved from <https://dictionary.cambridge.org/dictionary/english/bariatric>.

Campbell, B. (2019). Anesthesia. In J. Rothrock (Ed.), *Alexander's care of the patient in surgery* (16th ed., pp. 107–141). St. Louis, MO: Elsevier.

Chrimes, N. (2016). The Vortex: a universal 'high-acuity implementation tool' for emergency airway management. *British Journal of Anaesthesia, 117*(Suppl. 1): i20–i27. https://doi.org/10.1093/bja/aew175. Retrieved from <https://pubmed.ncbi.nlm.nih.gov/27440673/>.

Clinical Excellence Commission (CEC). (2020). CEC guidelines – COVID-19 infection prevention and control. Retrieved from <https://www.cec.health.nsw.gov.au/keep-patients-safe/COVID-19/infection-prevention-and-control>.

Cook, T. (2019). Airway management. In J. Thompson, I. Moppett, & M. Wiles (Eds.), *Smith and Aitkenhead's textbook of anaesthesia* (7th ed., pp. 456–506). Edinburgh: Churchill Livingstone.

Cook, T., & Harper, N. (2018). *Anaesthesia, surgery and life-threatening allergic reactions*. Report and findings of the Royal College of Anaesthetists' 6th National Audit Project. London: Royal College of Anaesthetists.

Dhesi, J., Moppett, I., & Partridge, J. (2019). Surgery under anaesthesia for the older surgical patient. In J. Thompson, I. Moppett, & M. Wiles (Eds.), *Smith and Aitkenhead's textbook of anaesthesia* (7th ed., pp. 666–681). Edinburgh: Churchill Livingstone.

Duff, J., Walker, K., Edward, K.-L., Ralph, N., Giandinoto, J.-A., Alexander, K., ... Stephenson, J. (2018). Effect of a thermal care bundle on the prevention, detection and treatment of perioperative inadvertent hypothermia. *Journal of Clinical Nursing, 27*(5–6), 1239–1249. https://dx.doi.org/10.1111/jocn.14171

Fawcett, D. (2019). Positioning the patient for surgery. In J. Rothrock & D. McEwen (Eds.), *Alexander's care of the patient in surgery* (16th ed., pp. 142–175). St. Louis, MO: Elsevier Saunders.

Gavel, G., & Walker, R. (2012). *Algorithm for management of laryngospasm*. Manchester: Royal Manchester Children's Hospital Manchester, UK.

Gillerman, R. (2020). Malignant hyperthermia. In F. Ferri (Ed.), *Ferri's clinical advisor*. Philadelphia, PA: Elsevier.

Haemoview Diagnostics. (2019). ROTEM. Retrieved from <https://www.haemoview.com.au>.

Heiner, J. (2018). Airway management. In J. Nagelhout & E. Sass (Eds.), *Nurse anesthesia* (6th ed., pp. 623–669). St. Louis, MO: Elsevier.

Hewson, D., & Hardman, J. (2019a). Regional anaesthetic techniques. In J. Thompson, I. Moppett, & M. Wiles (Eds.), *Smith and Aitkenhead's textbook of anaesthesia* (7th ed., pp. 527–557). Edinburgh: Churchill Livingstone.

Hewson, D., & Hardman, J. (2019b). Complications arising from anaesthesia. In J. Thompson, I. Moppett, & M. Wiles (Eds.), *Smith and Aitkenhead's textbook of anaesthesia* (7th ed., pp. 558–571). Edinburgh: Churchill Livingstone.

Higgins Roche, B. T., & Schwartz, P. (2018). Blood and blood component therapy. In J. Nagelhout & E. Sass (Eds.), *Nurse anesthesia* (6th ed., pp. 369–379). St. Louis, MO: Elsevier Saunders.

Hunter, J., & Shields, M. (2019). Muscle function and neuromuscular blockade. In J. Thompson, I. Moppett, & M. Wiles (Eds.), *Smith and Aitkenhead's textbook of anaesthesia* (7th ed., pp. 131–146). Edinburgh: Churchill Livingstone.

Ip, J., Walker, I., & Thomas, M. (2019). Paediatric anaesthesia. In J. Thompson, I. Moppett, & M. Wiles (Eds.), *Smith and Aitkenhead's textbook of anaesthesia* (7th ed., pp. 666–681). Edinburgh: Churchill Livingstone.

Jones, N., Long, L., & Zeitz, K. (2011). The role of the nurse sedationist. *Collegian (Royal College of Nursing, Australia), 18*(3), 115–123. https://dx.doi.org/10.1016/j.colegn.2011.04.001. Retrieved from <https://www.collegianjournal.com/article/S1322-7696(11)00023-0/abstract>.

Kasson, B. (2018). Obstetric anesthesia. In J. Nagelhout & E. Sass (Eds.), *Nurse anesthesia* (6th ed., pp. 1064–1091). St Louis, MO: Elsevier.

Kirkbride, D. (2019). The practical conduct of anaesthesia. In J. Thompson, I. Moppett, & M. Wiles (Eds.), *Smith and Aitkenhead's textbook of anaesthesia* (7th ed., pp. 441–455). Edinburgh: Churchill Livingstone.

Kossick, M. A. (2018). Clinical monitoring 1: Cardiovascular system. In J. Nagelhout & E. Sass (Eds.), *Nurse anesthesia* (6th ed., pp. 272–289). St. Louis, MO: Elsevier Saunders.

Krogh, M. A. (2018). Obesity and anesthesia practice. In J. Nagelhout & E. Sass (Eds.), *Nurse anesthesia* (6th ed., pp. 998–1014). St. Louis, MO: Elsevier Saunders.

Marley, R., & Clapp, T. J. (2018). Outpatient anesthesia. In J. Nagelhout & E. Sass (Eds.), Nurse anesthesia (6th ed., pp. 889–903). St. Louis, MO: Elsevier Saunders.

Marley, R. A., & Sheets, S. A. (2018). Preoperative evaluation and preparation of the patient. In J. Nagelhout & E. Sass (Eds.), Nurse anesthesia (7th ed., pp. 311–346). St. Louis, MO: Elsevier Saunders.

Millette, B., Athanassoglou, V., & Patel, A. (2018). High flow nasal oxygen therapy in adult anaesthesia. *Trends in Anaesthesia and Critical Care*, 18, 29–33. https://dx.doi.ord/10.1016/j.tacc.2017.12.001

Moore, E., Bergman, N., Anderson, G., & Medley, N. (2016). Early skin-to-skin contact for mothers and their healthy newborn infants. *Cochrane Library*. Retrieved from <https://www.cochrane.org/CD003519/PREG_early-skin-skin-contact-mothers-and-their-healthy-newborn-infants>.

Murphy, E. (2019). Patient safety and risk management. In J. Rothrock (Ed.), *Alexander's care of the patient in surgery* (16th ed., pp. 16–45). St. Louis, MO: Elsevier Saunders.

Nagelhout, J. (2018a). Local anesthetics. In J. Nagelhout & E. Sass (Eds.), *Nurse anesthesia* (6th ed., pp. 110–127). St. Louis, MO: Elsevier Saunders.

Nagelhout, J. (2018b). Neuromuscular blocking agents, reversal agents, and their monitoring. In J. Nagelhout & E. Sass (Eds.), *Nurse anesthesia* (6th ed., pp. 140–164). St. Louis, MO: Elsevier Saunders.

Nagelhout, J. (2018c). Inhalational anesthesia. In J. Nagelhout & E. Sass (Eds.), *Nurse anesthesia* (6th ed., pp. 80–92). St. Louis, MO: Elsevier Saunders.

Naguib, M., Lien, C., & Meistelman, C. (2015). Pharmacology of neuromuscular blocking drugs. In R. Miller (Ed.), *Miller's anesthesia* (8th ed., pp. 958–994). Philadelphia: Elsevier.

National Blood Authority. (2011). *Patient blood management guidelines*. Module 1 (under review). Retrieved from <https://www.blood.gov.au/pbm-module-1>.

National Blood Authority. (2013). Massive transfusion protocol template. Retrieved from <https://www.blood.gov.au/pbm-guidelines-transfusion-protocol-template>.

New Zealand Blood Service (NZBS). (2017). *Transfusion medicine handbook*. Auckland: NZBS.

New Zealand Nurses Organisation (NZNO). (2014). Registered nurse assistant to the anaesthetist. Knowledge and Skills Framework. Retrieved from <https://www.nzno.org.nz/groups/colleges/perioperative_nurses_college/resources/registerednurse_assistant_to_the_anaesthetist>.

Nightingale, C. E., Margarson, M. P., Shearer, E., Redman, J. W., Lucas, D. N., Cousins, J. M., & Griffiths, R. (2015). Perioperative management of the obese surgical patient 2015: Association of Anaesthetists of Great Britain and Ireland Society for Obesity and Bariatric Anaesthesia. *Anaesthesia*, 70(7), 859–876. https://dx.doi.org/10.1111/anae.13101

NSW Health. (2011). *PD2011_060: Central venous access device insertion and post insertion care*. Sydney: Author.

NSW Health. (2015). *GL2015_008: Standards for paediatric intravenous fluids* (2nd ed.). Sydney: Author.

NSW Health. (2017). PD2017_01. Infection prevention and control policy. Retrieved from <https://www1.health.nsw.gov.au/pds/ActivePDSDocuments/PD2017_013.pdf>.

Pandit, J., & Cook, T. (Eds). (2014). *Accidental awareness during general anaesthesia in the United Kingdom and Ireland*. NAPP5 Report and Findings. Royal College of Anaesthetists and the Association of Anaesthetists of Britain and Ireland. Retrieved from <https://www.nationalauditprojects.org.uk>.

Patty, A. (28 July, 2015). Cardiac arrest during cosmetic surgery: overdose of local anaesthetic likely. *Sydney Morning Herald*. Retrieved from <https://www.smh.com.au/nsw/cardiac-arrest-during-cosmetic-surgery-overdose-of-local-anaesthetic-likely-20150723-gijcn8.html#ixzz3hcudyFNU>.

Pellegrini, J. E. (2018). Regional anesthesia: spinal and epidural anesthesia. In J. Nagelhout & E. Sass (Eds.), *Nurse anesthesia* (6th ed., pp. 1015–1041). St. Louis, MO: Elsevier Saunders.

Pillai, A. (2019). Obstetric anaesthesia and analgesia. In J. Thompson, I. Moppett, & M. Wiles (Eds.), *Smith and Aitkenhead's textbook of anaesthesia* (7th ed., pp. 800–830). Edinburgh: Churchill Livingstone.

Rieker, M. (2018). Respiratory anatomy, physiology, pathophysiology and anesthetic management. In J. Nagelhout & E. Sass (Eds.), *Nurse anesthesia* (6th ed., pp. 563–623). St. Louis, MO: Elsevier Saunders.

Royal College of Anaesthetists and the Association of Anaesthetists of Great Britain and Ireland. (2014). 5th national audit project. Retrieved from <https://www.nationalauditprojects.org.uk/NAP5report>.

Schick, L. (2018). Assessment and monitoring of the perianesthesia patient. In J. Odom-Forren (Ed.), *Drain's perianaesthesia nursing: a critical approach* (7th ed., pp. 257–386). St. Louis, MO: Saunders.

Scott, S. (2019). Clinical measurement and monitoring. In J. Thompson, I. Moppett, & M. Wiles (Eds.), *Smith and Aitkenhead's textbook of anaesthesia* (6th ed., pp. 323–361). Edinburgh: Churchill Livingstone.

Sobey, R., & Tracy, A. (2018). Nonoperating room anesthesia. In J. Nagelhout & E. Sass (Eds.), *Nurse anesthesia* (6th ed., pp. 1194–1215). St. Louis, MO: Elsevier Saunders.

Tibble, R. (2019). Anaesthesia for day surgery. In J. Thompson, I. Moppett, & M. Wiles (Eds.), *Smith and Aitkenhead's textbook of anaesthesia* (7th ed., pp. 682–689). Edinburgh: Churchill Livingstone.

Tizani, A. (2017). *Harvard's nursing guide to drugs* (10th ed.). Sydney: Elsevier.

Trinsoon, C., & Patel, N. G. (2018). Fluid administration, perioperative goal-directed fluid therapy and electrolyte disorders. In J. Nagelhout & E. Sass (Eds.), *Nurse anesthesia* (6th ed., pp. 347–368). St. Louis, MO: Elsevier Saunders.

Welliver, M. (2018). Chemistry and physics of anesthesia. In J. Nagelhout & E. Sass (Eds.), *Nurse anesthesia* (6th ed., pp. 201–228). St. Louis, MO: Elsevier Saunders.

Whitman, Z., & Thompson, J. (2019). Local anaesthetic agents. In J. Thompson, I. Moppett, & M. Wiles (Eds.), *Smith and Aitkenhead's textbook of anaesthesia* (7th ed., pp. 90–98). Edinburgh: Churchill Livingstone.

Wong, J., Goh, Q. Y., Tan, Z., Lie, S. A., Tay, Y. C., Ng, S. Y., & Soh, C. R. (2020). Preparing for a COVID-19 pandemic: a review of operating room outbreak response measures in a large tertiary hospital in Singapore. *Canadian Journal of Anaesthesia/Journal Canadien d'Anesthesie*, 67, 732–745. https://dx.doi.org/10.1007/s12630-020-01620-9

World Health Organization (WHO). (2018). Factsheet: Obesity and overweight. Retrieved from <https://www.aihw.gov.au/getmedia/7c42913d-295f-4bc9-9c24-4e44eff4a04a/aihw-aus-221.pdf>.

World Health Organization (WHO). (2020). Infection prevention and control during health when COVID-19 is suspected. Retrieved from <https://www.who.int/publications/i/item/10665-331495>.

Wright, S. (2018). Assessment and management of the airway. In J. Odom-Forren (Ed.), *Drain's perianaesthesia nursing: a critical approach* (7th ed., pp. 417–430). St. Louis, MO: Saunders.

FURTHER READING

Acott, C. (2011). *Cricoid pressure: is there any evidence? ANZCA Australian Anaesthesia invited papers and selected continuing education lectures.* Melbourne: ANZCA.

Aitken, L., Marshall, A., & Chaboyer, W. (2012). *ACCCN's critical care nursing.* Melbourne: Australian College of Critical Care Nurses.

Al-Shaikh, B., & Stacey, S. (2019). *Essentials of equipment in anaesthesia, critical care and perioperative medicine* (5th ed.). London: Elsevier.

Australian and New Zealand College of Anaesthetists (ANZCA). (2014). Guidelines on checking anaesthesia delivery systems (PS31). Retrieved from <https://www.anzca.edu.au/resources/professional-documents/guidelines/ps31-guidelines-on-checking-anaesthesia-delivery-s>.

Australian Commission on Safety and Quality in Health Care (ACSQHC/the Commission) and Australian New Zealand Intensive Care Society (ANZICS). (2012). Central line insertion and maintenance guideline. Retrieved from <https://www.anzics.com.au/wp-content/uploads/2018/08/ANZICS_Insertionmaintenance_guideline2012_04.pdf>.

Bradley, P., Chapman. G., & Crook. B. (2016). *Airway assessment* [education statement]. Melbourne: ANZCA. Retrieved from <https://www.anzca.edu.au/getattachment/eff1ab5d-46cf-46db-95ef-5e65ecb88c26/PU-Airway-Assessment-20160916v1>.

Cadogan, M. (2019). Henry Edmund Gaskin Boyle. Life in the fastlane. Retrieved from <https://litfl.com/henry-edmund-gaskin-boyle/>.

Duff, J., Walker, K., Edward, K., Williams, R., & Sutherland-Fraser, S. (2014). Incidence of perioperative inadvertent hypothermia and compliance with evidence-based recommendations at four Australian hospitals: a retrospective chart audit. *ACORN Journal*, 27(3), 16–23.

Edelstein, S. B., & Metry, J. E. (2017). Anesthesia considerations for the geriatric patient. *Current Geriatrics Reports*, 6(3), 115–121. https://link.springer.com/article/10.1007/s13670-017-0206-0

Griffith, H., & Johnson, E. (1942). The use of curare in general anesthesia. *Anesthesiology*, 3(4), 418–420. doi:10.1097/00000542-194207000-00006.

Hagberg, C. (2017). *Benumof and Hagberg's airway management* (4th ed.). Philadelphia, PA: Saunders.

Lawyers and Legal Services Australia. (2010). *Shocking case of medical negligence.* Sydney: Lawyers and Legal Services Australia. Retrieved from <https://www.legallawyers.com.au/insurance-law/shocking-case-of-medical-negligence>.

MacGregor, K. (2013). A waking nightmare: how can we avoid accidental awareness during general anaesthesia? *Journal of Perioperative Practice*, 23(9), 185–190. https://dx.doi.org/10.1177%2F175045891302300902

Mulvey, D. (2019). Intravenous anaesthetic agents and sedatives. In J. Thompson, I. Moppett, & M. Wiles (Eds.), *Smith and Aitkenhead's textbook of anaesthesia* (7th ed., pp. 66–89). Edinburgh: Churchill Livingstone.

Munk, L., Anderson, L., & Gogenur, I. (2013). Emergence delirium. *Journal of Perioperative Practice*, 23(11), 251–254. https://dx.doi.org/10.1177/175045891302301103

Olsen, R., Pellegrini, J., & Movinsky, B. (2014). Regional anaesthesia: spinal and epidural anesthesia. In J. Nagelhout & K. Plaus (Eds.), *Nurse anesthesia* (5th ed., pp. 1070–1101). St. Louis, MO: Elsevier.

O'Shaughnessy, K. (2012). Cholinergic and antimuscarinic (anticholinergic) mechanisms and drugs. In P. Bennett, M. Brown, & P. Sharma (Eds.) *Clinical pharmacology* (11th ed., pp. 372–381). Edinburgh: Elsevier.

Pollock, W., & James, A. (2019). Pregnancy and postpartum considerations. In L. Aitken, A. Marshall, & W. Chaboyer, (Eds.), *ACCCN's critical care nursing* (4th ed., pp. 978–1022). Sydney: Elsevier.

Singh, A. (2014). Strategies for the management and avoidance of hypothermia in the perioperative environment. *Journal of Perioperative Practice*, 24(4), 75–78. https://dx.doi.org/10.1177%2F175045891602400403

CHAPTER 9

Intraoperative Patient Care

SHARON MINTON • MELISSA HALL • SIAN MITCHELL
EDITOR: BEN LOCKWOOD

LEARNING OUTCOMES

- Understand the anatomical and physiological concepts related to patient positioning
- Explore the neurovascular and integumentary consequences associated with anaesthesia and surgery, and ways to manage them
- Identify the nature and incidence of perioperative pressure injuries and ways to prevent them
- Examine several core nursing interventions aimed at ensuring patient safety, including the use of tourniquets, the WHO Surgical Safety Checklist and the surgical count
- Identify the different types of tissue specimens and discuss best practice when handling tissue specimens for pathology

KEY TERMS

accountable items

inadvertent perioperative hypothermia

patient positioning

patient safety

patient transfer

point of care testing

pressure injuries

skin integrity

surgical count

Surgical Safety Checklist

tissue specimen

tourniquets

venous thromboembolism (VTE)

INTRODUCTION

This chapter explores the intraoperative care provided to patients and covers issues that are directly relevant to patient safety during anaesthesia and surgery. Where feasible, these are discussed in the context of the patient scenarios presented in the Introduction at the beginning of this book. The chapter discusses the concepts of prevention of venous thromboembolism (VTE), maintenance of normothermia, and ensuring the correct patient and site of surgery. It also examines management of accountable items used during surgery – a primary nursing responsibility. Pertinent anatomical and physiological aspects associated with correct patient positioning for the intended surgery are discussed, along with nursing interventions aimed at keeping patients free from harm. The perioperative environment and related technologies, such as the use of tourniquets, pose their own unique risks; these are explored, along with methods to eliminate, reduce or control them. Finally, the chapter looks at correct identification and handling of specimens.

The risk that surgery poses should not be underestimated, with adverse events occurring more commonly among surgical patients than among other patient cohorts (World Health Organization [WHO], n.d.). Several of these adverse events originate in the perioperative environment.

ENSURING CORRECT PATIENT/SITE OF SURGERY

Surgery is not without risks and a safe environment for surgical patients requires a planned and systematic

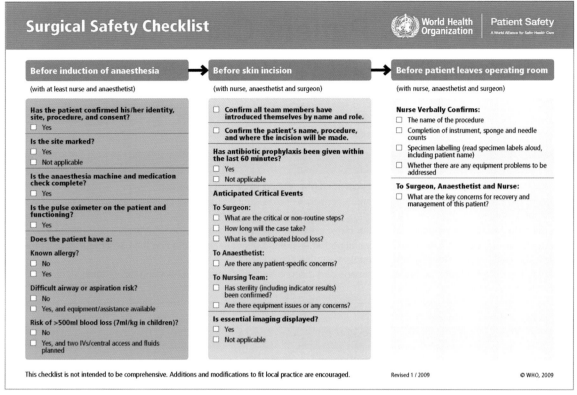

FIG. 9.1 WHO Surgical Safety Checklist. (Source: Adapted from World Health Organization. (2009). *Surgical Safety Checklist*. https://www.who.int/patientsafety/safesurgery/checklist/en.)

approach to perioperative care delivery. The WHO's **Surgical Safety Checklist** (SSC), discussed in earlier chapters, was developed to reduce the occurrence of unnecessary surgical deaths and avoidable complications (WHO, 2009). The SSC has been adapted and implemented in over 132 countries around the world. The correct implementation of a surgical checklist is one element to improve team communication and stimulate a culture in which safety is a priority (Abbott et al., 2017; Dias, 2018; Gillespie et al., 2018). A safety culture within hospitals is increasingly considered a crucial factor in the delivery of high-quality care (Alban et al., 2019; Australian Commission on Safety and Quality in Health Care [ACSQHC/the Commission], 2010; Lark, Kirkpatrick, & Chung, 2018; Odell et al., 2019). The SSC spells out critical activities that must occur at particular times during a surgical procedure. These times are:

- the period prior to induction of anaesthesia ('Sign In')
- the period after induction and before the surgical incision ('Time Out')
- the period during or immediately after wound closure ('Sign Out') (Fig. 9.1).

During Sign In, and in the presence of the patient, the anaesthetic nurse and anaesthetist verbally confirm:

- the presence of the correct patient
- the planned procedure
- the marking of the surgical site (when applicable)
- that consent has been obtained
- the patient's allergy status
- that the anaesthesia safety check (i.e. the anaesthetic machine and patient medications) is complete
- the availability and functionality of pulse oximetry
- whether the patient has a difficult airway or aspiration risk
- the risk of blood loss >500 mL (or 7 mL/kg in children)
- the availability of prosthesis/other special equipment, if required.

Ideally, the surgeon should be present for Sign In; however, their presence is not essential to complete this part of the SSC process, according to the WHO (2009).

Notwithstanding this, some Australian states have divided the responsibility of Sign In for level 3 procedures (those requiring an anaesthetist and proceduralist and usually occurring in the operating theatre) between the anaesthetist and surgeon. Each is required to confirm aspects of the above list that pertains to their area of care for the patient (Clinical Excellence Commission [CEC], 2017).

Time Out involves all members of the surgical team and occurs prior to skin incision. Staff must verbally confirm:

- that all team members have introduced themselves by name and role
- the patient's identification, the planned procedure and the operative site
- the anticipated critical events, which include:
  - surgeon review (e.g. anticipated blood loss, unexpected steps in procedure)
  - anaesthetist review (e.g. patient-specific issues)
  - nursing review (e.g. sterility of items confirmed, any equipment issues noted)
- prophylactic antibiotics administered within the last 60 minutes
- VTE prophylaxis ordered
- essential imaging displayed (as appropriate).

In Sign Out, the final stage of the SSC process, team members review and confirm:

- the nature of the surgical procedure completed
- that the count is correct and that all accountable items used during the procedure are accounted for
- that any surgical specimens obtained are correctly labelled
- that equipment malfunctions or issues that need addressing are identified
- that there is a review of PO care and any concerns are identified before the patient is transferred from the operating room.

The SSC is a useful, validated tool for patient identification, procedure matching and prevention of wrong-site surgery (Lark et al., 2018). It is simple, brief and quick to complete and is also adaptable (Anderson et al., 2018). Adaptations, however, must be done without sacrificing the primary focus on team function and communication. In Australia and New Zealand, the use of VTE prophylaxis and the availability of surgical prostheses/implants (items not included in the original SSC) form an integral part of the SSC ANZ edition (Royal Australasian College of Surgeons [RACS], 2009). The following critical items should not be removed from the SSC:

- patient involvement
- team introductions

- preoperative patient assessment
- preprocedural information sharing
- discussion of a treatment plan on completion of the surgery (Australian College of Operating Room Nurses [ACORN], 2020a).

The use of the trans-Tasman-endorsed SSC requires the participation of all members of the surgical team, who must be present and must cease all other activities to participate. It is important that the same team member leads and coordinates all stages of the checklist process; in most instances, this is the anaesthetic nurse.

Notwithstanding its utility and formal endorsement by key stakeholders, non-compliance with the use of the checklist remains problematic, with the presence and focus of the entire perioperative team being significant issues (Mahmood, Myopoulos, Bagli, Damignani, & Haji, 2019; Verwey & Gopalan, 2018).

PATIENT POSITIONING

To ensure **patient safety** and the safety of surgical team members during patient transfer and positioning, a planned approach with effective interprofessional communication is essential. This includes:

- identification and verification of the correct patient, correct site and correct procedure
- patient assessment
- consideration of the surgical position required
- the availability and preparation of support surfaces such as foam, gel, air-inflated or other pressure-reducing mattress overlays
- positioning equipment, and other medical devices or procedural equipment
- transfer method to be used.

Patient assessment should comprise patient and carer discussion, physical examination and review of the patient's medical records (Burlingame, 2017; Fawcett, 2019; Wang, Walker, & Gillespie, 2018a, 2018b).

Patient Transfer

Before **patient transfer** (lateral transfer) from a trolley or bed to the operating table (and vice versa), there must be consideration of the following two groups of factors:

Patient factors include:

- the patient's age, height, weight and body mass index (BMI)
- the patient's nutritional status
- the patient's history, including previous surgeries and comorbidities

- the patient's American Society of Anesthesiologist's (ASA) score and type of anaesthetic to be delivered
- the patient's mobility and range of motion
- the patient's skin integrity and pressure injury risk assessment
- areas of patient discomfort, both physical and psychological
- the presence of medical devices such as drains, catheters, intravenous lines or other items/equipment attached to the patient.

Team factors include:

- the surgical procedure to be undertaken
- the anatomical limitations of the position
- the exposure of the patient to protect both dignity and normothermia
- the length of time the patient is to remain in the position or if there are any potential changes to be made to the patient's position intraoperatively

- the requirements of the surgeon, the anaesthetist and others for access to the surgical site/airway
- the type and availability of transferring equipment
- the available team members (Burlingame, 2017; Fawcett, 2019; Goudas & Bruni, 2019; Spruce & Van Wicklin, 2016).

These factors will influence the team's preparation and the equipment required to carry out the transfer. The patient's age and mobility have a bearing on the resources required; for example, a mobile patient may be able to move to the operating table unaided. In contrast, an older (those over 80 years of age), frail or less mobile patient will require greater assistance from the surgical team and equipment. Particular care, planning and/or equipment are required to manage paediatric patients, frail older patients, obstetric patients and obese patients, especially the morbidly obese (Fawcett, 2019; O'Connor & Radcliffe, 2018); see Feature box 9.1 and Research box 9.2 later in the chapter.

FEATURE BOX 9.1
Transferring and Positioning the Obese Patient

The most commonly used measure to classify a patient's weight is body mass index (BMI). BMI is calculated by dividing weight in kilograms by height in metres squared (kg/m^2). An individual with a BMI of $\geq$30 kg/m^2 is considered obese and a BMI of $\geq$40kg/m^2 is morbidly obese (Fawcett, 2019). In 2017–18, two-thirds (67.0%) of Australian adults were classified as overweight or obese (12.5 million people), an increase from 63.4% in 2014–15 (Australian Bureau of Statistics [ABS], 2018), while in New Zealand, 32% of adults are considered obese. Among the Māori and Pacific Islander populations, the figures for obesity are 47% and 65%, respectively (New Zealand Ministry of Health, 2018). These data reflect an upward trend.

As an individual's BMI increases, so do the risks associated with anaesthesia and surgery. These include:

- difficulty accessing and controlling the airway, and reduced tolerance for positioning owing to decreased pulmonary function
- greater risk of peripheral nerve and pressure injuries
- increased risk of VTE
- increased risk of compartment syndrome from ill-fitting patient gowns, overly tight BP cuffs, calf compression devices and so forth
- risk of rhabdomyolysis where pressure injury sustained over extended periods can cause muscle fibre breakdown and the release of myoglobin into the bloodstream
- greater risk of a fall (Fawcett, 2019).

Obese patients require specialised lifting equipment such as mechanical patient lifters or air-assisted lateral transfer devices (e.g. HoverMatt) with adequate numbers of staff to perform the transfer safely (O'Connor & Radcliffe, 2018). Weight tolerance of beds and positional equipment needs to be ascertained and deemed appropriate for use prior to patient arrival. Patients may require modified positioning to minimise risk, such as 'ramping' the torso to achieve airway alignment and prevent hypoventilation (Carron, Safaee Fakhr, Ieppariello, & Foletto, 2020; Fawcett, 2019). Special care must be taken to ensure that skin folds are not trapped under the patient (Phillips, 2017). In addition, excess soft tissue can hamper exposure of the operative field and it may need to be retracted with adhesive tape. Depending on the particular needs of the obese patient, a practice session with team members may also be required to plan and orchestrate a safe and smooth experience for the patient (Croke, 2019; National Pressure Injury Advisory Panel [NPIAP], 2019).

As with all patients, privacy, respect and dignity are a must. The obese patient may be particularly self-conscious and psychologically vulnerable in relation to their body image. Planned and prepared intervention, non-judgemental and inclusive communication and care will not only result in physical safety for all involved but will also contribute necessary psychosocial support to the obese patient, encouraging them to feel safe and become more involved in their care (Carron et al., 2020; Fencl, Walsh, & Vocke, 2015).

Care must be taken when transferring patients with medical devices already in place. Their dislodgement can create discomfort (or worse) and resiting them delays progress. The planned procedure, the patient's condition, and staff and equipment availability will determine whether the initial transfer occurs while the patient is conscious or following induction of anaesthesia. Additionally, consideration must be given to patients who need repositioning intraoperatively (e.g. during minimally invasive surgery), as underprepared, disorganised or unplanned movements during repositioning increase the risk of:

- damage to the initial operative site
- airway compromise
- additional and unnecessary exposure to anaesthesia
- disconnection, displacement or dislodgement of anaesthetic tubing or monitoring
- falls and slips resulting in serious physical damage to the patient
- permanent disability or death (Soncrant et al., 2018).

Anaesthetist, surgeon and other staff requirements for patient access also need to be considered. At all times, the anaesthetist must be able to ensure ventilation adequacy, have IV access and address requirements for haemodynamic monitoring. The surgeon needs access to the surgical site and the instrument nurse needs to be able to maintain a critical aseptic field throughout the procedure (O'Connor & Radcliffe, 2018). Consequently, the patient's position is often a compromise between competing demands for surgical access balanced against the patient's need for safety and protection. The perioperative nurse's role within the surgical team is a crucial one. Continuous monitoring of the patient and patient advocacy are both required to help prevent positioning-related injuries. In order to achieve this, the perioperative nurse must have sound and up-to-date knowledge of correct positioning practices and comply with expected standards for practice (Croke, 2019; Crook, 2016; Davis, 2018; Fawcett, 2019; Spruce & Van Wicklin, 2016).

Transfer methods and rationales

Clear interprofessional communication and coordinated care are essential, with all surgical team members taking equal responsibility for maintaining safety of themselves, other team members and the patient during transfer. The duty of the perioperative nurse is to assess the surgical environment and the patient and to ensure that the most appropriate transfer equipment, positional aids and staff are available. The anaesthetist, who has responsibility for the patient's airway, generally co-ordinates the transfer (Fawcett, 2019) and directs the team, as well as the patient if the latter is conscious. When the patient is anaesthetised and/or unconscious, coordination of the transfer is managed by the anaesthetist in most instances, as maintenance of a patent airway, ventilation and cerebral circulation are the main priorities (Fawcett, 2019; O'Connor & Radcliffe, 2018).

When a conscious patient is able to participate in the move, interventions needed to secure a safe transfer include:

- giving clear directions and explanations
- ensuring there is a minimal gap between the trolley and the operating table
- using the brakes on both the trolley and the operating table
- making sure the patient's gown is loosened and not caught in the trolley/bed side rails
- placing team members on either side of the moving patient to assist with lateral transfer and to prevent the patient from sustaining a fall.

Patients should be instructed by a staff member who directs them to feel for the sides of the operating table as they move across, so that they can be confident they are centrally located. The trolley or bed should not be moved away until the patient is securely positioned and confirms this.

If the patient has reduced mobility and cannot move independently, then a lateral transfer device that runs the length of the patient, such as a patient slide board, patient slide sheet or mechanical device, such as an air-assisted lateral transfer device (e.g. HoverMatt), is needed (Fig. 9.2) (O'Connor & Radcliffe, 2018). These devices enable patient transfer while reducing the risk of injury to staff members. A minimum of four staff members is generally required for the safe transfer of these patients, using the safety precautions described above.

When transferring an unconscious or anaesthetised patient, the anaesthetist manages the patient's airway and supports the head. As the patient has no muscle control, their limbs need safeguarding so they do not overhang the operating table, predisposing them to injury. The patient's arms are secured across their chest or by their side and their legs are supported and moved in alignment with the body. These patients will have IV access and monitoring devices established and care must be taken not to obstruct or dislodge them. Use of an agreed-upon process is of particular value to assist with the coordination of the transfer, where instructions such as 'ready, steady, roll' tend to be less ambiguous than, 'one, two, three' (O'Connor & Radcliffe, 2018).

Once patient transfer has occurred the patient should be secured to the OR table with safety straps, and a staff member should remain with the patient

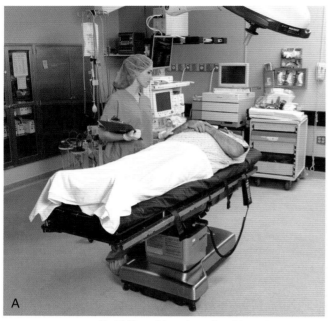
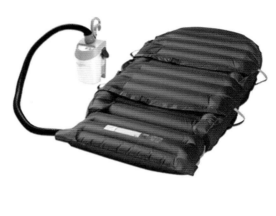

A   B

FIG. 9.2 (**A, B**) HoverMatt air-assisted lateral transfer device. (Source: Fawcett, D. L. (2019). Positioning the patient for surgery. In J. C. Rothrock & D. L. McEwen (Eds.), *Alexander's care of the patient in surgery* (16th ed., p. 163, Fig. 6.21A, B). St Louis, MO: Elsevier.)

during the lighter periods of anaesthesia (Fawcett, 2019; Soncrant et al., 2018).

Complications

Injuries associated with patient transfer include skin tears, joint dislocations, trauma to muscle and nerve tissue, obstruction or dislodgement of IV infusion tubing, catheters or drains, accidental extubation of artificial airways in unconscious patients, and patient falls (Mangham, 2017; O'Connor & Radcliffe, 2018). These complications can also occur when the patient is being positioned for surgery, or during the course of the surgery. Staff members are also at risk of injury, and many hospitals and other facilities have a 'no lift' policy in place, so nursing staff must familiarise themselves with the particular policy for their organisation.

Skin tears are a significant problem in healthcare and often occur during patient transfer and positioning, particularly in older, comorbid patients and those with a higher risk of pressure injury (LeBlanc & Baranoski, 2017). The International Skin Tear Advisory Panel (ISTAP) (2018) stresses the importance of assessing a patient's risk of skin tears prior to any manual handling procedure in addition to careful padding of positioning equipment. ISTAP (2018) also reinforces the importance

of healthcare staff maintaining short fingernails and removing jewellery when caring for patients, as these are well-documented causes of skin tears in patients (see Chapter 11 for further information on skin tears).

Complications are likely to arise if:
- surgical team members are too few in number
- staff members lack adequate training in the correct use of positioning equipment
- the appropriate patient-lifting/transfer device, positional aids and/or pressure-redistribution support devices are absent, incorrectly used or not used at all (Wang et al., 2018b).

The ACORN Standards note that perioperative staff must be aware of the potential adverse events associated with transferring and positioning patients so that they can enact prevention strategies and lessen the risk of such events, and that staff require training in manual handling and correct body mechanics, as well as in-service education when new mechanical devices are commissioned (ACORN, 2020b, 2020c, 2020d).

Correct **patient positioning** is essential to performing a safe and unconstrained surgical procedure while also protecting the patient from iatrogenic harm and preventing injury to staff assisting with transfer and positioning of patients (O'Connor & Radcliffe, 2018).

Patients are positioned so that:

- there is correct musculoskeletal alignment
- undue pressure on nerves, skin over bony prominences, earlobes, eyes, breasts and external genitalia is avoided
- there is provision for adequate thoracic excursion
- arteries and veins are not occluded
- other medical conditions, deformities and/or previous surgery are considered
- patient modesty is preserved (ACORN, 2020b; Van Wicklin, 2018).

Patients are immobile during surgery and unable to change and control their body position or complain of pain. Consequently, their risk of developing an injury and other complications, such as VTE or pulmonary dysfunction, is increased (O'Connor & Radcliffe, 2018; Phillips, 2017; Van Wicklin, 2018).

Anatomical and physiological considerations for patient positioning

A patient's tolerance of the stresses imposed by the surgical intervention depends significantly on the normal functioning of the vital body systems, all of which must be considered when planning the patient's position for surgery. The goals of positioning include mitigating the risk of injuries occurring from pressure, crushing, stretching, pinching or compression (Burlingame, 2017; Van Wicklin, 2018). The development of such injuries is influenced by patient-related factors (intrinsic) and environmental/procedure-related factors (extrinsic), which include the following:

Intrinsic factors include:

- patient's health status and physical condition – debilitated patients present greater positional challenges (O'Connor & Radcliffe, 2018)
- patient's age, for example the very young or the old, require special considerations
- obese patients irrespective of any other underlying pathophysiology (Kirkbride, 2019).

Extrinsic factors include:

- position required for the procedure – all positions pose a risk, some more so than others
- estimated length of time for the procedure and the associated immobility – surgery over 4 hours duration is associated with greater risk of pressure injury (O'Connor & Radcliffe, 2018; Spruce, 2017a)
- type of operating table used, mattress or overlay, and positioning aids required/available (Stanton, 2017; Wang et al., 2018b)
- type of anaesthetic given
- planned surgical procedure.

Integumentary system. The integumentary system can be injured as a result of the physical forces required to maintain the surgical position, in addition to the techniques and equipment used to move the patient into the position. These physical forces include pressure, shear and friction. The presence of moisture on the patient's skin may also contribute to causing injury (NPIAP, 2019). Additional risk factors for pressure injuries specific to individuals undergoing surgery include:

- pressure from medical devices to administer anaesthesia
- pressure from devices to secure the patient safely on the operating table and assist with surgery (Delmore & Ayello, 2017)
- increased hypotensive episodes during surgery
- low core temperature during surgery
- reduced mobility on day one postoperatively (NPIAP, 2019).

Injury to the skin and underlying tissues may be reduced with the use of prophylactic dressings applied to high-risk areas of the body prior to surgery – for example sacrum, heels, knees and elbows (Burlingame, 2017; Stanton, 2017). Specialist dressings are designed to control skin microclimate and provide a physical barrier between patients' skin and the medical devices used to support them (Burlingame, 2017). Although the NPIAP recommends the use of carefully selected and placed prophylactic dressings to reduce medical device-related pressure ulcers, further research is required to determine whether these dressings are effective in reducing the incidence of acquiring a pressure injury during the intraoperative period (NPIAP, 2019).

Pressure. Pressure is the force placed on the patient's underlying tissues. In order to avoid injury, normal capillary interface pressure (23–32 mmHg) must be maintained (Wang et al., 2018b). Above these levels, blood flow and tissue perfusion become restricted (Fig. 9.3A) and, if this pressure is unrelieved for a prolonged period, may result in tissue hypoxia and the development of more serious complications. Pressure is created by the patient's own body weight being forced downwards owing to gravity (Fig 9.3B). This can be mitigated by the use of pressure-redistribution support surfaces (Stanton, 2017). A high-specification reactive (constant low pressure) foam mattress or an active (alternating pressure) mattress is recommended on the operating table for high-risk patients (Wang et al., 2018b). Particular attention must be given to ensure that pressure on the heels is offloaded, with the knees in slight flexion, and all bony prominences are padded (NPIAP, 2019).

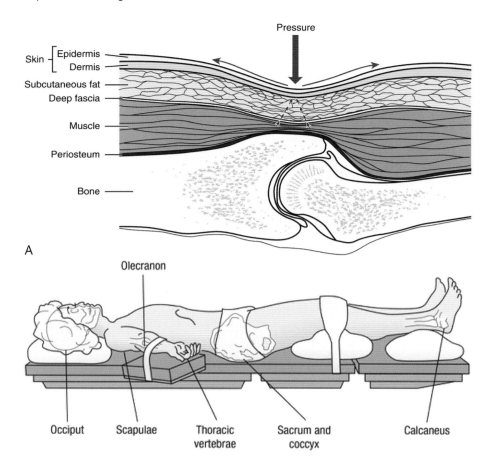

FIG. 9.3 (**A**) Tissues affected by pressure which causes deep tissue damage and necrosis. (**B**) Vulnerable pressure points when patients are positioned supine for surgery. (Source: (A) Phillips, N. (2017). *Berry and Kohn's operating room technique* (13th ed., p. 485, Fig. 26.1). St Louis, MO: Elsevier; (B) Spruce, L. (2017a). Preventing perioperative positioning and equipment injuries. In J. Sanchez, P. Barach, J. Johnson, & J. Jacobs (Eds.), *Surgical patient care (pp. 493–518).* Champaign, IL: Springer.)

Additional pressure can also come from the weight of devices that are placed in, on or against the patient, such as IV access devices, instruments, drills, Mayo stands, or surgical team members leaning on the patient. Likewise, bed attachments or positioning aids can compress tissues or pinch parts of the patient's body. These types of injuries are referred to as medical-device-related pressure injuries (MDRPIs) (Delmore & Ayello, 2017). This is a particular risk for obese patients

(Van Wicklin, 2018). Consequently, it is necessary for the surgical team to be vigilant when using any of these devices, as well as being mindful when assisting during surgery.

Shear. Shear is the movement of underlying tissue when the skeletal structure moves while the skin remains stationary. A parallel force creates shear. This occurs when, for example, the head of the operating table is lowered and the patient is placed in a head-down, supine position (Trendelenburg). As gravity pulls the skeleton down, the underlying tissues are stretched, folded or torn as they move with it. This can result in vascular occlusion as well as damaging the (static) skin (Fawcett, 2019).

Friction. Friction is the force produced when two surfaces rub against each other. Friction to the patient's skin occurs when the body is dragged across the operating table rather than lifted; this can abrade, burn or tear the patient's skin and encourage the development of pressure ulcers (NPIAP, 2019).

Moisture. The presence of moisture, such as skin preparation solution, blood, urine or surgical irrigation solutions, pooling underneath the patient can result in maceration of the skin and increase the likelihood of damage to it; hence measures to prevent such occurrences are required (Fawcett, 2019). Other factors related to moisture include the patient's level of continence, particularly in gynaecology and urology patients, and the patient's skin temperature in conjunction with contact with synthetic materials, which may induce excessive sweating. Hence, the microclimate of the patient's skin, which includes temperature, humidity and air flow, need to be considered relative to patient positioning. There is emerging evidence that suggests there is an association between elevated subdermal moisture, tissue inflammation and pressure injury development (O'Brien, Moore, Patton, & O'Connor, 2018; Oliveria, Moore, O'Connor, & Patton, 2017).

Pressure injury prevention. The NPIAP has developed evidence-based recommendations for the prevention and treatment of **pressure injuries**. Its clinical practice guideline was developed using a rigorous scientific methodology to appraise available research and make 575 evidence-based recommendations. Its recommendations for perioperative patients are listed in Research box 9.1.

The magnitude of the burden associated with pressure injuries should not be underestimated. In Australia, the rate of hospital-acquired pressure injuries was 9.7 per 10,000 hospitalisations in the year 2015–16, and many of these originated in the operating room (ACSQHC/the Commission, 2018a). Indeed, some postoperative injuries are clearly related to the patient's surgical position and the restraints or other medical devices used intraoperatively (NPIAP, 2019). In Australia, a number of state-based health departments are now initiating financial penalties for hospital-acquired pressure injuries, meaning their significance will have consequences for hospital expenditure (Goudas & Bruni, 2019). The imperative to reduce hospital-acquired pressure injury is reflected widely in current standards, with

---

RESEARCH BOX 9.1
NPIAP Recommendations for Perioperative Patients

1. Consider additional risk factors specific to individuals undergoing surgery.
2. Use a high specification reactive or alternating pressure support surface on the operating table for all individuals identified as being at risk of pressure ulcer development.
3. Position the individual in such a way as to reduce the risk of pressure ulcer development during surgery.
4. Ensure that the heels are free of the surface of the operating table. Ideally, heels should be free of all pressure – a state sometimes called 'floating heels'.
5. Use heel suspension devices that elevate and offload the heel completely in such a way as to distribute the weight of the leg along the calf without placing pressure on the Achilles tendon. Positioning the knees in slight flexion prevents popliteal vein compression and decreases the risk of perioperative deep vein thrombosis.
6. Position the knees in slight flexion when offloading the heels. This prevents popliteal vein compression and decreases the risk of perioperative deep vein thrombosis.

(Source: National Pressure Injury Advisory Panel. (2019). *Prevention and treatment of pressure ulcers: quick reference guide.* E. Haesler (Ed.). Perth: Cambridge Media.)

---

recommendations and guidelines requiring healthcare facilities to implement, maintain and audit processes to monitor, track and minimise the incidence and risk (ACORN, 2020b; ACSQHC/the Commission, 2017, NPIAP, 2019).

Perioperative nurses have a key role and responsibility related to pressure injury prevention. This involves the use of a validated pressure injury risk assessment tool that will assist in determining the degree of individual patient risk. The outcomes of pressure injury risk assessment subsequently inform the measures needed to prevent patient injury intraoperatively. However, there is limited evidence that perioperative nurses know about or use such tools (or other perioperative assessment activities) (Dalvand, Ebadi, & Ghenshlagh, 2018; Ebi, Hirko, & Mijena, 2019). There are, however, notable exceptions. Fig. 9.4 is an example of an electronic perioperative nursing care record that facilitates the assessment and documentation of **skin integrity** intraoperatively, as well as providing options to record information about patient positioning and the use of

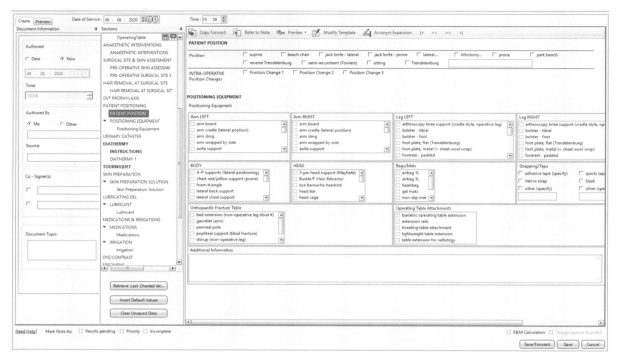

FIG. 9.4 Perioperative electronic nursing care record. (Source: Sunrise EMR, Noarlunga Hospital, South Australia. Allscripts Healthcare, Adelaide.)

pressure injury prevention devices. In fact, electronic medical records often required staff to assess and enter this kind of data as a forced function before they can proceed to other data entry activities.

Musculoskeletal system. During surgery and anaesthesia, normal protective reflexes (e.g. pain and pressure receptors) are depressed in the patient and muscle tone is lost as a result of the action of the pharmacological agents used. Consequently, patients are no longer able to respond normally if, during positioning and surgery, their muscles, tendons and/or ligaments are overstretched, twisted or strained; or body alignment (particularly for the patient's range of motion) is not maintained. Injury can also occur if dependent limbs fall over the edge of the operating table. It is advisable to use a body strap/safety belt to secure the patient to the operating table (Phillips, 2017). Obese patients may need additional straps, positioning aids or non-slip devices to prevent movement or slipping intraoperatively. This is particularly important during surgery involving the lithotomy or Trendelenburg positions.

Nervous system. Agents used to induce and maintain anaesthesia alter the patient's level of consciousness, which lies on a continuum from light sedation to general anaesthesia (Australian and New Zealand College of Anaesthetists [ANZCA], 2014; Hinkelbein et al., 2018). These agents also cause changes to sensation and protective reflexes. Together these effects increase the likelihood of nerve injury occurring during surgery because the patient is unable to respond normally to uncomfortable or painful stimuli. In most cases these injuries occur as a result of the formation of lesions secondary to damage incurred by undue pressure, stretching, twisting and pinching of nerves, which may be temporary or permanent depending on the severity of damage sustained. The ulnar nerve is the nerve most frequently injured during the perioperative period, followed by injury to the brachial plexus (Hewson & Hardman, 2019) and lumbosacral nerve roots (Fawcett, 2019; O'Connor & Radcliffe, 2018; Phillips, 2017; Spruce, 2018). Table 9.1 outlines nerves that are commonly injured and the causes (see Figs 9.5–9.10).

Neurophysiological monitors such as somatosensory evoked potential (SSEP) and transcranial electrical

TABLE 9.1
Peripheral Nerves at Risk of Injury

Nerve Involved	Cause of Damage
Median, radial and ulnar nerves	Pressure on the medial aspect of the patient's arm when devices used to secure the arm are unpadded or restraints are too tight (see Fig. 9.8) Poorly placed blood pressure cuff Patient's body weight on the lower (dependent) arm when in lateral position Patient positioned with flexed elbows and hands placed on the chest
Brachial plexus	Extending the arm beyond 90° angle when an arm board is used Pressure from shoulder braces (used in the Trendelenburg and steep Trendelenberg positions) – these should be avoided Patient's body weight on the lower (dependent) arm when in lateral position Arm unsecured and allowed to fall off the table Splitting of the sternum during cardiac surgery Over-rotation and lateral flexion of the patient's head (see Figs 9.9, 9.10)
Femoral and obturator nerves	Inappropriate positioning of abdominal, vaginal or anal retractors Inappropriate positioning of the patient in the lithotomy position, resulting in over-stretching of the nerve (see Fig. 9.5) Team members leaning against patient's thighs Slippage of pneumatic tourniquet cuff (see Fig. 9.24)
Sciatic nerve	Hyperflexion of the hip joint, particularly when the patient's legs are lifted incorrectly during surgery (see Fig. 9.6)
Pudendal nerve	Injury to the perineal and pudendal nerves, causing faecal incontinence and loss of perineal and penile sensation if a peroneal post is not well padded or places excess pressure on the pelvis while the patient is positioned on the traction table (see Fig. 9.21)
Common peroneal nerve	Pressure of the stirrups or leg-holding devices on the patient's calf when in the lithotomy position (especially hemi-lithotomy) (see Fig. 9.5) Failure to place a pillow between the patient's legs when lateral position used Incorrectly sized or inappropriate application of sequential compressive devices Pressure from devices placed under the patient's knees
Facial and nerves of the scalp	Too-tight placement of head strap Pressure from horseshoe-shaped head positioner (prone and sitting positions) – these should not be used Hyperextension, flexion or rotation of the neck Vigorous elevation of the mandible during airway support (see Fig 9.10)

(Sources: Fawcett, D. L. (2019). Positioning the patient for surgery. In J. C. Rothrock & D. L. McEwen (Eds.), *Alexander's care of the patient in surgery* (16th ed., pp. 142–175). St Louis, MO: Elsevier; Phillips, N. (2017). *Berry and Kohn's operating room technique* (13th ed.). St Louis, MO: Elsevier; Spruce, L. (2018). Back to basics: orthopedic positioning. *AORN Journal, 107*(3), 355–367.)

motor evoked potential (TCeMEP) modalities can be used to monitor electrophysiological conduction in the spinal cord, arm and brachial plexus nerves (Stanton, 2017). These monitors sound an alarm when nerves are compromised, giving the perioperative team a chance to perform corrective action before permanent injury occurs (Burlingame, 2017; Spruce, 2018; Stanton, 2017).

Cardiovascular system. Anaesthetic agents can affect the cardiovascular system by causing peripheral vasodilation and subsequent pooling of blood in the extremities, resulting in hypotension (Fawcett, 2019). Relaxation of muscle tone reduces the effectiveness of the skeletal muscle pump in returning blood to the heart, which further contributes to a reduction in cardiac output. Patient positioning can further exacerbate these effects; for example, reverse Trendelenburg orientation of supine, lateral or prone positions will cause blood to pool in the lower extremities, whereas lithotomy positioning results in blood pooling in the

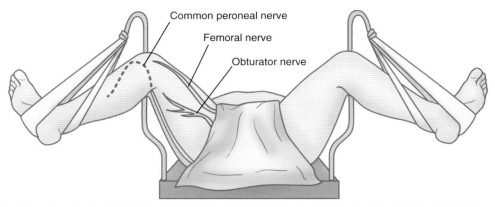

FIG. 9.5 Nerves of the inner thigh. (Source: Fawcett, D. L. (2019). Positioning the patient for surgery. In J. C. Rothrock & D. L. McEwen (Eds.), *Alexander's care of the patient in surgery* (16th ed., p. 154, Fig. 6.14). St Louis, MO: Elsevier.)

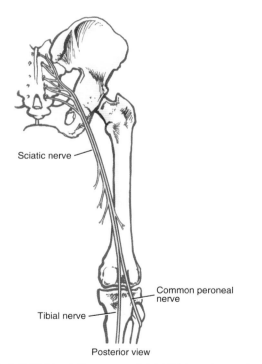

FIG. 9.6 Right sciatic nerve and right thigh and upper leg, posterior view. (Source: Fawcett, D. L. (2019). Positioning the patient for surgery. In J. C. Rothrock & D. L. McEwen (Eds.), *Alexander's care of the patient in surgery* (16th ed., p. 154, Fig. 6.12). St Louis, MO: Elsevier.)

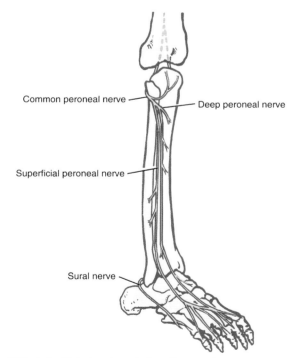

FIG. 9.7 Right leg, lateral view. (Source: Fawcett, D. L. (2019). Positioning the patient for surgery. In J. C. Rothrock & D. L. McEwen (Eds.), *Alexander's care of the patient in surgery* (16th ed., p. 154, Fig. 6.13). St Louis, MO: Elsevier.)

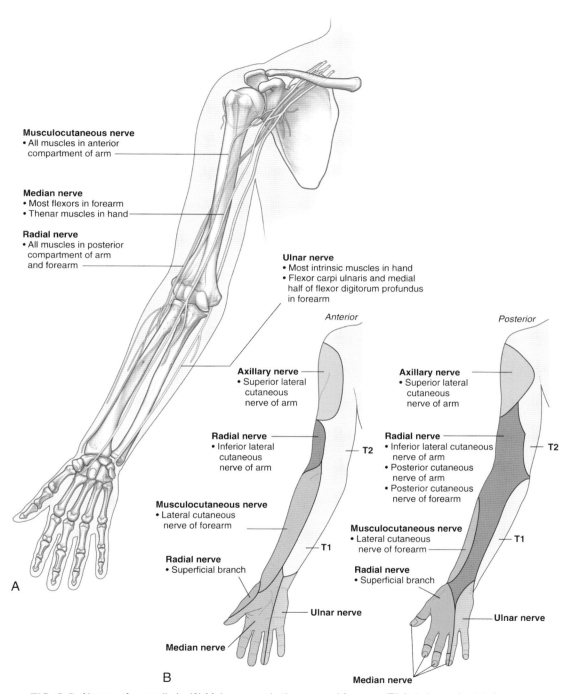

Musculocutaneous nerve
• All muscles in anterior
  compartment of arm

Median nerve
• Most flexors in forearm
• Thenar muscles in hand

Radial nerve
• All muscles in posterior
  compartment of arm
  and forearm

Ulnar nerve
• Most intrinsic muscles in hand
• Flexor carpi ulnaris and medial
  half of flexor digitorum profundus
  in forearm

Anterior

Posterior

Axillary nerve
• Superior lateral
  cutaneous
  nerve of arm

Axillary nerve
• Superior lateral
  cutaneous
  nerve of arm

Radial nerve
• Inferior lateral
  cutaneous
  nerve of arm

Radial nerve
• Inferior lateral cutaneous
  nerve of arm
• Posterior cutaneous
  nerve of arm
• Posterior cutaneous
  nerve of forearm

T2

T2

Musculocutaneous nerve
• Lateral cutaneous
  nerve of forearm

Musculocutaneous nerve
• Lateral cutaneous
  nerve of forearm

Radial nerve
• Superficial branch

Radial nerve
• Superficial branch

T1

T1

Ulnar nerve

Ulnar nerve

Median nerve

Median nerve

A

B

FIG. 9.8 Nerves of upper limb. (**A**) Major nerves in the arm and forearm. (**B**) Anterior and posterior areas
of skin innervated by major peripheral nerves in the arm and forearm. (Source: Drake, R. L., Vogl, W.,
Mitchell, A. W. M., Tibbitts, R., Richardson, P., Gray, H., & Horn, A. (2019). *Gray's anatomy for students*
(4th ed., International ed., p. 686, Fig. 7.16). Philadelphia: Elsevier.)

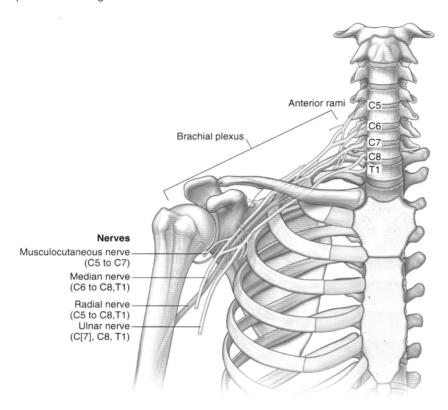

FIG. 9.9 Innervation of the upper limb. (Source: Drake, R. L., Vogl, W., Mitchell, A. W. M., Tibbitts, R., Richardson, P., Gray, H., & Horn, A. (2019). *Gray's anatomy for students* (4th ed., International ed., p. 684, Fig. 7.14). Philadelphia: Elsevier.)

lumbar region of the torso (Phillips, 2017). This leads to changes in the patient's blood pressure when they are initially placed into these positions and then subsequently returned to a supine position at the conclusion of surgery. Consequently, the movement of patients into and out of these positions must be carried out in a coordinated and unhurried way with good team communication throughout. Positioning should be postponed if the patient's blood pressure is unstable. Pregnant women, obese patients and patients with large abdominal masses are particularly at risk of supine hypotensive syndrome, owing to increased pressure on the aorta and inferior vena cava (IVC) (Cluver, Novilova, Hofmeyr, & Hall, 2013; Kirkbride, 2019). These patients should be positioned with a wedge under the right side to shift pressure off the underlying structures (Pillai, 2019). In obstetric surgery, a left lateral tilt of 10–15 degrees is recommended for women in the third trimester of pregnancy so as to reduce pressure on

the inferior vena cava (Aust, Koehler, Kuehnert, & Wiesmann, 2016).

Adequate arterial circulation is necessary to perfuse tissue, and occlusion of or pressure on peripheral vessels (such as might be caused by positioning devices or safety belts/straps) must be avoided (Phillips, 2017). For example, patients who are placed in the lithotomy position are at risk of compartment syndrome in their lower limb(s). This can occur when patients are in this position for extended periods of time. Compartment syndrome develops via a combination of prolonged tissue ischaemia and subsequent reperfusion of muscle within a tight osseofascial compartment and, if untreated, leads to necrosis and functional impairment (Fawcett, 2019; Phillips, 2017).

Additionally, there is increased potential for thromboembolic episodes. Different positions, such as lithotomy, the time spent in these positions and the devices used to maintain them (e.g. safety belts, stirrups

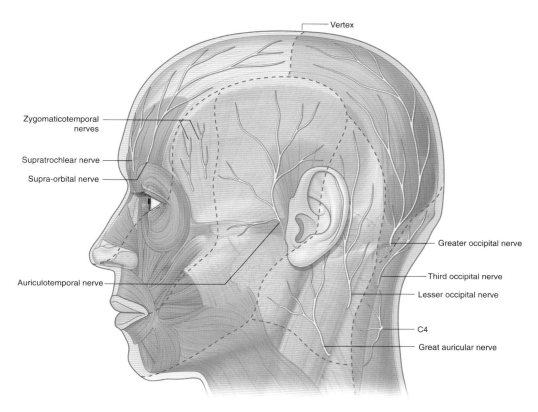

FIG. 9.10 Nerves of the scalp. (Source: Drake, R. L., Vogl, W., Mitchell, A. W. M., Tibbitts, R., Richardson, P., Gray, H., & Horn, A. (2019) *Gray's anatomy for students*. (4th ed., International ed., p. 913, Fig. 8.73). Philadelphia: Elsevier.)

or other leg-holding devices) contribute to venous stasis and the formation of thrombi (Bryant, Knights, Darroch, & Rowland, 2018).

Respiratory system. Respiratory function is compromised whenever movement of the patient's diaphragm is limited during positioning for anaesthetic and surgical procedures. Supine, lateral and prone positions requiring the patient to be in a horizontal plane result in reduced tidal volumes and changes to functional residual capacity of the lungs (Kirkbride, 2019; Phillips, 2017). Trendelenburg orientation further compromises respiratory function owing to the abdominal viscera shifting cephalad towards the diaphragm. These effects are exacerbated in patients who are obese, who smoke, who are pregnant or who have coexisting respiratory disease (Fawcett, 2019; Phillips, 2017). Prone and lateral positions further impede respiratory function resulting from asymmetrical ventilation of the lungs and

impaired gas exchange (Kirkbride, 2019). Ideally, patients should spend as little time as possible in these positions. Excessive pressure caused by positional aids or the placement of the patient's arms on the chest area should also be avoided (Fawcett, 2019).

Preparation for Safe Patient Positioning

The perioperative nurse has a significant role to ensure safe patient positioning. Upon scheduling of surgery, the perioperative nurse should consult with team members to identify and ensure the necessary equipment will be available. The equipment should be well maintained and checked to ensure good working order prior to use. Planning and preparation allows for all equipment to be gathered and assembled the day before or on the morning of surgery. Adequate numbers of staff should be allocated to ensure smooth and effective teamwork, with the perioperative nurse providing any necessary instruction, oversight or supervision of

TABLE 9.2
Supine Position – Nursing Interventions and Rationales

Nursing Intervention	Rationale
Select an appropriate pressure-redistributing surface or OR mattress, gel overlay or air support surface overlay	Pressure-redistributing surfaces such as pressure-relieving OR mattress or mattress overlays protect occiput, scapulae, olecranon, vertebrae, sacrum, coccyx, ischial tuberosities and calcaneus from undue pressure
Ensure appropriate padding or gel pads are placed on extensions or other positional aids as required (arm boards, J boards)	Protects the ulnar nerve from undue pressure
Heels should be offloaded, and knees slightly flexed at 5°–10°	Protects the heels from undue pressure and reduces the risk of venous thromboembolism, respectively. Prevents hyperextension of knees and resultant ligament and nerve damage
Keep arm board(s) level with the operating table and at an angle of 90° (or less); arm(s) must be loosely secured to the board and positioned with the palms facing up and fingers extended. If arms are to be tucked by the sides for surgical necessity, they must be secured to ensure they do not slide down the side of the OR table	Protects peripheral vasculature and nerves from damage, including the brachial plexus and ulnar nerve. Compartment syndrome and nerve damage can occur if arms are tucked too tightly by the patient's side
Ensure legs are positioned uncrossed at the ankle with a safety strap placed 5 cm above the knees, securely but without compromising the circulation	Relieves undue pressure, decreasing risk of venous thrombosis and reduces risk of patient falling from the OR table during lighter phases of anaesthesia

(Sources: Australian College of Perioperative Nurses. (2020b). *ACORN standards for perioperative nursing in Australia* (16th ed., Vol. 1). Clinical standards – patient positioning. Adelaide: Author; Burlingame, B. L. (2017). Guideline implementation: positioning the patient. *AORN Journal*, 106(3), 228–237; Fawcett, D. L. (2019). Positioning the patient for surgery. In J. C. Rothrock & D. L. McEwen (Eds.), *Alexander's care of the patient in surgery* (16th ed., pp. 142–175). St Louis, MO: Elsevier.)

support staff or orderlies who assist with positioning. When careful planning and preparation are implemented, unanticipated issues or concerns are able to be mitigated or managed, ensuring patient safety (ACORN 2020b; Croke, 2019).

Surgical Positions
There are several standard surgical positions, with a range of variations, and standard operating tables are designed to accommodate this range. Positions commonly used include:
- supine
- Trendelenburg and reverse Trendelenburg
- prone
- lateral
- lithotomy
- sitting: Fowler's and semi-Fowler's
- fracture table position.

Supine position
In the supine position, patients lie on their back with their arms either secured at their sides or placed out on an arm board. This commonly used position provides access to the abdominal, peritoneal and cardiothoracic cavities, the extremities and the head and neck. Table 9.2 shows nursing interventions and rationales for this position.

Trendelenburg and reverse Trendelenburg positions
These positions are variations of the supine position, with patients lying in a dorsal recumbent position (i.e. on their back). For the Trendelenburg position, which is used for lower abdominal or pelvic surgery, the patient is tilted head down (Fig. 9.11). In the reverse Trendelenburg position, the patient is head up, feet down, supine; this position is used for head and neck surgery and minimally invasive upper abdominal procedures (see Fig. 9.12). An important factor to consider for these positions is the potential for shearing forces to occur. These can be avoided by flexing the table at the position of the patient's knees, decreasing the gravitational pull towards the head in the Trendelenburg position. Shoulder braces previously used to

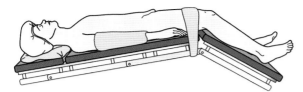

FIG. 9.11 Trendelenburg position. (Source: Phillips, N. (2017). *Berry and Kohn's operating room technique* (13th ed., p. 493, Fig. 26.17). St Louis, MO: Elsevier.)

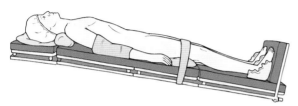

FIG. 9.12 Reverse Trendelenburg position. (Source: Phillips, N. (2017). *Berry and Kohn's operating room technique* (13th ed., p. 493, Fig. 26.18). St Louis, MO: Elsevier.)

prevent patient slippage should be avoided, as they are known to damage the brachial plexus (Fawcett, 2019). In the reverse Trendelenburg position, a padded table attachment can be fitted to the foot of the operating table on which the patient's feet rest. Tables 9.3 and 9.4 show nursing interventions and rationales for these positions.

Prone position

In the prone position, patients lie face down. This position is used when surgical access to the spine, rectum or dorsal areas of the extremities is required. It can be achieved on a standard operating table, or it may require a specially designed table or table fittings (e.g. a laminectomy frame); the choice is determined by the particular surgical intervention.

The patient is anaesthetised in the supine position prior to transfer, and the patient's airway is secured using a reinforced, flexible endotracheal tube (ETT), which will not kink. The ETT is secured with tape by the anaesthetist and eye protection implemented to prevent the risk of corneal abrasion. The patient is then lifted and placed with the abdomen down on the

---

TABLE 9.3
Trendelenburg Position – Nursing Interventions and Rationales

Nursing Intervention	Rationale
Observe the same precautions as for the supine position	This is a supine position variation; placement of the patient directly on a high friction coefficient surface, such as a gel overlay, prevents slippage
Break the table slightly at the position of the patient's knees	Helps prevent the effects of shearing forces as it counteracts gravitational pull
Observe respiratory function closely	Severely angled tilts diminish the patient's lung capacity owing to the pressure of the abdominal organs on the diaphragm, resulting in compression of the lung bases
Observe lower extremity circulation	May be diminished from blood pooling in the head and upper torso
Continue position only as long as necessary	Minimises the effects of compromised respiratory function and blood pooling in the upper torso
Tilt the patient in and out of the position slowly	Avoids sudden blood pressure shifts
Use safety straps, support strapping and lateral support posts when patient is to be placed in the steep Trendelenburg position or lateral tilt	Prevention of shear injury to the patient's skin, slips and falls of limbs and patient from the operating table

(Sources: Fawcett, D. L. (2019). Positioning the patient for surgery. In J. C. Rothrock & D. L. McEwen (Eds.), *Alexander's care of the patient in surgery* (16th ed., pp. 142–175). St Louis, MO: Elsevier; Soncrant, C. M., Warner, L. J., Neily, J., Paull, D. E., Mazzia, L., Mills, P. D., . . . Hemphill, R. R. (2018). Root cause analysis of reported patient falls in ORs in the Veterans Health Administration. *AORN Journal, 108*(4), 386–397.)

TABLE 9.4
Reverse Trendelenburg Position – Nursing Interventions and Rationales

Nursing Intervention	Rationale
Observe the same precautions as for the supine position	This is a supine position variation
Use of intermittent pneumatic compression devices and graduated compression stockings is recommended	Aids with lower limb venous return
Tilt the patient in and out of the position slowly	Avoids sudden blood pressure shifts
Ensure a padded footrest is secured to the foot of operating table	Prevents the patient slipping off the table

(Source: Fawcett, D. L. (2019). Positioning the patient for surgery. In J. C. Rothrock & D. L. McEwen (Eds.), *Alexander's care of the patient in surgery* (16th ed., pp. 142–175). St Louis, MO: Elsevier.)

operating table, and the face placed on a face pillow made of foam or gel. Head placement in the neutral position is recommended to minimise stress on the carotid and vertebral arteries and reduce the risk of cerebral vascular accident and nerve damage (Fawcett, 2019). Unless a mechanical patient lifter is available or a Jackson table is used, this transfer requires a minimum of four people to be executed safely, with one member of the team, usually the anaesthetist, supporting the patient's head and neck and safeguarding the patient's airway at all times. The position requires additional padding (often in the form of a specialised face pillow plus multiple pillows or rolls on the operating table) to protect vulnerable areas, such as the patient's eyes, ears, cheeks, lips and chin, breasts (females), genitalia (males), patellae and toes (Fig. 9.13). Table 9.5 shows nursing interventions and rationales for the prone position.

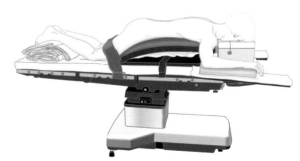

FIG. 9.13 Prone position using Wilson laminectomy frame for spinal procedures and face pillow head support. (Source: Fawcett, D. L. (2019). Positioning the patient for surgery. In J. C. Rothrock & D. L. McEwen (Eds.), *Alexander's care of the patient in surgery* (16th ed., p. 170, Fig. 6.32). St Louis, MO: Elsevier.)

TABLE 9.5
Prone Position – Nursing Interventions and Rationales

Nursing Intervention	Rationale
Use a latex-free foam or gel face pillow, or specialised head positioning frames (e.g. Mayfield headrest) – horseshoe headrest should not be used	Specialised positioning devices allow for the head and neck to be maintained in normal anatomical alignment and allow access to the patient's airway
Use a padded operating table mattress – gel mattress or pillows/rolls (or gel pad over laminectomy frame, if used)	Extra padding protects vulnerable areas, such as the cheeks, ears, chin, lips, breasts (female), genitalia (males), patellae and toes
Place padding on extensions as required (arm boards, J boards); arms should be secured loosely, palms down on padded arm boards and kept in natural alignment – they should not be allowed to hang over the edge of the operating table	Arms are moved down and forwards and placed on the arm board slowly and carefully to minimise the risk of damage to the brachial plexus; arms hanging over the table edge can sustain damage to the radial nerve
Place eye ointment in both eyes and ensure eyelids are securely taped closed; avoid direct pressure on the globe of the eye	The eyes are vulnerable to corneal abrasion, neuropathy and increases in intraocular pressure

(Sources: Fawcett, D. L. (2019). Positioning the patient for surgery. In J. C. Rothrock & D. L. McEwen (Eds.), *Alexander's care of the patient in surgery* (16th ed., pp. 142–175). St Louis, MO: Elsevier; National Pressure Injury Advisory Panel. (2019). *Prevention and treatment of pressure ulcers: quick reference guide*. E. Haesler (Ed.). Perth, Australia: Cambridge Media; Spruce, L. (2018). Back to basics: orthopedic positioning. *AORN Journal, 107*(3), 355–367.)

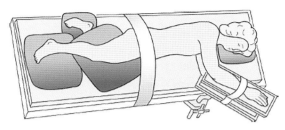

FIG. 9.14 Left lateral position with arm board. (Source: Spruce, L. (2018). Back to basics: orthopedic positioning. *AORN Journal, 107*(3), 355–367.)

Lateral position

In the lateral position, which is used for procedures involving the chest, kidney or hip joint, the patient lies on the non-operative (dependent) side, with the operative side uppermost. It requires a selection of positional aids to secure the patient because there is a risk of the patient rolling forwards or backwards intraoperatively or even falling off the table. The patient is anaesthetised in the supine position and then transferred or turned onto the dependent (non-operative) side. Positional aids include specially designed, padded arm rests (e.g. Carter Brain arm rest) to support the upper arm and keep it away from the operative area, plus table/safety straps and pliable bean bags, used to hold the patient securely to the operating table and to maintain the position throughout surgery (Figs 9.14 and 9.15). Alternatively, padded table attachments (lateral supports or kidney braces), one at the patient's back and a larger one supporting the abdomen, can be used. Table 9.6 shows nursing interventions and rationales for the lateral position.

Lithotomy position

For patients undergoing colorectal, gynaecological and urological surgery, the lithotomy position is required. This position involves the patient lying supine with their legs raised, abducted and secured in leg-positioning devices (stirrups) to expose the perineal area. Depending on the surgical access required, the patient's legs can be held at various angles to the trunk – in a low, standard or high lithotomy position. These positions are maintained with the use of a range of stirrups, which are chosen after considering the type of surgery and the proposed length of time for the procedure (Figs 9.16 and 9.17). Some stirrups feature hydraulic lift-assisted technology that provides easier movement of the leg into the desired position. They also permit adjustment of abduction and lithotomy while maintaining a critical aseptic field. The boots are padded, and some are extended on the lateral side to protect the head of the fibula and the peroneal nerve (e.g. Yellofins) (Fig. 9.18).

One of the most important precautions to consider when placing a patient in this position is the high risk

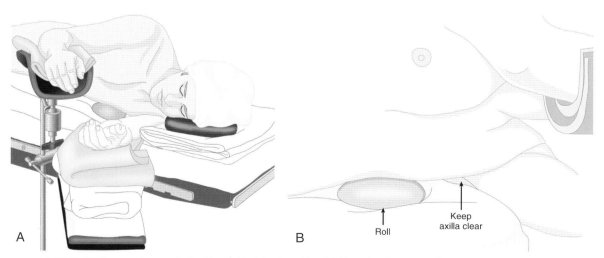

A   B   Roll   Keep axilla clear

FIG. 9.15 Proper placement of axillary roll in lateral position. (**A**) Note the placement of arms with additional padding under head to maintain alignment. Dependent eye is clear of the headrest. (**B**) The roll is placed under the chest wall, caudal to the axilla, leaving the axilla free to prevent compression of the brachial plexus. (Source: Fawcett, D. L. (2019). Positioning the patient for surgery. In J. C. Rothrock & D. L. McEwen (Eds.), *Alexander's care of the patient in surgery* (16th ed., p. 174, Fig. 6.38). St Louis, MO: Elsevier.)

TABLE 9.6
Lateral Position – Nursing Interventions and Rationales

Nursing Intervention	Rationale
Use padded operating table mattress and place padding on extensions as required (arm boards and arm supports)	Protects pressure points on the dependent side – ear, shoulder, hip, ankle
Place a pillow between the patient's knees with the bottom leg flexed at the knee and hip to assist in stabilising the patient on the operating table	Knees will rub against each other, damaging the skin; additionally, undue pressure can damage the peroneal nerve
Keep the head in alignment with the spine by placing a pillow under the patient's head	The spine is vulnerable to misalignment and twisting; this can place pressure on the dependent brachial plexus
Secure the patient using either lateral supports (kidney braces) (padded) at the abdomen and back, or devices such as beanbags or a vacuum beanbag positioner; additionally, a safety belt/table strap over the patient's upper thigh is required	Prevents the patient from falling off the operating table and ensures the patient does not move intraoperatively
Ensure the patient's shoulder on the non-operative (dependent) side is not over-extended and the lower arm is protected, usually by securing it to an arm board; place the upper arm on a lateral arm support; an axillary roll is placed under the chest posterior to the axilla	Prevents damage to the brachial plexus and ulnar nerve
Kidney surgery requires access to the retroperitoneal area of the flank – in this case, the patient is positioned so that the lower iliac crest is below the lumbar break where the kidney bridge is located on operating table; the latter is subsequently elevated (slowly) and the operating table flexed to lower the patient's upper torso and legs	Prevents the dependent flank area from compression and subsequent pooling of blood in the lower extremities

(Source: Fawcett, D. L. (2019). Positioning the patient for surgery. In J. C. Rothrock & D. L. McEwen (Eds.), *Alexander's care of the patient in surgery* (16th ed., pp. 142–175). St Louis, MO: Elsevier; National Pressure Injury Advisory Panel. (2019). *Prevention and treatment of pressure ulcers: quick reference guide*. E. Haesler (Ed.). Perth, Australia: Cambridge Media.)

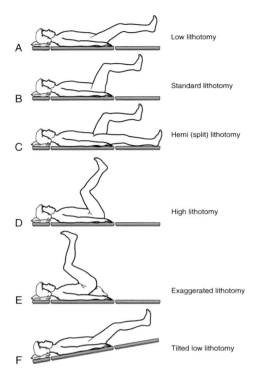

FIG. 9.16 (**A–F**) Commonly used lithotomy positions. (Source: Phillips, N. (2017). *Berry and Kohn's operating room technique* (13th ed., p. 485, Fig. 26.1). St Louis, MO: Elsevier.)

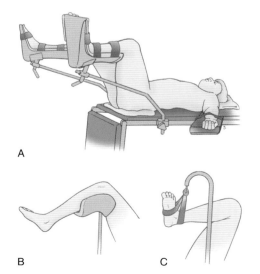

FIG. 9.17 (**A**) Lithotomy using boot-type stirrups. (**B**) Knee crutch stirrup. (**C**) Candy cane stirrup. (Source: Heizenroth, J. (2015). Positioning the patient for surgery. In J. Rothrock (Ed.) & D. McEwen (Assoc. Ed), *Alexander's care of the patient in surgery* (15th ed., Fig. 6.28). Elsevier Mosby, St Louis.)

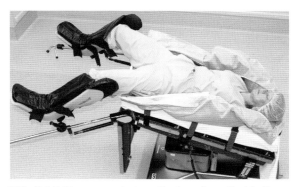

FIG. 9.19 Recommended positioning of a patient in the steep Trendelenburg position by using a vacuum-packed beanbag positioning device. (Source: Fawcett, D. L. (2019). Positioning the patient for surgery. In J. C. Rothrock & D. L. McEwen (Eds.), *Alexander's care of the patient in surgery* (16th ed., p. 165, Fig. 6.23). St Louis, MO: Elsevier.)

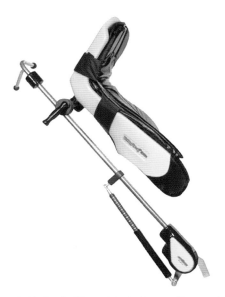

FIG. 9.18 Hydraulic lift-assisted stirrups. (Source: https://www.allenmedical.com/catalog/gyn—lapro—uro/gyn—lapro—uro-products/item/yellofins-elite-stirrups-with-lift-assist#!.)

of nerve damage and hip dislocation if the legs are not raised simultaneously, slowly and at the same angle and height at all times. The lithotomy and steep Trendelenburg (LST) position is used for some laparoscopic, colorectal, gynaecological and urological procedures, particularly when robotic-assisted surgery is undertaken. The LST incurs the same risks associated with both lithotomy and Trendelenburg positions, but with the additional risk of skin breakdown as a result of shear and friction. This is due to the steep head-down position, with a head-down tilt of between 30 and 45 degrees (Figs 9.19 and 9.20) (Fawcett, 2019; Mangham, 2017; Soncrant et al., 2018). Table 9.7 shows nursing interventions and rationales for the lithotomy position.

Sitting positions: Fowler's/semi-Fowler's position

The patient placed in the Fowler's/semi-Fowler's position is secured in an upright sitting position. This position is used for surgery involving the ears, nose, shoulders, abdomen and breasts and for some cranial procedures. In the latter case, the patient's head is held in a brace or supported with a head support attachment. Initially, the patient is placed in the supine position and, once anaesthetised, the table is manipulated so that the patient assumes a sitting position. The angle of this position (Fowler's or semi-Fowler's) will vary according to the type of surgery and the access

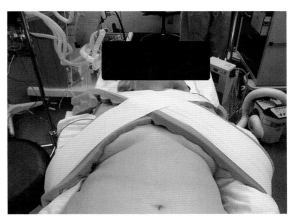

FIG. 9.20 Cross-chest safety strapping to prevent patient slippage on the OR table during steep Trendelenberg positioning. (Source: Fawcett, D. L. (2019). Positioning the patient for surgery. In J. C. Rothrock & D. L. McEwen (Eds.), *Alexander's care of the patient in surgery* (16th ed., p. 165, Fig. 6.24). St Louis, MO: Elsevier.)

required. The patient's arms must be secured so that they do not fall by the side of the body. They can rest on a pillow on the patient's lap. A padded footboard prevents foot drop. This position can cause pelvic pooling or venous stasis, resulting in cardiovascular instability, orthopaedic injury and/or tissue injury/necrosis (Fawcett, 2019). It can also cause an air embolus to enter the right atrium, necessitating immediate repositioning of the patient to a left lateral position, placement of the table into the steep

TABLE 9.7
Lithotomy Position – Nursing Interventions and Rationales

Nursing Intervention	Rationale
Secure stirrups/leg-holding devices at an equal level and height	Ensures stirrups do not dislodge during surgery, and that the patient's hips and legs are kept in alignment
Bring the patient's legs up into the stirrups simultaneously and slowly, keeping them at an equal height and angle at all times	Maintains hip alignment and prevents dislocation of the hip joint and overstretching of the femoral nerve; moving them slowly prevents blood pressure fluctuations
Ensure that the patient's buttocks remain on the table at all times and do not overhang it	Reduces the risk of lumbosacral strain and sciatic nerve damage
Ensure that the patient's fingers are not in the way of the stirrups or table break when adjusting equipment or the operating table	Fingers can be crushed in the stirrup joints and lower table break
Ensure that the stirrup poles and footrests are padded	Decreases the risk of thrombus formation or compartment syndrome and protects the posterior tibial and common peroneal nerves
Observe precautions for venous thromboembolism during longer procedures	Pressure on veins from the stirrups can increase the risk of thrombosis formation

(Source: Fawcett, D. L. (2019). Positioning the patient for surgery. In J. C. Rothrock & D. L. McEwen (Eds.), *Alexander's care of the patient in surgery* (16th ed., pp. 142–175). St Louis, MO: Elsevier; National Pressure Injury Advisory Panel. (2019). *Prevention and treatment of pressure ulcers: quick reference guide*. E. Haesler (Ed.). Perth, Australia: Cambridge Media.)

Trendelenburg position and insertion of a central venous catheter to withdraw the air bubble (Phillips, 2017).

Fracture table position

Some orthopaedic procedures require the use of a specialised fracture table. Indications for use include correcting a fractured neck of the femur, as well as performing some femoral procedures, because the table permits the necessary rotation and manipulation of the operative limb. Where possible, patients are anaesthetised prior to transfer onto this table. They are placed supine on the fracture table with the pelvis stabilised against a well-padded perineal post to protect against pudendal nerve and genital injury (Fig. 9.21). If needed, traction is achieved by restraining the injured limb in a well-padded, boot-like device that is part of the table's movable

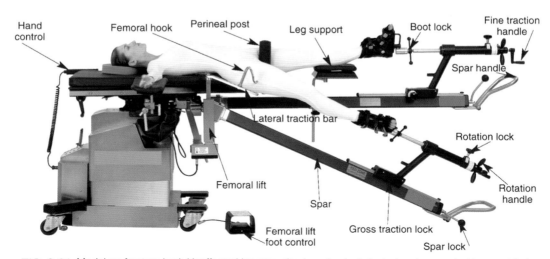

FIG. 9.21 Model on fracture bed. Unaffected leg may also be raised, abducted and supported in a padded leg rest. (Source: Fawcett, D. L. (2019). Positioning the patient for surgery. In J. C. Rothrock & D. L. McEwen (Eds.), *Alexander's care of the patient in surgery* (16th ed., p. 161, Fig. 6.17). St Louis, MO: Elsevier.)

TABLE 9.8
Recommended and Not Recommended Positioning Devices, Equipment and Support Surfaces

Recommended Practice	Not Recommended
POSITIONING DEVICES AND EQUIPMENT	
Viscoelastic gel products such as:	IV fluid bags
head rings	Towels
shoulder rolls	Bed sheets
chest rolls	Blankets
heel pads	Improvised products do not allow pressure to be redistributed
pillows	and can cause friction and shear injury
wedges	
Products designed to allow for redistribution of pressure	
Well-padded supports with secure table attachments:	Positioning devices used in vulnerable anatomical areas
arm boards	including:
J boards	shoulder supports
kidney supports	candy cane/pigtail stirrups
lateral supports	Wilson frame
boot stirrups	horseshoe head positioner
foot rests	
Appropriately positioned safety straps draw sheet	Circumferential wrist restraints
placement to tuck arms at patient's side	
Axillary rolls extending over at least 3 rib spaces	
SUPPORT SURFACES	
Viscoelastic gel overlays	Multiple layers of sheets and blankets
Convoluted foam	Towels
Vacuum-packed positioning device	Warming blankets

(Sources: Association of periOperative Registered Nurses (2017). Guideline summary: positioning the patient. *AORN Journal, 106*(3), 238–247; Crook, C. (2016). Advocacy: how far would you go to protect your patients? *AORN Journal, 103*(5), 522–525; Davis, S. S. (2018). The key to safety: proactive prevention. *AORN Journal, 108*(4), 351–353; Fawcett, D. L. (2019). Positioning the patient for surgery. In J. C. Rothrock & D. L. McEwen (Eds.), *Alexander's care of the patient in surgery* (16th ed., pp. 142–175). St Louis, MO: Elsevier.)

traction arm. The non-operative leg is placed on a support attachment and kept out of the way of the operative limb. The patient's arms are also secured away from the operative field. Nursing interventions associated with the supine position apply. Additionally, the distal lower extremity pulses should be assessed before, during and on completion of the procedure (Fawcett, 2019).

On completion of surgery, patient transfer to the bed or trolley requires the same care and considerations as highlighted earlier. Additionally, skin integrity needs reassessing, to ensure it has not changed during the intraoperative period, and the outcome documenting, to highlight continuity of patient care and to demonstrate that necessary preventative care was provided (Davis, 2018; Stanton, 2017).

Table 9.8 shows recommended and not recommended positioning devices, equipment and support surfaces.

PATIENT SCENARIOS

PATIENT SCENARIO 9.1: PATIENT POSITIONING

Reflect on our patient scenario of Mr Collins, a 78-year-old man who has been admitted to hospital for a right total knee replacement (TKR). (His full history and a brief description of the healthcare setting are provided in the Introduction to this book for readers to review when answering the questions in this unfolding scenario.) He will require a thorough risk assessment for the potential for pressure injury to occur during his surgery. He has a number of risk factors that will need to be considered carefully by the multidisciplinary team, including his age, the presence of comorbidities and the length of his surgery.

Critical Thinking Questions

- What position will Mr Collins be placed in for the surgical procedure?
- What planning and preparation are required to ensure that Mr Collins will be safely transferred to the OR table and positioned for his surgery?

- What special considerations need to be made for Mr Collins to ensure that he is kept safe and injury free on the OR table during his surgical procedure?

PREVENTION AND MANAGEMENT OF VENOUS THROMBOEMBOLISM

The development of venous thrombosis and subsequent pulmonary embolus (PE) make up two components of the condition of **venous thromboembolism (VTE)**. VTE is a mostly preventable surgical complication, yet remains a significant economic burden to the healthcare system by causing postoperative (PO) morbidity and mortality in the form of chronic venous insufficiency, recurrent thromboembolism and post-thrombotic syndrome (AORN, 2018; Tran et al., 2019). Despite extensive evidence to guide proper prophylaxis and treatment of VTE, therapies continue to be underutilised (ACSQHC/the Commission, 2018b; Kahn et al., 2018).

Venous thrombus formation is associated with systemic alterations in the coagulability of blood, venous stasis and damage to walls of blood vessels (Bryant et al., 2018). All surgical interventions pose some risk, but those patients with an increased susceptibility of developing VTE are shown in Box 9.1. It is important to note that there are additional intraoperative risks for the development of VTE. These include:

- length of surgery
- venous compression
- hypovolaemia/dehydration
- hypotension
- hypothermia
- use of a tourniquet, especially during prolonged inflation (AORN, 2018).

Prevention

Numerous professional groups have published guidelines regarding VTE prophylaxis, agreeing that all surgical patients should be assessed preoperatively as close to the time of admission as possible to determine their risk for VTE versus their risk of bleeding. This assessment should then guide decision making regarding the use of anticoagulant and/or mechanical prophylaxis (National Institute for Health and Care Excellence [NICE], 2018). Appropriate local VTE risk assessment guidelines which use a risk assessment tool that is easy to use and accurately identifies patients at risk are essential so that prophylactic measures are used in the correct at-risk group but are

---

BOX 9.1
Patients at Increased Risk of Developing VTE

- Aged >40 years
- Those undergoing major surgery, especially intra-abdominal and pelvic procedures
- Orthopaedic patients, especially those undergoing reconstructive surgery
- Older patients (>65 years)
- Patients with an acute inflammatory condition
- Smokers
- Obese patients (BMI > 30 kg/m^2)
- Those with a family history of thromboembolism
- Major trauma victims
- Those with metabolic disorders or blood dyscrasias (e.g. inherited thrombophilia disorders)
- Those with certain kinds of cancer
- Those on oral contraception and hormone replacement medications, tamoxifen, antipsychotics
- Prolonged bed rest or immobilisation (ACSQHC/the Commission, 2018b; AORN, 2018; Bryant et al., 2018)

---

avoided in low-risk groups (ACSQHC/the Commission, 2018b). Fig. 9.22 is an example of one such tool.

Both pharmacological therapies and non-pharmacological actions should be used to prevent VTE, with multimodal interventions being more efficacious than single therapies (Bryant et al., 2018; Saunders, Comerota, Ozols, Torrejon Torres, & Ho, 2018). VTE guidelines developed by groups such as NICE and the European Society of Anaesthesiology have specific recommendations regarding prophylaxis, depending on type of surgery and associated risk factors (European Society of Anaesthesiology, 2018; NICE, 2018). The optimum length of VTE prophylaxis, the timing of commencement and the duration of therapy should be determined for each individual patient, depending on their risk factors and type of surgery (NICE, 2018). Reassessment of VTE should occur when there is a change in clinical condition (level of mobility, after surgery), regularly (at least every 7 days), and on discharge (CEC, 2018). Documentation of VTE

NSW GOVERNMENT | Health

Facility:

FAMILY NAME		MRN	
GIVEN NAME		☐ MALE	☐ FEMALE
D.O.B. ____ / ____ / ____		M.O.	
ADDRESS			

VENOUS THROMBOEMBOLISM (VTE) RISK ASSESSMENT TOOL

LOCATION / WARD

COMPLETE ALL DETAILS OR AFFIX PATIENT LABEL HERE

SMR060250

For use in adult patients (>16 years) admitted to a NSW public hospital or health service.
For stroke or neurosurgery patients, seek specialist advice prior to completion

1. Assess VTE Risk and Allocate Patient into Risk Category

☐ Higher Risk

☐ Total hip replacement, total knee replacement, or hip fracture surgery
☐ Abdominal or pelvic surgery for cancer
☐ Multiple major trauma
☐ Acute spinal cord injury with paresis

☐ Moderate Risk

☐ Patients who are not in either the lower- or higher-risk group

☐ Lower Risk

☐ Ambulatory patient without **VTE risk factors**
☐ Non-surgical ambulatory patient with **VTE risk factors** BUT expected length of stay ≤ 2 days.
☐ Minor surgery* in patient without **VTE risk factors**
*same day surgery or operating time < 30 mins

→ Consider VTE Risk Factors →

VTE Risk Factors

☐ Age > 60 years
☐ Obesity (BMI > 30kg/m²)
☐ Moderate to major* surgery
    *operating time > 45 minutes and/or involves abdomen
☐ Prior history of VTE
☐ Known thrombophilia (including inherited disorders)
☐ Active malignancy or cancer treatment
☐ Myeloproliferative neoplasms
☐ Acute myocardial infarction
☐ Congestive heart failure
☐ Active or chronic lung disease
☐ Active infection
☐ Active rheumatic disease
☐ Acute inflammatory bowel disease
☐ Hormonal replacement therapy
☐ Oestrogen-based contraceptives
☐ Nephrotic syndrome
☐ Dehydration
☐ Varicose veins/chronic venous stasis
☐ Significantly reduced mobility relative to normal state
☐ Pregnant or < 6 weeks post-partum (Refer to Obstetrics Consultant / Team prior to commencing pharmacological and/or mechanical prophylaxis)
☐ Sickle cell disease

2. Identify Contraindications and Other Conditions to Consider with Pharmacological Prophylaxis

Absolute Contraindication

☐ Therapeutic anticoagulation e.g. with warfarin, dabigatran, rivaroxaban, fondaparinux, apixaban
☐ Active haemorrhage
☐ Thrombocytopenia (platelets < 50 x 10⁹/L) OR coagulopathy

☐ Other_____

Relative Contraindication
(Consider risk vs benefit)

☐ Intracranial haemorrhage within last year
☐ Craniotomy within 2 weeks
☐ Intraocular surgery within 2 weeks
☐ Gastrointestinal OR genitourinary haemorrhage within last month
☐ Active intracranial lesions/neoplasms
☐ Hypertensive emergency
☐ Post-operative bleeding concerns
☐ Use of antiplatelets (e.g. aspirin, clopidogrel, dipyridamole, prasugrel, ticagrelor)
☐ Inherited bleeding disorder
☐ High falls risk
☐ Severe trauma to head or spinal cord, with haemorrhage
☐ End stage liver disease (INR > 1.5)

Other Conditions

☐ Heparin-sensitivity or history of heparin-induced thrombocytopenia (HIT)
    (Consult Haematologist for alternative treatment e.g. danaparoid use)
☐ Insertion/removal of epidural catheter or spinal needle (lumbar puncture) (current or planned)
    (see other considerations overleaf)#
☐ Creatinine clearance <30mL/min
    (see recommendations overleaf)
☐ VTE prophylaxis for total body weight < 50kg or > 120kg or BMI ≥ 35: seek specialist advice regarding these patient groups. Evidence in extremes of body weight is limited and careful clinical consideration is required.

3. Identify Contraindications to Mechanical Prophylaxis

☐ Skin ulceration
☐ Severe peripheral vascular disease
☐ Severe dermatitis
☐ Lower leg trauma
☐ Severe lower leg deformity

☐ Recent lower limb DVT (anti-embolic stockings may be used)
☐ Massive leg oedema/pulmonary oedema due to congestive cardiac failure
☐ Where correct fitting of stocking cannot be achieved e.g. Morbid Obesity

☐ Peripheral neuropathy (Intermittent pneumatic compression can be used)
☐ Recent skin graft
☐ Stroke patients (avoid anti-embolic stockings)

VENOUS THROMBOEMBOLISM (VTE) RISK ASSESSMENT TOOL

SMR060.250

NO WRITING — Page 1 of 2

FIG. 9.22 Venous thromboembolism risk assessment tool. (Source: NSW Health, Clinical Excellence Commission. (2018). *Patient safety programs, VTE Risk Assessment Tool*, pp. 1–2. https://www.cec.health.nsw.gov.au/__data/assets/pdf_file/0010/458821/Venous-Thromboembolism-VTE-Risk-Assessment-Tool.pdf)

NSW GOVERNMENT | Health

Facility:

FAMILY NAME		MRN	
GIVEN NAME		☐ MALE	☐ FEMALE
D.O.B. _____ / _____ / _____		M.O.	
ADDRESS			

VENOUS THROMBOEMBOLISM (VTE) RISK ASSESSMENT TOOL

LOCATION / WARD

COMPLETE ALL DETAILS OR AFFIX PATIENT LABEL HERE

This tool does not preclude the use of clinical judgment, and should be used in conjunction with local policy and procedures where they exist.

4. Prescribe Appropriate Prophylaxis

☐ Higher Risk

Select one pharmacological option†   **AND**   **Select one or more mechanical device**

☐ Enoxaparin 40 mg subcutaneous once daily
☐ Enoxaparin 20 mg subcutaneous once daily if **Creatinine Clearance < 30 mL/min**
  (or use Heparin 5,000 units subcutaneous 8- or 12-hourly)§
☐ Dalteparin 5,000 units subcutaneous once daily
☐ Alternative agent for Orthopaedic Surgical patients (see below)**
☐ No pharmacological prophylaxis because of contraindication or not advised

† VTE prophylaxis dose for **total body weight < 50 kg or > 120 kg or BMI ≥ 35**: seek specialist advice regarding these patient groups. Evidence in extremes of body weight is limited and careful clinical consideration is required.

§ Note: In hip and knee replacement surgery, LMWH is preferred over heparin

☐ Graduated compression stockings / anti-embolic stockings
☐ Intermittent pneumatic compression
☐ Foot impulse device
☐ No mechanical prophylaxis because of contraindication

PLUS ☐ Early mobilisation   ☐ Patient education

☐ Moderate Risk

Select one pharmacological option†   **OR**   **If pharmacological prophylaxis is contraindicated or not advised, select one or more mechanical device:**

☐ Enoxaparin 40 mg subcutaneous once daily
☐ Enoxaparin 20 mg subcutaneous once daily if **Creatinine Clearance < 30 mL/min** (or use heparin)
☐ Dalteparin 5,000 units subcutaneous once daily
☐ Heparin 5,000 units subcutaneous 8- or 12-hourly
☐ No pharmacological prophylaxis because of contraindication or not advised

† VTE prophylaxis dose for **total body weight < 50 kg or > 120 kg or BMI ≥ 35**: seek specialist advice regarding these patient groups. Evidence in extremes of body weight is limited and careful clinical consideration is required.

☐ Graduated compression stockings / anti-embolic stockings
☐ Intermittent pneumatic compression
☐ Foot impulse device
☐ No mechanical prophylaxis because of contraindication

PLUS ☐ Early mobilisation   ☐ Patient education

☐ Lower Risk

☐ Prophylaxis not required   ☐ Early mobilisation   ☐ Patient education

Tool adapted with permission from the *San Diego Medical Center VTE Risk Assessment and Prophylaxis Orders*.

5. Other Considerations

#Prior to insertion or removal of epidural catheter or spinal needle (lumbar puncture), discuss with the anaesthetist. Section 5.9 of the Acute Pain Management: Scientific Evidence guideline produced by the Australian and New Zealand College of Anaesthetists and Faculty of Pain Medicine (2015) provides advice regarding timing of dosing.

**Orthopaedic Surgery: Alternative agents may include
☐ Hip replacement: dabigatran, rivaroxaban, apixaban or fondaparinux
☐ Knee replacement: dabigatran, rivaroxaban, apixaban or fondaparinux
☐ Hip fracture: fondaparinux, or aspirin in combination with LMWH
Note: These agents may be contraindicated or require dose adjustment depending on the degree of renal impairment; calculate **Creatinine Clearance** and refer to guidance in references (e.g. CEC NOAC Guidelines) before prescribing. Please check with your local pharmacy department regarding availability of NOACs and Fondaparinux

6. Consider Duration of Therapy

Medical patients:
☐ Duration of therapy will vary with ongoing risk. Continue prophylaxis until the patient is no longer at increased risk of VTE, for example until acute medical condition is stable and mobility returns to baseline or until hospital discharge

Surgical patients:
☐ Total hip replacement/hip fracture surgery: continue for 28 to 35 days
☐ Total knee replacement: continue for up to 14 days
☐ Lower leg immobilisation due to injury: until mobility returns to baseline
☐ Major general surgery: continue for up to 1 week or until mobility returns to baseline
☐ Abdominal or pelvic surgery for cancer: continue for up to 30 days

KEY:

LMWH = low molecular weight heparin e.g. enoxaparin, dalteparin

Date completed: ___/___/___ Name: _____ Signature: _____ Designation: _____

7. Reassess

Patients should be reassessed when clinical condition changes or regularly (every 7 days as a minimum)
Complete this section if the patient has been reassessed and no changes to risk have been identified (including risk factors). Complete a new form if there are changes to risk

☐ Date: ___/___/___ Name: _____ Signature: _____ Designation: _____
☐ Date: ___/___/___ Name: _____ Signature: _____ Designation: _____
☐ Date: ___/___/___ Name: _____ Signature: _____ Designation: _____

SMR060250

Holes Punched as per AS2828.1 : 2012
BINDING MARGIN - NO WRITING

FIG. 9.22, cont'd

risk assessment and prophylaxis must be recorded in the patient healthcare record; see Fig 9.22 for an example.

Anticoagulant prophylaxis

The main groups of anticoagulants include:

- heparin (unfractionated)
- low-molecular-weight heparins (LMWHs) (e.g. enoxaparin, dalteparin)
- warfarin
- various other novel drugs that act on specific factors that are part of the blood coagulation cascade (e.g. fondaparinux, dabigatran etexilate, apixaban and rivaroxaban) (Bryant et al., 2018).

Some of these novel anticoagulants are believed to have safer outcomes compared with traditional anticoagulants; however, heparin and the LMWHs are the mainstay of treatment when a rapid anticoagulant effect is required (Tritschler, Kraaijpoel, Le Gal, & Wells, 2018). Their use is contraindicated in patients who have active bleeding or who are at high risk of this (e.g. haemophiliacs) (Bryant et al., 2018; Queensland Health, 2018). Aspirin, which is an antiplatelet medication, is routinely used in Australia for patients undergoing hip and knee replacement surgery, in conjunction with mechanical prophylaxis where there are no additional risk factors for VTE or postoperative bleeding (Mirkazemi, Bereznicki, & Peterson, 2019). Research supporting aspirin's effectiveness is not definitive but there is also no clear evidence that it is ineffective (ACSQHC/the Commission, 2018b).

Mechanical prophylaxis

There are two main types of mechanical devices used in the prevention of VTE: graduated compression stockings and intermittent pneumatic compression devices. There are two distinct, non-interchangeable types of graduated compression stockings, and only those designed for protection against VTE which produce a calf pressure of 14–15 mmHg should be used as a prophylactic measure. The other type is used to treat chronic venous insufficiency (NICE, 2018). The correct use of graduated compression stockings is outlined in Box 9.2.

Intermittent pneumatic compression devices also reduce the incidence of deep vein thrombosis (DVT) and are more effective in high-risk patients when used in combination with anticoagulants; they can also be used when anticoagulants are contraindicated and are related to better patient compliance (Caprini, Arcelus, & Tafur, 2019). Recommendations for intermittent pneumatic compression device use for the purpose of prophylaxis are similar to those for the use of graduated compression stockings – namely, they should fit correctly and be used throughout the period of immobility until the patient returns to full ambulation, and their

---

BOX 9.2
Recommendations for the Use of Graduated Compression Stockings for VTE Prophylaxis

- Graduated compression stockings should be worn continuously during the period of immobility and until the return of full ambulation.
- The stockings must be measured and fitted for the individual patient.
- Patient compliance is essential, as the stockings must not be rolled down.
- Ideally, there should be pressure of 14–18 mmHg at the ankle when the patient is supine, with graduated compression to the knee and above.
- The stockings should be manufactured to a high standard, be independently tested, have a compression profile and be washable.
- Do not offer stockings to people who have:
  - critical limb ischaemia
  - peripheral neuropathy
  - peripheral bypass grafting
  - local conditions (e.g. fragile skin, dermatitis or recent skin graft)
  - severe oedema
  - major limb deformity or unusual leg shape causing ill-fitting
  - allergy to material of manufacture (NICE, 2018).

---

use should be avoided in the presence of limb ischaemia (NICE, 2018).

Complications with the use of either type of mechanical device are rare but include:

- compartment syndrome
- skin ulceration
- pressure injury
- common peroneal nerve palsy (AORN, 2018; Caprini et al., 2019).

Signs and Symptoms of VTE

Hospital-acquired VTE has an incidence of 9.7 per 1000 admissions. Surgical patients account for double that of medical patients (Stubbs, Assareh, Curnow, Hitos, & Achat, 2018). Many patients with VTE are asymptomatic (Benrashid, Youngwirth, Turley, & Mureebe, 2017), but the symptoms that may develop are summarised in Table 9.9. A greater risk to the patient occurs if a thrombus breaks off and travels via the venous system to the right ventricle and from there to the pulmonary artery or one of its branches, resulting in a PE, which can be life threatening. Most PEs originate in a lower limb or pelvic veins (AORN, 2018).

TABLE 9.9
Signs and Symptoms of Venous Thromboembolism

Venous Thromboembolism	Pulmonary Embolism[a]
Unilateral leg pain/calf tenderness	Tachycardia
Swelling and warmth of the affected limb	Dyspnoea
Dilation of superficial leg veins	Chest pain
Skin colour changes (erythema)	Hypotension
Can be difficult to distinguish from cellulitis, haematoma, thrombophlebitis, congestive heart failure	Hypoxaemia Acute decrease in end-tidal carbon dioxide concentration Haemoptysis Cardiovascular collapse/sudden death Presents similarly to myocardial infarction, congestive heart failure and other diseases

[a]Intraoperative and postoperative complications.

PATIENT SCENARIOS

PATIENT SCENARIO 9.2: VENOUS THROMBOEMBOLISM

Mrs Patricia Peterson is a 42-year-old Indigenous woman admitted for an emergency laparoscopic cholecystectomy. Mrs Peterson's full history and a brief description of the healthcare setting are provided in the Introduction to this book for readers to review when answering the questions in this unfolding scenario.

Critical Thinking Questions

- Considering the surgery she is about to undergo, what factors can you identify from Mrs Peterson's physical and medical conditions that may put her at risk of developing a VTE or secondary PE?
- What prophylactic measures do you think might be implemented for Mrs Peterson to help prevent a VTE from occurring during her surgery, and why?
- What are the nursing considerations for each potential preventative measure?

PREVENTION AND MANAGEMENT OF INADVERTENT PERIOPERATIVE HYPOTHERMIA

Inadvertent perioperative hypothermia (IPH) is defined as the unintended drop of a patient's core body temperature to below 36°C during the perioperative period (Collins, Budds, Raines, & Hooper, 2019; Williams, 2018). IPH is distinguished from *planned hypothermia*, which is deliberately employed as a neuroprotective technique in some cardiothoracic and neurosurgical procedures (Klein & Arrowsmith, 2019; Nathanson, 2019). IPH is a commonly reported complication in surgical patients, particularly in the intraoperative and immediate postoperative periods, with a reported prevalence ranging from 50% to 90% (Collins et al., 2019; Watson, 2018).

Two significant factors contribute to the development of a hypothermic state: anaesthesia and environmental effects (Collins et al., 2019; Ralph, Gow, & Duff, 2019).

As discussed in Chapter 8, anaesthesia medications inhibit the thermoregulatory system, resulting in the loss of normal physiological responses to temperature variations (e.g. shivering and vasoconstriction). This causes the redistribution of body heat to the peripheries, where it is more easily lost to the environment (Andrzejowski & Riley, 2019; Ousey et al., 2015). Indeed, a drop of up to 1°C –1.5°C in the first hour after induction of anaesthesia is commonly reported (Ralph et al., 2019; Williams, 2018). Environmental factors contribute to the loss of body heat through mechanisms of radiation, conduction, convection and evaporation (Collins et al., 2019; Williams, 2018). Examples of these include inadequately clothed patients and a low ambient operating room temperature; the use of cool IV, irrigating and skin-prepping fluids (Andrzejowski & Riley, 2019; Watson, 2018); movement of cool air over the patient's exposed skin and organs from laminar flow; and prolonged exposure of major abdominal/thoracic organs. Collins and colleagues (2019) report that a long procedural time is the most commonly identified risk factor in the development of IPH. If left unmanaged, the anaesthetic and environmental factors contributing to hypothermia can have a profound effect on patient outcomes.

Adverse Effects of IPH

The consequences of IPH can include:

- thermal discomfort and patient dissatisfaction
- postoperative shivering and increased oxygen consumption
- reduced hepatic blood flow and slower drug metabolism
- coagulopathy and increased blood loss requiring transfusion
- morbid cardiac events including DVT/PE
- impaired wound healing and increased surgical site infection
- prolonged recovery and hospital stay with associated costs (Andrzejowski & Riley, 2019; Ralph et al., 2019; Watson, 2018).

Patients at Risk of Developing IPH

Although all patients have some risk of developing IPH, there are certain patients at an increased risk:

- burns patients, in particular those with full-thickness burns to more than 10% of body surface area (BSA) or partial-thickness burns (>25% BSA)
- patients requiring major surgery
- immunocompromised patients
- patients with low body mass index (Andrezjowski & Riley, 2019)
- patients with impaired metabolism, diabetes mellitus or circulatory failure (Collins et al., 2019).

In addition, ACORN (2020e) identifies that the following groups of patients may have a higher risk of IPH where any *two* of the following risks apply:

- ASA Grade II–V (the higher the grade, the greater the risk) – see Chapter 8 (Torossian et al., 2015)
- a preoperative temperature <36°C within the hour prior to their surgical procedure
- procedural time >30 minutes (NICE, 2020)
- combined regional and general anaesthesia
- where the patient is at risk of cardiac complications (Torossian et al., 2015)
- hypothyroidism
- where patients are at the extremes of age – particularly children under 2 years old (Andrzejowski & Riley, 2019; Collins et al., 2019; NICE, 2020).

Reflect again on our patient scenario with Mr Collins, who is 78 years old and requiring a knee replacement. He is at risk of developing inadvertent perioperative hypothermia during his procedure. His age, physical condition and likely high ASA will all place him in an increased risk category. Combined with the anaesthesia techniques and the length of his surgery, he will need careful assessment and management regarding his thermal care.

Nursing Interventions and Management Strategies

Maintaining a baseline of normothermia is the goal for every perioperative patient. This requires that all patients are assessed for their risk of developing IPH prior to surgery so that preventative measures may be planned and implemented appropriately (AORN, 2019; Ralph et al., 2019). Educating patients about the importance of ensuring their own warmth prior to surgery is also recommended (NICE, 2020). Throughout the patient's perioperative journey, core (or near-core) temperature must be recorded at regular intervals (NICE, 2020; Sessler, 2016). Other than in an emergency, this should be within 1 hour prior to transfer to the OR, and the temperature should be 36°C or above. If it is not, active warming should be initiated preoperatively, particularly if the patient is identified as at higher risk of IPH (NICE, 2020).

Commonly used active warming devices include single use inflatable blankets that circulate warm air over the patient's skin during surgery, such as the Bair Hugger (Fig. 9.23). These are very effective if used in accordance with manufacturer instructions but are not without risk. Indeed, the practice known as 'hosing' – where the device's hose is placed under the sterile drapes or patient blankets without the inflatable blanket attached – is associated with traumatic burn injuries including third-degree burns (3M Company, 2016; Min, Yoon, Yoon, Bakh, & Seo, 2018; Zenoni & Smith, 2018), with temperatures in excess of 48°C being generated in some reports (Anaesthesia Key, 2019).

Both passive and active warming should be considered during anaesthesia preparation, as some anaesthetic procedures can take a considerable period of time for complex patients. This increases the risk of IPH, particularly if the room is cool and the patient is exposed for regional anaesthesia techniques or invasive monitoring (Watson, 2018; Williams, 2018). All patients having procedures where total operative time (i.e. from initiation of anaesthesia until arrival in the postanaesthesia care unit [PACU]) is expected to be greater than 30 minutes should also be considered for active warming methods. In procedures of shorter duration, only higher-risk patients should be actively warmed. Box 9.3 identifies ways to maintain or restore

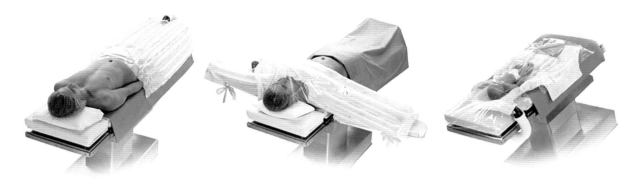

FIG. 9.23 Bair Hugger forced-air warming blankets. (Source: 3M Australia. https://www.3mnz.co.nz.)

BOX 9.3
ACORN Standards for the Management of Patient Normothermia

- Educate patients in the preoperative phase to keep themselves warm immediately prior to presenting for their surgery.
- Assess every patient for their risk of developing IPH. Identify those at high risk of IPH and plan and document care accordingly.
- Commence regular monitoring of the patient's temperature within 1 hour of surgery start, on arrival to the preoperative holding area, immediately prior to anaesthetic induction and then every 15 or 30 minutes thereafter, according to their care needs.
- Initiate warming interventions preoperatively and continue throughout the patient's surgery:
  - Ambient temperature of the OR should be maintained at 20°C–22°C
  - Minimise exposure of the patient during surgical preparation
  - Use cotton blankets and reflective sheets in conjunction with active warming

- Administer warm IV fluids and blood products in excess of 500 mL
- Use warmed irrigation fluids from a warming cabinet with thermostatic control to 38°C–40°C
- Use forced-air warming devices for all high-risk patients; where surgery is anticipated to be >30 minutes and commence with the maximum setting initially. Where forced-air warming is not possible, use under-body warming blankets. All active warming devices must be used in accordance with manufacturer's instructions.
- For those patients having surgery under sedation or regional anaesthesia techniques, assess patient comfort at regular intervals.
- Maintain postoperative warming strategies where indicated.
- Use a team approach to prevent and manage inadvertent perioperative hypothermia.

---

normothermia. Refer to Chapter 5 for further information on OR temperature control and Chapter 8 for additional information about maintaining normothermia during the induction of anaesthesia (ACORN, 2020e).

Intraoperatively, all patients should have their temperature routinely recorded every 30 minutes, and every 15 minutes for those patients with active warming technologies in use (NICE, 2020). Once the patient is admitted to PACU, their temperature should be recorded every 15 minutes until they are discharged to the ward (Collins et al., 2019; NICE, 2020; Watson, 2018). It is recommended that the same method (thermometer and route) is used to measure the patient's temperature throughout the patient's journey to enable accurate interpretation of any variations (Watson, 2018) or, where this is not possible, a device that measures core or near-core temperature is used (Sessler, 2016). If a patient is hypothermic postoperatively, active warming should be initiated and discharge from the PACU delayed until the patient's temperature is >36°C (Watson, 2018).

Despite the availability of cost-effective and easily implemented evidence-based guidelines aimed at preventing or treating IPH, they are frequently under-utilised, both intra- and postoperatively (Ralph et al., 2019). The reasons for poor compliance with guidelines seems to be related to a lack of awareness among nurses and anaesthetists about the availability of evidence-based guidelines relating to thermal care of patients (Boet et al., 2017; Munday, Delaforce, Forbes, & Deoghh, 2019). Further education targeted at the multidisciplinary teams is recommended as a means of reducing this gap between theory and practice (Munday et al., 2019).

SURGICAL COMPLICATIONS AND THE OLDER PATIENT

Demographic data show that life expectancy is steadily increasing, with a male born in Australia between 2014 and 2016 predicted to live to be just over 80 years of age and a female to almost 85 (ABS, 2018). People's expectations of healthcare combined with advances in anaesthesia and surgical techniques mean there is a subsequent increase in the number of older patients having surgery for common and age-related conditions such as atherosclerosis, cancer, arthritis and prostatism (Betelli, Cucinotta, & Neuner, 2018; Partridge, Sbai, & Dhesi, 2018). Increasingly, complex surgery is performed on patients over the age of 80 with higher levels of success (Betelli et al., 2018). Not only do older patients present for surgery with their primary complaint, but also they can bring with them one or more coexisting chronic conditions or comorbidities owing to physiological decline related to age (Partridge et. al., 2018; Tommasino & Corcione, 2018). The human body can to some extent compensate for age-related changes, but the physiological reserve of the older person is more limited and can be exceeded when subjected to stressors such as surgery (Betelli et al., 2018). The expected age-related physiological changes in the older person and the associated perioperative implications are summarised in Table 9.10, and Feature box 9.2 explores perioperative implications of surgery in older patients with fractured hips (see Chapter 8 for further details on age-related aspects of anaesthesia).

TOURNIQUETS

Tourniquets are often used during surgery on limbs and digits to constrict their blood flow, resulting in a bloodless field at the distal surgical site. These devices may be mechanical (e.g. a blood pressure cuff), electronic or pneumatic (utilising a heavier, more secure type of blood pressure cuff for use on the arms or legs) (Phillips, 2017). Pneumatic tourniquets consist of an inflatable cuff connected via double or single tubing to a pressure regulator, compressed gas supply and display unit (Fig. 9.24). Electronic units contain digital pressure settings, alarms and adjustable timing settings. Simpler devices, such as purpose-made rubber tubing or tourniquet bands, are used on digits (AORN, 2020a; McEwin, 2017). Sometimes, improvised devices such as rubber gloves, rubber bands or drainage tubes are used on digits; however, resultant digit ischaemia and necrosis have been reported when such items have inadvertently been left in place and concealed under dressings or casts. This has caused considerable pain and distress for the patient, and in some instances digit amputation (Hidalgo Diaz et al., 2018). Development of purpose-made devices such as the 'ForgetMeNot' digit tourniquet have gained popularity as a result. Users report more-consistent achievement of digit exsanguination and control over tourniquet pressure during procedures. These devices are reusable and are accounted for at the end of the procedure, minimising the risk of being left on the patient (Hidalgo Diaz et al., 2018).

Recommendations for the safe use of tourniquets include:
- staff training, education and competency assessment
- checking and maintenance of all equipment immediately prior to use and at regularly scheduled intervals
- patient identification, verification and operative limb marking
- comprehensive patient assessment and identification of contraindications
- correct application of the cuff
- use of the correct amount of pressure
- observance of minimum required inflation time and monitoring of maximum inflation time
- accurate patient observation, monitoring and documentation of use
- directions for cleaning and decontamination of cuffs (ACORN, 2020f; Croke, 2020; Jensen, Hicks, & Labovitz, 2019).

As there are several different (and complex) types of tourniquets, the specific manufacturer's recommendations should guide use, in conjunction with departmental policy and procedures. The use of tourniquets is associated with significant risk, as tourniquets compress underlying soft tissue, as well as depriving the area of blood supply. Consequently, they have been linked to soft-tissue injuries involving skin, muscle,

TABLE 9.10
Expected Age-related Physiological Changes in the Older Patient

Physiological Changes	Perioperative Implications
CARDIOVASCULAR SYSTEM	
<ul><li>↓ Myocytes = relative</li><li>↑ Fibroblasts = ↑ collagen and collagen crosslinking between adjacent fibres and changes in elastin</li><li>Fibrotic areas throughout the myocardium = ↓ ventricular compliance</li><li>↑ Stiffening of peripheral vasculature</li><li>↑ Atherosclerosis</li><li>↓ Cardiac output</li><li>↓ Baroreceptor sensitivity</li><li>Conducting system fibrosis</li></ul>	<ul><li>Labile blood pressure</li><li>Susceptibility to hypotension</li><li>Susceptibility to fluid overload</li><li>↑ Chance of cardiac failure</li><li>↓ Peripheral circulation<ul><li>↑ risk of pressure areas and VTE</li></ul></li><li>↓ Ability to adapt to blood pressure changes</li><li>↑ Susceptibility to arrhythmias</li></ul>
PULMONARY SYSTEM	
<ul><li>↓ Muscle mass and lung elasticity</li><li>↓ Cough reflex and swallowing function</li><li>↓ Response to hypoxia and hypercarbia</li><li>↓ Respiratory muscle strength and functional alveolar surface area</li></ul>	<ul><li>↓ Lung capacity</li><li>↑ Susceptibility to residual anaesthetic gases</li><li>↑ Aspiration risk</li><li>Susceptibility to hypoxia and hypercarbia</li><li>Ventilation/perfusion mismatch and ↑ risk of hypoxaemia and atelectasis</li></ul>
NERVOUS SYSTEM	
<ul><li>↓ Neurotransmitters</li><li>Cognitive decline/impairment (e.g. dementia/Alzheimer's)</li></ul>	<ul><li>↑ Risk of postoperative delirium and cognitive dysfunction</li><li>Possible impaired ability to give consent</li><li>Advance Care Directives perioperative implementation</li></ul>
HEPATIC/RENAL SYSTEM	
<ul><li>↓ Renal function</li><li>↓ Renal mass</li><li>↓ Hepatic blood flow</li></ul>	<ul><li>↓ Speed of drug excretion from kidneys<ul><li>↑ sensitivity to drugs</li></ul></li><li>Altered drug metabolism</li></ul>
MUSCULOSKELETAL SYSTEM	
<ul><li>↓ Bone calcium<ul><li>osteoporosis, spinal curvatures</li></ul></li><li>↓ Tissue elasticity</li><li>↓ Muscle mass</li><li>Arthritic joint changes</li></ul>	<ul><li>Difficulties with positioning for surgery and spinal anaesthesia</li><li>↓ Mobility and flexibility of tendons and ligaments affecting range of motion of joints</li><li>↑ Risk of pressure areas</li><li>↑ Risk of hypothermia</li><li>Pain, joint deformities that can cause positioning challenges</li></ul>
INTEGUMENTARY SYSTEM	
<ul><li>↑ Fragility of epidermis</li></ul>	<ul><li>↑ Risk of skin tears</li></ul>
SENSORY SYSTEM	
<ul><li>↓ Acuity of visual and auditory senses<ul><li>cataract development</li><li>hearing loss</li></ul></li></ul>	<ul><li>↑ Communication difficulties</li></ul>

(Sources: Ghironzi, G., Canet Capeta, J., Fernandez Cortes, A., & Betelli, G. (2018). Aging and age-related functional changes. In G. Betelli (Ed.), *Perioperative care of the elderly: clinical and organisational aspects* (pp. 3–8). Cambridge: Cambridge University Press; Howlett, S. E. (2017). Effects of ageing on the cardiovascular system. In *Brocklehurst's textbook of geriatric medicine and gerontology* (8th ed., pp. 96–100). Philadelphia: Elsevier; Lin, H. S., McBride, R. L., & Hubbard, R. E. (2018). Frailty and anaesthesia – risks during and post surgery. *Local and Regional Anaesthesia, 11*, 61–73. https://dx.doi.org/10.2147/LRA.S142996.)

FEATURE BOX 9.2
Perioperative Implications of Surgery in Elderly Patients With Fractured Hips

Hip fractures are a common and serious injury sustained by older people. There are considerable costs associated with the treatment and rehabilitation of these patients. For the individual, a hip fracture impacts on mobility, function, living arrangements and even survival.

The Australian and New Zealand Hip Fracture Registry (ANZHFA) was established in 2015 to collect data to improve hip fracture care, improving outcomes for patients. It provides a means to track performance and drive change.

Data from both the ANZHFA and the ACSQHC show that women make up approximately 70% of hip fracture patients, with people over 90 making up 25%. Māori and Pacific Islander people make up only 3.8% of data reported from New Zealand, while Indigenous populations make up less than 1% of Australian data. In 2016, the ACSQHC developed the Hip Fracture Clinical Care Standard. It contains seven quality statements describing the care a patient should be offered.

The Hip Fracture Clinical Care Standard notes that timing of surgery, cognitive assessment and pain management are particularly relevant to perioperative services.

POSTOPERATIVE DELIRIUM/COGNITIVE IMPAIRMENT

Interestingly, data from ACSQHC show that 38% of patients had known cognitive impairment or known dementia, but only 35% of patients in Australia and 50% in New Zealand had a documented cognitive assessment prior to surgery. There is some suggestion in the literature that prolonged surgical wait times in this cohort are associated with an increase in the risk of developing postoperative delirium (Ravi et. al., 2019). ACSQHC states that surgery should occur within 48 hours of hospital presentation if there is no clinical contraindication and it is the patient's preference. In 2018, 82% and 76% of patients in Australia and New Zealand respectively were operated on within this timeframe, the average being 34–37 hours. Surgical fixation of most fractured hips is the expectation because it optimises function and/or alleviates pain (ANZHFR, 2019).

PAIN

Pain is to be assessed on admission and regularly throughout the hospital stay using multimodal analgesia as appropriate. ACSQHC noted that 72% of hospitals had a pathway for the management of pain in these patients, which is a significant improvement from the 2017 figure of 56%. 2018 also saw an increase in the use of nerve blocks to manage pain.

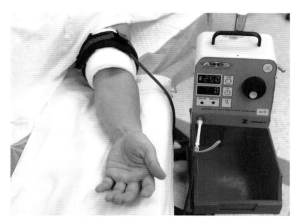

FIG. 9.24 Pneumatic tourniquet.

nerves and vasculature; additionally, their use can have systemic sequelae (Jensen et al., 2019). Complications include:
- allergic reactions, such as latex allergy
- pressure injuries, skin bruising, abrasion, blistering and chemical burns (from skin preparation solutions pooling or soaking beneath the tourniquet)
- nerve injury
- fatal or near-fatal PE and DVT after deflation
- toxic reactions as with reperfusion syndrome
- post-tourniquet syndrome (sustained PO swelling, stiffness and painful limb)
- compartment syndrome
- impaired wound healing
- subcutaneous fat necrosis
- digital necrosis
- rhabdomyolysis (ACORN, 2020f; Jensen et al., 2019; Spruce, 2017b).

Tourniquet Use

When selecting a cuff, the length and width should be individualised for each patient (ACORN, 2020f; Phillips, 2017). This will depend on the shape and diameter of the extremity and the particular procedure the patient is undergoing (Spruce, 2017b). The widest cuff possible within any given length should be selected because wider cuffs occlude blood flow at lower pressures. Contoured cuffs are recommended for obese patients, in whom limbs tend to be conical in shape. These prevent the risk of neurovascular damage, cuff slippage and subsequent underlying soft-tissue damage. The length of the cuff also needs to be considered; it should overlap itself by at least 7.5 cm but no more than 15 cm, as excessively long cuffs increase pressure on the underlying tissue and wrinkle the underlying skin. Additionally, the need for a latex-free cuff and selection of a single-use versus reusable cuff needs to be determined (ACORN, 2020f). Cuffs should be located at the point of maximum circumference of the extremity – that is, the upper arm or the proximal third of the thigh (Phillips, 2017).

Prior to tourniquet inflation, the operative limb requires exsanguination to prevent intravascular thrombosis and formation of embolus. Exsanguination of the limb may be achieved by either elevating the limb for 3–5 minutes or wrapping an Esmarch's (rubber) bandage from the distal part of the limb to the proximally located cuff. Recent evidence supports the use of limb elevation as the preferred exsanguination method for patients undergoing surgery without general anaesthesia use (Croke, 2020). Patients subsequently reported decreased levels of limb pain post procedure. Use of the hand-over-hand method for limb exsanguination should never be considered as an option.

To avoid skin damage, soft, wrinkle-free padding is wrapped around the limb before applying the tourniquet cuff (see Fig. 9.24). To prevent skin preparation solution from collecting under the cuff and causing skin maceration or burns, an impervious U-shaped drape is placed around the cuff. The requisite cuff (or inflation) pressure varies, depending on the patient's limb occlusion pressure (LOP) and other factors including limb circumference (Table 9.11). Inflation pressure should always be confirmed with the medical officers prior to inflation, and set at the lowest possible setting to minimise risk of postoperative complications such as reduced pain and limb swelling (AORN, 2020b; Croke, 2020). Cuff inflation should be rapid to allow arteries and veins to occlude simultaneously (Phillips, 2017).

The use of pneumatic tourniquets is contraindicated in patients with the following:

- diabetes mellitus
- McArdle disease (glycogen storage disease)
- hypertension, particularly in those taking antihypertensives
- coronary artery disease
- raised intracranial pressure
- neuropathy
- sickle cell disease
- rheumatoid arthritis
- open injuries of the limbs
- infection
- extremity pain
- chronic lymphoedema
- tumour in the operative limb
- arterial and venous disease, including a history of VTE
- compartment syndrome
- arteriovenous access fistula or vascular access port (Bowen, 2019; Jensen et al., 2019; Phillips 2017; Spruce, 2017b).

Complications from tourniquet use arise from excessive cuff pressures and/or length of inflation time. However, as there is a paucity of evidence to determine safe duration, inflation pressure or reperfusion periods, time should be kept to a minimum (Spruce, 2017b). ACORN guidelines (2020f) recommend 60 minutes of inflation time for upper limbs and 60–90 minutes for lower limbs. Once the tourniquet inflation time is reached, the surgeon and anaesthetist must be notified and the tourniquet should be deflated with a 10–15-minute release of pressure before re-inflation (ACORN, 2020f).

Wang and colleagues (2017) describe short-duration tourniquet usage during total knee arthroplasty, where the tourniquet is inflated just prior to cement application and released immediately after cement hardening. The short-duration tourniquet use resulted in more blood loss for patients in the intraoperative phase of surgery, but decreased evidence of postoperative and hidden blood loss into the tissues. Patients also reported less limb swelling, less pain and an early return to rehabilitation in the initial postoperative period (Wang et al., 2017).

Perioperative nurses must possess sound knowledge of the indications and contraindications for tourniquet use. They must demonstrate an ability to check, maintain and operate all associated equipment and supplies. Patient safety is potentiated when accurate and comprehensive assessment is performed and planning and care delivery

TABLE 9.11
Tourniquet Inflation Pressures (Adults)

Limb Occlusion Pressure (LOP)	Pneumatic Cuff Pressure
Upper limb	Add 50–75 mmHg above systolic arterial blood pressure. Most common pressure is 200–250 mmHg
Lower limb	Add 100–150 mmHg above systolic arterial blood pressure Most common pressure is 300–350 mmHg

For paediatric patients, adding 50–100 mmHg above systolic blood pressure is recommended (Tredwell, Wilmink, Inkpen, & McEwen 2001)

are coordinated and communicated among the team (Jensen et al., 2019).

Prior to use the intraoperative nursing team should undertake the following checks:
- Ensure the tourniquet battery is fully charged.
- Inspect cuffs, tubing and connectors for damage or flaws.
- Test the tourniquet unit for accuracy and functionality, and calibrate as necessary (AORN, 2020b).

During use the circulating nurse should assess the the pneumatic tourniquet regularly to:
- monitor the inflation pressure to detect fluctuations
- monitor and record the duration of inflation and inform the surgical team when the cuff has been inflated for 1 hour, and every 15 minutes thereafter (Phillips, 2017)
- document the use of a tourniquet, including cuff location, name of the staff member who applied and removed it, devices used for skin protection, cuff pressure, and times of inflation and deflation
- continuously monitor the patient for signs of normothermia, respiratory acidosis (paediatric patients) and pain tolerance (during local and regional anaesthetic procedures) (AORN, 2020b; Croke, 2020)
- assess skin integrity under the cuff before and after use (ACORN, 2018e).

Table 9.12 summarises pre-, intra- and postoperative nursing interventions for the use of tourniquets.

TABLE 9.12
Pre-, Intra- and Postoperative Nursing Interventions for the Use of Tourniquets

Nursing Intervention	Rationale
Check that equipment and a range of sizes are available	Each patient presents with unique needs and risk factors. Selection of a suitable tourniquet device and cuff will prevent harm to the patient and facilitate use of lowest inflation pressure to achieve a bloodless operative field
Assess the need for padding beneath the tourniquet	Significant pressure injury and tissue damage can occur if suitable padding is not applied to the patient's skin
Ascertain the need and method for exsanguination, e.g. gravity or Esmarch bandage	Exsanguination enhances a bloodless field, minimises risk of intravascular thrombus and embolus formation and may minimise pain associated with tourniquet use
Check required pressure settings	Minimal inflation pressures are recommended to reduce the risk of complications due to high inflation pressures
Check tourniquet alarm settings (60 and 90 minutes)	Nerve injury, venous engorgement, hyperaemia or ischaemia may result after prolonged tourniquet inflation time
Assess skin integrity under the cuff before use	To establish a baseline of the patient skin and tissue integrity for comparison after tourniquet use
Monitor the inflation pressure intraoperatively to detect fluctuations	To ensure continuous and controlled pressure
Monitor and record the duration of inflation and inform the surgical team when the cuff has been inflated for 1 hour, and every 15 minutes thereafter (Phillips, 2017)	To prevent injury associated with prolonged tourniquet inflation
Document the use of a tourniquet, including cuff location, name of the staff member who applied and removed it, devices used for skin protection, cuff pressure, and times of inflation and deflation	To ensure accurate documentation in the medical record and adherence to legal requirements
Continuously monitor the patient's vital signs throughout the procedure	Tourniquet use can affect the patient's blood pressure, respiration, body temperature and pain tolerance. Any changes should be reported and recorded immediately
Assess skin integrity under the cuff after use	To detect and report any inadvertent injury

(Sources: Australian College of Perioperative Nurses. (2020f). *ACORN standards for perioperative nursing in Australia* (16th ed., Vol. 1). Clinical standards – pneumatic tourniquet. Adelaide: Author; Croke, L. (2020). Guideline for pneumatic tourniquet safety. *AORN Journal, 111*(4), 8–10; Phillips, N. (2017). *Berry and Kohn's operating room technique* (13th ed.). St Louis, MO: Elsevier.)

PATIENT SCENARIOS

PATIENT SCENARIO 9.3: TOURNIQUET USE

Consider our patient Mr Collins, who is to undergo TKR surgery, which may require tourniquet use. The surgeon will need to determine whether Mr Collins' history of hypertension, use of antihypertensive medication, extent of coronary artery disease and extremity pain serve as contraindications for tourniquet use.

RN Rob Cohen is the circulating nurse caring for Mr Collins during his TKR. The surgeon, Dr Slattery, has requested a tourniquet cuff be placed on Mr Collins' right thigh.

> **Critical Thinking Questions**
>
> - Outline the risks associated with each of the following and the steps RN Cohen should take to minimise injury to Mr Collins. Provide rationales for your answers.
>   - Tourniquet cuff selection and placement
>   - Cuff inflation pressure and duration
>   - Patient assessment during the intraoperative period.

THE MANAGEMENT OF ACCOUNTABLE ITEMS USED DURING SURGERY

To ensure that all items used during a surgical procedure are removed from the patient (unless intentionally retained) a systematic and standardised approach is required. This is necessary to reduce the risk of injury associated with inadvertent retention of a surgical item (RSI) (ACORN 2020g). As discussed in Chapter 3, the management of accountable items is the primary responsibility of the instrument and circulating nurses, one of whom must be an RN, and it is achieved by undertaking a **surgical count** (the count). **Accountable items** are instruments, sharps, absorbent items such as sponges and gauze swabs, and small miscellaneous items and device fragments that by their nature and usage may be retained. Due to continuous technological advances, there is no definitive list of accountable items, and perioperative nurses must remain alert, as practice and surgical items continue to evolve. Broadly speaking, however, those items that must be counted include, but are not limited to:

- instruments recorded on the tray list
- absorbent items, including sponges, swabs, patties, cherries, peanuts, eye swabs (strolls), gauze strips, cotton wool balls and skin preparation swabs
- sharps, including needles, detachable blades, disposable scalpels and diathermy tips
- vascular items, comprising vessel loops ('ligaloops'), 'snuggers', cardiac snares, tapes, ligature reels, 'ligaboots', clip cartridges and disposable bulldog clips
- disposable retraction instruments such as fishhooks and visceral retractors
- items that are identified in the local count policy
- additional items opened during the procedure and deemed at risk of being inadvertently retained.

Other items can be counted at the discretion of the RN in charge and/or the instrument nurse (ACORN 2020g). Though an uncommon occurrence, the persistence of RSIs and errors in the count suggests counting is not always sufficient to prevent RSIs (Whitehorn, 2019). Other ways to prevent these adverse events are evolving as attempts to identify their causes are explored. Research in the early 2000s highlighted that patient-specific characteristics (obesity) and case-specific characteristics (emergencies, unanticipated change in procedure) increased the risk; however, more recent research indicates that OR culture, team attentiveness and communication may be more significant (Steelman, Shaw, Shine, & Hardy-Fairbanks, 2019b; Steelman, Thenuwara, Shaw, & Shine, 2019c).

Other ways to prevent RSIs by taking a systems approach to error reduction are continuing to be developed and trialled. These include the use of information technologies such as barcoding and radiofrequency identification systems in surgical sponges, UV fluorescent needles and other items (Steelman, Schaapveld, Storm, Perkhounkova, & Shane, 2019a; Whitehorn, 2019), and the implementation of surgical team behavioural changes (Steelman et al., 2019b & c). Notwithstanding the use of evolving technologies, they remain adjuncts to completing the surgical count. No technology can replace the manual count process, which remains paramount but should be used in conjunction with traditional counting methods to improve the success of both processes (ACORN 2020g; Agrawal, 2012; Whitehorn, 2019).

The Count

Perioperative nursing standards guide the conduct of the count. These standards identify roles and responsibilities, spell out a detailed process for conducting the count and provide rationales. They also describe actions to take in emergency surgery or in the event of an incorrect surgical count being recorded (ACORN

2020g). In Australia, the ACORN standard *Accountable items* has been established in common law as the standard for the practice of counting (Cockburn, Davis, & Osborne 2019; Staunton & Chiarella, 2020).

The standards should be used in conjunction with respective state/territory or national health department policies or guidelines (if evident) (ACORN 2020g). It is acknowledged that the risk of items being retained unintentionally can vary depending on the nature of the surgical procedure (among other things). Consequently, those procedures that require the management of accountable items should be defined and items that must be counted should be determined by each hospital or facility's multidisciplinary perioperative management committee, who must also ensure that their surgical teams comply with any locally developed policy (ACORN, 2020g; Agrawal, 2012).

General principles and roles and responsibilities of staff are as follows:

- The circulating and instrument nurses are responsible for ensuring that the count is accurate and documented in the patient's intraoperative nursing record and the count sheet. They also work collaboratively with other members of the surgical team to ensure that all surgical items are retrieved on completion of surgery.
- The nurses use instrument tray lists to establish a reference point for ascertaining that all instrumentation is accounted for at the end of the procedure.
- Individual instruments opened throughout the procedure are included in the list of instruments to be checked.
- The surgeon must allow sufficient time for the instrument and circulating nurses to conduct the count before, during and on completion of the surgical procedure.
- The surgeon must carry out a manual and visual search of the operative field to ensure that all instruments and equipment are removed prior to completion of the surgical procedure.
- If the anaesthetic team opens an accountable item during the surgical procedure, it is the responsibility of that team member to inform the instrument nurse and/or the circulating nurse, who must sight the item and ensure that it is documented on the count sheet.

The procedure for completing the count is highlighted in Box 9.4. Research box 9.2 describes perioperative nurses' perceptions of the barriers and enablers to undertaking the count.

Loan Instruments

Numerous surgical procedures require the use of loan instrumentation from medical companies or other hospitals. The number of trays in a loan set utilised for some procedures (e.g. revision arthroplasty) can easily number more than 10. Hence, accounting for all the contents of these trays can add additional time, complexity and stress to the counting process. Measures that could be implemented to mitigate the risk of an RSI when using loan sets may include ensuring that nurses are experienced in the surgical procedure or are supervised by someone who is, enlisting the assistance of medical representatives to provide clinical support throughout the procedure, and the provision of education regarding the surgical technique and loan instrumentation prior to the procedure. Local policies may require medical companies to provide illustrated tray lists to assist not only in the completion of the count but also with the processing of trays through sterilising departments (ACORN, 2020h).

Incorrect Count

An incorrect count occurs when the items recorded on the count sheet do not match the actual number of items evidenced in the closing count(s). If there is a discrepancy, the instrument nurse must notify the surgeon/proceduralist immediately and ask for a thorough search of the surgical site (Steelman et al., 2019b). If this is unsuccessful, an immediate search of the surgical environment, including the surgical drapes and linen, the floor and rubbish containers should be completed, and the anaesthetist and the perioperative nurse leader in charge of the department notified. If the missing item is one that is X-ray detectable, an X-ray should be taken prior to the patient leaving the operating room (unless contraindicated by the patient's condition) and the outcome documented. If a non-X-ray-detectable item is missing, an appropriate thorough visual and manual search is required. A missing microneedle that is not X-ray detectable (as determined by the health service organisation in conjunction with the radiology department) may require the use of a microscope and/or magnet to locate (ACORN, 2020h; CEC, 2013). If the missing item remains unaccounted for, the intraoperative nursing record must reflect this. Additionally, a record of the incident, including actions taken to address it, is necessary, in line with local policy (ACORN, 2020h). There are many more cases where an 'incorrect' count is in fact a miscount and/or an error of documentation and these are associated with complacency and/or failure to adhere to recommended guidelines (Steelman et al., 2019b).

Emergency Situations

In an emergency and when the patient's condition is critical, normal counting procedures may be waived and

BOX 9.4
Undertaking the Surgical Count

- The count is performed whenever accountable items are used during a surgical procedure.
- It is carried out by two nurses, one of whom must be an RN, with both nurses counting aloud together.
- A minimum of two counts of all accountable items should be completed. Where a body cavity is entered, an additional count is undertaken when the body cavity is closed.
- The initial count is performed immediately prior to the commencement of the surgical procedure. After the completion of the first count, all accountable items must remain in the operating room until the completion of the surgery and the final count.
- Additional counts can be undertaken at any time during the surgical procedure, at the discretion of the instrument nurse and/or if local policy dictates this.
- The third or final count is performed and documented on commencement of the closure of the skin or an equivalent closure.
- The surgeon is informed of the outcome of each count.
- A progressive 'counting away' technique is used.
- If it is necessary to relieve one or both nurses (e.g. as part of a fatigue management plan for lengthy surgical procedures), the name(s) of the relieving nurse(s) and relieving times must be documented on patient's intraoperative nursing record.

- The tray list is used to check that all instruments in the tray are accounted for prior to the commencement of the surgical procedure. This list is signed by the instrument nurse prior to the return of the tray for cleaning and sterilisation.
- The surgeon is notified immediately of any discrepancy in the count and appropriate interventions are undertaken to rectify this situation (see the section on 'Incorrect count').
- All accountable items remain in their packing until counted. All items are then separated and counted. When counting swabs and sponges, each is opened so that both nurses can see the X-ray detectable marker.
- Additional items added during the surgical procedure are counted and recorded.
- Those nurses responsible for the count must sign the count sheet.
- If the count is interrupted, counting of that item is recommenced.
- On completion of the surgical procedure, the surgeon also documents the outcome of the count in accordance with local policy.
- The completed original copy count sheet is included in the patient's medical record.
- All accountable items are removed from the operating room only at the end of the surgical procedure and completion of the final count, and prior to the commencement of the next surgical procedure.

(Sources: Australian College of Perioperative Nurses. (2020g). *ACORN standards for perioperative nursing in Australia* (16th ed., Vol. 1). Clinical standards – accountable items used during surgery and procedures. Adelaide: Author; Clinical Excellence Commission. (2013). *Management of instruments, accountable items and other items used for surgery or procedures policy directive*. PD2012_034. https://www1.health.nsw.gov.au/pds/ActivePDSDocuments/PD2013_054.pdf.)

RESEARCH BOX 9.2
The Patient, Case, Individual and Environmental Factors That Impact on the Surgical Count Process: an Integrative Review

The objective of this research was to identify empirical data regarding nurses' knowledge and practices in relation to the surgical count. Literature was reviewed from 2013 to 2018, yielding 215 studies, which were systematically excluded and critically appraised using validated tools, resulting in 10 articles included in the final sample.

The studies identified several groups of factors that impact on the surgical count process, causing deviation from procedure or an inability to follow correct processes:

- **patient-related factors** – high BMI or deep cavities
- **case-related factors** – emergency or unplanned surgery, increased length of surgery, multiple teams and staff performing multiple roles

- **individual factors** – adherence to policy, type of leadership in the OR, impact of hierarchy, respectful communication, disparate views on correct processes and untidy instrument trolleys
- **environmental factors** – location of procedure in a rural or teaching facility, loud music or talking, fast pace and time constraints.

The literature review notes that the evidence supports the fact that human error in relation to the surgical count is prevalent, and although considered onerous, undertaking the surgical count accurately and correctly is pivotal to patient safety and preventing retained surgical items.

(Source: Warwick, V., Gillespie, B. M., McMurray, A., & Clark-Burg, K. (2019). The patient, case, individual and environmental factors that impact on the surgical count process: an integrative review. *Journal of Perioperative Nursing, 32*(3), 9–19.)

an X-ray performed at the end of the surgical intervention (or when the patient's condition is sufficiently stable) (ACORN, 2020h). This is a long-standing practice, which continues in many operating rooms and remains a recommended standard. This is notwithstanding the limitation of X-rays and/or their interpretation and the resultant failure to detect many surgical items used in practice currently (Steelman et al., 2019a). The surgeon must be informed when a count is not completed and participate in actions to redress the consequences (ACORN, 2020h). Additionally, the perioperative nurse must document when a count is not completed.

PATIENT SCENARIOS

SCENARIO 9.4: LOAN INSTRUMENT MANAGEMENT

Mr Collins' surgeon has requested a loan set of instruments that the nursing team has not used before. This means that the instrument nurse EN Noakes will have multiple extra trays of loan instruments on her set-up for TKR surgery.

> **Critical Thinking Question**
>
> - List the steps the nursing team will undertake to manage this situation to ensure that Mr Collins does not have a retained surgical item (RSI).

SCENARIO 9.5: THE SURGICAL COUNT

Mrs Janine Clark is a 35-year-old pregnant woman admitted for an elective lower segment caesarean section (LSCS). Mrs Clark's full history and a brief description of the healthcare setting is provided in the Introduction to this book for readers to review when answering the questions in this unfolding scenario.

RN Sandy Pereira is the instrument nurse when Mrs Clark is scheduled for her caesarean section.

> **Critical Thinking Questions**
>
> - Considering the anatomy involved, how many counts will RN Pereira be performing during this procedure? When will she be completing them and why?
> - The final count reveals that a sponge is missing; outline the steps RN Pereira would take and provide rationales for her actions.

COLLECTION OF SPECIMENS

The perioperative nurse must adhere to best practice and strive to prevent errors when managing specimens to ensure patient safety and best outcomes, especially considering that the perioperative environment can be a complex workplace with distractions continuously arising from patient needs (Martin, Metcalfe, & Whichello, 2015; Van Wicklin, 2015; Yu, Lee, & Mills, 2019).

The removal of a **tissue specimen** frequently necessitates an invasive process and it can be potentially devastating if mishandling/loss of the specimen occurs. Cases of specimen mishandling have resulted in misdiagnoses and, in some instances, patients have been required to undergo additional surgery to remove more tissue for pathology. In other cases, patients have had necessary treatment withheld or received inappropriate or aggressive forms of treatment as a consequence (ACORN, 2020i; Martin et al., 2015). Mismanagement of specimens has cost implications for healthcare facilities, legal ramifications for hospitals and surgical team members, and results in distress for all involved. So, it is imperative to establish clear and unambiguous processes for the identification, collection and transportation of specimens. To this end, specimen handling is a component of the WHO SSC, whereby all team members are required to identify and verify patient and specimen information prior to the patient leaving the OR (ACORN, 2020i; WHO, 2009). Table 9.13 outlines the different types of specimens collected in the OR.

Specimen management errors occur when incorrect patient identification or inadequate patient verification procedures are performed, interprofessional communication is unclear or absent, and specimen collection and recording procedures are not followed (Zervakis Brent, 2016). Critical periods during intraoperative care delivery have been identified where excessive workload or distraction and disruption strongly correlate with risk of adverse events; hence specimen management should be performed with effective coordination, communication and accountability, and without interruption (Wright, 2016; Yu et. al., 2019).

Recommended practices provide guidance for the handling, containment, identification, labelling and transporting of specimens within the perioperative environment and beyond, and these are outlined in Table 9.14 for our patient Mrs Peterson in Scenario 9.2 undergoing a laparoscopic cholecystectomy and removal

TABLE 9.13
Specimens Collected in the OR

Microbiology	Typically, specimens are collected via a sterile culture tube and swab dispensed to the sterile field. Suspected anaerobic microorganisms are aspirated into a sterile disposable syringe, all air is expelled and the syringe is promptly capped. Cultures should be refrigerated or sent to the laboratory immediately.
Cytology	Solid tissue is excised or fluid is removed via aspiration to allow study of the cells obtained. Fine-needle aspiration biopsies can also be taken to obtain cells from solid lesions in the breast, thyroid, neck, lymph nodes or soft tissues.
Histology	Dissected or aspirated tissue is examined to determine a diagnosis. Tissue may be excised (a mass or entire structure is removed from the body) or sampled via incisional biopsy (a portion of a mass is removed). Tissue is frequently prepared for examination by being placed in a preservative, e.g. 10% buffered formalin solution.
Frozen section	Used to determine whether the specimen tissue and the surrounding lymph nodes collected are malignant. The removed tissue is placed in a sterile specimen container without any added preservative, such as formalin or normal saline solution. The tissue is sent directly to the pathology department where it is quick frozen, sliced, stained and examined under a microscope. When the tissue examination is complete, the pathologist will report the results directly to the surgeon in the operating room.
Foreign bodies	A removed foreign body should be carefully handled according to policy, and a record kept for legal purposes. A foreign body may be taken by the police as evidence or requested by the patient. A clear chain of custody should be recorded, documenting all persons handling the specimen.
Breast tissue	Breast tissue must be handled carefully to preserve genetic and molecular markers used to determine patient prognosis and treatment options. Breast cancer specimens should be kept moist and not come into contact with any dry or absorbent materials. Excision to fixation time for these specimens should not exceed 1 hour and these times should be accurately recorded in the perioperative patient record.
Forensic evidence	Forensic evidence, such as bullets or knife blades removed from the patient, should not come into contact with metal forceps, instruments and receptacles as this may alter ballistic evidence. Chain of custody documentation should always accompany the specimen to protect the evidence.
Amputated limbs	Amputated extremities are double plastic bagged before sending to the laboratory or morgue. A patient may wish the amputated extremity to be preserved or returned for burial with their body after death; this is common in Indigenous and Māori populations. Indeed, the New Zealand Code of Health and Disability Services Consumers' Rights has a statement that every consumer has the right to make a decision about the return of any body part removed during their healthcare.

(Sources: Kinlaw, T. S. & Whiteside, D. (2019). Surgical specimen management in the preanalytic phase: perioperative nursing implications. *AORN Journal, 110*(3), 238–247; Murphy, E. (2019). Patient safety and risk management. In J. C. Rothrock & D. L. McEwen (Eds.), *Alexander's care of the patient in surgery* (16th ed., pp. 15–36). St Louis, MO: Elsevier; New Zealand Health and Disability Commissioner (2020) . The Code of Health and Disability Services Consumers' Rights (the Code) Regulations 1996. Retrieved from <https://www.hdc.org.nz/your-rights/about-the-code/code-of-health-anddisability-services-consumers-rights/>; Phillips, N. (2017). *Berry and Kohn's operating room technique* (13th ed.). St Louis, MO: Elsevier.)

of her gallbladder. While such guidelines are useful, they must be used in conjunction with other practices, such as those associated with infection control and the use of personal protective equipment, and the management of specimens must be subjected to regular audit.

Point of Care Testing (PoCT)

Point of care testing refers to the performance of pathology assessment located immediately near to the patient. This sometimes occurs in the OR (e.g. breast specimen X-ray) as it has the advantage of rapid delivery of test results, ensuring timely or immediate intervention and treatment. However, major risks to patient safety can occur if theatre staff are not sufficiently educated and trained to use the diagnostic equipment; if the equipment is not tested, calibrated and maintained adequately; and when results are misinterpreted or not acted on appropriately (New South Wales Health, 2015).

CONCLUSION

This chapter provided information pertinent to patient safety within the perioperative setting. It outlined a range of nursing activities along with their rationales

TABLE 9.14
Correct Handling and Transportation of Gall Bladder Specimen for Mrs Peterson's Laparoscopic Cholecystectomy Surgery

Recommended Practice	Process
Undertake assessment for specimen-handling requirements	Confirm with surgeon Mrs Peterson's gallbladder is to be collected as a histology specimen. Confirm the use of formalin as preservative agent for the containment of the specimen. Determine whether any other specimens are to be collected during the procedure and how they are to be managed – or how the surgeon would like to manage any gallstones found present in Mrs Peterson's gallbladder. Collect and prepare an appropriately sized specimen container to allow for specimen size and appropriate volume of formalin preservative.
Ensure an accurate patient and specimen identification procedure is undertaken	At the time her gallbladder is removed from her body, confirm that the labels to be used for specimen identification contain Mrs Peterson's correct name, date of birth and unique hospital identifier and have been cross-checked against her ID bracelet, operative list and consent form. The instrument nurse receives the specimen from surgeon, who identifies the specimen as 'gallbladder' and confirms that formalin preservative is required. The instrument nurse verifies information using 'repeat back' technique with the surgeon. The instrument nurse confirms specimen information with the circulating nurse. The circulating nurse verifies information using 'repeat back' technique with the instrument nurse. The circulating nurse documents specimen information on Mrs Peterson's verified labels as 'gallbladder', 10% buffered formalin as fixative agent used, and date and time of collection. The instrument nurse and the circulating nurse reconfirm Mrs Peterson's name and specimen information using a 'write down, read back' process and visual confirmation. The circulating nurse dons the necessary personal protective equipment and the specimen is safely transferred to the labelled specimen container. The instrument and circulating nurse ensure that the gallbladder is the only specimen handled on the critical aseptic field at the one time to avoid mishandling and misidentification. In addition to the specimen container, the circulating nurse documents the verified patient and specimen details for Mrs Peterson on the perioperative nursing record, pathology request form and pathology register. A final team check is conducted of all specimens and associated documentation prior to Mrs Peterson leaving the operating room.
Provide accurate preparation and labelling of the specimen container	The circulating nurse prepares the contained gallbladder in preparation for transfer to pathology by ensuring that: • the specimen container is leakproof and has a tight-fitting lid • verified patient identification labels with specimen details are securely attached to the specimen container • all labels are placed on the container and not the lid, to ensure that the information is not lost when the lid is removed in the pathology department.
Establish accurate communication and documentation of the collection, and chain of custody	At the end of the procedure, the nurse records in the specimen register Mrs Peterson's details, number and type of specimen(s), diagnosis, studies required, date and time of collection, the surgeon's name and contact details, and the name of the nurse who prepared the specimen for transport. The documentation logged should establish a clear chain of custody from time of specimen removal to arrival in the pathology department.
Ensure safe and appropriate transportation of specimen to pathology laboratory	The specimen register contains a place for the signature of the pathology technician, who takes custody of Mrs Peterson's gallbladder specimen upon arrival at the pathology department.

(Sources: Australian College of Perioperative Nurses. (2020i). *ACORN standards for perioperative nursing in Australia* (16th ed., Vol. 1). Clinical standards – specimen identification, collection and handling. Adelaide: Author; World Health Organization. (2009). *Surgical Safety Checklist*. https://www.who.int/patientsafety/safesurgery/checklist/en.)

aimed at ensuring that the patient is provided with the safest possible care. The chapter explored the basic anatomical and physiological considerations related to patient transfer and positioning, the potential sequelae for incorrectly positioned patients and the interventions necessary to avoid them. Common complications related to surgery, such as inadvertent perioperative hypothermia and VTE, and the measures used to prevent or ameliorate them, were also explored and their limitations in practice noted. This chapter also examined the policies, procedures and standards that underpin correct site surgery and the surgical count. Finally, best practice related to the care and handling of tissue specimens was addressed.

RESOURCES

Agency for Clinical Innovation
https://www.aci.health.nsw.gov.au
Association for Perioperative Practice
https://www.afpp.org.uk
Association of periOperative Registered Nurses
https://www.aorn.org
Australian and New Zealand College of Anaesthetists
https://www.anzca.edu.au
Australian College of Operating Room Nurses
https://www.acorn.org.au
International Federation of Perioperative Nurses
https://www.ifpn.org.uk
Operating Room Nurses Association of Canada
https://www.ornac.ca
Royal Australasian College of Surgeons
https://www.surgeons.org

Video Resources

AfPP. (2016, 19 Jul). AfPP – how to – the surgical instrument count [video]. Retrieved from <https://youtu.be/rR3H7m85vDc>.

AORN. (2016, 31 Aug). Guideline essentials – prevention of retained surgical items: timing of the count [video]. Retrieved from <https://youtu.be/r—1a_9HQj8>.

Freelance Surgical. (2014, 20 August). Correct placement of tourniquet cuffs [video]. Retrieved from <https://www.youtube.com/watch?v=IGHX5iDrAac>.

Health Quality and Safety Commission New Zealand. (2014, 26 February). Perioperative harm – WHO surgical safety checklist [video]. Retrieved from <https://www.youtube.com/watch?v=UoYOdmDX4rA>.

HoverTech International. (2017, 24 January). HoverMatt training video [video]. Retrieved from <https://www.youtube.com/watch?v=wbI_zgXyyzQ>.

TechnologicHolita. (2012, 17 May). Trident specimen radiography system [video]. Retrieved from <https://www.youtube.com/watch?v=C8OwsXmRcHA>.

REFERENCES

3M Australia (2020). Online accessed at https://www.3mnz.co.nz

3M Company. (2016). Hosing risks – misuse puts patients at risk. Retrieved from <http://safepatientwarming.com/spw/hosingreusecommingling/hosing/risks/index.html>.

Abbott, T. E. F., Ahmad, T., Phull, M. K., Fowler, A. J., Hewson, R., Biccard, B. M., . . . Pearse, R. M. (2017). The surgical safety checklist and patient outcomes after surgery: a prospective observational cohort study, systematic review and meta-analysis. *British Journal of Anaesthesia, 120*(1), 146e155. https://dx.doi.org/ 10.1016/j.bja.2017.08.002.

Agrawal, A. (2012). Counting matters: lessons from the root cause analysis of a retained surgical item. *Joint Commission Journal on Quality and Patient Safety, 38*(12), 566–574.

Alban, R. F., Anania, E. C., Cohen, T. N., Fabri, P. J., Gewertz, B. L., Jain, M., . . . Sax, H. C. (2019). Performance improvement in surgery. *Current Problems in Surgery, 56*(6), 211–246.

Anaesthesia Key. (2019). Patient warming devices [webpage]. Retrieved from <https://aneskey.com/patient-warming-devices/>.

Anderson, K. T., Bartz-Kurycki, M. A., Masada, K. M., Abraham, J. E., Wang, J., Kawaguchi, A. L., . . . Tsao, K. (2018). Decreasing intraoperative delays and meaningful use of the surgical safety check list. *Surgery, 163*, 259–263.

Andrezjowski, J., & Riley, C. (2019). Metabolsim, the stress response to surgery and perioperative thermoregulation. In Thompson, J. P., Moppett, I. J., & Wiles, M., (Eds.), *Smith and Aitkenhead's textbook of anaesthesia* (7th ed., pp. 248–236). Edinburgh: Churchill.

Association of periOperative Registered Nurses (AORN). (2017). Guideline summary: positioning the patient. *AORN Journal, 106*(3), 238–247.

Association of periOperative Registered Nurses (AORN). (2018). Guideline for prevention of venous thromboembolism. In Guidelines for perioperative practice. Denver, CO: Author.

Association of periOperative Registered Nurses (AORN). (2019). Guideline for prevention of hypothermia. In Guidelines for perioperative practice. Denver, CO: Author. Retrieved from <https://aornguidelines.org/guidelines/content?sectionid=173731777&view=book>.

Association of periOperative Registered Nurses (AORN). (2020a). Guideline for pneumatic tourniquet safety. In Perioperative standards and recommended practices. Denver, CO: Author. Retrieved from <https://aornguidelines.org/guidelines/content?sectionid=173719470&view=book>.

Association of periOperative Registered Nurses (AORN). (2020b). Guideline quick view: pneumatic tourniquets. *AORN Journal, 111*(6), 720–723.

Aust, H., Koehler, S., Kuehnert M., & Wisemann, T. (2016). Guideline – recommended 15° left lateral table tilt during cesarean section in regional anaesthesia – practical aspects: an observational study. *Journal of Clinical Anesthesia, 32*, 47–53.

Australian and New Zealand College of Anaesthetists (ANZCA). (2014). Guidelines on sedation and/or analgesia for diagnostic and interventional medical, dental or surgical procedures, 2014. Retrieved from <https://www.anzca.edu.au>.

Australian and New Zealand Hip Fracture Registry (ANZHFR). (2019). *Annual report of hip fracture care 2019*. Australian and New Zealand Hip Fracture Registry.

Australian Bureau of Statistics (ABS). (2018). *National health survey: first results, 2017–18*. Cat. no. 4364.0.55.001. Retrieved from <https://www.abs.gov.au/ausstats/abs@.nsf/mf/4364.0.55.001>.

Australian College of Perioperative Nurses (ACORN). (2020a). *ACORN standards for perioperative nursing in Australia* (16th ed., Vol. 1). Clinical standards – surgical safety. Adelaide: Author.

Australian College of Perioperative Nurses (ACORN). (2020b). *ACORN standards for perioperative nursing in Australia* (16th ed., Vol. 1). Clinical standards – patient positioning. Adelaide: Author.

Australian College of Perioperative Nurses (ACORN). (2020c). *ACORN standards for perioperative nursing in Australia* (16th ed., Vol. 1). Clinical standards – new equipment and instrumentation. Adelaide: Author.

Australian College of Perioperative Nurses (ACORN). (2020d). *ACORN standards for perioperative nursing in Australia* (16th ed., Vol. 1). Clinical standards – manual Handling. Adelaide: Author.

Australian College of Perioperative Nurses (ACORN). (2020e). *ACORN standards for perioperative nursing in Australia* (16th ed., Vol. 1). Clinical standards – hypothermia. Adelaide: Author.

Australian College of Perioperative Nurses (ACORN). (2020f). *ACORN standards for perioperative nursing in Australia* (16th ed., Vol. 1). Clinical standards – pneumatic Tourniquet. Adelaide: Author.

Australian College of Perioperative Nurses (ACORN). (2020g). *ACORN standards for perioperative nursing in Australia* (16th ed., Vol. 1). Clinical standards – accountable items used during surgery and procedures. Adelaide: Author.

Australian College of Perioperative Nurses (ACORN). (2020h). *ACORN standards for perioperative nursing in Australia* (16th ed., Vol. 1). Clinical standards – loan sets and trial reusable medical devices. Adelaide: Author.

Australian College of Perioperative Nurses (ACORN). (2020i). *ACORN standards for perioperative nursing in Australia* (16th ed., Vol. 1). Clinical standards – specimen identification, collection and handling. Adelaide: Author.

Australian Commission on Safety and Quality in Health Care (ACSQHC/the Commission). (2010). Australian safety and quality framework for health care. Retrieved from <https://www.safetyandquality.gov.au/sites/default/files/migrated/ASQFHC-Guide-Policymakers.pdf>.

Australian Commission on Safety and Quality in Health Care (ACSQHC/the Commission). (2016). *Hip fracture care clinical standard*. Sydney: ACSQHC. Retrieved from <https://www.safetyandquality.gov.au>.

Australian Commission on Safety and Quality in Health Care (ACSQHC/the Commission). (2017). *National safety and quality health service standards* (2nd ed.). Comprehensive care standard. Sydney: ACSQHC. Retrieved from <https://www.safetyandquality.govt.au>.

Australian Commission on Safety and Quality in Health Care (ACSQHC/the Commission). (2018a). Selected best practices and suggestions for improvement for clinicians and health system manager. Hospital-acquired complication: Pressure injury. Retrieved from <https://www.safetyandquality.gov.au>.

Australian Commission on Safety and Quality in Health Care (ACSQHC/the Commission). (2018b). *Venous thromboembolism prevention clinical care standard*. Sydney: ACSQHC. Retrieved from <https://www.safetyandquality.gov.au>.

Benrashid, E., Youngwirth, L. M., Turley, R. S., & Mureebe, L. (2017). Venous thromboembolism: prevention diagnosis and treatment. In J. Cameron & A. Cameron (Eds.), *Current surgical therapy* (12th ed., pp. 1091–1098). Philadelphia: Elsevier.

Bettelli, G., Cucinotta, D., & Neuner, B. (2018). Introduction: aging, healthcare systems and surgery. In G. Bettelli (Ed.), *Perioperative care of the elderly: clinical and organisational aspects* (pp. 1–2). Cambridge: Cambridge University Press.

Boet, S., Patey, A. M., Baron, J. S., Mohamed, K., Pigford, A. E., Bryson, J. C., . . . Grimshaw, J. M., (2017). Factors that influence effective perioperative temperature management by anaesthesiologists: a qualitative study using the Theoretical Domains Framework. *Candadian Journal of Anaesthesia/Journal canadien d'anaesthesie, 64*(6), 581–596.

Bowen, B. A. (2019). Orthopedic surgery. In J. C. Rothrock & D. L. McEwen (Eds.), *Alexander's care of the patient in surgery* (16th ed., pp. 666–754). St. Louis, MO: Elsevier.

Bryant, B., Knights, K., Darroch, S., & Rowland, A. (2018). *Pharmacology for health professionals* (5th ed.). Sydney: Mosby Elsevier.

Burlingame, B. L. (2017). Guideline implementation: positioning the patient. *AORN Journal, 106*(3), 228–237.

Caprini, J. A., Arcelus, J. I., & Tafur, A. J. (2019). Venous thromboembolic disease: mechanical paharmacologic prophylaxis. In *Rutherford's vascular surgery and endovascular therapy* [e-book] (9th ed., pp. 1927–1935). Philadelphia, PA: Elsevier.

Carron, M., Safaee Fakhr, B., Ieppariello, G., & Foletto, M. (2020). Perioperative care of the obese patient. *British Journal of Surgery, 107*(2), e39–e55. https://dx.doi.org/ 10.1002/bjs.11447

Clinical Excellence Commission [CEC]. (2013). *Management of instruments, accountable items and other items used for surgery or procedures policy directive*. PD2012_034. Retrieved from <https://www1.health.nsw.gov.au/pds/ActivePDSDocuments/PD2013_054.pdf>.

Clinical Excellence Commission [CEC]. (2017). *Clinical procedure safety policy directive*. PD2017_032. Retrieved from <https://www1.health.nsw.gov.au/pds/Pages/doc.aspx?dn=PD2017_032>.

Clinical Excellence Commission [CEC]. (2018). Patient safety programs, VTE risk assessment tool. Retrieved from <http://www.cec.health.nsw.gov.au/__data/assets/pdf_file/0010/458821/Venous-Thromboembolism-VTE-Risk-Assessment-Tool.pdf>.

Cluver, C., Novilova, N., Hofmeyr, G. J., & Hall, D. R. (2013). Maternal position during caesarean section for preventing maternal and neonatal complications. *Cochrane Database of Systematic Reviews, 3*, CD007623. https://dx.doi.org/10.1002/14651858.CD007623.pub3

Cockburn, T., Davis, J., & Osborne, S. (2019). Retained surgical items: lessons from Australian case law of items unintentionally left behind in patients after surgery. *Journal of Law and Medicine, 26*(4), 841–848.

Collins, S., Budds, M., Raines, C., & Hooper, V. (2019). Risk factors for perioperative hypothermia: a literature review. *Journal of Perianesthesia Nursing, 34*(2), 338–346.

Croke, L. (2019). Essential strategies for safe patient positioning. *AORN Journal, 110*(5), 11–15.

Croke, L. (2020). Guideline for pneumatic tourniquet safety. *AORN Journal, 111*(4), 8–10.

Crook, C. (2016). Advocacy: how far would you go to protect your patients? *AORN Journal, 103*(5), 522–525.

Dalvand, S., Ebadi, A., Ghenshlagh, G. (2018). Nurses' knowledge on pressure injury prevention: a systematic review and meta-analysis based on the Pressure Ulcer Knowledge Assessment Tool. *Clinical, Cosmetic and Investigational Dermatology, 11*, 613–620.

Davis, S. S. (2018). The key to safety: proactive prevention. *AORN Journal, 108*(4), 351–353.

Delmore, B. A., & Ayello, E. A. (2017). Pressure injuries caused by medical device and other objects: a clinical update. *American Journal of Nursing, 117*(12), 36–45.

Dias, M. (2018). Evidence summary: surgical safety checklist: effectiveness (clinical outcomes). The Joanna Briggs Institute EBP Database, JBI@Ovid. 2018; JBI11274.

Drake, R. L., Vogl, W., Mitchell, A. W. M., Tibbitts, R., Richardson, P., Gray, H., & Horn, A. (2019). *Gray's anatomy for students* (4th ed., International ed.). Philadelphia: Elsevier.

Ebi, W. E., Hirko, G. F., & Mijena, D. A. (2019). Nurses' knowledge to pressure ulcer prevention in public hospitals in Wollega; a cross-sectional study design. *NMC Nursing. 18*(20). https://dx.doi.org/10.1186/s12912-019-0346-y

European Society of Anaesthesiology. (2018). Guidelines on venous thromboembolism prophylaxis. Retrieved from <https://www.esahq.org/guidelines/guidelines/published>.

Fawcett, D. L. (2019). Positioning the patient for surgery. In J. C. Rothrock & D. L. McEwen (Eds.), *Alexander's care of the patient in surgery* (16th ed., pp. 142–175). St. Louis, MO: Elsevier.

Fencl, J. L., Walsh, A., & Vocke, D. (2015). The bariatric patient: an overview of perioperative care. *AORN Journal, 102*(2), 116–128.

Ghironzi, G., Canet Capeta, J., Fernandez Cortes, A., & Betelli, G. (2018). Aging and age-related functional changes. In G. Betelli (Ed.), *Perioperative care of the elderly: clinical and organisational aspects* (pp. 3–8). Cambridge: Cambridge University Press.

Gillespie, B. M., Harbeck, E. L., Lavin, J., Hamilton, K., Gardiner., Withers, T. K., & Marshall, A. P. (2018). Evaluation of a patient safety programme on Surgical Safety Checklist compliance: a prospective longitudinal study. *British Medical Journal Open Quality, 7*, e000362. https://dx.doi.org/10.1136/bmjoq-2018-000362.e

Goudas, L., & Bruni, S. (2019). Pressure injury risk assessment and prevention strategies in operating room patients – findings from a study tour of novel practices in American hospitals. *ACORN Journal, 32*(1), 33–38.

Heizenroth, J. (2015). Positioning the patient for surgery. In J. Rothrock (Ed.) & D. McEwen (Assoc. Ed), *Alexander's care of the patient in surgery* (15th ed.). Elsevier Mosby, St Louis.

Hewson, D., & Hardman, J. (2019). Complications arising from anaesthesia. In J. P. Thompson, I. J. Moppett, & M. Wiles (Eds.), *Smith and Aitkenhead's textbook of anaesthesia* (7th ed., Ch. 26, pp. 558–571). Edinburgh: Elsevier.

Hidalgo Diaz, J. J., Muresan, L., Touchal, S., Bahlouli, N., Liverneaux, P., & Facca, S. (2018). The new digit tourniquet ForgetMeNot. *Orthopaedics & Traumatology: Surgery & Research, 104*, 133–136.

Hinkelbein, J., Lamperti, M., Akeson, J., Santos, J., Costa, J., De Robertis, E., . . . Fitzgerald, R. (2018). European Society of Anaesthesiology and European Board of Anaesthesiology Guidelines for procedural sedation and analgesia in adults. *European Journal of Anaesthesiology, 35*, 6–24.

Howlett, S. E. (2017). *Effects of ageing on the cardiovascular system in Brocklehurst's textbook of geriatric medicine and gerontology* (8th ed., pp. 96–100). Philadelphia: Elsevier.

International Skin Tear Advisory Panel (ISTAP). (2018). Best practice recommendations for the prevention and management of skin tears in aged skin. *Wounds International.* Retrieved from <https://www.woundsinternational.com>.

Jensen, J., Hicks, R. W., & Labovitz, J. (2019). Understanding and optimizing tourniquet use during extremity surgery. *AORN Journal, 109*(2), 172–182.

Kahn, S. R., Morrison, D. R., Diendéré, G., Piché, A., Filion, K. B., Klil-Drori, A., . . . Geerts, W. (2018). Interventions to increase the use of measures to prevent the development of blood clots in hospitalized medical and surgical patients. *Cochrane Database of Systematic Reviews, 4*, CD008201. https://dx.doi.org/10.1002/14651858.CD008201.pub3

Kinlaw, T. S., & Whiteside, D. (2019). Surgical specimen management in the preanalytic phase: perioperative nursing implications. *AORN Journal, 110*(3), 238–247.

Kirkbride, D. (2019). The practical conduct of anaesthesia. In J. P. Thompson, I. J. Moppett, & M. Wiles (Eds.), *Smith and Aitkenhead's textbook of anaesthesia* (7th ed., pp. 441–455). Edinburgh: Churchill Livingstone.

Klein, A W., & Arrowsmith, J. (2019). Anaesthesia for cardiac surgery. In J. P. Thompson, I. J. Moppett, & M. Wiles (Eds.), *Smith and Aitkenhead's textbook of anaesthesia* (7th ed., pp. 799–813). Edinburgh: Churchill Livingstone.

Lark, M. E., Kirkpatrick, K., & Chung, K. C. (2018). Patient safety movement: history and future directions. *Journal of Hand Surgery, 43*(2), 174–178.

LeBlanc, K., & Baranoski, S. (2017). Skin tears: finally recognized. *Advances in Skin & Wound Care, 30*(2), 62–63.

Lin, H. S., McBride, R. L., & Hubbard, R. E. (2018). Frailty and anaesthesia – risks during and post surgery. *Local and Regional Anesthesia, 11*, 61–73. https://dx.doi.org/10.2147/LRA.S142996

Mahmood, T., Myopoulos, M., Bagli, D., Damignani, R., & Haji, F. A. (2018). A mixed methods study of challenges in the implementation and use of the surgical safety checklist. *Surgery, 165*(2), 832–837.

Mangham, M. (2017). Positioning of the anaesthetized patient during robotically assisted surgery: perioperative staff experiences. *ACORN Journal, 30*(1), 20–22.

Martin, H., Metcalfe, M. H., & Whichello, R. (2015). Specimen labeling errors: a retrospective study. *On-Line Journal of Nursing Informatics, 19*(2), 1–9.

McEwin, J. (2017). Equipment preparation: tourniquets. Retrieved from <https://tourniquets.org/equipment-preparation/>.

Min, S., Yoon, S., Yoon, J., Bakh, J., & Seo, J. (2018). Randomised trial comparing forced-air warming to upper or lower body to prevent hypothermia during thorascopic surgery in the lateral decubitus position. *British Journal of Anaesthesia, 120*(3), 555–562.

Mirkazemi, C., Bereznicki, L. R., & Peterson, G. M. (2019). Comparing Australian orthopaedic surgeons' reported use of thromboprophylaxis following arthroplasty in 2012 and 2017. *BMC Musculoskeletal Disorders, 20*, 57. https://dx.doi.org/10.1186/s12891-019-2409-3

Munday, J., Delaforce, A., Forbes., G., & Deoghh, S. (2019). Barriers and enablers to the implementation of perioperative hypothermia prevention practices from the perspectives of the multidisciplinary team: a quality study using the Theoretic Domains Framework. *Journal of Multidisciplinary Healthcare, 12*, 395–417.

Murphy, E. (2019). Patient safety and risk management. In J. C. Rothrock & D. L. McEwen (Eds.), *Alexander's care of the patient in surgery* (16th ed., pp. 15–36). St. Louis, MO: Elsevier.

Nathanson, M. (2019). Neurosurgery anaesthesia. In J. P. Thompson, I. J. Moppett, & M. Wiles (Eds.), *Smith and Aitkenhead's textbook of anaesthesia* (7th ed., pp. 769–787). Edinburgh: Churchill Livingstone.

National Institute for Health and Care Excellence (NICE). (2018). Venous thromboembolism in over 16s: reducing the risk of hospital-acquired deep vein thrombosis or pulmonary embolism (NICE Guideline NG89). Retrieved from <https://www.nice.org.uk/guidance/ng89/resources/venous-thromboembolism-in-over-16s-reducing-the-risk-of-hospitalacquired-deep-vein-thrombosis-or-pulmonary-embolism-pdf-1837703092165>.

National Institute for Health and Care Excellence (NICE). (2020). Inadvertent perioperative hypothermia overview. Retrieved from <https://pathways.nice.org.uk/pathways/inadvertent-perioperative-hypothermia>.

National Pressure Ulcer Advisory Panel, European Pressure Ulcer Advisory Panel and Pan Pacific Pressure Injury Alliance. (NPUAP-EPUAP-PPPIA). (2019). *Prevention and treatment of pressure ulcers: Quick reference guide*. E. Haesler (Ed.). Osborne Park, Australia: Cambridge Media.

New Zealand Health and Disability Commissioner. (2020). The Code of Health and Disability Services Consumers' Rights (the Code) Regulations 1996. Retrieved from <https://www.hdc.org.nz/your-rights/about-the-code/code-of-health-and-disability-services-consumers-rights/>.

New Zealand Ministry of Health. (2018). Tier 1 statistics 2017/18: New Zealand health survey. Retrieved from <https://www.health.govt.nz/nz-health-statistics/health-statistics-and-data-sets/obesity-statistics U4233-012edit.doc>.

NSW Health. (2015). Point of care testing (PoCT) policy. PD2015_028. Retrieved from <https://www1.health.nsw.gov.au/pds/ActivePDSDocuments/PD2018_028.pdf>.

O'Brien, G., Moore, Z., Patton, D., & O'Connor, T. (2018). The relationship between nurses assessment of early pressure ulcer damage and sub epidermal moisture measurement: a prospective explorative study. *Journal of Tissue Viability, 27*(4), 232–237.

O'Connor, D., & Radcliffe, J. (2018). Patient positioning in anaesthesia. *Anaesthesia and Intensive Care Medicine, 19*(11), 585–590. https://dx.doi.org/10.1016/j.mpaic.2018.08.019

Odell, D. D., Quinn, C. M., Matulewicz, R. S., Johnson, J., Engelhardt, K. E., Stulberg, J. J., . . . Bilimoria, K. Y. (2019). Association between hospital safety culture and surgical outcomes in a statewide surgical quality improvement collaborative. *Journal of the American College of Surgeons, 229*(2), 175–183. https://dx.doi.org/10.1016/j.jamcollsurg.2019.02.046

Oliveira, A. L., Moore, Z., O'Connor, T., & Patton, D. (2017). Accuracy of ultrasound, thermography and subepidermal moisture in predicting pressure ulcers: a systematic review. *Journal of Wound Care, 26*(5), 199–215.

Ousey, K. J., Edward, K. L., Stephenson, J., Duff, J., Walker, K. N., & Leaper, D. J. (2015). Perioperative warming therapy for preventing surgical site infection in adults undergoing surgery (protocol). *Cochrane Database of Systematic Reviews, 6*, CD011731. https://dx.doi.org/ 10.1002/14651858.CD011731

Partridge, J., Sbai, M., & Dhesi, J. (2018). Proactive care of older people undergoing surgery. *Aging Clinical and Experimental Research, 30*, 253. https://dx.doi.org/10.1007/s40520-017-0879-4

Phillips, N. (2017). *Berry and Kohn's operating room technique* (13th ed.). St. Louis, MO: Elsevier.

Pillai, A. (2019). Obstetric anaesthesia and analgesia. In J. P. Thompson, I. J. Moppett, & M. Wiles (Eds.), *Smith and Aikenhead's textbook of anaesthesia* (7th ed., pp. 800–830). Edinburgh: Churchill Livingstone.

Queensland Health. (2018). *Guidelines for the prevention of venous thromboembolism (VTE) in adult hospitalized patients*. State of Queensland (Queensland Health), December 2018. Retrieved from <https://www.health.qld.gov.au/__data/assets/pdf_file/0031/812938/vte-prevention-guideline.pdf>.

Ralph, N., Gow, J., & Duff, J. (2019). Preventing perioperative hypothermia is clinically feasible and cost effective. *Journal of Perioperative Nursing. 32*(1), 1. Retrieved from <https://www.journal.acorn.org.au>.

Ravi, B., Pincus, D., Choi, S., Jenkinson, R., Wasserstein, D., & Redelmeir, D. A. (2019). Association of duration of surgery with postoperative delirium among patients receiving hip fracture repair. *JAMA Network Open, 2*(2), e190111. https://dx.doi.org/10.1001/jamanetworkopen.2019.0111

Royal Australasian College of Surgeons (RACS). (2009). Surgical Safety Checklist. Retrieved from <https://www.surgeons.org/member-services/college-resources/#surgicalsafety>.

Saunders, R., Comerota, A. J., Ozols, A., Torrejon Torres, R., & Ho, K. M. (2018). Intermittent pneumatic compression is a cost-effective method of orthopedic postsurgical venous thromboembolism prophylaxis. *ClinicoEconomics and Outcomes Research*, 10, 231–241. https://dx.doi.org/10.2147/CEOR.S157306

Sessler, D., I. (2016). Perioperative thermoregulation and heat balance. *Lancet*, 387(10038), 2655–2664.

Soncrant, C. M., Warner, L. J., Neily, J., Paull, D. E., Mazzia, L., Mills, P. D., . . . Hemphill, R. R. (2018). Root cause analysis of reported patient falls in ORs in the Veterans Health Administration. *AORN Journal*, 108(4), 386–397.

Spruce, L. (2017a). Preventing perioperative positioning and equipment injuries. In J. Sanchez, P. Barach, J. Johnson, & J. Jacobs. (Eds.), *Surgical patient care* (pp. 493–518). Champaign, IL: Springer.

Spruce, L. (2017b). Back to basics: pneumatic tourniquet use. *AORN Journal*, 106(3), 220–226.

Spruce, L. (2018). Back to basics: orthopedic positioning. *AORN Journal*, 107(3), 355–367.

Spruce, L., & Van Wicklin, S. A. (2016). Back-to-basics: positioning the patient. *ACORN Journal*, 29(2), 14–17.

Stanton, C. (2017). Guideline for positioning the patient. *AORN Journal*, 105(4), 8–10.

Staunton, P., & Chiarella, M. (2020). *Law for nurses and midwives* (9th ed.). Sydney: Elsevier.

Steelman, V. M., Schaapveld, A. G., Storm, H. E., Perkhounkova, Y., & Shane, D. M. (2019a). The effect of radiofrequency technology on time spent searching for surgical sponges and associated costs. *AORN Journal*, 19(6), 718–727.

Steelman, V. M., Shaw, C., Shine, L., & Hardy-Fairbanks, A. J. (2019b). Unintentionally retained foreign objects: a descriptive study of 308 sentinel events and contributing factors. *Joint Commission Journal on Quality and Patient Safety*, 45, 249–258.

Steelman, V. M., Thenuwara, K., Shaw, C., & Shine, L. (2019c). Unintentionally retained guidewires: a descriptive study of 73 sentinel events. *Joint Commission Journal of Quality and Patient Safety*, 45, 81–90.

Stubbs, J. M., Assareh, H., Curnow, J., Hitos, K., & Achat, H. M. (2018). Incidence of in-hospital and post-discharge diagnosed hospital-associated venous thromboembolism using linked administrative data. *Internal Medicine Journal*, 48(2), 157–165. https://dx.doi.org/ 10.1111/imj.13679

Tommasino, C., & Corcione, A. (2018). Anesthesia for the elderly patient. In A. Crucitti, (Ed.), *Surgical management of elderly patients* (pp. 9–29). Champaign, IL: Springer.

Tran, H. A., Gibbs, H., Merriman, E., Curnow, J. L., Laura Young, L., Bennett, A., . . . Nandurkar, H. (2019). The diagnosis and management of venous thromboembolism – guidelines of the Thrombosis and Haemostasis Society of Australia and New Zealand. Retrieved from <https://www.thanz.org.au/documents/item/411>.

Tredwell, S. J., Wilmink, M., Inkpen, K., & McEwen, J. A. (2001). Pediatric tourniquets: analysis of cuff and limb interface, current practice, and guidelines for use. *Journal of Pediatric Orthopaedics*, 21(5), 671–676.

Tritschler, T., Kraaijpoel, N., Le Gal, G., & Wells, P. S. (2018). Venous thromboembolism: advances in diagnosis and treatment. *Journal of the American Medical Association*, 320(15), 1583–1594. https://dx.doi.org/10.1001/jama.2018.14346

Torossian, A., Brauyer, A., Höcker, J., Berthold, B., Wulf, H., & Horn, E.-P. (2015). Preventing inadvertent perioperative hypothermia. *Deutsche Arzteblatt International*, 112(10), 166–172. https://dx.doi.org/10.3238/arztebl.2015.0166

Van Wicklin, S. A. (2015). Back to basics: specimen management. *AORN Journal*, 101(5), 558–564.

Van Wicklin, S. A. (2018). Challenges in the operating room with obese and extremely obese surgical pattients. *International Journal of Safe Patient Handling and Mobility*, 8(3), 120–131.

Verwey, S., & Gopalan, P. D. (2018). An investigation of barriers to the use of the World Health Organization Surgical Safety Check List in theatres. *South African Medical Journal*, 108(4), 336–341.

Wang, I., Walker, R., & Gillespie, B. M. (2018a). Pressure injury prevention for surgery: results from a prospective, observational study in a tertiary hospital. *ACORN Journal of Perioperative Nursing*, 31(3), 25–28.

Wang, I., Walker, R., & Gillespie, B. M. (2018b). Pressure injury prevention in the perioperative setting: an integrative review. *ACORN Journal of Perioperative Nursing*, 31(4), 27–35.

Wang, K., Ni, S., Li, Z., Zhong, Q., Li, R., Li, H., . . . Lin, J. (2017). The effects of tourniquet use in total knee arthroplasty: a randomized, controlled trial. *Knee Surgery Sports Traumatology Arthroscopy*, 25(9), 2849–2857.

Warwick, V., Gillespie, B. M., McMurray, A., & Clark-Burg, K. (2019). The patient, case, individual and environmental factors that impact on the surgical count process: an integrative review. *Journal of Perioperative Nursing*, 32(3), 9–19.

Watson, J. (2018). Inadvertent postoperative hypothermia prevention: passive versus active warming methods. *Journal of Perioperative Nursing*, 31(1), 43–46. https://dx.doi.org/10.26550/2209-1092.1025

Whitehorn, A. (2019). Evidence summary. Operating room: surgical counts. The Joanna Briggs Institute EBP Database, JBI@Ovid. 2019; JBI5504.

Williams, K. (2018). Benefits of passive warming on surgical patients undergoing regional anesthetic procedures. *Journal of Perianesthesia Nursing*, 33(6), 928–934.

World Health Organization (WHO). (2009). Surgical Safety Checklist. Retrieved from <https://www.who.int/patient-safety/safesurgery/checklist/en>.

World Health Organization (WHO). (n.d.). Safe surgery. Retrieved from <https://www.who.int/patientsafety/safesurgery/en>.

Wright, M. I. (2016). Implementing no interruption zones in the perioperative environment. *AORN Journal*, 104(6), 536–540.

Yu, M., Lee, T., & Mills, M. E. (2019). The effect of barcode technology use on pathology specimen labeling errors. *AORN Journal*, 109(2), 183–191.

Zenoni, S., & Smith, S. (2018). *Perioperative hypothermia prevention in burn patients*. Surgical Critical Care Evidence-Based Medicine Guidelines Committee, Orlando. Retrieved from <https://www.surgicalcriticalcare.net/Guidelines/Hypothermia%20in%20burn%20patients%202018.pdf>.

Zervakis Brent, M. A. (2016). OR specimen labeling. *AORN Journal, 103*(2), 164–176.

FURTHER READING

Evered, L., Scott, D. A., & Silbert, B. (2017). Cognitive decline associated with anaesthesia and surgery in the elderly: does this contribute to dementia prevalence? *Current Opinion in Psychiatry, 30*(3), 220–226.

Mouser, J. G., Dankel, S. J., Jessee, M. B., Mattocks, K. T., Buckner, S. L., Counts, B. R., & Loenneke, J. P. (2017). A tale of three cuffs: the hemodynamics of blood flow restriction. *European Journal of Applied Physiology, 117*, 1493–1499.

Stankiewicz, M., & Wyland, M. (2017). A review of suspected intra-operative antiseptic burns: a quality improvement review. *ACORN Journal of Perioperative Nursing, 30*(4), 25–29.

Woodfin, K. O., Johnson, C., Parker, R., Mikach, C., Johnson, M., & McMullin, S. P. (2018). Use of a novel memory aid to educate perioperative team members on proper patient positioning technique. *AORN Journal, 107*(3), 325–332.

CHAPTER 10

Surgical Intervention

TINA BORIC • DEBORAH BURROWS • PENNY SMALLEY
EDITOR: BEN LOCKWOOD

LEARNING OUTCOMES

- Discuss the instrument categories/functions, including the names of at least two instruments from each category
- Outline the stages of surgery and discuss the rationale for having a surgical sequence
- Discuss the two insertion techniques used in minimally invasive abdominal surgery
- Identify advances in techniques and technology

KEY TERMS

bipolar	neutral zone
diathermy	operating room (OR) layout
electrosurgical devices	robotic surgery
instrumentation	surgical instruments
laser	surgical plume evacuation
minimally invasive surgery	surgical sequence
monopolar	

INTRODUCTION

The perioperative nurse plays an important role in the surgical intervention of patients. Underpinning this role is a sound knowledge of anatomy, the physiological response to surgery, aseptic technique, safety, and legal and ethical aspects. Importantly, in order to provide appropriate assistance to the surgical team, nurses also require knowledge of the sequence of surgery, the **instrumentation** required and the wound closure materials used. This chapter discusses the instrumentation, equipment and methodologies of surgical intervention. It also provides a historical overview of surgery along with an outline of the principles of surgical intervention and the sequence of surgery. The chapter concludes with an examination of some of the innovations associated with minimally invasive and robotic surgery.

Consider the patient scenarios (detailed in the Introduction to this book) of Mrs Patricia Peterson, admitted for an emergency laparoscopic cholecystectomy, Mr James Collins, scheduled for a right total knee replacement, and Thanh Nguyen, admitted for an orchidopexy, as you read this chapter.

HISTORICAL SURGICAL PERSPECTIVE

Surgery is as old as human beings, with archaeologists finding skulls with evidence of having had a surgical procedure performed dating back to 350,000 BCE (Sullivan, 1996). Prior to anaesthesia and anaesthetic technique, surgery was performed only if absolutely necessary. Surgery developed along with knowledge in microbiology, disinfection and anaesthetics.

Today surgery incorporates a holistic approach to patient care, encompassing all aspects of pre- and postoperative preparation and intervention. As a discipline, surgery combines physiological management with an interventional aspect of treatment, which may be restorative, corrective, diagnostic or palliative (see

TABLE 10.1
Common Indications for Surgical Procedures

Indication for Surgical Procedure	Example
Aesthetics	Facelift
Augmentation	Breast implants
Bypass/shunt	Vascular rerouting
Debulking	Decreasing the size of a mass
Diagnostics	Biopsy tissue sample
Diversion	Creation of a stoma for urine
Drainage/evacuation	Incision into abscess
Excision	Remove tissue or structure by sharp dissection
Exploration	Invasive examination
Extraction	Removal of a tooth
Harvest	Autologous skin graft
Incision	Open tissue or structure by sharp dissection
Palliation	Relief of obstruction
Parturition	Caesarean section
Procurement	Donor organ
Reconstruction	Creation of a new breast
Removal	Foreign body
Repair	Closing of a hernia
Stabilisation	Repair of a fracture
Staging	Checking of cancer progression
Termination	Abortion of a pregnancy
Transplant	Placement of a donor organ or tissue

(Source: Phillips, N. (2017). *Berry & Kohn's operating room technique* (13th ed., p. 2). St Louis, MO: Elsevier.)

Table 10.1). All surgery has clearly defined principles of operative technique (Phillips, 2017). These principles are illustrated in Fig. 10.1.

Historically, the perioperative environment has been viewed as being 'daunting' to the novice. However, the perioperative setting continues to progress towards an environment focused on teamwork and transparency, with the common goal of optimised patient safety. This evolution also makes the transition for newcomers an easier one today (Hartman & Kovoussi, 2018).

Advancements in technology continue to influence the perioperative specialty; consequently, surgical interventions occur in a wide variety of forms. In any given setting, perioperative patient presentation and operative technique may vary from an incision and drainage of an abscess to a robotic total knee replacement (Cuming, 2019). Subsequently, the skill set required of today's perioperative nurse is necessarily dynamic and diverse, including knowledge of the procedure, potential risks and complications, as well as the ability to anticipate and advocate to enable holistic care of the perioperative patient (Cuming, 2019).

SEQUENCE OF SURGERY

Every surgical procedure, no matter how simple or complex, follows a defined **surgical sequence**. This generalised sequence is adapted for the specific surgical procedure being performed. Knowledge of the stages of surgical intervention, instrumentation and suture material assists the perioperative nurse in ensuring safe patient outcomes. A working knowledge is required of the sequential steps for a specific surgical procedure, based on four concepts that should be considered for any surgical event:

- procedure to be undertaken
- approach used
- possible complications to be encountered
- closure technique.

Understanding these steps and being able to apply them to an individual patient's procedure are important skills for the perioperative nurse. These concepts are illustrated in Fig. 10.2.

Stages of the Surgical Procedure

There are five sequential stages of a surgical procedure (Fig. 10.3). The instrument nurse must have an in-depth knowledge of each stage of the surgical sequence in order to anticipate the surgeon's requirements. The focus for the circulating nurse is the provision of support to the surgical team, and management and coordination of the operating room. Refer to Chapter 1 for more information.

- Stage I Open refers to the initial incision made by the surgeon with a scalpel blade or electrocautery device.
- Stage II Dissection and exposure is the process of separating tissues or structures (often with scissors) in order to gain access and adequate visualisation of the surgical field. Exposure is sometimes assisted by the use of retraction devices.
- Stage III Exploration and isolation is the process of investigating the structures to be operated on, as well as the surrounding structures, to eliminate

Aseptic technique
Plan the incision
• Use correct instrumentation
• Gentle tissue retraction and even pressure prevents damage
Handle tissues gently
• Maintain tissue hydration
• Minimise trauma and tissue tension to prevent capillary compromise and reduce postoperative pain
Preserve blood supply
• Control bleeding, achieve haemostasis
• Remove blood clots and haematomas to reduce surgical site infections and improve healing
Debride devitalised tissue
• Remove necrotic tissue
• Wound irrigation or lavage
• Prepare wound edge
Careful tissue approximation
• Eliminate dead space and gaps between tissue layers in which haematomas and serum can collect
• Immobilise the wound
Promotes wound healing

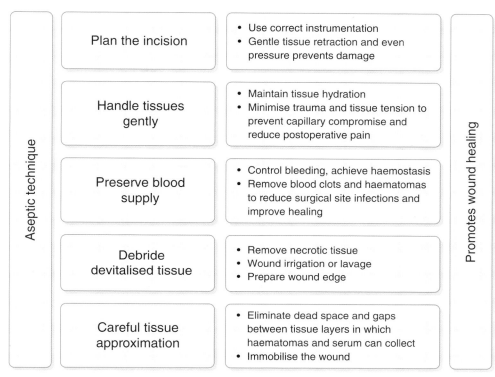

FIG. 10.1 Principles of operative technique. (Source: Adapted from Fuller, J. K. (2018). *Surgical technology: principles and practice* (7th ed., p. 428). St Louis, MO: Elsevier Saunders.)

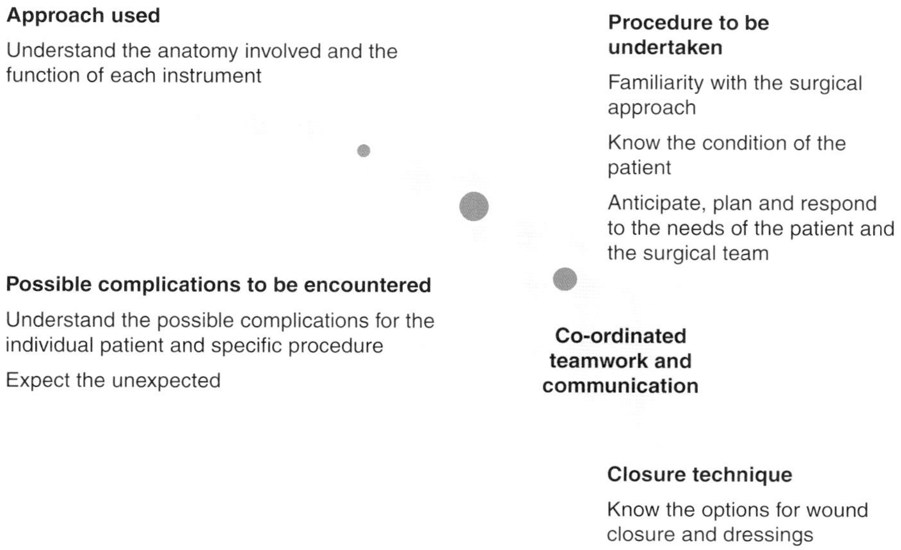

Approach used
Understand the anatomy involved and the function of each instrument
Procedure to be undertaken
Familiarity with the surgical approach
Know the condition of the patient
Anticipate, plan and respond to the needs of the patient and the surgical team
Possible complications to be encountered
Understand the possible complications for the individual patient and specific procedure
Expect the unexpected
Co-ordinated teamwork and communication
Closure technique
Know the options for wound closure and dressings

FIG. 10.2 The four concepts that should be considered for any surgical event. (Source: Adapted from Phillips, N. F. and Hornacky, A. (2021). *Berry & kohn's operating room technique* Fourteenth edn. St. Louis, Missouri: Elsevier.)

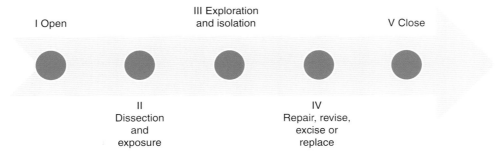

FIG. 10.3 Sequential stages of a surgical procedure. (Source: Adapted from Fuller, J. K. (2018). *Surgical technology: principles and practice* (7th ed., p. 405). St Louis, MO: Elsevier Saunders.)

differential diagnoses, plan the best approach or technique to employ, and to physically isolate the operative structures from the surrounding anatomy.
• Stage IV Repair, revise, excise or replace refers to the actions required to complete the surgery as indicated.

• Stage V Close refers to the process of restoring functional or anatomical alignment of structures, ensuring haemostasis, suturing or securing the layers of the wound closed and applying a wound dressing.

PATIENT SCENARIOS

Mrs Patricia Peterson is a 42-year-old Indigenous woman admitted for an emergency laparoscopic cholecystomy. Mrs Peterson's full history and a brief description of the healthcare setting is provided in the Introduction at the front of the book for readers to review when answering the questions in this unfolding scenario.

SCENARIO 10.1: INSTRUMENT NURSE'S ROLE – PREPARATION FOR SURGERY

A third-year student nurse, Rose Cheng, has been assigned by RN Sandy Pereira to double scrub with EN Noakes as the instrument nurse for Mrs Peterson's surgery. Student Nurse Cheng is not sure of all the steps involved in a laparoscopic cholecystectomy. After the preparation of instrumentation and equipment has been completed, RN Pereira tells student nurse Cheng that she has an hour to prepare for the case before it will commence.

> **Critical Thinking Questions**
>
> • Where could Rose go to source the necessary information to assist her with this case?
> • Identify the sequence of surgery for Mrs Peterson's procedure.

INSTRUMENTS

Surgical instruments are critical to the surgical procedure. There are many elements to learn regarding **instrumentation**, such as names, handling, function, intended use, cleaning, sterilisation and reassembly. All are very important; however, for many new nurses the most important element is to follow the progression of an operation and, through observation, learn which instruments are required for the various steps in the procedure, their function and names. This knowledge enhances the nurse's performance and leads to an ability to anticipate the surgeon's requirements throughout the operative procedure. In preparing instrumentation for an operation, the instrument nurse should check the sterility, working condition and completeness of the instruments being used. Instruments should only ever be used for their intended purpose.

Instrument Categories

Some basic manoeuvres are common to all surgical procedures. The surgeon dissects, resects or alters tissue and/or organs to restore or repair body functions or body parts (Phillips, 2017). Surgical instruments are designed to act as the tools that the surgeon needs for each manoeuvre and are categorised into the following groups:
• cutting and dissecting instruments

- debulking instruments
- grasping and holding instruments
- clamping and occluding instruments
- retracting and exposing instruments
- closure and approximation instruments
- scopes and viewing instruments
- powered surgical instruments
- micro instruments
- robotic instruments
- miscellaneous/ancillary/accessory: dilating, probing, measuring and aspiration instruments.

Anatomy of a ring-handled instrument

Some hinged instruments are ring handled to enable ease of holding, with the option of a ratchet to secure them in the closed position. The features of a ring-handled instrument are outlined below (see also Fig. 10.4).

- Tips should mesh together evenly when the instrument is closed.
- Jaws hold tissue or perioperative materials securely and the pattern of the jaws dictates its purpose. Artery clamps/forceps have a serrated pattern, whereas needle holders have a cross-hatched pattern.
- The box lock has a pin that holds the two sides of the instrument together.
- The shank is the area between the box lock and ring handles; the length is appropriate to the wound depth.
- Ratchets interlock to keep the jaws locked when the instrument is closed.
- Ring handles are for ease of holding.

Cutting and dissecting instruments

Sharp dissection. Sharp dissection is the process of tissue division by a sharp instrument that causes the least tissue damage (Myint & Kirk, 2019). Scalpels and scissors are used for sharp dissection (Myint & Kirk, 2019). Dissection can also be achieved by using a range of other technologies such as diathermy (electricity), laser (light waves), ultrasound dissection and cavitron ultrasonic surgical aspirator (CUSA) (sound waves), ligasure (vibration) and argon beam coagulation (gas-generated plasma beam) (Myint & Kirk, 2019), which are discussed under the electrosurgical equipment section of this chapter.

Scalpels. Various scalpel blades are available with configurations for different uses. The Bard Parker (BP) and Beaver scalpel handles hold disposable scalpel or knife blades. The Fischer tonsil, Smillie cartilage and myringotome scalpel handles incorporate the blade into the handle.

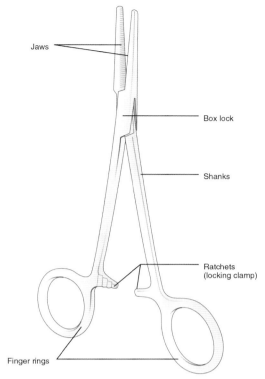

FIG. 10.4 Anatomy of a ring-handled clamp. (Source: Adapted from Fuller, J. K. (2018). *Surgical technology: principles and practice* (7th ed., Fig. 11.4, p. 225). St Louis, MO: Elsevier Saunders.)

Scalpel blades (and other sharp instruments) are a potential sharps hazard (refer to Chapter 5) and therefore should not be passed from hand to hand, and all handling of sharps should be reduced to a minimum to assist in the prevention of injury and infection to the healthcare worker (National Health and Medical Research Council [NHMRC], 2019). This can be achieved by strategies including providing verbal announcements when passing sharps and using a basin and neutral zone to pass sharps (the management of sharps is discussed later in this chapter, and in more detail in Chapter 5). The **neutral zone** is a designated area created to hold any sharp instrumentation in a receptacle or magnetic pad and is accessed by only one scrubbed person at a time (Cromb, 2019). The Australian College of Perioperative Nurses (ACORN) Standard for 'Sharps and preventing sharps-related injury' details the responsibility of healthcare workers to use these strategies when handling and passing sharp instruments as part of a multi-tiered approach to prevent sharps injuries in the perioperative environment (ACORN, 2020a). In certain surgical specialities, such as cardiac, vascular and neurosurgery, it is not possible to pass scalpel blades and atraumatic needles in this manner; hence, the instrument nurse should grasp the top of the scalpel handle and pass the scalpel with the handle towards the surgeon and the blade pointing downwards and back towards the instrument nurse. In such cases, a modified neutral zone should be used; the sharp is placed in the surgeon's hand and the surgeon returns the sharp to the neutral zone (Association of periOperative Registered Nurses [AORN], 2017).

Scissors. Scissors may open and close or have a spring action. The spring action provides better control and more precision, which is important when dissecting delicate tissues, such as those within the eye. Handles can be short or long, with blades straight or angled. Four basic types of scissors are available (Fig. 10.5):

- *Dissecting scissors* must have sharp edges, are commonly curved, and are available in several types. The curvature, weight and size vary according to the intended use. The two most commonly utilised are the Mayo (for dissection of heavy tissue, such as the fascia) and the much finer Metzenbaum scissors (for dissection of delicate tissue, such as intestine or blood vessels). There are various styles of scissors designed for each surgical specialty; for example, Potts scissors for vascular surgery have sharp-angled jaws.
- *Suture scissors* have round tips to prevent trauma to the delicate surrounding structures; the blades are most commonly straight. When holding suture scissors, the ring finger and thumb are placed into the ring handles, and the index finger is placed along the outside of the blade below the fulcrum (box join) to stabilise the scissors. If more stability is needed while cutting sutures, the fingers of the opposite hand may be placed under the box joint.
- *Dressing scissors* are heavier to prevent damage to the scissors themselves. They are designed to cut wound dressing, and should never be used for tissue dissection.
- *Wire cutters* are used to cut stainless steel wires; the blades are short and heavy similar to pliers.

Some other instruments that belong under the heading of sharp dissection instruments include bone-cutting instruments, such as chisels, gouges, rasps, osteotomes, files, drills, saws, rongeurs and bone nibblers. Curettes, biopsy forceps, punches, snares and dermatomes are also included in this category.

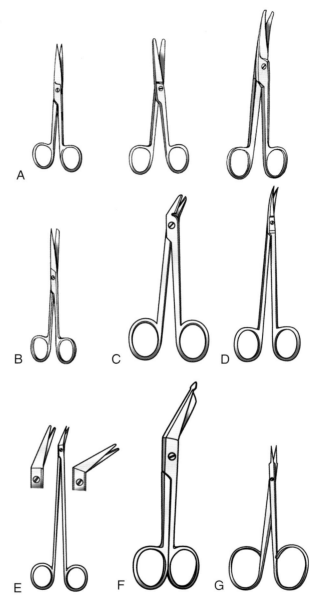

FIG. 10.5 Types of surgical scissors. (**A**) Tissue scissors. Blades may be straight or curved and either tip can be sharp or blunt. (**B**) Joseph nasal scissors. (**C**) Tenotomy scissors. (**D**) Wire suture scissors. (**E**) Lister bandage scissors. (**F**) Suture scissors. (**G**) Potts angled scissors. (Source: Phillips, N. (2017). *Berry & Kohn's operating room technique* (13th ed., Fig. 19.5, p. 327). St Louis, MO: Elsevier Mosby.)

Blunt dissection. Another form of separating tissues is blunt dissection. This involves separating or splitting tissues along a tissue plane without actively cutting. This allows the surgeon to follow a natural path, in contrast to sharp dissection, which creates a path. A range of instrumentation can be used in a blunt dissection technique, including scissors, 'peanuts' or gauze on a forcep, fingertips or even inserting closed dissectors and allowing them to open for a gentle blunt dissection technique. Blunt dissection can also be performed by a sponge-covered finger or the blunt edge of an instrument (Myint & Kirk, 2019).

Debulking instruments
Sharp dissection instruments such as curettes, osteotomes and files fall under the debulking category. Debulking instruments are used with the intent of decreasing the mass of firm tissue (Phillips, 2017).

Grasping and holding instruments
Grasping and holding instruments are used to grasp or hold onto tissue, sutures, swabs or drapes. They include:
• dissecting/tissue forceps
• towel clips
• sponge-holding forceps.
    When preparing instrumentation, the points of forceps should be checked to ensure that they are of equal length and that the teeth or serrations mesh smoothly and evenly when gently closed. The surgeon will grip the dissecting forceps like a pencil, with the tips pointing down. The instrument nurse should pass these forceps by holding the tips or the base of the forceps, allowing the surgeon to place his or her hand in the middle, ready for use.

Dissecting/tissue forceps. Dissecting/tissue forceps hold tissue to stabilise it so that the surgeon can perform a manoeuvre, such as dissecting or suturing, without injuring the surrounding tissues (Fig. 10.6A, B). One group of dissecting forceps have a tweezer-like action; they vary in length and are available as toothed or non-toothed (Fig. 10.6C–K). Toothed dissecting forceps have opposing 'spurs' or 'teeth' on either side of the jaws, which interlock to provide extra grip. Toothed dissecting forceps are most commonly used on thick, strong tissues, such as skin, muscle, cartilage and fascia. The size of the 'spurs' or 'teeth' on the forceps indicates the type of tissue each would be used for. For example, the Gillies forceps have finer teeth and are more likely to be used on the skin, whereas the thick heavy teeth of Bonney's forceps means that they are likely to be used for the fascia, cartilage or muscle. A common version of

the non-toothed variety is the DeBakey forceps, which are routinely used on delicate tissues, such as blood vessels, bowel, nerves and ureters.
    The other group of tissue forceps are ring handled and have a scissor action. They can be either *traumatic* or *atraumatic*. The Allis forceps have a row of teeth (traumatic) at the end to hold tissue gently but securely. The Babcock forceps have a smooth rounded end (atraumatic) that is designed to fit around a structure or to grasp tissue without injury, and are commonly used on the bowel or appendix. Other ring-handled forceps may be straight or curved (e.g. stone forceps), have sharp points (e.g. Lahey forceps) or have curved or angled points on the ends of the jaws (e.g. tenaculum, bone-holding forceps).

Towel clips. To secure drapes, diathermy quivers or other items in order to prevent them falling off or below the level of the aseptic field, towel clips are used. Care must be taken not to coil an active electrosurgical lead through the handles of the towel clip (or any metal instrument) to prevent current leakage through the lead (Pfiedler Education, 2018), which presents a patient safety risk as there is potential for a fire or a burn to the patient (Phillips, 2017). Some disposable drapes have loops for attaching the diathermy leads or the sucker tubing to the drapes without the need for towel clips.

Sponge-holding forceps. Sponge-holding forceps have several functions. Their most common use is to pick up swabs for skin preparation. Gauze squares can be wrapped around the tips to make what is referred to as a 'swab on a stick', which can be used to soak up fluid in a small space, for blunt dissection or for gentle retraction of tissues. The gauze squares used for a 'swab on a stick' must contain a radio-opaque marker that will show up on X-ray in the case of an incorrect count.

Clamping and occluding instruments
Clamps occlude, manipulate, crush or hold tissue and other material. Between the ring handles is a ratchet that is designed to lock the jaws onto tissue or other material. Within this category are artery clamps/forceps, and crushing and non-crushing clamps.

Artery clamps/forceps. Artery clamps/forceps occlude or clamp blood vessels and other tissue with minimal trauma because of the deep transverse serrations within the jaws. They come in different sizes and styles – straight, curved, short and long. The serrations should be cleanly cut and mesh together evenly as

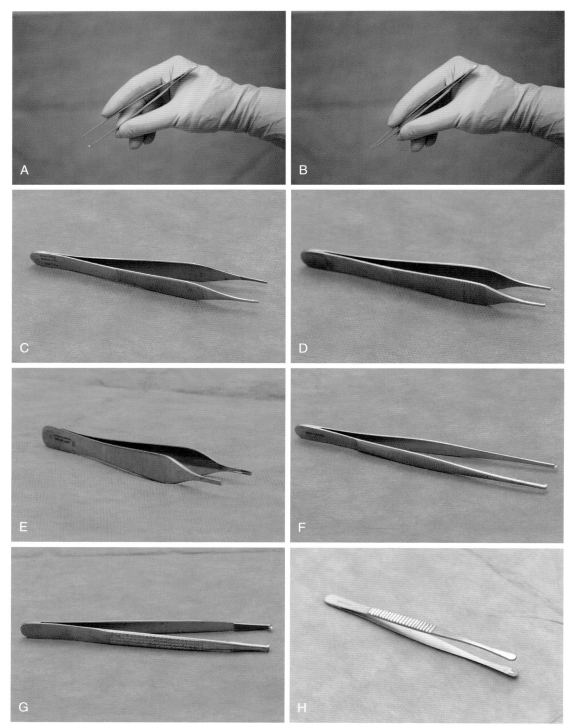

FIG. 10.6 Tissue graspers and forceps. (**A, B**) Proper technique to hold surgical graspers. (**C**) Adson forceps. (**D**) Forceps with teeth. (**E**) Adson forceps with teeth. (**F**) Bonney forceps. (**G**) Brown–Adson forceps. (**H**) Russian forceps.

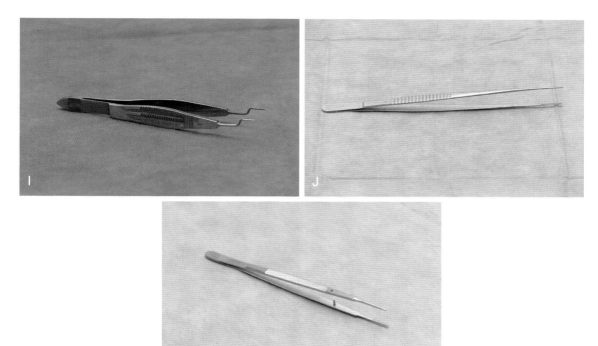

FIG. 10.6, cont'd (**I**) DeBakey forceps. (**J**) Bayonet Cushing forceps with teeth. (**K**) Gerald forceps. (Source: Hartman, C. J., & Kovoussi, L. R. (2018). *Handbook of surgical sequence* (Figs 5.1–5.10, p. 47). Philadelphia, PA: Elsevier.)

these serrations hold the tissues within the jaws of the clamp. Artery clamps/forceps must not be used for any reason other than that they are designed for. This rule applies to all instruments.

Crushing clamps. There are many variations of crushing clamps, all designed for a specific purpose. The jaws may be straight, curved or angled, and the serrations may be horizontal, diagonal or longitudinal. The tip may be pointed or rounded or have a tooth along the jaw, such as on a hysterectomy clamp. Some clamps are designed for use on specific organs, such as bowel clamps, which are used on bowel tissue that is diseased and requires dissection and removal.

Non-crushing clamps. Non-crushing clamps are designed to gently occlude a structure without causing injury to that structure. Non-crushing vascular clamps are used to occlude peripheral or major blood vessels temporarily (e.g. non-crushing vascular DeBakey clamps), which minimises tissue trauma. The jaws of

these clamps have opposing rows of finely serrated teeth and may be straight, curved, angled or S-shaped. Non-crushing bowel clamps are atraumatic and hold healthy bowel tissue without causing damage. These non-crushing clamps enable the bowel tissue and blood vessels to be re-anastomosed.

Retracting and exposing instruments
Retractors hold back wound layers and anatomical structures to allow visualisation of the operative site; they can be manual hand-held or self-retaining (Figs 10.7 and 10.8). There are two types of self-retaining retractors: those that attach to a frame, such as the Bookwalter, Omni-Tract and Lone Star retractors; and those that are held in place by a ratchet, such as the Weitlander and Gelpi retractors. Self-retaining retractors should be handed to the surgeon in the closed position. Hand-held retractors usually come in pairs and can be single or double ended, traumatic or atraumatic, with a variety of shapes and sizes (e.g. skin hooks, cat's paw, rakes, Czerny, Langenbeck and Deaver retractors).

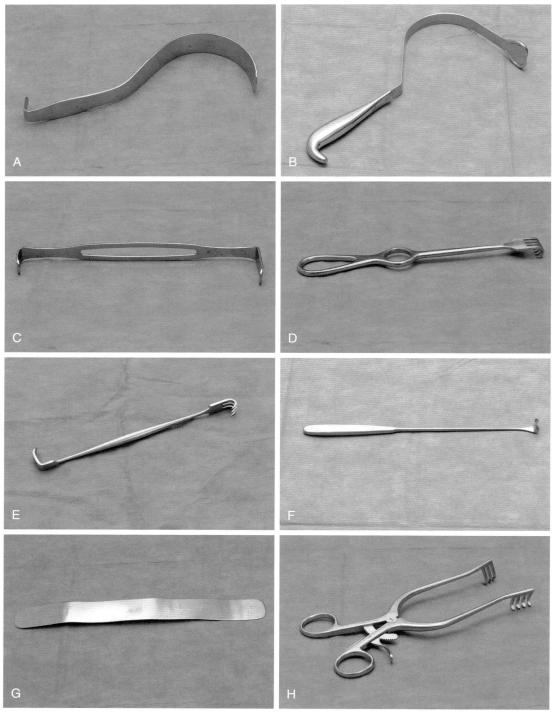

FIG. 10.7 Manual retractors. (**A**) Deaver retractor. (**B**) Volkman (rake) retractor. (**C**) Harrington (sweetheart) retractor. (**D**) Senn retractor. (**E**) Army–navy retractor. (**F**) Cushing vein retractor. (**G**) Weitlaner retractor. (**H**) Ribbon (malleable) retractor.

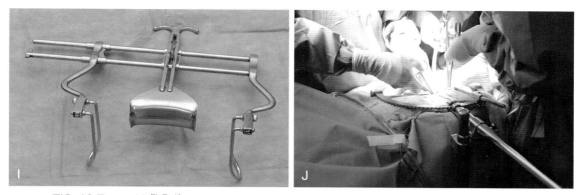

FIG. 10.7, cont'd **(I)** Balfour retractor with centre blade attached . **(J)** Bookwalter retractor system. (Source: Hartman, C. J., & Kovoussi, L. R. (2018). *Handbook of surgical sequence* (Figs 5.48–5.58, pp. 56–58). Philadelphia, PA: Elsevier.)

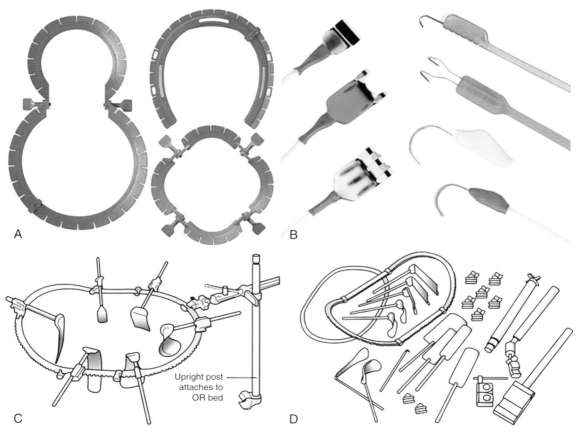

FIG. 10.8 Self-retaining retractors. **(A)** Lone Star retractor. **(B)** Lone Star retractor stays. **(C)** Bookwalter retractor assembled. **(D)** Bookwalter retractor disassembled. (Sources: (A, B) Reproduced with permission of Cooper Surgical https://www.coopersurgical.com/detail/lone-star-self-retaining-retractors-disposable-2/; (C, D) Phillips, N. (2017). *Berry & Kohn's operating room technique* (13th ed., Fig. 19.28, p. 334). St Louis, MO: Elsevier Mosby.)

At the beginning and end of the surgical count, any retractor with screws or extra blades must be checked and accounted for to ensure that no items or loose parts are retained within the patient. Recommendations based on a review of sentinel events due to retention of materials in surgery by the Victorian Surgical Consultative Council (2019) state that 'All detachable components of an instrument/retractor should be included in the surgical count'. Staff need to ensure they are familiar with the counting procedures/guidelines for their healthcare facility.

Closure and approximation instruments
Needle holders. Needle holders grasp a suture needle securely so that it can be passed through tissues without moving (Fig. 10.9). The pattern is cross-hatched rather than grooved, and provides a smoother surface to enable a good grip on the needle. This pattern also

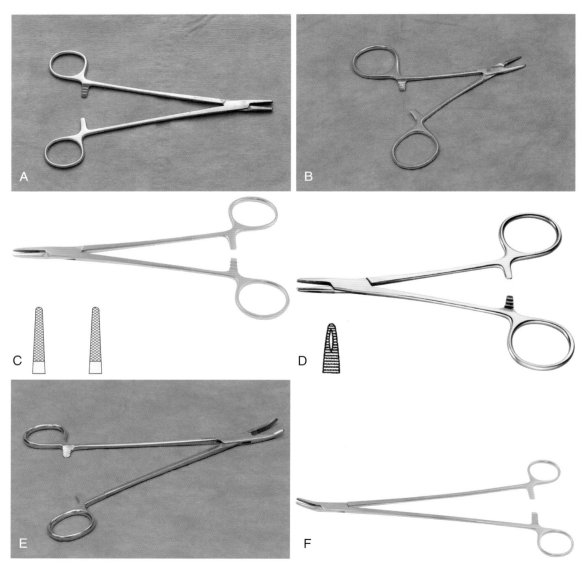

FIG. 10.9 Needle holders. (**A**) Mayo–Hegar needle holder. (**B**) Webster needle holder. (**C**) Crile–Wood needle holder. (**D**) Olsen–Hegar needle holder. (**E**) Collier needle holder. (**F**) Finochietto needle holder.

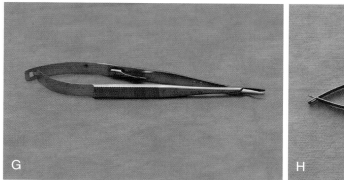
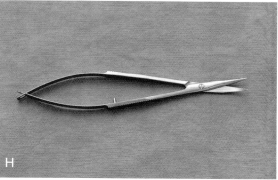

FIG. 10.9, cont'd (**G**) Heaney needle holder. (**H**) Castroviejo needle holder. (Source: Hartman, C. J., & Kovoussi, L. R. (2018). *Handbook of surgical sequence* (Figs 5.31–5.38, pp. 52–53). Philadelphia, PA: Elsevier.)

prevents rotation and flattening of the needle, which inhibits damage to the needle. Needle holders can be straight or curved. Most have a ratchet; however, in some surgical specialties (e.g. cardiac, ophthalmology and vascular surgery) they have spring-action handles. The spring-action handle on a needle holder provides a much smoother, gentler motion for the surgeon. Another style of non-ratcheted needle holder incorporates scissors within the shaft of the needle holder for ease of cutting sutures. This style is often favoured by plastic surgeons, who use these needle holders when there are many individual sutures needed to approximate a wound, thus minimising surgical time.

The general rule of thumb is: the length of the needle holder is determined by the depth of the wound, and the physical size of the suture needle indicates the size of the jaws of the needle holder required. For example, a fine needle requires small jaws and a large needle needs larger jaws. Inappropriate selection of the needle holder will damage either the instrument or the needle being used.

Sutures and needles. Sutures, needles and their associated properties and usages are discussed in detail in Chapter 11.

Staplers and clip appliers. A reusable clip applicator (Fig. 10.10) can be used to load single clips to mark or occlude vessels and structures. Preloaded multi-clip applicators are also available (Phillips, 2017).

Surgical staplers can be used to cut, resect, anastomose and connect structures, and are commonly used in gastrointestinal, thoracic and gynaecological surgery (Cromb, 2019) (Fig. 10.11). Surgical staplers can be

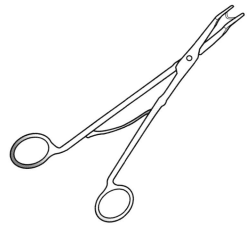

FIG. 10.10 A reusable clip applicator. (Source: Phillips, N. (2017). *Berry & Kohn's operating room technique* (13th ed., Fig. 19.32, p. 339). St Louis, MO: Elsevier Mosby.)

designed for both laparoscopic and open procedures and can be classified as circular, end-to-end anastomosis (EEA), linear GIA (Medtronic) or NTLC (Ethicon linear cutter), terminal end, L-shaped (used for closing the end of stomach or bowel) and contour curve (Ethicon), a curved L-shaped stapler designed for lower pelvic transection (Ethicon, 2019; Medtronic, 2020; Phillips, 2017).

Internal anastomosis staplers are used to connect two hollow organs which are aligned side by side; one end of the stapler is inserted into each tube and, as the stapler is activated, some styles have a blade that cuts as it staples and anastomoses the two structures (Phillips, 2017).

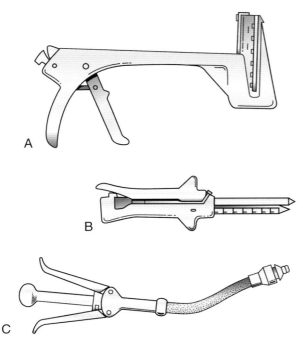

FIG. 10.11 Internal staplers. (**A**) Terminal end stapler. (**B**) Internal anastomosis stapler. (**C**) End-to-end stapler. (Source: Phillips, N. (2017). *Berry & Kohn's operating room technique* (13th ed., Fig. 19.33, p. 340). St Louis, MO: Elsevier Mosby.)

End-to-end staplers are often circular staplers which anastomose two hollow tubular structures end to end, and are used most commonly for bowel anastomosis. The ends of the stapler are inserted into the tubular structures from both the proximal and distal ends. As the ends of the stapler close, a double row of staples is fired, and a blade in the stapler trims the rim from both ends of bowel. Once the stapler is separated, both of the rims (known as donuts) – one from the proximal end and one from the distal end – are sent to pathology (Phillips, 2017). Further advances in technology have seen staplers such as the Signia, which transects, resects and anastomoses using adaptive firing technology (Medtronic 2020) and which is responsive to the force applied.

Scopes and viewing instruments
Viewing instruments allow the surgeon to examine hollow structures, organs and cavities, with some viewing instruments allowing operative procedures to be performed through them. Examples of viewing instruments include endoscopes (which can be rigid or flexible) and speculums (used to hold open and view a canal such as the ear or vagina) (Phillips, 2017).

Powered surgical instruments
Powered instruments are primarily used to saw, drill and shape bone, or in plastic surgery to harvest skin grafts (Phillips, 2017).

Micro-instruments
Micro-instruments are miniature instruments designed to function with precision on the delicate tissue in microsurgery. Many micro-instruments are spring loaded, the design of which enables ease of handling and activation by the surgeon, as well as optimising the view of the surgical field (Phillips, 2017).

Robotic instruments
Robotic instrumentation has the same function and tips as minimally invasive laparoscopic instrumentation. Above the tip is the 'wrist' of the instrument, which robotically articulates in response to movements and inputs from the surgeon (Cromb, 2019) (Figs 10.12 and 10.13). Robotic instruments are used in the da Vinci robotic system and Mako robotic-arm assisted surgery, discussed later in this chapter.

Miscellaneous/ancillary/accessory instruments
The miscellaneous category contains instruments that do not fit into any other category by virtue of their function. These include suction and aspiration tips – for example, Poole suckers, Yankauer suckers and Fraser suckers with trocars (obturators and sheathes). Other accessory instruments include dilators and probes, measuring instruments, mallets and screwdrivers (Phillips, 2017).

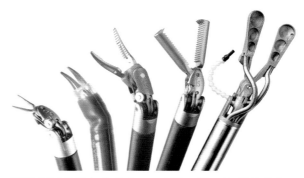

FIG. 10.12 Robotic instrumentation. (Source: Ball, K. A. (2019). Surgical modalities. In J. C. Rothrock & D. L. McEwen (Eds.), *Alexander's care of the patient in surgery* (16th ed., Fig. 8.35, p. 219). St Louis, MO: Elsevier.)

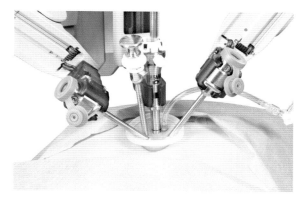

FIG. 10.13 Robotic single-incision port for multiple instruments. (Source: Ball, K. A. (2019). Surgical modalities. In J. C. Rothrock & D. L. McEwen (Eds.), *Alexander's care of the patient in surgery* (16th ed., Fig. 8.36, p. 219). St Louis, MO: Elsevier.)

Instrument Handling and Passing

Instrument exchange occurs with the instrument nurse focusing on the instrument to be handed and passing the instrument directly into the surgeon's hand, leaving the surgeon to focus on the surgical field (Table 10.2 and Fig. 10.14). The position of the instrument nurse and instrument table/trolley depends on the **operating room (OR) layout** and subsequent traffic patterns (Fig. 10.15). OR designs are discussed in Chapter 5. Other determinants include:

- the positioning of the set-up in an area with minimal traffic flow
- the position of other members of the perioperative team (e.g. surgeon, anaesthetist)
- the site and side of the surgical procedure to be performed.

As a general rule, the instrument nurse stands opposite the surgeon and beside the assistant for ease of instrument passing and maximum visibility.

TABLE 10.2
Instrument Passing Techniques to Consider

Skill	Considerations for Instrument Nurse	Rationale
Passing instruments with adequate pressure	Pass in a deliberate and committed manner Use a small amount of pressure	Weak pressure when passing an instrument creates a distraction of uncertainty and the potential for the surgeon to unnecessarily look away from the aseptic field
Providing a slight pause when passing an instrument	Provide a slight pause as the surgeon takes the instrument to ensure the surgeon has a proper grasp of the instrument	No pause technique can lead to unstable transfer and the likelihood of dropping the instrument A grabbing technique can lead to injury Allows the instrument nurse to remove the passing hand from the transfer zone
Minimising handling of instruments	Count and place instruments where they will be needed for the duration of the operation Place instruments in the surgeon's hand ready for use without repositioning	Deliberate planned movements decrease handling, ensure that instruments can be retrieved quickly and decrease the potential for dropping the instruments Instruments are passed in a way that they are ready for immediate use and do not have to be repositioned
Passing sharps	Transfer sharps using an established neutral zone or designated receptacle If the type of surgery prevents this practice, place one hand over the scalpel handle with the blade facing down and back towards the nurse	This establishes safe practices for all the surgical team and decreases the potential for needle-stick injury A risk assessment appropriate to the specialty surgery will determine the technique most appropriate for safe transfer of sharps
Passing ring-handled instruments	Hold instruments by the box joint with the tips facing up and the curve of the instrument ready to face towards the centre of the surgeon's hand	The instrument curve is passed so that it is positioned ready for immediate use The instrument is held at the box joint so that the surgeon can grasp it easily by the ring handles, ready to use

Continued

TABLE 10.2
Instrument Passing Techniques to Consider—cont'd

Skill	Considerations for Instrument Nurse	Rationale
Selecting the correct instruments	Select the type and length of the instrument that will be suitable for the task	Using large instruments for delicate surgery is more likely to cause tissue damage Using delicate instruments for dense tissue is more likely to lead to instrument damage Short instruments will not reach deep wounds Long instruments are unstable on superficial wounds
Recognising and passing complementary instruments together	Some instruments may require a complementary instrument (e.g. scissors *and* forceps, needle holder *and* forceps) If the surgeon asks for an instrument automatically hand the complementary instrument as well	Assists in reducing operating time
Two-handed passing (ambidextrous)	When using complementary instrumentation, place one instrument in one hand and the other in the other hand Use both hands to pass the instruments simultaneously to the surgeon Do not cross over hands on passing	Passing two instruments at the same time: • decreases the instrument nurse's impact on the surgical space • decreases instrument handling and movement • decreases the surgical time

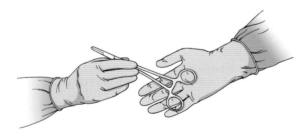

FIG. 10.14 Passing an instrument. (Source: Phillips, N. (2017). *Berry & Kohn's operating room technique* (13th ed., Fig. 19.46, p. 343). St Louis, MO: Elsevier Mosby.)

The layout of the instrument table will vary depending on the operation, the hospital's practice and the teaching staff within the perioperative environment. A key consideration is to strive for standardisation so that the nurse always knows where the instruments are for every case. The relevant instruments needed for the procedure should be prioritised so that those used most frequently are placed in closest reach (Fig. 10.16). Points to consider are as follows:

• The Mayo table (if used) should contain those instruments that are used frequently (Fig. 10.17).
• Although the Mayo table is placed in close proximity to the surgical field, it is the instrument nurse who manages the flow of instruments to and from the Mayo table. Self-selection from the Mayo table by the surgical team should be discouraged owing to the risk of sharps injury and/or misplacement of items. A neutral zone on the Mayo table will be of benefit to the team, particularly if the instrument nurse is unable to assist.
• Similar instruments should be placed together (e.g. varying sizes of artery clamps, various tissue forceps).
• The tips of instruments should face the centre of the Mayo table so that all the tips can be easily seen; the tips should not face out to prevent inadvertent injury. Box joints should be more towards the centre of the table for ease of grasp.
• Instruments that are not commonly needed should be placed on the instrument tray and table furthest away to allow more room for surgical items that are needed more frequently (e.g. sponges, sutures, wet sponge for cleaning instruments).
• More instrument tables may be required for more-complex procedures or if it is necessary to have clean and contaminated areas to demarcate any contaminated instruments (e.g. in bowel surgery).

Care of Instrumentation

Instruments are very expensive, but they can last a long time if they are properly cared for and maintained.

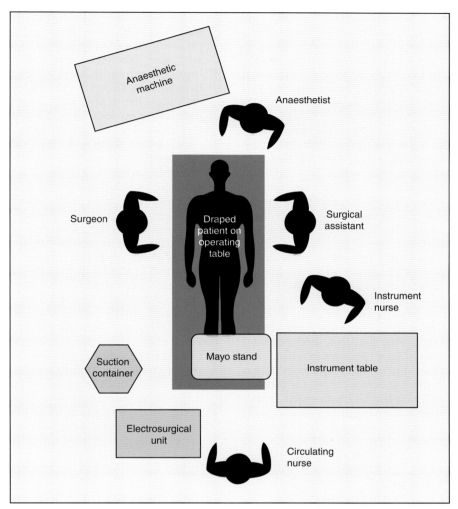

FIG. 10.15 Layout of the operating room showing sterile field, team members and unsterile equipment.

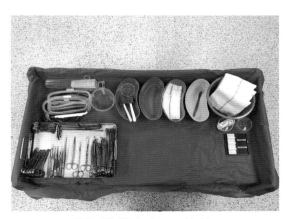

FIG. 10.16 Instrument table.

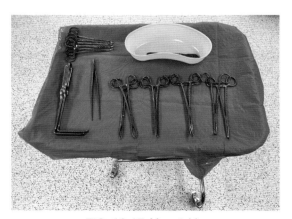

FIG. 10.17 Mayo table.

Patients deserve the best possible care and this care extends to the provision of clean, functioning instruments (Spear, 2018).

General rules apply to the care of instrumentation that are particularly relevant to the scenario of Mr James Collins, undergoing a right TKR (see the following Scenario). The instrument nurse for Mr Collins should ensure the following:

- Forceps, clamps and other hinged instruments are inspected at the beginning and end of the procedure to ensure that the jaws or teeth align, and they have no defects and function properly.
- Instruments are used for their intended purpose only. Scissors or clamps that are misused can be forced out of alignment and break. Curved tissue scissors that are used to cut sutures or dressings will soon become blunt.
- Blood and/or tissue is wiped off instruments, including powered tools, intraoperatively using a moistened sponge (Goodman & Spry, 2017). Bone fragments should be removed from reamers after each use. Excess tissue should be cleaned out of reamers and broaches between each use (Fuller, 2018). Blood or tissue that dries, becomes hard on the serrations of jaws or blades of scissors and impairs the function of the instrument makes cleaning more difficult postoperatively and causes instruments to become stiff and damaged. Instruments with lumens or channels (e.g. Frazier suckers) should be irrigated periodically, intraoperatively, to prevent blockages.

- Powered instruments used in Mr Collins' case are heavy and must be stored and passed with caution to avoid injury and inadvertent activation. The safety switch should be activated when not in use.
- Instruments used in Mr Collins' surgery should have the least amount of visible soil as possible at the conclusion of the case and should be sent for reprocessing as soon as possible after surgery. If there is a delay in this occurring, an enzymatic spray, gel or foam may be used to treat the instruments to prevent biofilm forming on them (Goodman & Spry, 2017).
- Damaged or blunt instruments should be set aside for repair or replacement (Goodman & Spry, 2017).
- Lighter instruments should always be kept on top of heavier instruments (Goodman & Spry, 2017).
- Sharp instruments should be separated (Spear, 2018). Sharp edges and pointed tips should be protected so that staff members responsible for cleaning are not injured.
- Instruments should be handled gently at all times and should not be thrown, bounced or dropped.

Additionally, for cases using delicate instruments and cables:

- Delicate or microsurgery instruments should be kept separate from other instrumentation. Heavy instruments should never be placed on top of delicate or microsurgery instruments.
- Fibreoptic cables should be coiled loosely and placed on top of or separated from other instrumentation.

PATIENT SCENARIOS

SCENARIO 10.2: INSTRUMENT NURSE'S ROLE – INSTRUMENT HANDLING

Surgical instruments are described as the 'tools of the trade'.

Critical Thinking Questions

- Why is it important for the instrument nurse to have in-depth knowledge of the design, structure and anatomy of surgical instruments?
- If a surgeon asks RN Pereira to pass them a scissor, what factors would she consider in selecting an appropriate type of scissor to pass? Consider when curved scissors may be used and when straight scissors would be used.

Electrosurgical Equipment

Electrosurgical devices work either by converting energy from a high-frequency electrical current into heat that can cut and cauterise tissue or by using light, sound or vibration to achieve the same effect. These devices have specific hazards associated with their use, and are often governed by safety standards, which are outlined in Chapter 5. The most common electrosurgical device used in perioperative practice is the electrosurgical unit (ESU, or **diathermy** machine). The ESU generates an electrical current at extremely high frequency, which cuts or coagulates tissue (as well as variations of the latter, such as tissue desiccation or fulguration), controlling blood loss in the surgical field (Aminimoghaddam, Pahlevani, & Kazemi, 2018; Golpaygani, Movahedi, & Reza, 2016). There are two main types of diathermy: monopolar and bipolar, both of which have unique applications (Ball, 2019).

Monopolar diathermy

In **monopolar** diathermy, the current is usually applied to the tissue through the use of a small hand-held electrode, termed the 'active' electrode. This may be in the form of a 'diathermy' pencil, blade, forceps, needlepoint, loop or ball depending on the surgery being performed (Ball, 2019). The surgeon activates the current to cut or coagulate tissue by means of a switch on the 'pencil', or using a foot pedal during closed urology or laparoscopic surgery, for example. The current then flows through the patient and exits via the patient return electrode, which is in contact with the patient's body, returning it to the ESU to complete the electrical circuit (Fig. 10.18). The patient return electrode may be an adhesive pad, which contains conductive gel (Fig. 10.19), or a large mat placed under the patient (Fig. 10.20) (Ball, 2019). Feature box 10.1 details the patient return electrode, and Feature box 10.2 summarises information on safe use of electrosurgery.

Bipolar diathermy

Bipolar diathermy uses a pair of fine forceps controlled by the surgeon via a foot pedal (Ball, 2019). It is commonly used for coagulation of minor blood vessels in neurosurgery, plastic surgery or paediatric surgery. In this mode, the current flows down one tine of the forceps across the tissue that is grasped between the forceps and returns to the ESU through the opposing tine

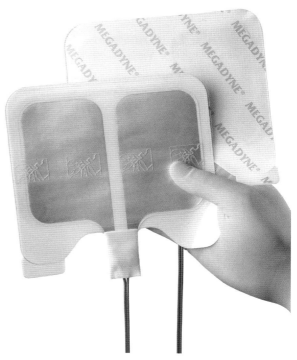

FIG. 10.19 Single-use patient return electrode split pad. (Source: Ball, K. A. (2019). Surgical modalities. In J. C. Rothrock & D. L. McEwen (Eds.), *Alexander's care of the patient in surgery* (16th ed., Fig. 8.44, p. 225). St Louis, MO: Elsevier.)

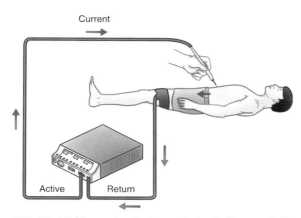

FIG. 10.18 Monopolar electrosurgical unit. (Source: Ball, K. A. (2019). Surgical modalities. In J. C. Rothrock & D. L. McEwen (Eds.), *Alexander's care of the patient in surgery* (16th ed., Fig. 8.41, p. 223). St Louis, MO: Elsevier.)

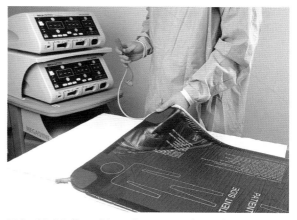

FIG. 10.20 Reusable patient return electrode capacitive pad. (Source: Ball, K. A. (2019). Surgical modalities. In J. C. Rothrock & D. L. McEwen (Eds.), *Alexander's care of the patient in surgery* (16th ed., Fig. 8.45, p. 225). St Louis, MO: Elsevier.)

FEATURE BOX 10.1
Application of the Patient Return Electrode

Patient return electrodes (also known as dispersive electrodes or diathermy plates) may be single-use adhesive plates (see Fig. 10.19) or reusable mats also known as capacitive pads (see Fig. 10.20). Depending on local policy, the patient return electrode may be positioned by a patient care assistant (PCA) or an orderly. In this circumstance, the nurse is responsible for confirming the correct placement of the electrode (or patient contact with mat) and the condition of the patient's skin following removal of the electrode.

The following safety points must be followed when positioning the patient on a capacitive pad:

- Place a sheet between the patient and the capacitive pad.
- Avoid pooling of fluids, such as antiseptic or alcoholic skin preparations and solutions, and remove any damp materials prior to draping.

The following safety points must be followed when positioning the patient return electrode:

- Select an appropriate patient return electrode for the patient's age and size.
- Ensure skin is dry and free of hair to enable good contact between skin and patient return electrode.
- Select well-vascularised tissue such as muscle (e.g. outer thigh or buttock) and avoid bony protuberances, scar tissue and implants as these do not provide a sufficient safe area of vascularised tissue.
- Place the patient return electrode as close as possible to the site of surgery.
- Apply the patient return electrode after patient positioning whenever possible and re-assess if the patient is re-positioned.
- Avoid pooling of fluids, such as antiseptic or alcohoiic skin preparations and solutions, and remove any damp materials prior to draping.

(Source: Australian College of Perioperative Nurses. (2020b). *Standards for perioperative nursing in Australia* (16th ed., Vol. 1) Clinical standards – electrosurgical equipment. Adelaide: Author.)

FEATURE BOX 10.2
Safe Use of Electrosurgery Devices

Due to the potential risk of injury and fire when using electrosurgery equipment, the perioperative nurse should follow these safety considerations:

DO:
- Ensure all staff using the equipment are trained in the use of the specific device.
- Minimise the risks of exposure to the hazards of surgical plume by using appropriate evacuation equipment and techniques whenever energy-based devices are activated (see Fig. 10.22).
- Use the lowest required power setting.
- Ensure alarm settings remain audible at all times.
- Place foot pedals in an impervious cover when the risk of fluid exposure is high (e.g. closed urology surgery).
- *Always* inspect and confirm adequacy of the insulation when using minimally invasive surgical instruments.
- *Always* use cannula systems made from the same material, either all metal or all plastic.
- Place the electrosurgical device in the holster/quiver when not in use.
- Use separate holsters/quivers for each device.
- Clean the active electrode regularly to prevent build-up of blood, tissue or eschar.
- Be cautious using the electrosurgical device in the presence of flammable liquids (e.g. alcoholic prep solutions) and anaesthetic gases.

DO NOT:
- Place any fluids on the ESU.
- Tightly coil or loop the cable of the electrosurgical device.
- Use combined metal and plastic cannula systems.

(Source: Australian College of Perioperative Nurses. (2020b). *Standards for perioperative nursing in Australia* (16th ed., Vol. 1) Clinical standards – electrosurgical equipment. Adelaide: Author.)

(Fig. 10.21). This mode does not require a patient return electrode.

Related electrosurgical equipment

Additional electrosurgical devices are available that incorporate enhanced haemostatic features – for example, an argon beam coagulator. This device combines argon gas with electrosurgery to improve the effectiveness of the coagulation mode by producing rapid haemostasis that creates a thinner, more flexible eschar, allowing the surgeon greater visibility (Phillips, 2017).

Alongside electricity, the use of ultrasonic technology to achieve haemostasis is now commonplace within the OR. Ultrasonic technology uses high-frequency sound waves to cut and coagulate tissue (Ball, 2019). A handpiece held by the surgeon converts electrical energy into a mechanical vibration, at a range of 20–25 kHz to 55,000 kHz, depending on the type of tissue to be treated. Tissue is vaporised in a very precise manner, resulting in less damage to surrounding tissue, with none of the dangers associated with electrical currents used in electrosurgery because no

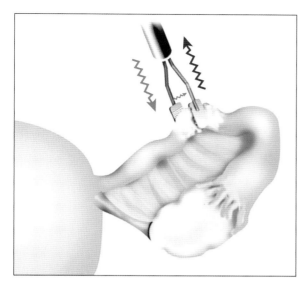

FIG. 10.21 The current form in the electrosurgical unit (ESU) flows through an insulated conductor of the bipolar forceps to exert its thermal action on the tissue. The current flows from the active jaw (electrode) to the inactive (neutral) jaw of the electrode. The current flows back to the ESU via the insulated neural limb of the bipolar forceps. Note that current flow to tissue is limited to that which is enclosed between active and neutral electrodes (forceps jaws). (Source: Baggish, M. S., & Karram, M. M. (2016). *Atlas of pelvic anatomy and gynecologic surgery* (4th ed.). Philadelphia, PA: Elsevier.)

electricity passes to or through the patient (Ball, 2019). Other ultrasonic devices such as the cavitron ultrasonic surgical aspirator (CUSA) combine irrigation and aspiration into the handpiece to facilitate dissection and removal of specific coagulated tissue. This selective dissection is advantageous when removing tumours from surrounding structures such as vessels and nerves (Hao et al., 2016). Ultrasonic energy is advantageous because it produces only a small amount of aerosolisation, no surgical plume or odour and no stray energy (Ball, 2019).

Laser

Laser is a unique form of light energy that is concentrated into a narrow beam of a single wavelength, with specific characteristics that allow it to cut, coagulate, vaporise or disrupt tissue. The effects of the laser on tissue depend on its wavelength, its absorption in water, melanin or haemoglobin, power output, focal length and size of the beam, as well as the type of device used to deliver the energy to the surgical field.

Lasers can pose numerous safety hazards. Stringent national and professional standards for laser safety provide means for controlling the associated hazards and, therefore, help to minimise risks to perioperative personnel; these are discussed in detail in Chapter 5.

Surgical Plume and Evacuation Devices

Surgical plume is produced when biological tissue is disrupted or vaporised by energy-based surgical equipment such as electrosurgical and ultrasonic devices, lasers (ACORN, 2020c; Smalley, 2019; Tan & Russell, 2017) and high-speed surgical drills and saws (Ministry of Health, NSW, 2015). The resultant plume is hazardous to staff and patients, so must be evacuated from the surgical field (ACORN 2020c). The specific hazards of surgical plume are outlined in Chapter 5.

Surgical plume evacuation units (Fig. 10.22) extract, capture and filter the plume via an array of systems, each designed to be compatible with a variety of surgical procedures and instrumentation. It is important to obtain devices that are appropriate for each facility's surgical services. Plume evacuation systems should be positioned in every room, and used in every case where an energy-based device is to be used (ACORN, 2020c; Ball, 2019). The capture inlet (hand-held tubing, diathermy pencil, active or passive laparoscopy filters, etc.) should be positioned no more than a few centimetres from where the plume is being generated, and without interfering with visibility or access to the surgical site (Standards Australia, 2015). Wall suction, floor canisters, fluid capture devices or standard suction tips (e.g. Yankauer suction tips) must never be used to suction surgical plume. If wall suction must be used, an in-line filter with ultra-low particulate air (ULPA) filtration (0.12 μm) must be installed between the wall outlet and the canister system (Standards Australia, 2015).

SHARPS SAFETY

Policies to minimise the risk of sharps injuries for healthcare workers are discussed in detail in Chapter 5. Considerations for sharps safety in the perioperative environment include the following:
- Use safety needles/devices wherever possible.
- Use puncture-resistant containers and/or a neutral zone within the aseptic field when transferring sharps (e.g. scalpels, sutures and other sharp equipment) from the instrument nurse to the surgeon.
- Do not recap needles after use.
- Remove scalpel blades in accordance with AS/NZS 3825: 1998 (Standards Australia, 1998).

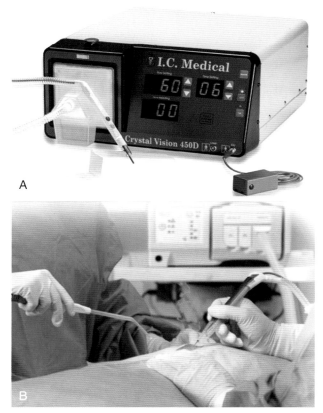

A

B

FIG. 10.22 (**A**) Surgical plume evacuator and diathermy pencils. (**B**) Atmos surgical plume evacuator in use. (Sources: (A) Big Green Surgical Company, Crystal Vision Model 450-D brochure. https://651daef9-40d5-41a8-b777-d6993c7ff55f.filesusr.com/ugd/8bd03c_67cf27f6db524dd8a6717a54f9299f1f.pdf; (B) Medica https://www.medica.de.)

- Dispose of blades as soon as possible and as close to the point of use as possible. Blades should not be removed by hand or using the resheathing method. Instead, they should be removed from the instrument using a safety-engineered medical device and in accordance with the manufacturer's advice (ACORN, 2020a).
- Use magnetic needle mats to store and dispose of needles and blades.
- Surgeons should use designated instruments for retracting tissue, rather than their hands, to prevent accidental sharps injuries, and blunt suture needles and disposable stapling equipment to minimise the risks involved in using hand-held sutures to anastomose tissue.
- Encourage good communication between surgical team members to ensure that sharps are not left unattended within the aseptic field (ACORN, 2020a).

- Wear two sets of gloves (double gloving) to minimise sharps injuries. Wearing a second pair of gloves has been shown to provide added protection against puncturing the inner gloves (ACORN, 2020a; Cromb, 2019; Wilson, 2019).

NEW TECHNOLOGY IN THE OPERATING THEATRE

Technology is constantly evolving and enhancing new surgical procedures, which require specific medical devices and products. Indeed, surgical innovations and advances in imaging technology over the past 50 years have revolutionised the way that diagnostic and surgical procedures are being carried out (Hughes-Hallett, Mayer, Pratt, Vale, & Darzi, 2015). Surgery is becoming less invasive, faster, more automated and technically

FEATURE BOX 10.3
Technological Advances in the Operating Suite

Clinical practice is changing with the progression of surgical tools and the increase of data available for the surgeon to replace traditional techniques with minimally invasive surgery (MIS), single-incision laparoscopic surgery (SILS), natural-orifice transluminal endoscopic surgery (NOTES), robotic surgery and telesurgery. A wide variety of surgical systems such as robots, navigation, 3D imaging, radiology and ultrasonography will integrate together in the future and provide increased quality and throughput of healthcare (Bernado, 2017). Robotic technology is also being used as part of routine cleaning regimens, which can take 1 to 3 hours to complete depending on the size of the room and can be performed during the night when the room is not in use (King & Spry, 2019).

With the introduction of new technology in the operating room (OR), there can be additional patient safety risks to be managed such as those related to robotic-assisted surgery (RAS) (see section on advances in minimally invasive surgery later in this chapter). When working with robotic technology, the surgeon is physically separated from the rest of the team and, in this setting, communication is extremely important to ensure good teamwork and coordination of care. Perioperative nurses should also seek to play an active role in evaluations of new products and devices to help ensure safe, quality care and intended patient outcomes are met (Saletnik, 2018). Education and training in the use of all new technology is important for perioperative nurses. This should be combined with an awareness that the patient's safety will always be the central nursing consideration, whether the workplace is an ageing facility, an outlying area with minimal resources and limited technology or an increasingly technical environment such as a hybrid OR (Luck & Gillespie, 2017).

gynaecological; ear, nose and throat; urological; cardiovascular/thoracic; plastic; orthopaedic and neurosurgery (Ball, 2019). MIS uses small incisions or no incisions, telescopes, cameras and fibreoptic light leads to assist the surgeon to visualise the procedure. The incisions are so small that they are typically closed with one or two sutures.

MIS has progressed immensely over the past decade and will continue to change as more surgical procedures are performed in this manner. The advantages of MIS for patients are considered to outweigh those of open surgery and include:
- smaller surgical scars
- less trauma to the body
- decreased postoperative pain and thus less requirement for pain relief
- shorter recovery period
- quicker return to normal activities (Ball, 2019).

Consequently, many complex cases such as hysterectomy, nephrectomy and hemi-colectomy can now be undertaken either completely laparoscopically or laparoscopically assisted. However, minimally invasive surgical procedures are not without their risks to the patient. The length of operating time is frequently longer than the equivalent 'open' surgical procedure, thereby increasing anaesthesia time, which may have an impact on patient outcomes (Ball, 2019). Serious complications of endoscopy include perforation of a major vessel or organ, bleeding from a biopsy site or any area where tissue has been cut or when endoscopic sutures or clips have become dislodged, and moderate or severe hypothermia (Phillips, 2017). There are also some significant disadvantages for the surgeon, which, on occasion, can lead to the procedure becoming an open surgical procedure. These include:
- restricted vision
- difficulty handling the instruments
- restricted mobility of tissues.

In the case of abdominal MIS, all patients should be prepped and draped and instrumentation and consumables readily available for conversion to an open surgical procedure when warranted because of recognised or potential complications (Ball, 2019).

Sequence of Surgery for Abdominal MIS
As with open surgery, MIS follows a generalised sequence of surgery. The three broad sequences involved are shown in Fig. 10.23.

Access and Exposure
Pneumoperitoneum is the introduction of carbon dioxide into the peritoneal cavity: filling the cavity with

more advanced than ever before, with the ability to image, navigate and visualise with increasing accuracy and definition. Feature box 10.3 outlines some of the recent technological advances in perioperative practice.

MINIMALLY INVASIVE SURGERY
The development of **minimally invasive surgery** (MIS) has been one of the most dramatic advancements in surgery over the past few decades and has evolved from a diagnostic modality to a widespread surgical technique (Ball, 2019). MIS can be referred to as endoscopic, telescopic, laparoscopic or keyhole surgery. MISs are prevalent in all fields of surgery on almost all anatomical areas, including bariatric; general;

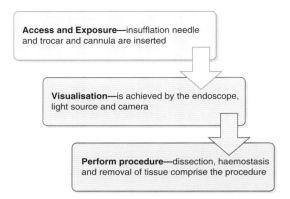

Access and Exposure—insufflation needle and trocar and cannula are inserted

↓

Visualisation—is achieved by the endoscope, light source and camera

↓

Perform procedure—dissection, haemostasis and removal of tissue comprise the procedure

FIG. 10.23 Sequence of surgery for an abdominal MIS. (Source: Adapted from Phillips, N. (2017). *Berry & Kohn's operating room technique* (13th ed., p. 632). St Louis, MO: Elsevier Mosby.)

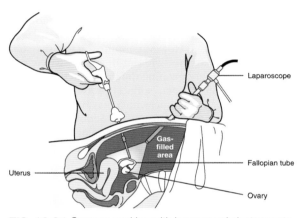

FIG. 10.24 Surgeon working with laparoscopic instruments within a CO_2-filled pneumoperitoneum. (Source: Phillips, N. (2017). *Berry & Kohn's operating room technique* (13th ed., Fig. 32.2, p. 624). St Louis, MO: Elsevier Mosby.)

gas pushes the abdominal wall away from the organs/structures. By doing so the organs/structures within the cavity are not damaged when the trocar/cannula is inserted, and the surgeon is able to visualise the contents of the peritoneal cavity. Pneumoperitoneum is achieved via the first cannula introduced or by the insertion of an insufflation needle (commonly referred to as a Veress needle). Sterile tubing is attached to either the insufflation needle or a three-way tap on the cannula; the end of the tubing is passed off the aseptic field and connected to the gas insufflator (Fig. 10.24).

In the open insertion technique, a cannula with a blunt obturator and an insufflation needle with an

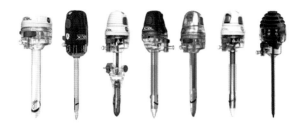

FIG. 10.25 Disposable trocars and cannulae. (Source: Endopath Xcel Trocars https://www.jnjmedicaldevices. com/en-EMEA/product/endopath-xcel-trocars.)

expandable sleeve attached can be used to accomplish intra-abdominal access, resulting in less trauma to the abdominal wall and smaller fascial defects as the muscles are spread, not cut (Ball, 2019). Once insufflation is achieved, the needle is withdrawn, leaving the sleeve in place, through which the instrumentation can be introduced (Phillips, 2017). The closed or blind technique involves the insertion of an insufflation needle, filling the abdominal cavity with carbon dioxide first, and then insertion of the first trocar and cannula. Sharp (self-piercing) trocars are used in this technique as they puncture the skin on the way through the peritoneum. In both techniques, the initial cannula is inserted at the inferior aspect of the umbilicus; however, alternative sites may be chosen depending of the type of surgery or if the patient has had previous abdominal surgery, as there can be a risk that loops of bowel or adhesions have adhered to the previous incision site.

The number and type of cannulae or trocars inserted will depend on the surgical procedure. For example, in an appendicectomy, three cannulae are inserted, but a cholecystectomy or bowel resection requires four or five cannulae as more instrumentation is needed to help retract surrounding structures and possibly apply suction at the same time. All cannulae have taps, which can be used to attach gas tubing to allow for insufflation of the peritoneal cavity and smoke evacuation tubing to remove any excessive smoke plume, which can interfere with the surgeon's visual field.

Trocars come in a range of shapes and sizes and differ in the functionality of their tips, with options such as clear visualising, bladeless, dilating, blunt and balloon (Figs 10.25–10.27). Depending on the manufacturer, the trocar tips can be retractable or have a shield that covers the sharp tip once entry has been achieved. The bladeless trocar separates tissue without cutting or stretching the tissue and provides the option of visualising the insertion of this type of trocar. Recent advancements

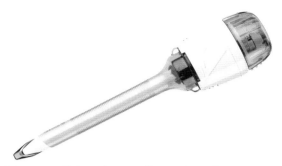

FIG. 10.26 Balloon tip trocar. (Source: https://www.medline. com/media/catalog/sku/fog/FOGCTB33_PRI02.JPG. © Applied Medical Resources Corporation.)

relating to the design of cannulae have resulted in a newer version of cannula with a better grip and balloon occlusion, which prevent accidental removal or movement of the cannula during surgery (see Fig. 10.26) (Ball, 2019; Phillips, 2017).

Visualisation

Visualisation requires four elements: the laparoscope, the camera, the light cable and the control unit. Many types of laparoscopes are available and their size (diameter) and length depend on the access required to visualise the area (Ball, 2019). Flexible telescopes provide a panoramic view, whereas rigid telescopes provide either a direct (0 degrees) scope or angled (30 degrees, 70 degrees or 120 degrees) view. Fig. 10.28 shows examples of rigid endoscopes and Fig. 10.29 shows the camera and video set-up for a laparoscopic procedure.

The heat from the light source is not transmitted down the length of the telescope, which prevents tissue from being inadvertently damaged. However, it should be noted that the end of the fibreoptic cable is often very hot. Once disconnected from the telescope, the light source should be switched to standby or off to prevent accidental burning of the patient and/or the drapes (see Chapter 5 for more information on fire safety).

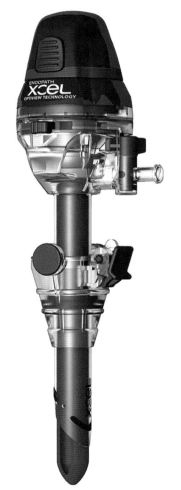

FIG. 10.27 Blunt tip trocar. (Source: https://www.med-line.com/media/catalog/sku/eth/ETH2H12LP_PRI02.JPG.)

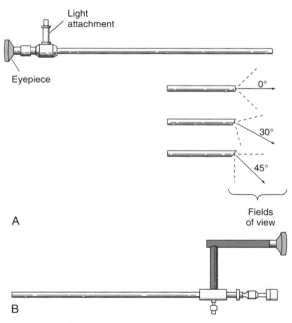

FIG. 10.28 Basic rigid endoscopes. (Source: Phillips, N. (2017). *Berry & Kohn's operating room technique* (13th ed., Fig. 32.46, p. 626). St Louis, MO: Elsevier Mosby.)

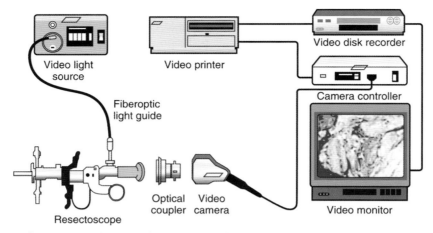

FIG. 10.29 Camera and video setup for endoscopy. (Source: Phillips, N. (2017). *Berry & Kohn's operating room technique* (13th ed., Fig. 32.6, p. 627). St Louis, MO: Elsevier Mosby.)

Performing the Procedure

In order to perform an operative procedure using minimally invasive technique, the surgeon's hands must be free to manipulate the instrumentation, and the assistant and instrument nurses must also be able to see the operative field. This can be achieved by the introduction of a video camera. The video camera enlarges the images from the telescope and projects them onto a television screen, which means that all members of the surgical team can observe the procedure. Fig. 10.30 shows a typical video laparoscopic cart, which can also be ceiling mounted in some facilities, as shown in Fig. 10.31 (see Chapter 5 for more information on theatre design and hybrid operating theatres).

When tissues such as the appendix, ovary and gall bladder are removed, a specially designed laparoscopic specimen bag can be used to prevent spillage of their contents. In the case of laparoscopic bowel resection, once the segment of bowel has been resected, a slightly larger incision is made through which the segment of bowel will be removed. A wound edge protector can be used to protect the wound from contamination from the diseased bowel.

Equipment

Advances continue to be made in MIS, with different surgical specialisations developing new techniques. Although the types of instruments available for MIS are similar to those used for open surgery and can be classified according to the five instrument categories, adaptations have been made to allow their use via a laparoscope. Fig. 10.32 shows a variety of laparoscopic instruments.

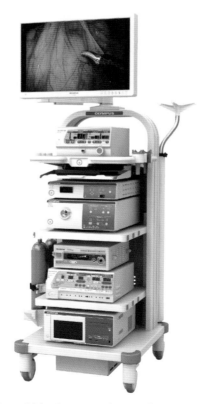

FIG. 10.30 Video laparoscopic cart. (Source: Ball, K. A. (2019). Surgical modalities. In J. C. Rothrock & D. L. McEwen (Eds.), *Alexander's care of the patient in surgery* (16th ed., Fig. 8.32, p. 217). St Louis, MO: Elsevier.)

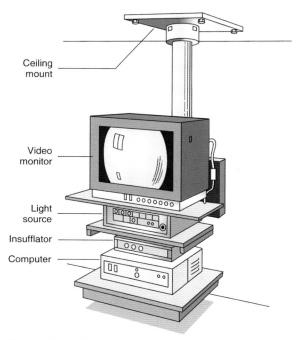

Ceiling mount

Video monitor

Light source

Insufflator

Computer

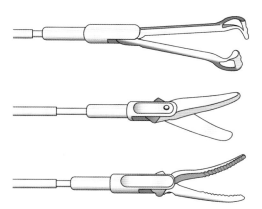

All instrumentation is available in reusable and disposable form and some instruments are available in obese sizes. The following are some of the most common instruments available:

- Telescope: 30 degrees 10 mm and 0 degrees 5 mm.
- Graspers: bowel grasper (DeBakey-like forceps) and/or a bull nose grasper. Both types are considered

atraumatic, which means that the surgeon can handle both the bowel and the appendix without causing any damage.
- Diathermy: preference depends on the surgeon and can be either a hook (monopolar) or a Marylands style (bipolar).
- Irrigator/suction device: single nozzle through which both suction and irrigation can be performed, but not simultaneously.
- Endoloops: these snare-like loops of suture material are pre-knotted within an introducer sleeve. Once the suture loop is around the designated tissue, the existing suture knot is pushed down the introducer sleeve until it is tightly secured around the tissue.
- Endocatch bag: this is quite simply a specimen bag (it looks a bit like a butterfly net) which allows the tissue to be removed without any spillage of its contents into the peritoneal cavity. Endocatch bags come in 10 mm or 15 mm sizes (Fig. 10.33).
- Expander balloons: these balloons are used as dissectors to create the space for surgery to be performed (Fig. 10.34)

A more recent advance in the field of abdominal laparoscopic surgery is single-incision laparoscopic surgery (SILS), also known as single-port access surgery. SILS uses one entry point, typically in the umbilical site, allowing for the introduction of a single port that incorporates a number of lumen to reduce the number of incisions (Assali et al., 2018; Ball, 2019).

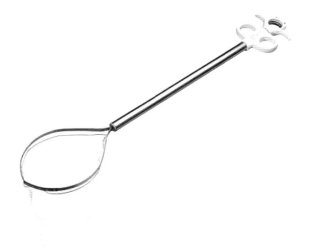

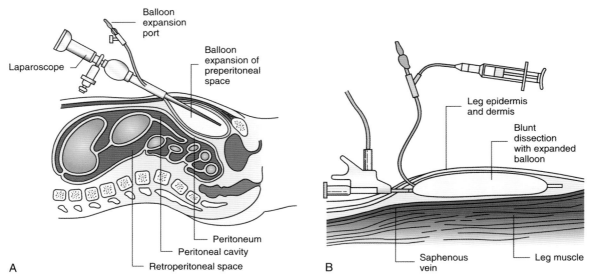

FIG. 10.34 Balloon expansion of surgical planes. (Source: Phillips, N. (2017). *Berry & Kohn's operating room technique* (13th ed., Fig. 32.3, p. 625). St Louis, MO: Elsevier Mosby.)

FEATURE BOX 10.4
Gelpoint Access Platform by Applied Medical

The GelPoint access platform is designed for use in laparoscopic-assisted abdominal and transanal minimally invasive surgical procedures. In laparoscopic-assisted procedures, three to four ports are inserted initially and once the dissection and ligation have been performed a small open incision is created to enable the specimen to be retrieved. Using this device (see Fig. 10.35), a small open incision is performed at the beginning of the procedure, the device is inserted into the open incision and the surgery begins – hence the patient has one small incision only. Essentially, the GelPOINT access platform is an Alexis wound protector that has an airtight seal; it enables the surgeon to insert the laparoscopic ports through the airtight seal in locations that suit the surgeon and or/ the type of bowel resection being performed. Once the laparoscopic part of the procedure has been performed, the airtight seal and laparoscopic ports are removed; what is left is an Alexis wound protector and the open incision through which the specimen is retrieved.

(Source: Applied Medical (2019).)

The GelPOINT advanced access platform facilitates triangulation of standard instrumentation through a single incision (Feature box 10.4 and Fig. 10.35).

Hand-assisted surgery is an extension on MIS whereby the surgeon makes an additional small incision in the patient's abdomen, along with the small incisions for the laparoscopic instrumentation, at the beginning of the surgery. This technique then utilises an access sleeve placed into the additional incision to maintain the pressures in the abdomen and allows the surgeon to insert their hand to grasp, palpate or remove the organs; it is especially useful for bowel surgery or splenectomy, where the specimen is large (Ball, 2019; Gulcu, Isik, Ozturk, & Yilmazlar, 2018).

Paediatric Considerations

While paediatric minimally invasive surgical procedures have advantages similar to those of adult procedures – such as less pain, better cosmetic outcomes, reduced heat and water loss and shorter hospital stays – there are some serious physiological effects that need to be considered (Pelizzo et al., 2017). The creation of a pneumoperitoneum means an increase in intra-abdominal pressure, which causes significant changes in the cardiopulmonary and respiratory systems. This, plus extreme positioning (reverse Trendelenburg), creates significant risk to paediatric patients. Studies have indicated that low pneumoperitoneum and intra-abdominal pressures of between 8 and 12 mmHg should be used in infants and children (McHoney, Kiely, & Mushtaq, 2017). In addition, paediatric instrumentation needs to be shorter and the diameter of cannula/trocars needs to be smaller (3 mm as opposed to 5 mm, 10 mm and 15 mm used in adults) as the paediatric abdomen is smaller than in adults.

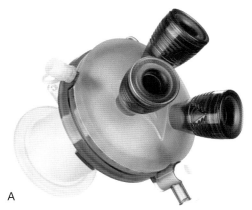
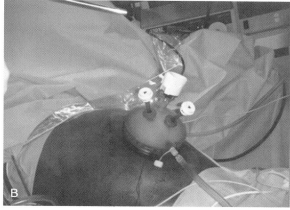

FIG. 10.35 (**A**) Single entry access platform that facilitates triangulation of laparoscopy instruments. (**B**) Single access platform in situ. (Source: Ball, K. A. (2019). Surgical modalities. In J. C. Rothrock & D. L. McEwen (Eds.), *Alexander's care of the patient in surgery* (16th ed., Fig. 8.13, p. 206). St Louis, MO: Elsevier.)

PATIENT SCENARIOS

SCENARIO 10.3 : MINIMALLY INVASIVE INVESTIGATION

Consider our paediatric patient, Thanh Nguyen, who will undergo an orchidopexy to resolve his unde-scended testicle.

The paediatric surgeon may choose to use a minimally invasive approach to investigate the groin or lower abdomen so as to ascertain the location of the undescended testicle before performing the orchidopexy.

Operating Room Set-up for Minimally Invasive Surgery

Each surgeon will have individual requirements regard-ing the layout of equipment in the operating room, but there are general guidelines to set up for minimally invasive surgical procedures. In general surgery, most procedures are performed with the camera stack/trolley on the patient's side and towards the patient's head (see Fig. 10.36). In gynaecological/obstetric surgery, most procedures are performed with the camera stack/trolley towards the patient's feet or between the pa-tient's legs. In urological surgery, most procedures are performed with the camera stack/trolley on either the right or the left side (depending on the room) and to-wards the patient's head. Fig. 10.37 shows surgeons performing MIS with camera and screens towards the patient's head.

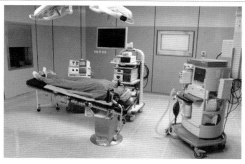

FIG. 10.36 Basic room set-up for minimally invasive surgical procedure. (Source: Pignata, G., Bracale, U., & Lazzara, F. (Eds.). (2016). *Laparoscopic surgery: key points, operating room setup and equipment* (Fig 4.2, p. 44,). Champaign, IL: Springer.)

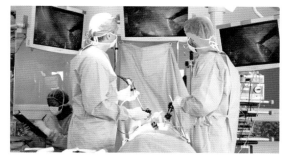

FIG. 10.37 Performing laparoscopic surgery. (Source: https://www.shutterstock.com/de/video/clip-30269893-laparoscopic-surgical-training-operation-transmitted-on-hospital.)

PATIENT SCENARIOS

SCENARIO 10.4: LAPAROSCOPIC SURGERY

Laparoscopic surgery is the type of surgical technique our scenario patient, Mrs Patricia Peterson, will be undergoing as a result of her diagnosis of acute cholecystitis. She has arrived for her emergency laparoscopic cholecystectomy, and the nurses are preparing the theatre and equipment. It is noted that Mrs Peterson has a BMI of 28 and a previous medical history of an endoscopic retrograde cholangiopancreatography (ERCP).

Critical Thinking Questions

- Identify at least three laparoscopic instruments required to perform the cholecystectomy, not including the telescope, camera and light lead. Provide the rationale for your choice.
- With Mrs Peterson's weight in mind, what other considerations should be taken into account when setting up the instrumentation? Provide the rationale for your answers.
- Reflect on the access type most suitable for Mrs Peterson, considering her past history and BMI. Give reasons for your decision.
- Consider why Mrs Peterson's procedure may be converted to an open procedure.
- Reflect on how the operating room would be configured for Mrs Peterson's surgery in your facility. What factors could impact on the configuration?

Advances in Minimally Invasive Surgery

One of the most advanced technologies in the perioperative environment is **robotic surgery**. Robotic surgery was first developed in the 1990s to address some of the limitations of MIS, although it has been suggested that the term used should be computer-enhanced surgical devices. With the addition of a robot, the surgeon sits at an operative console with three-dimensional (3D) imaging and hand-held controls (Fig. 10.38). Robotic surgery provides enhanced 3D visualisation of the anatomy.

Some of the advantages of robotic systems include decreased length of stay, reduced complications and faster recovery (Carlos & Saulan, 2018). With all the advantages, there remains some disadvantages such as the cost of the equipment, the amount of space required to set up the system, the extensive training and education required, and the additional staff required (Carlos & Saulan, 2018). Robotic arms do not have tremors and can stabilise telescopes and long instruments better than an assistant. Robotic arms also have smaller hand movements, enabling them to work better in a small workspace and tolerate two-dimensional visibility; however, hand dexterity is missing.

The da Vinci robot is considered the biggest advancement in robotic surgery. In the latest trend, known as natural orifice transluminal endoscopic surgery (NOTES), flexible endoscopes enter via the gastrointestinal, urinary or reproductive tracts and traverse the wall of the structure to enter the peritoneal cavity, mediastinum or chest.

Surgical navigation systems

Neurosurgery imaging and surgical navigation is another advance in the use of technology. The StealthStation navigation system (Fig. 10.39) enables surgeons to visualise the patient's anatomy in 3D prior to and during surgery, while also seeing the exact location of their surgical instrumentation. StealthStation navigation enables surgeons to:
- enhance tumour boundary recognition
- determine the optimal placement and size of the craniotomy
- account for brain shift during the procedure
- plan the least-invasive surgical path (Medtronic, 2019).

Computer-assisted knee replacement surgery allows surgeons to operate with smaller incisions and greater precision:
- Surgeons can align a patient's bones and knee replacement implants with a degree of accuracy not possible with the naked eye.
- Smaller incisions offer the potential for faster recovery, less bleeding and less pain for patients.
- Computers used during orthopaedic surgery offer visual mapping to help doctors make crucial decisions before and throughout the knee replacement operation. The key is to combine the precision and accuracy of computer technology with the surgeon's skill to perform surgery.
- Advanced imaging technology provides a computer-generated representation of a patient's knee joint, allowing the surgeon to operate with smaller openings and with more precision. In addition, this technology provides surgeons with greater 'vision' during the surgery (Hart & Sierra, 2018).

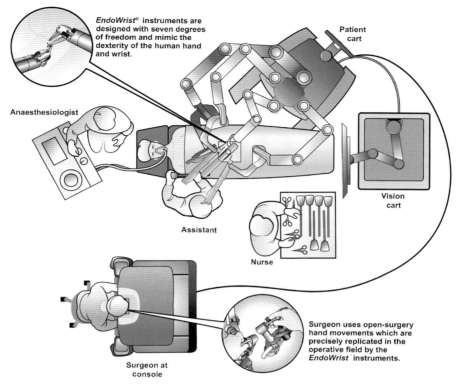

EndoWrist® instruments are designed with seven degrees of freedom and mimic the dexterity of the human hand and wrist.

Patient cart

Anaesthesiologist

Vision cart

Assistant

Nurse

Surgeon uses open-surgery hand movements which are precisely replicated in the operative field by the *EndoWrist* instruments.

Surgeon at console

FIG. 10.38 Robotic instruments and hand controls. (Source: Ball, K. A. (2019). Surgical modalities. In J. C. Rothrock & D. L. McEwen (Eds.), *Alexander's care of the patient in surgery* (16th ed., Fig. 8.34, p. 219). St Louis, MO: Elsevier.)

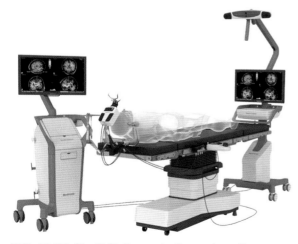

FIG. 10.39 StealthStation navigation system. (Source: https://legacymedsearch.com/medtronic-expands-surgical-synergysm-with-fda-clearance-of-the-stealth-autoguide-system-for-cranial-procedures/.)

The Mako is an orthopaedic robot used for partial and total knee replacements and total hip replacement surgery. The patient undergoes a preoperative CT scan, which is used to create a 3D reconstruction of the patient's knee/hip anatomy. This reconstruction model is then loaded into the Mako system software to create a personalised preoperative plan. Intraoperatively, the Mako system guides the surgeon to operate within defined boundaries to provide accurate alignment and placement of prostheses (Hampp et al., 2019). Early clinical findings indicate that the Mako is associated with increased accuracy, precision and protection of soft tissue, as well as reported patient satisfaction and improved ergonomics for the surgeon in comparison with open joint replacement (Khlopas et al., 2018). Other benefits such as reduced postoperative pain, improved recovery and reduced hospital time prior to discharge have also been reported (Kayani, Konan, Tahmassebi, Pietrzak, & Haddad, 2018).

CONCLUSION

This chapter has focused on assisting perioperative nurses to understand the process of surgical intervention and their role in this process. Every surgical procedure, including MIS, follows a generalised sequence of steps. By researching and understanding this sequence, the instrument and circulating nurses make judgements with regards to the instrumentation required to complete the surgical procedure. This is of particular importance in circumstances where the patient's anatomy, BMI or age require specialised instrumentation or equipment to ensure a safe surgical outcome. This chapter has aimed to give a greater understanding of the core elements of instrumentation, as well as an overview of new and innovative surgical approaches in order to assist the perioperative nurse to make an informed assessment of the needs of the patient, as well as those of the attending surgical team. Advances in technology notwithstanding, it is important for the perioperative nurse to always remember that the patient is the centre of focus and consideration for their safety and the risks and hazards involved in surgery is paramount (see Chapters 3 and 5 for further details on risks and hazards).

RESOURCES

Covidien
https://www.medtronic.com/covidien/en-us/products/surgical-stapling.html
Echelon
https://www.jnjmedicaldevices.com/en-US/product-family/surgical-stapling
Mako robotic-arm partial knee replacement
https://patients.stryker.com/knee-replacement/options/mako-robotic-arm-assisted-total-knee
StrykerMako robotic-arm assisted total hip replacement
https://patients.stryker.com/hip-replacement/options/mako-robotic-arm-assisted

Video Resources

Knee arthroscopy
https://www.youtube.com/watch?v=xwYrx8BA18o
Lap cholecystectomy
https://www.youtube.com/watch?v=qNEbypney3w
Laparoscopic sleeve gastrectomy for morbidly obese patients
https://www.youtube.com/watch?v=KM6UQzMwbWU&feature=share
Robotic surgery
https://www.youtube.com/watch?v=WhDQqRDOA4k
Surgical instruments
https://www.youtube.com/watch?v=XDTWRMs07XU

REFERENCES

Aminimoghaddam, S., Pahlevani, R., & Kazemi, M. (2018). Electrosurgery and clinical applications of electrosurgical devices in gynecologic procedures. *Medical Journal of the Islamic Republic of Iran, 32*, 90. https://dx.doi.org/10.14196/mjiri.32.90

Applied Medical. (2019). GelPOINT access platform. Retrieved from <https://www.appliedmedical.com/Products/Gelpoint>.

Assali, S., Eapen, S., Carman, T., Horattas, S., Daigle, C., & Paranjape, C. (2018). Single-port laparoscopic appendicectomy: beyond the learning curve: a retrospective comparison with multi-port laparoscopic appendicectomy. *Surgical Laparoscopy, Endoscopy and Percutaneous Techniques, 28*(5), 291–294.

Association of periOperative Registered Nurses (AORN). (2017). Guideline at a glance: sharps safety. *AORN Journal, 106*(1), 87–89.

Australian College of Perioperative Nurses (ACORN). (2020a). *ACORN standards for perioperative nursing in Australia* (16th ed., Vol. 1). Clinical standards – sharps and preventing sharps-related injury. Adelaide: Author.

Australian College of Perioperative Nurses (ACORN). (2020b). *ACORN standards for perioperative nursing in Australia* (16th ed., Vol. 1). Clinical standards – electrosurgical equipment. Adelaide: Author.

Australian College of Perioperative Nurses (ACORN). (2020c). *ACORN standards for perioperative nursing in Australia* (16th ed., Vol. 1). Clinical standards – surgical plume. Adelaide: Author.

Baggish, M. S., & Karram, M. M. (2016). *Atlas of pelvic anatomy and gynecologic surgery* (4th ed.). Philadelphia, PA: Elsevier.

Ball, K. A. (2019). Surgical modalities. In J. C. Rothrock & D. R. McEwen (Eds.), *Alexander's care of the patient in surgery* (16th ed., pp. 201–243). St. Louis, MO: Elsevier Mosby.

Bernardo, A. (2017). The changing face of technologically integrated neurosurgery: today's high-tech operating room. *World Neurosurgery, 106*, 1001–1014. http://dx.doi.org/10.1016/j.wneu.2017.06.159

Carlos, G., & Saulan, M. (2018). Robotic emergencies: are you prepared for a disaster? *AORN Journal, 108*(5), 493–501.

Cromb, M. (2019). Sutures, sharps and instruments. In J. C. Rothrock (Ed.), *Alexander's care of the patient in surgery* (16th ed., Ch. 7, pp. 176–200). St. Louis, MO: Elsevier Mosby.

Cuming, R. G. (2019). Concepts basic to perioperative nursing. In J. C. Rothrock (Ed.), *Alexander's care of the patient in surgery* (16th ed., Ch. 1, pp. 1–14). St. Louis, MO: Elsevier Mosby.

Ethicon. (2019, Feb 20). Surgical stapling: backed by a body of evidence [webpage]. Retrieved from <https://www.jnjmedicaldevices.com/en-US/product-family/surgical-stapling>.

Fuller, J. K. (2018). *Surgical technology: principles and practice* (7th ed.). St. Louis, MO: Elsevier Saunders.

Golpaygani, A. T., Movahedi, M. M., & Reza, M. (2016). A study on performance and safety tests of electrosurgical equipment. *Journal of Biomedical Physics & Engineering, 6*(3), 175–182.

Goodman, T., & Spry, C. (2017). *Essentials of perioperative nursing* (6th ed.). Burlington, MA: Jones & Bartlett Learning.

Gulcu, B., Isik, O., Ozturk, E., & Yilmazlar, T. (2018). Hand-assisted laparoscopy: expensive but considerable step between laparoscopic and open colectomy. *Surgical Laparoscopy, Endoscopy & Percutaneous Techniques, 28*(4), 214–218.

Hampp, E. L., Chughtai, M., Scholl, L. Y., Sodhi, N., Bhowmik-Stoker, M., Jacofsky, D. J., & Mont, M. A. (2019). Robotic-arm assisted total knee arthroplasty demonstrated greater accuracy and precision to plan compared with manual techniques. *Journal of Knee Surgery, 32*(3), 239–250. https://dx.doi.org/10.1055/s-0038-1641729

Hao, M., Wang, Z., Wei, F., Wang, J., Wang, W., & Ping, Y. (2016). Cavitron ultrasonic surgical aspirator in laparoscopic nerve-sparing radical hysterectomy: a pilot study. *International Journal of Gynecological Cancer, 26*(3), 594–599. https://dx.doi.org/ 10.1097/IGC.0000000000000628

Hart, A., & Sierra, R. J. (2018). Computer-assisted surgery for total knee replacement: navigating toward improved outcomes. *Journal of Bone and Joint Surgery, 100*(15), 105. https://dx.doi.org/ 10.2106/JBJS.18.00352

Hartman, C. J., & Kovoussi, L. R. (2018). *Handbook of surgical sequence.* Philadelphia, PA: Elsevier.

Hughes-Hallett, A., Mayer, E. K., Pratt, P. J., Vale, J. A., & Darzi, A. W. (2015). Quantitative analysis of technological innovation in minimally invasive surgery. *British Journal of Surgery, 102*(2), 151–157. https://dx.doi.org/10.1002/bjs.9706

Kayani, B., Konan, S., Tahmassebi, J., Pietrzak, J. R. T., & Haddad, F. S. (2018). Robotic-arm assisted total knee arthroplasty is associated with improved early functional recovery and reduced time to hospital discharge compared with conventional jib-based total knee arthroplasty. *Bone & Joint Journal, 100-B*(7), 930–937. https://dx.doi.org/ oi:10.1302/0301-620X.100B7

Khlopas, A., Sodi, N., Sultan, A. A., Chughtai, M. C., Molloy, R. M., & Mont, M. A. (2018). Robotic arm-assisted total knee arthroplasty. *Journal of Arthroplasty, 33,* 2002–2006. https://dx.doi.org/10.1016/j.arth.2018.01.060

King, C. A., & Spry, C. (2019). Infection prevention and control. In J. C. Rothrock & D. L McEwen (Eds.), *Alexander's care of the patient in surgery* (16th ed., pp. 54–106). St. Louis, MO: Elsevier Mosby.

Luck, E. S., & Gillespie, B. M. (2017). Technological advancements in the OR: do we need to redefine intraoperative nursing roles? *AORN Journal, 106*(4), 4279–4281 http://dx.doi.org/10.1016/j.aorn.2017.08.012

McHoney, M., Kiely, E., & Mushtaq, I. (2017). *Color atlas of pediatric anatomy, laparoscopy, and thoracoscopy.* Berlin: Springer.

Medtronic. (2019). Neurosurgery navigation, StealthStation™ S8 Surgical Navigation System [webpage]. Retrieved from <https://www.medtronic.com/us-en/healthcare-professionals/products/neurological/surgical-navigation-systems/stealthstation/cranial-neurosurgery-navigation.html>.

Medtronic. (2020). Signia™ stapling system[webpage]. Retrieved from <https://www.medtronic.com/covidien/en-us/support/products/surgical-stapling/signia-stapling-system.html>.

Ministry of Health, NSW. (2015). GL2015_002. *Work health and safety – controlling exposure to surgical plume.* Sydney: Author. Retrieved from <https://www1.health.nsw.gov.au/pds/ActivePDSDocuments/GL2015_002.pdf>.

Myint, F., & Kirk, R. M. (2019). *Kirk's basic surgical techniques* (7th ed.). Edinburgh: Elsevier.

National Health and Medical Research Council (NHMRC). (2019). *Australian guidelines for the prevention and control of infection in healthcare.* Canberra: Author. Retrieved from <https://www.nhmrc.gov.au/about-us/publications/australian-guidelines-prevention-and-control-infection-healthcare-2019>.

Pelizzo, G., Carlini, V., Iacob, G., Pasqua, N., Maggio, G., Brunero, M., . . . Calcaterra, V. (2017). Pediatric laparoscopy and adaptive oxygenation and hemodynamic changes. *Pediatric Reports, 9*(7214), 21–25.

Pfiedler Education. (2018). *Electrosurgery* [CE online]. Denver, CO: Author. Retrieved from <https://www.pfiedlereducation.com/diweb/catalog/item/id/4963770/q/q=Electrosurgery&c=514>.

Phillips, N. F., & Hornacky, A. (2021). *Berry & kohn's operating room technique* (14th ed.). St Louis, Missouri: Elsevier.

Pignata, G., Bracale, U., & Lazzara, F. (Eds.). (2016). *Laparoscopic surgery: key points, operating room setup and equipment* Champaign, IL: Springer.

Saletnik, L. (2018). Technology in the perioperative environment. *AORN Journal, 108,* 488–490. https://dx.doi.org/10.1002/aorn.12414

Smalley, P. (2019). Are you ready to take control of surgical plume? [unpublished conference paper]. The 9th Conference of the European Operating Room Nurses Association, 16–19 May 2019, The Hague, Netherlands.

Spear, J. M. (2018). Contaminated instruments present patient safety issues: the role of the perioperative team. *AORN Journal, 108*(4), 438–444. http://dx.doi.org/10.1.1002/aorn.12375

Sullivan, R. (1996). The identity and work of the Ancient Egyptian surgeon. *Journal of the Royal Society of Medicine, 89*(8), 469.

Standards Australia. (1998). *AS 3825:1998 Procedures and devices for the removal and disposal of scalpel blades from scalpel handles.* Homebush: Author.

Standards Australia. (2015). AS *16571:2015 Systems for evacuation of plume generated by medical devices* (ISO 16571:2014, MOD). Homebush: Author.

Tan, E., & Russell, K. P. (2017). Surgical plume and its implications: a review of the risk and barriers to a safe work place. *Journal of Perioperative Nursing, 30*(4), Article 2. Retrieved from <https://dx.doi.org/10.26550/2209-1092.1019>.

Victorian Surgical Consultative Council. (2019). *Retained materials in surgery.* Victorian Government. Retrieved from <https://bettersafercare.vic.gov.au/sites/default/files/2019-01/INFORMATION%20BULLETIN_Retained%20materials%20in%20surgery_FINAL.pdf>.

Wilson, J. (2019). *Infection control in clinical practice* (3rd ed., Ch. 7, pp. 237–278). London: Elsevier.

FURTHER READING

Agcaoglu, O., Sengun, B., Senol, K., Gurbuz, B., Ozoran, E., Carilli, S., & Tezelman, S. (2019). Comparison of technical details and short term outcomes of single incision versus multiport laparoscopic adrenalectomy. *Surgical Laparoscopy, Endoscopy & Percutaneous Techniques, 29*(1), 49–52.

AS/NZS 4187. (2014). *Reprocessing of reusable medical devices in health service organizations* (4th ed.). Sydney: SAI Global.

Cheng, Z., Wang, Y., Chen, L., Gong, J., & Zhang, W. (2018). Effects of different levels of intra-abdominal pressure on the postoperative hepatic function of patients undergoing laparoscopic cholecystectomy: a systematic review and meta-analysis. *Surgical Laparoscopy, Endoscopy & Percutaneous Techniques, 28*(5), 275–281.

Esen, E., Aytac, E., Agcaoglu, O., Zenger, S., Balik, E., Baca, B., . . . Bugra, D. (2018). Totally robotic versus totally laparoscopic surgery for rectal cancer. *Surgical Laparoscopy, Endoscopy & Percutaneous Techniques, 28*(4), 245–249.

Hu, A., Menon, R., Gunnarsson, R., & de Costa, A. (2017). Risk factors for conversion of laparoscopic cholecystectomy to open surgery – a systematic literature review of 30 studies. *American Journal of Surgery, 214*, 920–930.

Mannino, M., Toro, M., Teodoro, M., Sartelli, M., Ansaloni, L., Catena, F., & Di Carlo, I. (2019). Open conversion for laparoscopically difficult cholecystectomy is still valid solution with unsolved aspects. *World Journal of Emergency Surgery, 14*, 7.

Melklor, K., Powell, A., & Lewis, W. (2018). Laparoscopic surgery's 100 most influential manuscripts: a bibliometric analysis. *Surgical Laparoscopy, Endoscopy & Percutaneous Techniques, 28*(1), 13–19.

Nicklin, J. (2017). The future of robotic-assisted laparoscopic gynaecological surgery in Australia – a time and place for everything. *Obstetrics and Gynaecology, 57*, 493–498.

Vilaca, J., Leite, M., Correia-Pinto, J., Hogemann, G., Costa, P., & Leao, P. (2018). The influence of 3D in single-port laparoscopy surgery: an experimental study. *Surgical Laparoscopy, Endoscopy & Percutaneous Techniques, 28*(4), 261–266.

CHAPTER 11

Wound Healing, Haemostasis and Wound Closure

LOUISE WEBBER • ERIN WAKEFIELD
EDITOR: BRIGID M GILLESPIE

LEARNING OUTCOMES

- Briefly discuss the anatomy of the skin and associated structures
- Explain the physiology of wound healing and how this relates to patients with surgical wounds
- Differentiate between acute wounds and chronic wounds
- Describe a system used to classify surgical wounds
- Discuss methods for wound closure, dressings and drainage

KEY TERMS

atraumatic needle	maturation
blunt point taper needle	needles
debridement	proliferation
drains	surgical incision
dressings	suture
embolisation	taper cut needle
haemostasis	wound closure
inflammation	wound healing

INTRODUCTION

Wound healing is a complex, interlinked chain of events. Wounds occur as a result of surgery or trauma and bring about an immediate healing response (Carville, 2017). Knowledge of the anatomy of the skin and the physiology of wound healing is essential to care competently for patients with wounds. Effective wound management requires an understanding of the wound-healing process including physiology of healing and factors affecting wound healing. Knowledge of the common surgical incisions, wound closure methods and the materials used is important in perioperative practice. The perioperative nurse also requires knowledge of the various dressings and drains available and their rationale for use. Further understanding and knowledge of the basic concepts

of wound healing and wound care will provide the new practitioner with confidence in caring for patients in the perioperative setting.

This chapter sequentially discusses the anatomy of the skin, wound types and classification systems and wound-healing processes applied to surgical patients, through to surgical incisions, methods of haemostasis, sutures, wound closure, and dressings and drains commonly used.

SKIN ANATOMY

The skin is the largest organ in the human body (Sorg, Tilkorn, Hager, Hauser, & Mirastschijski, 2017). As such, knowledge of the anatomy of the skin and its associated structures is important for the perioperative nurse. Understanding skin anatomy, and the physiology of wound healing, allows for planning and delivery of appropriate patient-centred care.

The most superficial layer of the skin is the epidermis. This avascular layer renews itself every 2 weeks. It provides a physical, bacterial and chemical barrier to the outside world (Sorg et al., 2017), and prevents dehydration of deeper skin layers and loss of body fluid (McCance & Huether, 2019). The epidermis consists of many overlapping layers of epidermal cells and it receives its nutrients from blood vessels in the underlying dermis (Phillips, 2017). It contains melanocytes (which prevent ultraviolet radiation from penetrating and provide skin colour), and also Langerhans cells, which provide an immune defence (McCance & Huether, 2019).

Beneath the epidermis, the dermis contains connective tissues such as collagen and elastin. The dermis provides the skin with a supportive layer, and the ability to move and stretch (McCance & Huether, 2019). The structures associated with the skin, including hair shafts and muscles, sweat glands, sebaceous glands, nerve endings, veins and arteries (McCance & Huether, 2019), are located here (Fig. 11.1).

The next layer of tissue is the subcutaneous layer. It is also known as the hypodermis (McCance & Huether, 2019). It consists of adipose or fatty tissue, which is yellow, greasy and slippery to touch. Adipose tissue provides cushioning, insulation and also a reserve of energy. Large blood vessels, lymphatics and nerves are also found within the hypodermis (McCance & Huether, 2019).

Underneath this lies the fascia: a thin membrane that fully encapsulates muscle. It is transparent and glossy in appearance. It separates the subcutaneous layer from muscles, tendons and bones. The fascia provides the muscle with protection and helps it adhere to bony prominences; it also provides structure for a network of nerve fibres, blood vessels, and lymphatic channels (McCance & Huether, 2019).

WOUND TYPES AND WOUND HEALING

A wound is an interruption to the tissue and underlying structures. It may occur with or without tissue loss, and may be intentional (surgical) or unintentional (traumatic) (Turrentine et al., 2015).

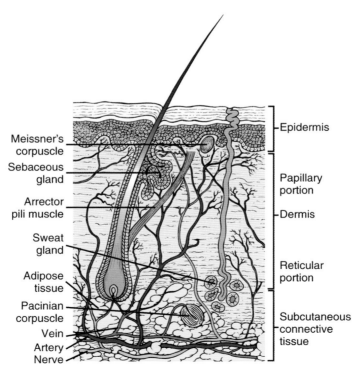

FIG. 11.1 Anatomy of the skin. (Source: Phillips, N. (2017). *Berry & Kohn's operating room technique* (13th ed., p. 531, Fig. 28.1). St Louis, MO: Elsevier.)

Wounds may be classified as acute wounds, which proceed through the normal repair process, or chronic wounds, which fail to heal through a normal healing trajectory.

Surgical Wounds

Surgical site incisions and/or excisions constitute intentional wounds; an *incision* is a cut or an opening into intact tissue, whereas an *excision* is the removal of tissue. Other types on intentional wounds include occlusions. Examples include applying a band to haemorrhoids in order to reduce the blood flow and viability of the tissue. Fallopian tubes can also be occluded with plastic clips to prevent movement of the ovum to the uterus.

Traumatic Wounds

Traumatic wounds can be classified by cause – mechanical, thermal or chemical destruction. For example, wounds can occur following trauma (mechanical), as a result of being burnt (thermal) or from contact with chemicals such as acid (chemical) (Turrentine et al., 2015). These wounds may require surgical intervention – owing to the nature of the injury, contamination and tissue damage – to facilitate wound healing. There are many types of traumatic wounds; these include bites, burns and skin tears. Feature box 11.1 describes skin tears, which most commonly occur in older adults.

FEATURE BOX 11.1
Skin Tears

Skin tears are traumatic wounds caused by mechanical forces such as friction, shearing or trauma, and result in shearing of the skin layers (LeBlanc, Campbell, Wood, & Beeckman, 2018). A skin tear results in separation of the epidermis from the dermis (a partial thickness wound) or the epidermis and dermis from the underlying structures (a full thickness wound) (Van Tiggelen et al., 2021). Development and psychometric property testing of a skin tear knowledge assessment instrument (OASES) in 37 countries. Journal of Advanced Nursing, 77(3), 1609-1623). Perioperative patients are at increased risk of skin tears owing to mechanical forces during surgery (e.g. use of positioning equipment and medical devices).

(Sources: LeBlanc K., Campbell, K. E., Wood, E., & Beeckman D. (2018). Best practice recommendations for prevention and management of skin tears in aged skin: an overview. *Journal of Wound Ostomy and Continence Nursing, 45*(6), 540–542. https://dx.doi.org/10.1097/WON.0000000000000481; Van Tiggelen, H., Alves, P., Ayello, E., Bååth, C., Baranoski, S., Campbell, K., . . . Beeckman, D. (2021). Development and psychometric property testing of a skin tear knowledge assessment instrument (OASES) in 37 countries. *Journal of Advanced Nursing*, 77(3), 1609–1623.)

Chronic Wounds

Chronic wounds fail to heal in a timely manner and do not progress beyond one of the phases of healing (Carville, 2017). They are complicated by underlying pathology where healing is delayed by intrinsic and extrinsic factors (Carville, 2017). Examples of chronic wounds are pressure injuries that result from compromised circulation over a bony prominence or a venous ulcer that develops due to chronic venous insufficiency. Wounds that do not heal within a reasonable period (4–6 weeks) are considered chronic wounds.

THE PHASES OF WOUND HEALING

Fig. 11.2 illustrates the wound-healing continuum.

Wound healing is a series of physiological events divided into four phases:

Haemostasis (1–3 Days)

Haemostasis occurs immediately during injury. Following injury, blood vessels will briefly constrict, and platelets accumulate at the damaged site, adhere to one another and form a platelet plug composed of fibrin (Camp, 2014).

Inflammation (3 Days to 3 Weeks)

Inflammation is identified as the presence of heat, swelling, erythema, pain and decreased function and should not be confused with the symptoms of infection. During the inflammatory phase the wound produces exudate, which is essential to the healing as it maintains a moist wound environment, supports the diffusion of growth factors across the process wound bed and supplies essential nutrients for cell metabolism. Wound exudate is usually high during the inflammatory phase and decreases as healing progresses (World Union of Wound Healing Societies (WUWHS), 2019).

Proliferation (3 Weeks to 1 Year)

The **proliferation** phase occurs 3–4 days after injury and lasts for about 2 weeks. It is an intense phase during which there is formation and deposition of new tissue in the form of granulation, epithelialisation and contraction of the wound.

Maturation

Maturation is the final phase, commencing approximately 3 weeks after injury and continuing for up to 2 years. Collagen tissue produced in the proliferative phase is remodelled, giving better tensile strength. At the same time there is a decrease in vascularity, leaving a pale, flatter scar. The new tissue regains only about 80% of its original tensile strength (Doughty & Sparks, 2016).

Healing responses

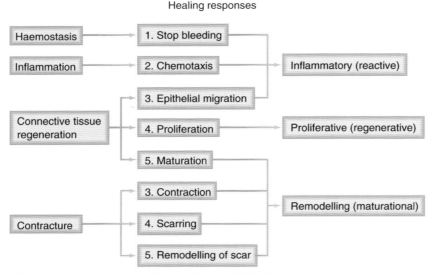

FIG. 11.2 Wound-healing continuum. (Source: Bak, J. (2015). Wound healing, dressings and drains. In J. C. Rothrock, & D. R. McEwen (Eds.), *Alexander's care of the patient in surgery* (15th ed., pp. 253–269). St Louis, MO: Elsevier Saunders.)

These phases overlap and the time for each phase will vary.

WOUND-HEALING PROCESS

The three mechanisms by which surgical wounds may be closed and subsequently heal are primary intention, secondary intention and tertiary intention or delayed primary closure (Fig. 11.3).

Primary Intention

Surgically clean wounds heal by a process of collagen synthesis, which effectively seals the wound (McCance & Huether, 2019). This is facilitated by minimal tissue loss and approximation of wound edges, with sutures, clips or tapes. There is no dead space on closure, and minimal contamination because of adherence to aseptic technique in the operating theatre. Very little epithelialisation is required for healing and little wound edge contraction occurs (McCance & Huether, 2019).

Secondary Intention

Secondary intention healing occurs in open wounds where approximation of wound edges is impossible and there is loss of tissue (McCance & Huether, 2019). Some examples may include a surgical wound where there has been dehiscence, or an intentionally left-open surgical wound (Chetter, Oswald, Fletcher, Dumville, & Cullum, 2017) where there is gross infection and the wound edges are not approximated. Healing occurs over a longer time by granulation. There is eventual re-epithelialisation, scar formation and wound contraction (McCance & Huether, 2019). Research box 11.1 describes the impact of chronic wounds on patients' well-being.

Tertiary Intention

When approximation and suturing are delayed intentionally by three or more days due to gross infection, or where extensive tissue has been removed, then healing by tertiary intention/delayed primary closure occurs (Phillips, 2017). This method is controversial with regards to reduction of infection rates in contaminated abdominal wounds. Some research shows that this method reduces infection rates (Singh, Young, & McNaught, 2017), whereas results of other studies suggest there are no differences in outcomes (Krpata, 2019).

FACTORS AFFECTING WOUND HEALING

There are numerous factors that affect wound healing, including:

- the patient's age and physical status
- pre-existing conditions such as diabetes
- tissue oxygenation levels

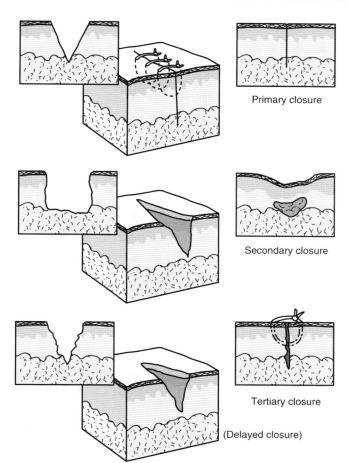

Primary closure

Secondary closure

Tertiary closure

(Delayed closure)

FIG. 11.3 Mechanism of wound healing. (Source: Phillips, N. (2017). *Berry & Kohn's operating room technique* (13th ed. p. 560, Fig. 29-1). St Louis, MO: Elsevier.

RESEARCH BOX 11.1
Secondary Intention Wound Healing

Recent studies from the UK found that wounds healing by secondary intention account for up to 28% of surgical wounds (Chetter, Oswald, Fletcher, Dumville, & Cullum, 2017; McCaughan, Sheard, Cullum, Dumville, & Chetter, 2018). Wounds healing by secondary intention are costly to treat, may result in a longer hospital stay, and will impact on the psychosocial care required of the patient.

(Sources: Chetter, I. C., Oswald, A. V., Fletcher, M., Dumville, J. C., & Cullum, N. A. (2017). A survey of patients with surgical wounds healing by secondary intention; an assessment of prevalence, aetiology, duration and management. *Journal of Tissue Viability, 26*(2), 103–107; McCaughan, D., Sheard, L., Cullum, N., Dumville, J., & Chetter, I. (2018). Patients' perceptions and experiences of living with a surgical wound healing by secondary intention: a qualitative study. *International Journal of Nursing Studies, 77*, 29–38.)

- nutritional status and body mass index (BMI)
- normothermia (Bak, 2015).

Delayed primary healing in a surgical wound is commonly caused by a surgical site infection (SSI). Wound healing can also be impaired by poor surgical technique: rough handling of tissue may cause trauma that can lead to bleeding and other conditions conducive to infection (Bak, 2015).

Obese patients are at increased risk of poor wound healing, with increased risk of infection, wound dehiscence and breakdown, and this is coupled with the potential for poor nutrition and poor vascularity of adipose tissue to further challenge the wound-healing potential.

SCENARIO 11.1: RISK FACTORS FOR WOUND BREAKDOWN

Mrs Patricia Peterson is a 42-year-old Indigenous woman admitted for an emergency laparoscopic cholecystectomy. Mrs Peterson's full history and a brief description of the healthcare setting are provided at the front of the book for readers to review when answering the questions in this unfolding scenario.

Critical Thinking Question

• Considering the surgery Mrs Peterson is about to have, identify clinical factors from her medical history that may put her at increased risk of surgical wound breakdown. Provide rationales for your answers.

SURGICAL INCISIONS

A **surgical incision** to the skin, allowing access into the tissues of the body to expose the underlying tissue, bone or organs, is required to perform surgery. The direction of the incisional line is determined by the anatomical plane in the body. When planning a surgical incision, the surgeon needs to take several issues into consideration – for example:

• access and adequate exposure to the necessary anatomical structures (allowing for extension of the incision if required)
• minimising interference with the function of the skin and appendages by preserving important structures such as nerves and blood vessels
• strong wound closure, minimising the risk of wound dehiscence or incisional hernia
• whether rapid entry is required
• cosmesis.

The perioperative nurse must be aware of the type of incision planned, as this will assist in setting up the necessary instrumentation. For example, if muscles are to be split or incised there is likely to be more bleeding, requiring haemostats and use of diathermy. The location, size and depth of the planned surgical incision will also guide the nurses' selection of needle holders and retractors, for example, and dressings.

Langer's Lines

Anatomist Karl Langer (1819–87) was an Austrian professor whose work used cadavers to demonstrate the effects of different incisions and wound retraction techniques in skin. He described how the skin has cleavage or tension lines, which are a result of the skin's relationship with the underlying musculature (Phillips, 2017). In 1861, he wrote a seminal paper on the physical and mechanical properties of skin (Abyaneh, Griffith, Falto-Aizpurua, & Nouri, 2014). He found that incisions healed with less scarring if natural cleavage lines were followed. Nowadays these are known as Langer's lines (Abyaneh et al., 2014).

Abdominal Incisions

The primary reference point for abdominal incisions is the umbilicus, while secondary surface landmarks include the xiphoid, the symphysis pubis and the iliac crests (see Fig. 11.4). Incisions may be vertical, horizontal or oblique (Phillips, 2017). Fig. 11.5 shows anterior surface incisions. Fig. 11.6 illustrates the abdominal muscles and Table 11.1 outlines common abdominal incisions applicable to open abdominal and pelvic procedures (Phillips, 2017).

WOUND CLASSIFICATION

Table 11.1 shows the classification system applied to surgical wounds as reflected in the Centers for Disease Control and Prevention (CDC) guidelines (Berríos-Torres et al., 2017).

SCENARIO 11.2: WOUND CLASSIFICATIONS

Mr James Collins is a 78-year-old man, who has been admitted for an elective right total knee replacement (TKR). Mr Collins' full history and a brief description of the healthcare setting are provided in the Introduction to this book for readers to review when answering the questions in this unfolding scenario.

Critical Thinking Question

• How would you classify Mr Collins' wound? Please give a rationale for your answer.

Management of Non-viable Tissue – Surgical Debridement

Debridement is the removal of dead or necrotic tissue from the wound bed. The wound-healing process is

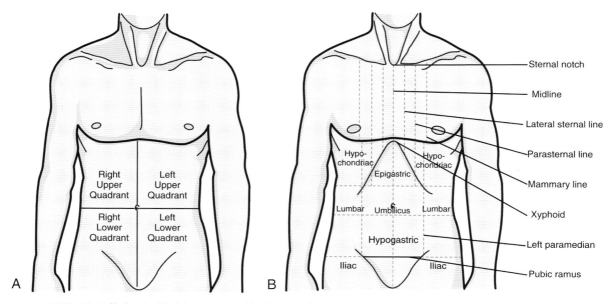

FIG. 11.4 Abdominal incisions; surgical landmarks. (Source: Phillips, N. (2017). *Berry & Kohn's operating room technique* (13th ed., p. 534, Fig. 28.4). St Louis, MO: Elsevier.

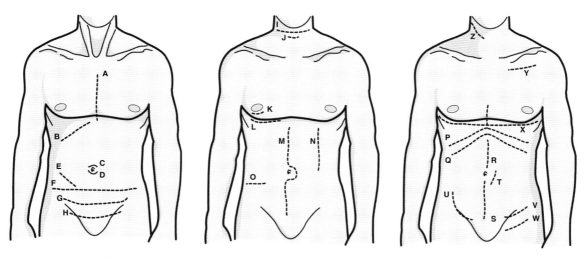

Anterior Surface Incisions

A. Sternotomy
B. Kocher (Subcostal)
C. Supraumbilical
D. Infraumbilical
E. McBurney's appendectomy
F. Transverse
G. Maylard transverse muscle-cutting
H. Pfannenstiel

I. Thyroidectomy
J. Tracheotomy
K. Infraareolar
L. Inframammary
M. Midline
N. Paramedian
O. Rockey-Davis

P. Mercedes
Q. Chevron
R. Epigastric (upper midline)
S. Lower midline
T. Pararectus
U. Gibson (hand-assisted laparoscopy)
V. Inguinal
W. Femoral
X. Clamshell
Y. Subclavicular
Z. Carotid

FIG. 11.5 Anterior surface incisions. (Source: Phillips, N. (2017). *Berry & Kohn's operating room technique* (13th ed., p. 536, Fig. 28.7). St Louis, MO: Elsevier.

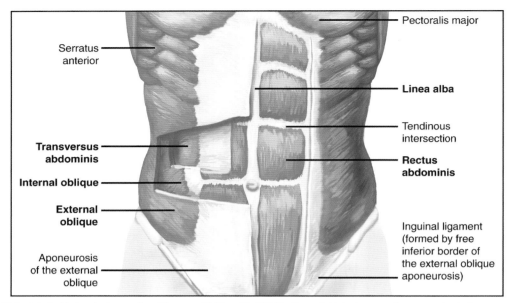

FIG. 11.6 Abdominal muscles. (Source: Phillips, N. (2013). *Berry & Kohn's operating room technique* (13th ed.). St Louis, MO: Elsevier.)

delayed because of the increased risk of infection and increased inflammatory activity in the wound bed. The aim of debridement is to remove necrotic tissue from the wound bed, reduce the pressure, facilitate wound assessment and address the inflammatory status of the wound favourable to new cell growth (White & Asimus, 2014). Methods of debridement include:

- mechanical debridement
- conservative sharp wound debridement
- dressing wound debridement
- biosurgical wound debridement
- enzymatic wound debridement
- surgical wound debridement (White & Asimus, 2014).

Surgical wound debridement occurs in the operating room and is non-selective removal of devitalised tissue using sharp instruments to obtain a clean wound bed (White & Asimus, 2014). However, it may also include removal of viable tissue to obtain a clean tissue margin for closure, grafting or negative-pressure wound therapy. The choice of debridement method should be made with consideration of the patient, suitability of available methods and the treating clinician (Ramundo, 2016).

SURGICAL HAEMOSTASIS

Surgical haemostasis is the deliberate halting of blood flow. Haemostasis is necessary to prevent the patient experiencing the physiological effects of excessive blood loss and ensure optimal visibility for the surgeon. It also plays a role in infection prevention. Retained blood may create dead space, preventing approximation of tissues, and may create a focus for infection (Phillips, 2017). Bleeding does not just occur from pulsating arteries; generally it is more insidious, involving capillary or venous oozing that needs to be proactively managed intraoperatively (Phillips, 2017). There are many methods of haemostasis, and the perioperative nurse must have a good working knowledge of the handling and mechanism, safe use, risks and benefits of the required instrumentation.

Methods of Surgical Haemostasis

Surgical haemostasis methods can be classed in many ways.

Mechanical haemostasis

Mechanical haemostasis is achieved by compressing the ends of severed vessels, temporarily slowing the flow of blood until the patient's own normal clotting mechanisms have sealed the vessel. Examples include:

- instruments
- ligatures/ties
- ligating clips
- bone wax

TABLE 11.1
Wounds Classified Into Four Types, as Described in the CDC Guidelines

Classification	Wound Type	Key Descriptors	Examples
I	Clean Expected infection rate: 1%–5%	Elective procedure with wound made under ideal operating room conditions Primary closure, wound not drained No break in sterile technique during surgical procedure No inflammation present Alimentary, respiratory or genitourinary tract or oropharyngeal cavity not entered	Eye surgery Hernia repair Breast surgery Neurosurgery (non-traumatic) Cardiac and peripheral vascular surgery
II	Clean-contaminated Infection rate: 3%–11%	Primary closure, wound drained Minor break in aseptic technique occurred No inflammation or infection present Alimentary, respiratory or genitourinary tract or oropharyngeal cavity entered under controlled conditions without significant spillage or unusual contamination	Gastrectomy, cholecystectomy (without spillage) Elective appendicectomy, cystoscopy and/or cystoscopy/transurethral resection (negative urine cultures) Total abdominal hysterectomy, dilation and curettage of the uterus, caesarean section Tonsillectomy (not infected at time of surgery) (Ortega et al., 2012)
III	Contaminated Infection rate: 10%–17%	Open, fresh traumatic wound of less than 4 hours duration Major break in aseptic technique occurred Acute, non-purulent inflammation present Gross spillage/contamination from gastrointestinal tract Entrance into genitourinary or biliary tracts with infected urine or bile present	Rectal surgery, laparotomy (with significant spillage) Traumatic wounds (e.g. gunshot, stab wounds – non-perforation of viscera) Acute inflammation of any organ without frank pus present (e.g. acute appendicitis or cholecystitis) (Ortega et al., 2012)
IV	Dirty (infected) wound Infection rate: above 27%	Old traumatic wound of more than 4 hours duration from dirty source or with retained necrotic tissue, foreign body or faecal contamination Organisms present in aseptic field before procedure Existing clinical infection: acute bacterial inflammation encountered, with or without purulence; incision to drain abscess Perforated viscus	Debridement Incision and drainage of an abscess Total evisceration, perforated viscera Amputation or patients with positive preoperative blood (Ortega et al., 2012)

(Sources: Adapted from Berríos-Torres, S., Umscheid, C., Bratzler, D., Leas, B., Stone, E., Kelz, R., … Schecter, W. (2017). Prevention of surgical site infection. *Journal of the American Medical Association Surgery, 152*(8), 784–791; Phillips, N. (2017). *Berry & Kohn's operating room technique* (13th ed.). St Louis, MO: Elsevier.)

- packing
- pledgets
- patties
- balloon catheters
- tourniquets
- simple digital pressure (Harkin & Dunlop, 2018).

Instruments. Instruments such as artery forceps or the smaller mosquito forceps clamp to hold a small amount of tissue or the end of a blood vessel. Often, the pressure of clamping a blood vessel is sufficient to achieve haemostasis (Phillips, 2017).

Ligating clips. Ligating clips are small, V-shaped, staple-like devices. When placed on a blood vessel and closed shut, ligating clips occlude the lumen and stop the bleeding. Ligating clips are available in small plastic carriers preloaded with multiple clips which require individual loading onto a sterile, reusable instrument (Fig. 11.7). The perioperative nurse must double check that the clip is seated securely into the applicator. Metal clips are considered a sharp, and may be difficult to locate if they fall away from the device. It is also prudent for the instrument nurse to have two clip applicators prepared for the surgeon. Often, during dissection, when using this device for haemostasis, the surgeon will 'clip, clip, cut' the vessel in rapid succession. All clips, regardless of material, are an implant and must be documented in the perioperative nursing notes. Laparoscopic ligating clips are also available in a disposable, preloaded instrument that delivers and closes the clips (Phillips, 2017).

Bone wax. Bone wax is comprised of sterile, processed beeswax. It is smeared along the open edge of the bone, working as a barrier to stop oozing from the cut bone surface. It is helpful for the surgeon if the instrument nurse warms the bone wax to a pliable consistency prior to handing over for use. Wax is contraindicated if infection is present, and it can remain in situ for many years, preventing union of bones (Phillips, 2017). It is also considered to be a foreign body, and some patients may be sensitive to it (Phillips, 2017).

Packing. Surgical sponges or packs can be used for packing a wound site intraoperatively, and effectively

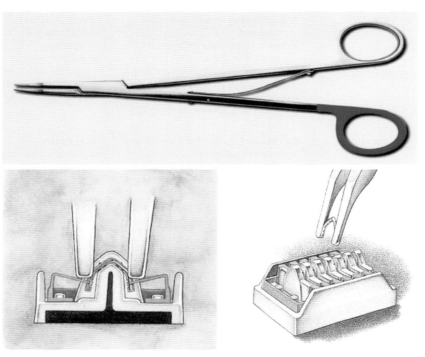

FIG. 11.7 Loading a clip applicator. (Source: Fuller, J. (2013). *Surgical technology principles and practice* (6th ed.). St Louis, MO: Elsevier.)

place pressure on the wound edges or in a body cavity to reduce bleeding. The surgeon may require the packs to be moistened with a warm, sterile irrigating solution. The instrument nurse must declare to the circulating nurse when a countable item, such as a surgical pack, is placed inside the abdominal cavity for haemostasis, and then again when it is removed. A pack soaked in blood can easily become hidden in a surgical field. Packs are also effective in keeping the surgical site free of blood. The best way for the scrub nurse to assist with this task is to blot or dab at the site with the pack, not wipe; this may remove small clots (Phillips, 2017).

Pledgets. Pledgets are small pieces of felt material that are used to reinforce a suture line where bleeding may occur through the needle hole, or when the tissue is very fragile and might tear (Phillips, 2017). They are often used in cardiac surgery and remain in place as part of the suture.

Patties. Compressed, absorbent, radio-opaque cotton-oid patties look like a small piece of felt with a string attached, and are available in various sizes. They are used to absorb blood from delicate areas such as the brain and spinal cord (Phillips, 2017). The instrument nurse counts the patties, moistens them with normal saline, presses out excess moisture and keeps them flat before use.

Balloon catheters. Postpartum haemorrhage (generally considered to be a blood loss of >1000 mL (Royal Australian and New Zealand College of Obstetricians and Gynaecologists [RANZCOG], 2017) is a leading cause of maternal mortality worldwide (Wang et al., 2018). In Australia, the postpartum haemorrhage rate is between 5% and 15% (RANZCOG, 2017). Many women with this condition can be managed with intravenous oxytocics and active management of the third stage of labour (placenta delivery). However, when the patient needs resuscitation and is brought to the operating room, insertion of a Bakri balloon may be required (Fig. 11.8). The balloon tamponade effect is very successful in providing haemostasis (Wang et al., 2018).

Tourniquets. A tourniquet compresses the underlying vessels, restricting blood flow to a limb or digit and creating a bloodless field for the procedure (Phillips, 2017). A pneumatic tourniquet (Fig. 11.9) is used when compression is required to reduce blood flow to a limb (e.g. during an open reduction and internal fixation of a fractured ankle). Generally, the appropriate pressure

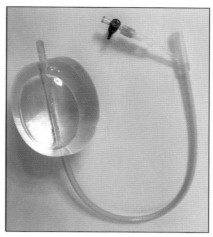

FIG. 11.8 A Bakri balloon. (Source: Suarez, S., Conde-Agudelo, A., Borovac-Pinehiro, A., Suarez-Rebling, D., Eckardt, M., Theron, G., & Burke, T. (2020). Uterine balloon tamponade for the treatment of postpartum haemorrhage: a systematic review and meta analysis. *American Journal of Obstetrics and Gynaecology, 222*, 293e1–52.)

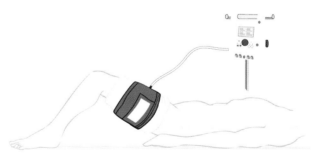

FIG. 11.9 Pneumatic tourniquet. (Source: Fuller, J. (2013). *Surgical technology principles and practice* (6th ed.). St Louis, MO: Elsevier.)

for an adult leg is less than 350 mmHg, and an arm 250 mmHg, but is determined at the discretion of the surgeon. The pressure applied to the patient's limb, the name of the person responsible for applying the tourniquet and the length of time the tourniquet is inflated must be documented in the perioperative procedure record.

The surgeon may exsanguinate the limb prior to tourniquet insufflation and prior to skin preparation. After protecting the skin with a soft bandage, the patient's limb is raised and an inflatable rubber 'exsanguinator' is applied. The tourniquet is then inflated to prevent blood returning to the limb. This task may also

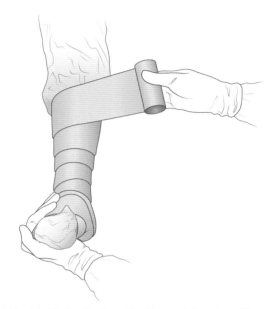

FIG. 11.10 Application of an Esmarch bandage. (Source: Fuller, J. (2013). *Surgical technology principles and practice* (6th ed.). St Louis, MO: Elsevier.)

be performed (using a sterile Esmarch bandage) by the instrument nurse when skin preparation and draping are complete (Fig. 11.10). See Chapter 9 for further information about care of patients when tourniquets are in use.

Applying an elastic band or clamping a Penrose drain or the finger of a glove firmly around the base of an extremity such as a finger can reduce blood flow. Again, use of and application time of this tourniquet must be documented on the perioperative nursing notes.

Adjuncts to mechanical haemostasis
Several products are available to provide an adjunct to mechanical haemostasis. The effect of these products is to speed the formation of a blood clot. Some examples of the most commonly used products are outlined below.

Absorbable gelatin. Absorbable gelatin (Gelfoam) is a haemostatic agent made from porcine gelatin, which is compressed into a pad. It is available in many sizes, and can be cut to the desired shape without crumbling. The gelatin sponge absorbs up to 45 times its own weight in blood when it deposits fibrin into the bleeding site and forms a clot (Phillips, 2017). It can be soaked in thrombin or adrenaline

solution at the surgeon's request. The instrument nurse must be careful not to handle the gelatin foam with damp gloves, as it may become unsuitable for use. Use of non-toothed forceps with a dry pair of scissors is the most efficient method for obtaining the desired shape.

Absorbable cellulose. Absorbable oxidised cellulose is available in the form of a knitted fabric (Surgicel) and is applied as a dry product to bleeding areas. As the oxidised cellulose reacts with blood, it increases in size to form a gel-like clot. This alone may stop the bleeding or can act as a scaffold for the body to enlarge the clot (Anwar, Nofal, & Elmalt, 2017). Due to its ease of movement, the knitted fabric can be rolled and inserted into the operative site via a laparoscopic port. It can stop bleeding in areas where ooze is difficult to control by other means of haemostasis, such as the underside of the liver during a laparoscopic cholecystectomy or in a postadenoidectomy bleed (Anwar et al., 2017). On oozing surfaces, oxidised cellulose can absorb 10 times its own weight (Phillips, 2017).

Pharmacological and chemical haemostasis
There are several pharmacological and chemical agents commonly available to achieve haemostasis in surgery.

Thrombin. Topical thrombin (Thrombostat) is an enzyme that is extracted from dried beef blood, and is one of the most common haemostatic agents in the world, having been in use since the 1940s (Park, Suk, & Park, 2018). Thrombin accelerates coagulation of blood by converting fibrinogen to fibrin and precipitates clot formation (Phillips, 2017).

Floseal. Floseal is a biodegradable matrix haemostatic sealant, made from gelatin and human thrombin (Wakelam, Dimitriadis, & Stephens, 2017). When applied to a bleeding site, it works in two ways: the gelatin absorbs fluid to create a clot and tamponade effect, and the thrombin converts fibrinogen to fibrin, accelerating clot formation (Ramirez et al., 2018). It is applied in a gel form, and is often used in surgery when applying absorbable gelatin and thrombin separately has not provided the required level of haemostasis (Ramirez et al., 2018). It is effective not only in the perioperative arena to achieve haemostasis, but also in the emergency department, where research shows it is a cheap and easily tolerated haemostatic agent for halting uncontrolled epistaxis (Wakelam et al., 2017).

Oxytocin. Oxytocin is a hormone produced in the pituitary gland which can also be prepared synthetically for therapeutic injection. It is commonly used in obstetric and gynaecological surgery. It is safe for use, and has minimal side effects (Swapnika, Priya, Priya, & Allirathinam, 2018) . Oxytocin has an important use in the final stage of labour. It enhances contractions, promotes the delivery of the placenta and prevents bleeding from the 'raw' area of uterine wall of previous placental attachment (McCance & Huether, 2019).

Adrenaline. Adrenaline is a naturally occurring hormone, produced by the adrenal glands. It is also produced commercially for its vasoconstricting properties, and is used in many surgeries to reduce the flow of blood to the surgical site. Local anaesthetic often contains adrenaline. It is important for the perioperative nurse to remember that local anaesthetic with adrenaline should never be administered to the peripheries (hands, nose, penis and toes). Use of local anaesthetic must be documented in the patient's perioperative nursing notes; the patient must further be monitored for potential side effects.

Fibrin glue. Fibrin glue is a biological adhesive and haemostatic agent. It is composed of fibrinogen, cryoprecipitate from human plasma, calcium chloride and reconstituted thrombin of bovine origin (Phillips, 2017). Upon application directly to tissues, thrombin converts fibrinogen to fibrin to produce a clot. Fibrin glue is commonly known by its brand name of Tisseal in Australia and requires a specific method to mix the provided substances to create a useable product. It needs to be prepared immediately prior to use to prevent it congealing (Phillips, 2017). Tisseal is different from other fibrin-based products in that it does not contain bovine derivatives (Phillips, 2017).

Tranexamic acid. Tranexamic acid (TXA) is a synthetic substance which has antifibrinolytic properties and is gaining in popularity worldwide. The results of a 2010 multinational, randomised placebo-controlled trial of TXA indicated significant reductions in postoperative complications: TXA reduced the risk of death from haemorrhage by approximately one-sixth (Goobie, 2017). It is now on the World Health Organization's list of essential medicines for trauma, bypass or postpartum bleeding. Ongoing research needs to be undertaken with regards to the optimal dose and side effects (Goobie, 2017). Prothrombotic and proconvulsant effects have been documented (Myles et al., 2017).

Energy-based methods of securing haemostasis

There are several modalities that use energy to provide haemostasis throughout a surgical procedure.

Electrosurgery. Electric current can be used to cut or coagulate most tissues, including fat, fascia, muscle, internal organs and vessels. Electrosurgery is used to a greater or lesser extent in all surgical specialties, and the electrosurgical unit (ESU) can be seen in all operating rooms. The machine comes with a range of disposable 'tools' that surgeons can use to achieve ongoing haemostasis. See Chapter 6 for further information on ESUs and other energy-based surgical modalities.

Laser. Laser light is used for controlling bleeding or for the ablation and excision of tissues – such as in benign hypertrophy of the prostate. Each operating suite must comply with strict safety rules while using laser (as discussed in Chapter 6) (ACORN, 2020b).

Ultrasonic scalpel. There are many names for the ultrasonic scalpel – ultrasonic shear and harmonic scalpel are just two (Ai et al., 2018). The titanium blades of the scalpel move by a rapid ultrasonic motion which cuts and coagulates tissue simultaneously. It generates less heat than the ESU and therefore does not cause as much damage to adjacent tissues (Okhunov et al., 2018). Vibrations from the tool denature protein molecules, producing a coagulum that seals bleeding vessels. The continuous vibration of the denatured protein generates heat within the tissue to cause deeper coagulation. Because electricity is not required to produce coagulative effects on tissue, a diathermy grounding pad is not required (Phillips, 2017). This device is growing in popularity, and is able to provide superior vessel occlusion in both laparoscopic and open surgeries (Ai et al., 2018).

Haemostatic scalpel. The blade of the haemostatic scalpel seals blood vessels as it cuts through the tissue (Phillips, 2017). When the surgeon activates the scalpel handle, the blade transmits thermal energy (heat) to tissues as the sharp edge cuts through them. The surgeon can alter the temperature to suit the tissue being cut; this can range between 110°C and 270°C (Phillips, 2017). Rapid haemostasis with minimal tissue damage occurs, making the haemostatic scalpel a popular choice. As electric current from the microcircuitry does not pass through the tissues, a grounding pad is not required (Phillips, 2017).

Gyrus PlasmaKinetic SuperPulse generator. The Gyrus haemostatic device uses plasma kinetic energy, which provides high-current but very-low-voltage energy to the tissues. This is delivered to the tissues through a handset via rapid pulses and then rapid cooling (Tu, Chang, Wu, & Sheu, 2019). Less thermal spread damage to the tissues occurs compared with the traditional ESU method of haemostasis, and surgical plume is not created (Phillips, 2017). A recent study found that use of the Gyrus was more effective than using clips, sutures and staples in achieving haemostasis in laparoscopic-assisted vaginal hysterectomy (Tu et al., 2019). This study also found that the blood loss was 35% less in the Gyrus group than in the control group (Tu et al., 2019).

Additional methods of haemostasis

Embolisation. Embolisation is a procedure which blocks blood flow to a targeted area in the body. It can be used to prevent blood flow (e.g. to starve a tumour) (Weinberg et al., 2017) or to stop bleeding. Various substances can be used to block the blood vessel, including medical glue (Mohr-Sasson et al., 2018), medical putty, tiny metal coils (Lv, Cao Song, He, Jiang, & Youxiang Li, 2017), plastic beads or absorbable gelatin (Sawada, Kawarada, & Yasuda, 2018). The technique is often used in neurosurgery to embolise a cerebral aneurysm or the blood supply to an arteriovenous malformation, thereby negating the need for open surgery (Lv et al., 2017). Embolisation is also used to help the surgeon control bleeding during – or even after – the surgical procedure (Van Den Heever, Barrett, Webb, Spruyt, & Louw, 2015).

NovaSure. The NovaSure® is an endometrial ablation device used in the treatment of abnormal uterine bleeding when other non-surgical treatments have been tried. It is especially useful in the treatment of patients with adenomyosis, and research shows that the recurrence rate of pain and abnormal bleeding is lessened in both the short and the long term after NovaSure application (Philip et al., 2018).

SUTURES, LIGATURES AND NEEDLES
Sutures

A **suture** is a thread of material used to approximate tissue or ligate blood vessels (Alshomer, Madhavan, Pathan, & Song, 2017). Suturing is used as a form of wound closure, but it can also be used for intraoperative haemostasis, stabilisation of anatomy or traction (Phillips, 2017). It is important that the surgeon uses

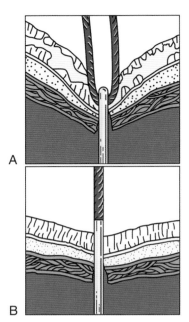

FIG. 11.11 A Eyed needle. B Atraumatic needle. (Source: Phillips, N. (2017). *Berry & Kohn's operating room technique* (13th ed., p. 548, Fig. 28.15). St Louis, MO: Elsevier.)

the correct suture not only for tissue approximation without tissue injury, but also to maximise wound healing and minimise ischaemia and scarring (Byrne & Aly, 2019; Kim et al., 2018).

Currently, needle and suture material are joined as a continuous unit referred to as an **atraumatic needle**, which is individually packaged and presterilised. Atraumatic needles cause less tissue trauma because only one strand of suture material is pulled through the tissues, rather than two as with an eyed needle (Fig. 11.11). Eyed needles such as the Mayo needle still have use nowadays, but are declining in popularity.

Sutures are categorised in many ways – for example, according to their absorbent qualities (or lack thereof), their origins (such as synthetic nylon or bovine-derived gut) (Alshomer et al., 2017), the material they are made from (e.g. silk), their size and other properties (Fig. 11.12).

Absorbable/non-absorbable sutures

Absorbable sutures are derived from animal or synthetic polymer (Phillips, 2017). Animal collagen-based sutures are broken down by the body's enzymes, while synthetic polymers are broken down by a process called hydrolysis: water is absorbed into the suture and

Each packet is color-coded by type of suture composition for ease of identification when selectiong for a procedure. The package colors are similar between manufacturers for type and chemical makeup of suture.

METHOD TO SELECT A SUTURE FOR A SURGICAL PROCEDURE
1. Identify by color (Trade name)
2. Gauge of suture (more zeros indicate smaller gauge)
3. Size and configuration of needle/tip (actual needle and tip image)
   Double needle image indicates a needle on each end
4. Number of strands/needles per pack (Most packs have one needle/suture combination) (some packs have 3 or 8 swaged-on needles) (Ties can be single, very long, or 12 precut strands)

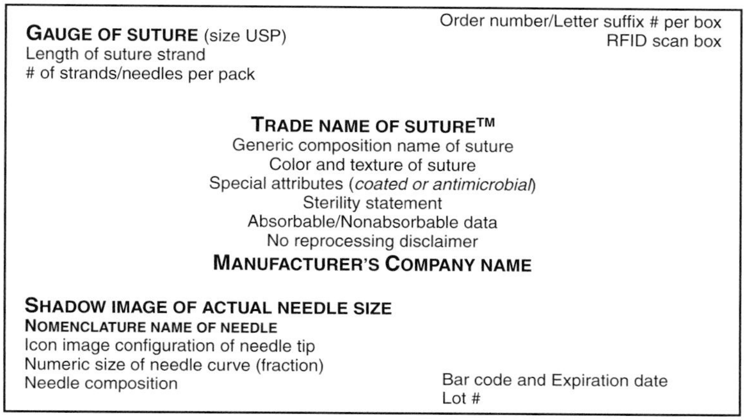

GAUGE OF SUTURE (size USP) Length of suture strand # of strands/needles per pack	Order number/Letter suffix # per box RFID scan box
<div align="center">**TRADE NAME OF SUTURE**™ Generic composition name of suture Color and texture of suture Special attributes (*coated or antimicrobial*) Sterility statement Absorbable/Nonabsorbable data No reprocessing disclaimer **MANUFACTURER'S COMPANY** name</div>	
SHADOW IMAGE OF ACTUAL NEEDLE SIZE **NOMENCLATURE NAME OF NEEDLE** Icon image configuration of needle tip Numeric size of needle curve (fraction) Needle composition	Bar code and Expiration date Lot #

FIG. 11.12 Image of a suture packet. (Source: Phillips, N. (2017). *Berry & Kohn's operating room technique* (13th ed., p. 541, Fig. 28.12). St Louis, MO: Elsevier.)

causes a breakdown of its structure over time (Byrne & Aly, 2019). These processes can be affected by a patient having protein deficiency, or in the presence of infection; wound dehiscence may occur if the suture strength is lost too rapidly (Byrne & Aly, 2019).

Non-absorbable sutures are composed of synthetic or natural material. They are not broken down by the body, but rather encapsulated – that is, fibroblast cells form a fibrous capsule around the suture (Byrne & Aly, 2019). Over time, suture extrusion may occur because of a biofilm formation or seeding of the suture, and the patient may need to return to theatre for its removal, possibly years after the initial surgery (Beidas & Gusenoff, 2019, p. S86). Fig. 11.13 shows a suture extrusion.

Natural and synthetic materials

Natural suture materials are derived from sources such as animal (collagen and gut) and silk. Synthetic sutures are artificially derived from materials such as nylon, polypropylene, polyethylene, polyester, polyglactin and surgical steel (Phillips, 2017).

Diameter or size of suture material

In Australia, suture sizes are classified according to the United States Pharmacopeia (USP) system. This is a unique classification system and starts with the 0 (pronounced 'zero') size suture. Suture diameters that are larger are progressively bigger – for example, a 1 vicryl is a 'heavier' and thicker suture, commonly used for closure of the peritoneum. A size 2 Ticron is an even thicker suture material, which may be used for shoulder joint stabilisation. Conversely, as sutures become smaller in diameter, the pronunciation changes. For example, a size 2-0 (pronounced two-oh) suture is narrower, and would be appropriate for a superficial muscle layer, perhaps near the ankle. Further, as the suture diameter becomes smaller, so too do the corresponding numbers. A suture the size of an eyelash, for eye or cardiac surgery, may be an 8-0 (pronounced eight-oh) (Byrne & Aly, 2019).

The diameter of the suture material and the size of the atraumatic needle attached are chosen according to the type, size and density of the tissue being approximated (Fig. 11.14). It is important for the instrument nurse always to handle sharps in a safe manner according to hospital policy, and to choose a needle holder that is appropriate for the size of the needle and the depth/position of the surgical site.

Monofilament and multifilament sutures

There are many considerations when choosing to use a mono- or multifilament suture. Monofilament sutures

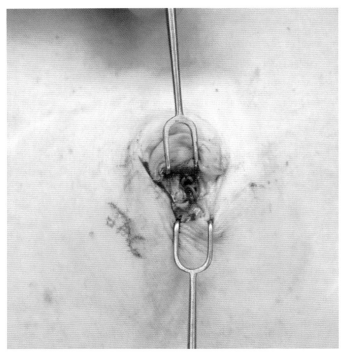

FIG. 11.13 Image is of a suture extrusion. (Source: Beidas, O., & Gusenoff, J. (2019). Deep and superficial closure. *Aesthetic Surgery Journal, 39*(Suppl 2), p. S86.)

SMALLER GAUGE										ZERO									LARGER GAUGE		
12-0	11-0	10-0	9-0	8-0	7-0	6-0	5-0	4-0	3-0	2-0	0	1	2	3	4	5	6	7	8	9	10

FIG. 11.14 Image of suture diameters. (Source: Phillips, N. (2017). *Berry & Kohn's operating room technique* (13th ed., p. 540, Box 28.1). St Louis, MO: Elsevier.)

have less resistance on passing through the tissue and are less likely to hold foreign organisms, potentially leading to infection. However, they can be easily weakened by crushing when handled. Multifilament sutures are generally stronger and, due to their braided or twisted nature, more flexible and pliable (Byrne & Aly, 2019). Current research is focusing on the effects of coating sutures – particularly multifilament – in an antimicrobial substance (Baygar, Sarac, Ugur, & Karaca, 2019) for prevention of potential SSI. Fig. 11.15 illustrates a multifilament and a monofilament suture.

Elasticity or memory
Elasticity or memory is the ability of the suture strand to retain its original 'packet' shape after being stretched (Phillips, 2017). Once removed from their packaging,

gut, nylon and prolene suture materials remain coiled. It is important for the instrument nurse to remove the elasticity of the suture material, to allow for ease of use by the surgeon. The atraumatic needle is loaded within the jaws of a needle holder in the usual way. The instrument nurse, taking much care not to pull the suture from the swaged end of the needle, must grasp the suture near the swaged end with thumb and forefinger. With the other hand, the distal end of the suture must be pulled taut until the elasticity is reduced.

Tensile strength
The amount of force exerted on the suture material to make it break is known as its tensile strength. Tensile strength also takes into consideration the time for which the suture retains its integrity before breaking down.

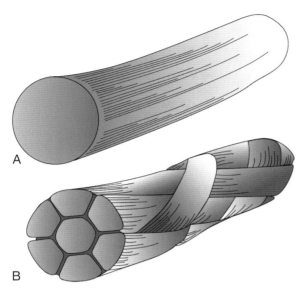

FIG. 11.15 A Monofilament suture. B. Multifilament suture. (Source: Adapted from McCarthy, J. (2015). Sutures, needles and instruments. In J. C. Rothrock, & D. R. McEwen (Eds.), *Alexander's care of the patient in surgery* (15th ed., pp. 189–210). St Louis, MO: Mosby.)

Ligature/Ties

Ligatures are made from suture material and are available in prepackaged standard lengths, in precut lengths or as ligature reels, in which the material is wound around a spool. Ties may be passed to the surgeon in several ways, depending on the surgery being performed and the individual preference of the surgeon. Standard length ties may be divided and cut into halves, thirds or quarters, depending on the depth of the tissue being ligated. Ties can be grasped within the jaws of an artery or tissue forceps, or simply handed to the surgeon.

Needles
Anatomy of a needle

Needles vary greatly depending on the type and location of tissue being sutured. While some needles are straight, most are curved, and are described according to degrees of a circle (e.g. $\frac{1}{4}$, $\frac{1}{2}$, $\frac{3}{4}$, $\frac{5}{8}$). The size of the circle depends on how wide or large a 'bite' is required and how much room there is to insert the needle. Fig. 11.16 shows the different types of needles.

- The *point* is the extreme tip of the needle which penetrates the tissue; many types are used in current practice.
- The *body* is the part of the needle that is grasped by the needle holder. It can be rounded, triangular, rectangular or trapezoidal, depending on the type of tissue the needle is expected to penetrate.
- The *swaged end* is where the suture material and the needle are joined to become one unit (Phillips, 2017).
- The *eye* of the needle is the segment of the needle where the suture material attaches to the needle. Atraumatic or swaged needles do not have this eye. A surgeon may request the instrument nurse to load a Mayo needle with a specific length or diameter of suture.

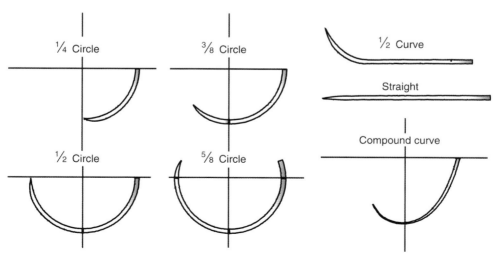

FIG. 11.16 Shapes of needle bodies. (Source: Phillips, N. (2017). *Berry & Kohn's operating room technique* (13th ed., p. 547, Fig. 28.12). St Louis, MO: Elsevier.)

Types of needle points

Both the body and the point of a needle determine which tissues the needle will penetrate. Within each classification, numerous types of needles are available. Figs 11.17 and 11.18 show the different needle types and shapes of suture tips.

Cutting edge. Cutting-edge needles have two or more opposing edges, which slice through the tissues (Phillips, 2017). They can be divided into two main types – conventional and reverse needles – which are determined by the location of the cutting edge. A conventional cutting-edge needle has its cutting edge on the concave (inside edge) side of the needle, whereas the cutting edge of the reverse cutting-edge needle lies on the convex (outside edge) side of the needle. Cutting-edge needles are predominantly used on skin; however, special types have been designed specifically for individual surgical specialties, such as ophthalmology and plastic surgery (Phillips, 2017).

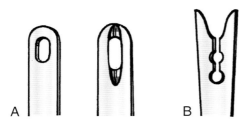

FIG. 11.17 A Mayo needle eyes. B Swaged needle. (Source: Phillips, N. (2017). *Berry & Kohn's operating room technique* (13th ed., p. 547, Fig. 28.13). St Louis, MO: Elsevier.)

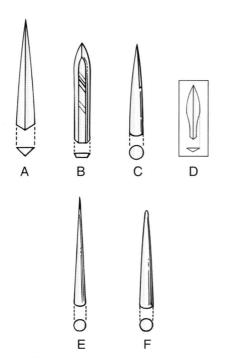

FIG. 11.18 Shapes of suture tips. (Source: Phillips, N. (2017). *Berry & Kohn's operating room technique* (13th ed., p. 546, Fig. 28.11). St Louis, MO: Elsevier.)

Taper point. The point of a taper needle pierces the tissue while the flattened/rounded body of the needle spreads tissue without cutting. The taper point is used in softer tissue that offers less resistance to the needle as it passes through and is considered less traumatic because of the way in which it separates the tissues and causes less bleeding. Taper needles can be used on all tissues except skin (i.e. blood vessels, muscle, viscera, peritoneum and fat) (Phillips, 2017).

A **blunt point taper needle** is designed to pass through friable tissue, such as liver or kidney. It is often used to prevent needlestick injuries and is commonly requested in hepatobiliary and gynaecological surgery (Phillips, 2017).

The **taper cut needle** was designed for vascular/cardiothoracic surgery, particularly for use with calcified, fibrotic blood vessels or prosthetic grafts. The cutting edges extend only a short distance from the needle tip and blend into a rounded, tapered body. Hence, the cutting edges pass through the hard, calcified portion of the blood vessel, while the remaining rounded taper body passes through the friable section of the blood vessel. Table 11.2 shows the different types of needles, wire types and their uses.

Body of the needle

The gauge of the wire and the length, shape and finish determine the 'body' of the needle. Factors to consider when choosing a needle body include the following:

- Tough tissue will require a heavier-gauge needle, whereas microsurgery will require a fine-gauge needle.
- The depth of bite required to penetrate the tissue determines the needle length.
- The circumference of the needle body may be round, oval or triangular (Phillips, 2017).

Loading needles

It is the role of the scrub nurse to choose an appropriate-sized needle holder with an appropriate width of tip. A needle holder has specifically designed jaws to

TABLE 11.2
Needle Types and Their Uses

Needle Type	Wire Type	Tissue	Surgery Examples
Taper	Fine	Soft	Bowel, vascular
	Medium	Fibrous	Fascia
	Heavy	Tough	Gynaecological
Blunt	—	Fibrous	Fascia, gynaecological
Cutting	Fine	Tough	Plastic
	Medium	—	Skin closure
	Heavy	—	Orthopaedics
Taper cutting	Fine	Vessels	Vascular
	Medium	Tough	Gynaecological
Spatula	Fine	Delicate	Ophthalmic

(Source: Adapted from Phillips, N. (2017). *Berry & Kohn's operating room technique* (13th ed.). St Louis, MO: Elsevier.)

grasp the needle securely; check these are in good working order prior to use. The gauge of the needle determines the appropriate-sized jaws; fine, small needles are loaded onto fine-tipped needle holders. The length of the needle holder will depend on the depth of wound closure required; use a longer needle holder when working in deep cavities and a short one for skin closure (Phillips, 2017). Feature box 11.2 provides practical tips for loading needles onto a needle holder.

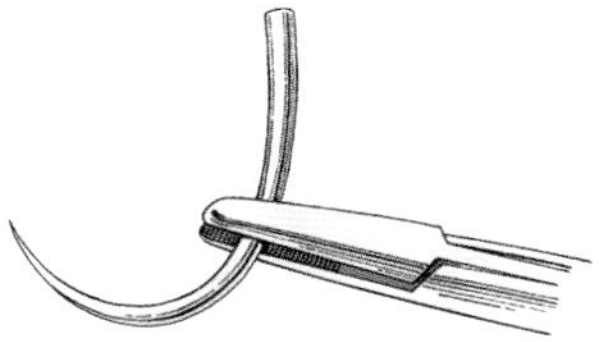

FIG. 11.19 A needle in a holder. (Source: Phillips, N. (2017). *Berry & Kohn's operating room technique* (13th ed. p. 548, Fig. 28.16). St Louis, MO: Elsevier.)

FEATURE BOX 11.2
Practice Tips

Safety of the instrument nurse is paramount when loading needles; ensure you have a clean and tidy workspace, where you will not be accidentally bumped. Load the needle one-third of the distance from the swaged end, at a 90° angle. The needle should never be clamped over the swaged area, as this weakens the attachment. Ensure that the needle is grasped firmly in the jaws by tightening the jaws one or two 'ratchet' clicks (see Fig. 11.19). It is vital that the suture is handed to the surgeon in a neutral zone, such as a yellow sharps dish, and in accordance with the ACORN standards (2020a) and hospital policy. These standards have been created to reduce the risk of sharps injury to both nursing and medical staff. In some specialty surgeries (e.g. vascular), surgeons may alter the angle of the needle to suit the area they are suturing. Remember to check whether your surgeon is right- or left-handed.

(Source: Australian College of Perioperative Nurses (ACORN). (2020a) Sharps and preventing sharps related injuries. In *ACORN standards for perioperative nursing in Australia* (16th ed., Vol. 1). Adelaide: Author.)

WOUND CLOSURE

The goal of **wound closure** is to decrease wound morbidity and the effect this has on patients (Krpata, 2019). Approximating the wound edges, eliminating dead space and distributing tension evenly along the suture line are all important considerations. Adequate haemostasis prior to commencing closure and appropriate selection of suture materials also affect the patient's outcome. Wound closures often include deep and superficial sutures but may also include staples, clips, tapes or glues. Selection of skin sutures for closure is dependent on patient-related factors, and surgeons' preferences. Research box 11.2 highlights the findings of a systematic review of literature reviews.

Wound Closure Methods

There are many methods of suturing wounds; the most common are described below. The method chosen by the surgeon will take many individual patient characteristics into account, alongside, of course, surgeon preference. It is important that the perioperative nurse

RESEARCH BOX 11.2
Absorbable Versus Non-absorbable Sutures for Skin Closure

A recent review of systematic reviews (Sheik-Ali & Guets, 2018) sought to provide an overview of the currently available evidence comparing absorbable with non-absorbable sutures for the closure of surgical incisions. The authors analysed data from 25 randomised control trials, which included 5781 patients. Their findings showed that there were no significant differences in surgical site infections, postoperative complications or risk of wound dehiscence between the use of absorbable and non-absorbable sutures.

(Source: Sheik-Ali, S., & Guets, W. (2018). Absorbable vs non absorbable sutures for wound closure. Systematic review of systematic reviews. *Wound Medicine, 23*, 35–37.)

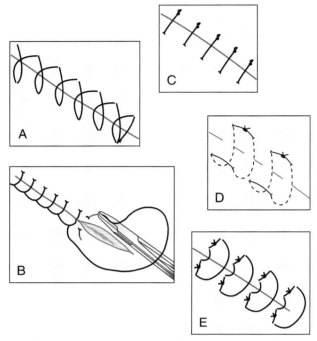

FIG. 11.20 Examples of suturing techniques: A Simple continuous. B Continuous locking. C Simple interrupted. D Horizontal mattress. E Vertical mattress. (Source: Phillips, N. (2017). *Berry & Kohn's operating room technique* (13th ed. p. 538, Fig. 28.8). St Louis, MO: Elsevier.)

has a good understanding of suture material and needle types to provide the best possible outcome for the patient. Examples of different suturing techniques are illustrated in Fig. 11.20.

Simple continuous sutures
In this method, the suture is anchored at one end of the wound and proceeds towards the opposite end, taking even bites of tissue. The suture is then anchored at the other end of the wound. This method is often used for a large wound closure, such as of the peritoneum, and may incorporate multiple layers (Phillips, 2017).

Simple interrupted sutures
Here each suture is placed and tied individually. Using this method, the surgeon may require the instrument nurse to cut the ends of the suture after each knot is complete. It is important to communicate with the surgeon to determine the best place (length) to cut the suture. The instrument nurse should stabilise the suture scissors with the index finger (known as the 'tripod stance') and the suture should be cut only with the tips of the scissors facing away from the patient (Phillips, 2017), ensuring the skin is never injured.

Continuous running/locking (blanket stitch)
Here a single suture is passed in and out of the tissue layers and looped through the free end before the needle is passed through the tissue for another stitch. Each new stitch locks the previous stitch (Phillips, 2017). The surgeon may require assistance to keep the 'tail' of the suture held firmly out of the way while the next stitch is placed, prior to locking. This method is commonly used for closure of the uterus.

Subcutaneous sutures
Subcutaneous sutures are placed under the epidermis, and provide a popular method of wound closure. Neat cosmetic results occur, as there is no skin perforation from the needle. Absorbable, undyed sutures are used.

Retention sutures
In this method, interrupted, non-absorbable retention or 'stay' sutures are placed alongside the primary suture line to relieve lateral tension on the suture line; this has been proved to reduce the risk of wound dehiscence (Ito et al., 2018), particularly in laparotomies. A 'heavy' suture is used, and a bolster (soft plastic tube) may be threaded over the suture to protect the skin (Phillips, 2017).

Drain sutures
Drains are often anchored to the skin by a suture to prevent accidental dislodgement. Silk sutures are the most used drain stitch material.

Laparoscopic sutures

Suturing laparoscopically is an important skill for the surgeon, and one that requires much training (Peker, Biler, Hortu, & Şendağ, 2019). For the perioperative nurse, however, there are only two choices. In Australia, a small number of laparoscopic sutures are available as preknotted loops, in prepackaged lengths, which are preloaded into a delivery mechanism. The nurse must take care to account for all parts of this device. After the surgeon has pulled the distal end of the suture to tighten it, a narrow 1 cm plastic component is removed from the external part of the delivery device; care must be taken for this to be removed from the operative site. Laparoscopic scissors are used to cut the tie. These preloaded sutures are most commonly used in laparoscopic appendicectomies to tie off the pedicle (Phillips, 2017).

The second method commonly used requires three laparoscopic instruments: the needle holder, the knot pusher and the laparoscopic scissors. This method can be difficult for the surgeon; it is a challenge to work from an image on a screen, as there is a lack of tactile feedback via the laparoscopic instruments, and a need for great dexterity in managing the instrumentation (Peker et al., 2019).

Given that the perioperative nurse must use a neutral zone to pass all sharps, this method may require extra planning preoperatively, and clear communication with the operating surgeon is essential to ensure safety of all scrubbed staff and the patient.

Other Methods of Wound Closure

Skin staples

These preloaded disposable devices provide the benefit of reducing tissue handling, thereby reducing the length of the procedure. Skin staples are used to close the skin layer of an incision, and are made from non-corroding metal (Fig. 11.21). Recent research, however, has shown that electively choosing skin staples over subcuticular suturing may leave the patient at greater risk of infection (Fox et al., 2018).

Tissue adhesives

Tissue adhesives such as 'skin glue' have been available since 1949 (Tacconi, Spinelli, & Signorelli, 2019) and have been used most commonly in the emergency room, particularly for children with minor traumatic wounds. Tissue adhesives provide good closure; current formulations of tissue adhesives set rapidly, have a greater breaking strength and are flexible. They provide painless closure and even have antimicrobial, bacteriostatic properties (Tacconi et al., 2019). Patients

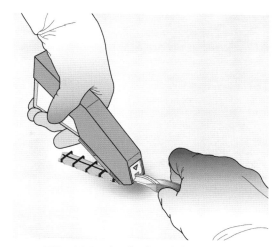

FIG. 11.21 Application of skin staples.

can shower because the adhesive also provides a waterproof barrier. Synthetic adhesives are glue-like adhesives that polymerise to bind tissue edges together. Biological and synthetic adhesives, such as fibrin glue compound, have great application in haemostasis (Phillips, 2017). Tissue adhesives may be used for microsurgical anastomoses of blood vessels, nerves and fallopian tubes.

Drains

Drains are often inserted during surgery to provide a pathway allowing blood, lymph, intestinal secretions, bile, pus, air or urine to be transported away from the surgical site. Drains can be used prophylactically or therapeutically. A drain is inserted prophylactically to remove unwanted fluid, air or secretions from around the surgical site, to decrease dead space in the wound (Anker et al., 2019), to promote wound healing, to provide a mechanism to observe for haemorrhage or leakage of fluids such as bile (Hokuto et al., 2016) and to potentially reduce postoperative pain. The presence of a collection of fluid, air or secretions has historically been thought to act as a medium in which microbes can grow, leading to an SSI (Wu, Tian, Kubilay, Ren, & Li, 2016). However, researchers also argue the presence of a drain may be a conduit for ascending infections and other complications (Gavriilidis, Hidalgo, de'Angelis, Lodge, & Azoulay, 2017), such as failure to prevent formation of a haematoma (Anker et al., 2019).

The use of prophylactic drains in surgery has been controversial for many years, with inconclusive support

RESEARCH BOX 11.3
Use of Prophylactic Drains

A systematic review and meta-analysis of four randomised control trials including 796 patients was undertaken to assess the effectiveness of prophylactic drains in reducing postoperative complications (Xu & Tao, 2019). Clinical outcomes in patients who underwent laparoscopic cholecystectomy for acute cholecystitis were compared across those patients who had a prophylactic drain inserted versus those who did not receive a prophylactic drain (Xu & Tao, 2019). Results showed no difference in patient length of stay or infection rates, and those patients with a drain reported higher pain levels.

(Source: Xu, M. & Tao, Y. L. (2019). Drainage versus no drainage after laparoscopic cholecystectomy for acute cholecystitis: a meta-analysis. *American Surgeon, 85*(1), 86–91.)

in the research literature, as described in Research box 11.3.

The presence of a drain may result in an inflammatory reaction which can affect healing (Wu et al., 2016). Many patient-centred factors must be considered when selecting and inserting a drainage system.

A drain that is inserted therapeutically is used to reduce the amount of an already present collection, which may be necrotic or purulent material. Drains are usually inserted at the time of surgery, primarily through a small stab incision near the operative site or, in the case of a peripheral open purulent wound, placed centrally and then affixed gently to the wound edges.

Drains may or may not be sutured to the skin. The most common suture used is a 2-0 silk stitch on a cutting edge. The perioperative nurse must document the use of this drain stitch in the intraoperative record; it is vital information for the nurse who will be removing the drain later. Some drains work by directing the fluid away through the lumen of the tube itself; other drains have a small fenestration at the tip, which drains into a closed system; yet other drains act by 'wicking' the fluid away by capillary action into an absorbent dressing or drainage bag. It is important also to document the type of drain used and whether the tip of the drain has been shortened. Again, this is important information for the ward nurse who may be removing the drain. Many commonly used drains, such as the Redivac or Hemovac, have a rounded tip, which is inspected on removal. If the drain has been shortened with scissors

and the tip is blunt, the ward nurse will need evidence that the drain has not broken off inside the patient. It is also important to check its location and whether the drain is sutured in place and is patent, with its attachments secure, before the patient leaves the operating room.

Drain types

Passive drains. Passive drains use gravity and the body's own capillary action to move unwanted fluids away from the operative site (Marchegiani et al., 2018). A Penrose drain is a soft latex tube, of varying size, often used for the superficial drainage of abscesses. It can be modified for multiple uses, particularly during hand surgery (Sano, Kimura, Hashimoto, & Ozeki, 2013).

A Yeates drain is a soft, multi-lumen silicone corrugated drain, which also uses capillary action and gravity to drain into a dressing (such as a folded combine pad) or drainage bag. It has been used in the operating theatres since the 1960s (Yeates, 1962). The perioperative nurse must note any modification in size or shape to this drain in the perioperative nursing records.

Active drains. Active drains are attached to an external source of vacuum to create suction under a negative pressure in the wound (Marchegiani et al., 2018). Active drains are detailed below.

Closed wound drainage systems. Closed drainage systems, such as the Hemovac or Redivac drains, are sterile, self-contained drainage units. The closed unit minimises the pathway of pathogens to the wound site. Closed units may be used with or without suction; that is, they can be active or passive drains. The negative pressure in the reservoir acts to draw fluid gently away from the wound site.

The Jackson-Pratt drain is a flat, soft silicone drainage stem with multiple fenestrations and is packaged as a separate, single item. It can be attached into the closed drainage system of the Redivac or the Hemovac system. This drain is often used for breast surgery, but can also have use in cardiac surgery as it is softer and more easily tolerated by patients (Mirmohammad-Sadeghi, Pourazari, & Akbari, 2017).

The Blake's drain is similarly packaged as a separate item and attaches onto the Redivac or the Hemovac suction system. It is almost an X shape, providing four channels along the peripheries, and has a silastic centre. It is commonly used for general surgeries, such as colorectal. A study recently found that insertion of a subcuticular Blake's drain was effective in drawing away potentially contaminated abdominal fluid post bowel surgery (Watanabe et al., 2017), although more research is required.

Chest drains. In cardiac surgery, harvesting of the left internal thoracic artery and associated pleural tissue damage creates the need for chest drains (Mirmoham-mad-Sadeghi et al., 2017). Drainage of the pleural cavity ensures complete expansion of the lungs after surgery, preventing complications such as atelectasis, infection and tamponade, and providing a means of assessing for bleeding (Mirmohammad-Sadeghi et al., 2017). Air and fluid must be evacuated from the pleural space after surgical procedures within the chest cavity (Fig. 11.22). One or more chest tubes are inserted. If the surgeon inserts two, the upper tube evacuates air and the lower

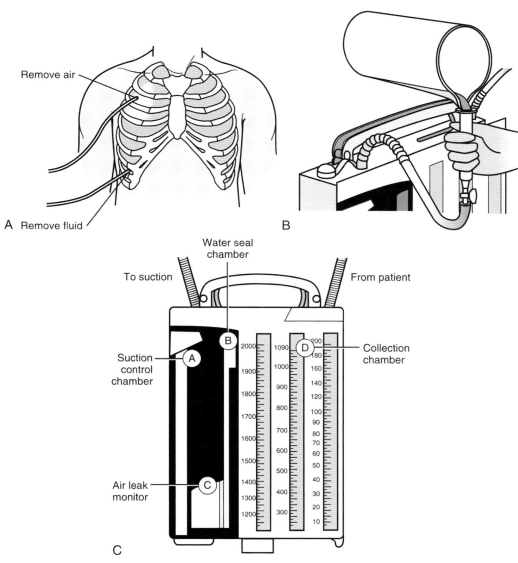

FIG. 11.22 A Placement of drains. B Scrub person pours sterile water into the unit to create a water seal. C Tubing attachment to three-chamber collection unit. (Source: Phillips, N. (2017). *Berry & Kohn's operating room technique* (13th ed., p. 576, Fig. 29.4). St Louis, MO: Elsevier.)

tube drains fluid (Phillips, 2017). Care must be taken when moving and transferring the patient to ensure that the drain is kept below chest height.

Specialised drains
- T-tube is a T-shaped, soft latex drain that is inserted into the common bile duct, allowing bile to be drained away. It is most commonly used after a complicated laparoscopic cholecystectomy (Phillips, 2017).
- Pezzer drain is a bulb-shaped drain commonly used for rectoanal fissures (Aparíício et al., 2019).
- Mini-vac is a small, low-suction drain, commonly used in procedures on the finger, in which the estimated drainage is small.

SURGICAL DRESSINGS
Dressings are applied to a surgical incision or wound site for the first 48 hours to provide the best environment for wound healing to occur (Carville, 2017). Surgical wounds healing by secondary intention should require minimal intervention other than protection and monitoring for complications (Carville, 2017). A surgical dressing ideally:
- protects the wound from pathogenic contamination
- absorbs exudate
- maintains thermal insulation
- may provide support and immobilisation of the incisional area (Carville, 2017; Graça, Miguel, Cabral, & Correia, 2020).

The choice of dressing should be made after assessing the wound, the needs of the patient and the wound requirements (Graça et al., 2020).

Types of Dressings
Dressings are classified in several ways according to their actions, such as moisture retention, moisture donation, exudate management, haemostatic or antimicrobial (Swanson, 2014). They may also be classified as primary or secondary dressings. Primary dressings are applied directly over the wound to absorb exudate and maintain a moist wound-healing environment; secondary dressings are placed over the primary dressing to absorb further exudate or provide added protection from trauma (Bak, 2015).

Recommended dressings for wounds healing by primary intention include (Carville, 2017):
- simple dressings: dry non-adherent/island dressings/ semi-permeable films
- silicone dressings
- hydrocolloids
- foams.

Simple dressings
Dry non-adherent dressings. These dressings have low absorbency and are used for protective measures. The non-adherent pad prevents sticking to the wound surface, minimising trauma on removal (Morris, 2006). These non-adherent dressings are used as the contact layer in island dressings.

Island dressings. Island dressings consist of a central non-adherent pad with a secondary layer that is adherent (Carville, 2017). The secondary layer secures the dressing to the skin and may be permeable, semi-permeable or occlusive. Due to their low absorbency capacity, these dressings are used on wounds healing by primary intention.

Semi-permeable films. Film dressings are transparent, adhesive membranes that allow the movement of moisture vapour and oxygen across the dressing but are impermeable to bacterial contaminants (Swanson, 2014). This property is known as the moisture vapour transfer rate (MVTR), and may vary among products. The MVTR allows the wound environment to remain moist, clean and warm (Jones & Milton, 2000). Film dressings may allow for inspection of the wound and surrounding skin without dressing removal. They are often used as a secondary dressing for fixation.

Silicone dressings
These dressings have historically been used for scar management to improve cosmetic appearance (Swanson, 2014). However, with new technology they are now widely used as a primary dressing to provide moist wound healing with atraumatic removal. They may be used for low to moderately exudative wounds. Silicone dressings are used where there is a need to protect fragile skin and prevent trauma to the wound interface.

Hydrocolloid dressings
Hydrocolloid dressings originated from stoma products. The dressings are made of a base of polymers that are gel forming, including carbomethoxycellulose (CMC), pectins, gelatin and elastomers (Carville, 2017; Swanson, 2014). The base has an adhesive film or foam backing to adhere to the body of the dressing to provide a protective moist wound environment. These dressings have low to moderate absorbency, depending on the product brand.

Foams
Polyurethane foams are absorbent dressings that may be adhesive with a waterproof backing or

non-adhesive (Morris, 2006). They may also be combined with other dressings such as hydrocolloids, films or hydrofibres to enhance properties, and with variants such as antimicrobials, surfactants, antiseptics and medications to improve healing outcomes (Swanson, 2014).

Pressure dressings

These are bulky dressings added to the immediate layer of a three-layer dressing. This type of dressing acts to eliminate dead space and prevent haematoma or oedema. It also distributes pressure evenly, absorbs extensive drainage, encourages wound healing and minimises scarring by influencing wound tension, and immobilises a body area or supports soft tissues when muscles have been moved. A pressure dressing helps to provide comfort to the patient postoperatively. These dressings are often used in plastic, knee and breast surgery (Phillips, 2017).

Stent dressings

A stent dressing is a method of applying pressure and stabilising tissues when it is impossible to dress an area, such as on the face or neck.

Bolster/tie-over dressings

Dressing materials may be sutured in place to exert an even pressure over autografted wounds to prevent haematoma or seroma formation.

Antimicrobial/antiseptic dressings

There are several antimicrobial dressings available that include silver or polyhexamethylene biguanide (PHMB). These dressings are usually applied to wounds that are infected or heavily contaminated with a high bacterial load and healing by secondary intention. They are not indicated for surgical wounds closed by primary intention but may be applied postoperatively. The effectiveness of these dressings in preventing surgical site infection remains equivocal. A Cochrane systematic review investigating the use of topical antibiotics for preventing SSI in wounds healing by primary intention was inconclusive (Heal, Banks, Lepper, Kontopantelis, & van Driel, 2016).

Negative-pressure wound therapy (NPWT)

The application of negative-pressure wound therapy (NPWT) (or vacuum therapy) to closed surgical wounds is becoming increasingly common. The negative-pressure system provides a sterile, closed system using foam or gauze dressings to support wound healing through:
- reducing local oedema
- increasing tissue perfusion and stimulating formation of new granulation tissue
- decreasing bacterial load and subsequent risk of infection
- managing wound exudate (WUWHS, 2016).

NPWT may also be used for secondary closure if primary closure cannot be achieved, such as in abdominal surgery (Stevens, 2009), for stabilising sternal wounds to reduce movement to facilitate healing (Brega, Calvi, & Albertini, 2021; De Martino et al., 2020) or for prevention of surgical site infections (Webster et al., 2019).

Research box 11.4 summarises a Cochrane review of the effectiveness of negative-pressure wound therapy in prevention of wound complications.

RESEARCH BOX 11.4
Effectiveness of Negative-pressure Wound Therapy in Prevention of Wound Complications

A Cochrane review of negative-pressure wound therapy (NPWT) for surgical wounds healing by primary closure included 44 studies with 7447 surgical patients (Norman et al., 2020). Review findings suggested there was inconclusive evidence to support the use of NPWT for prevention of surgical site infection. There was also inconclusive evidence on the incidence of seroma development, haematoma, hospital re-admission and cost effectiveness. The authors concluded that higher-quality independently funded trials are needed.

(Source: Norman, G., Goh, E. L., Dumville, J. C., Shi, C., Liu, Z., Chiverton, L., … Reid, A. (2020). Negative pressure wound therapy for surgical wounds healing by primary closure. *Cochrane Database of Systematic Reviews*, 6(6), CD009261.)

PATIENT SCENARIOS

SCENARIO 11.3: NEGATIVE-PRESSURE WOUND THERAPY (NPWT)

Ms Janine Clark, a 35-year-old multipara, is scheduled to have an elective lower segment caesarean section (LSCS). Ms Clark has a BMI of 39.1 kg/m² and has had two previous LSCSs with difficult wound healing. Ms Clark's full history and a brief description of the healthcare setting are provided in the Introduction to this book for readers to review when answering the questions in this unfolding scenario.

At the conclusion of the caesarean procedure, consultant surgeon Dr Emma Tan requests a negative-pressure wound therapy dressing be applied to the suture line.

Critical Thinking Question
- Explain the rationale for Dr Tan's choice of dressing for Ms Clark.

CONCLUSION
Wound healing is a complex process that involves the activation and synchronisation of intracellular, intercellular and extracellular elements. This chapter has explored types of wound healing, surgical haemostasis and wound closure. The perioperative nurse must show sound assessment, planning, implementation and evaluation of all aspects of wound management during the perioperative period to provide the best patient-centred care.

ACKNOWLEDGEMENTS
We acknowledge the contributions of Ann Parkman and Dr Marilyn Richardson-Tench, who were co-authors of Chapter 11 in the second edition of this textbook.

RESOURCES
NHMRC Australian Guidelines for the Prevention and Control of Infection in Healthcare (2019)
https://www.nhmrc.gov.au/about-us/publications/australian-guidelines-prevention-and-control-infection-healthcare-2019
Wounds Australia
htttps://www.woundsaustralia.com.au
Wounds International
htttps://www.woundsinternational.com

VIDEO RESOURCES
Burn management in the OR
https://youtu.be/lFPHYjjKJVs
Wound debridement
https://youtu.be/2DBWtPwcNag

REFERENCES
Abyaneh, M., Griffith, R., Falto-Aizpurua, L., & Nouri, K. (2014). Famous lines in history – Langer lines. *Journal of the American Medical Association: Dermatology, 10*, 1087. https://dx.doi.org/10.1001/jamadermatol.2014.659

Ai, X., Ho, L., Yang, N., Han, L., Lu, J., & Yue, X. (2018). A comparative study of ultrasonic scalpel (US) versus conventional metal clips for closure of the cystic duct in laparoscopic cholecystectomy (LC): a meta-analysis. *Medicine, 97*(51), e13735.

Alshomer, F., Madhavan, A., Pathan, O., & Song, W. (2017). Bioactive sutures: a review of advances in surgical suture functionalisation. *Current Medicinal Chemistry, 24*(2), 215–223. https://dx.doi.org/10.2174/0929867324666161118141724

Anker, A. M., Miranda, B. H., Prantl, L., Kehrer, A., Strauss, C., Brébant, V., & Klein, S. M. (2019). 50 shades of red: the predictive value of closed suction drains for the detection of postoperative bleeding in breast surgery. *Aesthetic Plastic Surgery, 43*(3), 608–615. https://dx.doi.org/10.1007/s00266-019-01345-1

Anwar, M., Nofal, A., & Elmalt, A. (2017). Surgicel use in control of primary postadenoidectomy bleeding. *Ear, Nose and Throat Journal, 96*(9), 372.

Aparíício, D., Leichsenring, C., Sobrinho, C., Pignatelli, N., Geraldes, V., & Nunes, V. (2019). Supralevator abscess: new treatment for an uncommon aetiology: case report. *International Journal of Surgery Case Reports, 59*, 128–131. https://dx.doi.org/10.1016/j.ijscr.2019.05.016

Australian College of Perioperative Nurses (ACORN). (2020a). Sharps and preventing sharps related injuries. In *ACORN standards for perioperative nursing in Australia* (16th ed., Vol. 1). Adelaide: Author.

Australian College of Perioperative Nurses (ACORN). (2020b). Laser safety. In *ACORN standards for perioperative nursing in Australia* (16th ed., Vol. 1). Adelaide: Author.

Bak, J. (2015). Wound healing, dressings and drains. In J. C. Rothrock, & D. R. McEwen (Eds.), *Alexander's care of the patient in surgery* (15th ed., pp. 253–269). St. Louis, MO: Elsevier Saunders.

Ball, K. (2015). Surgical modalities. In J. C. Rothrock, & D. R. McEwen (Eds.), *Alexander's care of the patient in surgery* (15th ed., pp. 211–252). St. Louis, MO: Elsevier Saunders.

Baygar, T., Sarac, N., Ugur, A., & Karaca, I. (2019). Antimicrobial characteristics and biocompatibility of the surgical sutures coated with biosynthesized silver nanoparticles. *Bioorganic Chemistry, 86*, 254–258.

Beidas, O., & Gusenoff, J. (2019). Deep and superficial closure. *Aesthetic Surgery Journal, 39*(Suppl 2), S85–S93.

Berríos-Torres, S., Umscheid, C., Bratzler, D., Leas, B., Stone, E., Kelz, R., … Schecter, W. (2017). Prevention of surgical site infection. *Journal of the American Medical Association: Surgery, 152*(8), 784–791. https://dx.doi.org/https://dx.doi.org/10.1001/jamasurg.2017.0904

Brega, C., Calvi, S., & Albertini, A. (2021). Use of a negative pressure wound therapy system over closed incisions option in preventing post-sternotomy wound complications. *Wound Repair and Regeneration, 29* Mar. https://dx.doi.org/10.1111/wrr.12914. Online ahead of print.

Byrne, M., & Aly, A. (2019). The surgical suture. *Aesthetic Surgery Journal, 39*(Suppl. 2), S67–S72

Camp, M. A. (2014). Hemostatic agents: a guide to safe practice for perioperative nurses. *AORN Journal, 100*(2), 131–147. https://dx.doi.org/10.1016/j.aorn.2014.01.024

Carville, K. (2017). *Wound care manual* (7th ed.). Osborne Park: Silver Chain Foundation.

Chetter, I. C., Oswald, A. V., Fletcher, M., Dumville, J. C., & Cullum, N. A. (2017). A survey of patients with surgical wounds healing by secondary intention; an assessment of prevalence, aetiology, duration and management. *Journal of Tissue Viability, 26*(2), 103–107. https://dx.doi.org/10.1016/j.jtv.2016.12.004

De Martino, A., Del Re, F., Falcetta, G., Morganti, R., Ravenni, G., & Bortolotti, Y. (2020). Sternal wound complications: results of routine use of negative pressure wound therapy. *Brazilian Journal of Cardiovascular Surgery, 35*(1),50-57. https://dx.doi.org/10.21470/1678-9741-2019-0242

Doughty, D., & Sparks, B. (2016). Wound-healing physiology and factors that affect the wound repair process. In R. A. Bryant, & D. P. Nix (Eds.), *Acute and chronic wounds: current management concepts* (5th ed., pp. 63–81). St. Louis, MO: Elsevier.

Fox, N., Melka, S., Miller, J., Bender, S., Silverstein, M., Saltzman, D., & Rebarber, A. (2018). Suture compared with staple closure of skin incision for high-order cesarean deliveries. *Obstetrics and Gynecology, 131*(3), 523–528. https://dx.doi.org/10.1097/AOG.0000000000002484

Fuller, J. (2013). *Surgical technology principles and practice* (6th ed.). St. Louis, MO: Elsevier.

Gavriilidis, P., Hidalgo, E., de'Angelis, N., Lodge, P., & Azoulay, D. (2017). Re-appraisal of prophylactic drainage in un-complicated liver resections: a systematic review and meta-analysis. *HPB, 19*(1), 16–20.

Goobie, S. (2017). Tranexamic acid: still far to go. *British Journal of Anaesthesia, 118*(3), 293–295. https://dx.doi.org/10.1093/bja/aew470

Graça, M., Miguel, S., Cabral, C., & Correia, I. (2020). Hyaluronic acid-based wound dressings: a review. *Carbohydrate Polymers, 241*, 116364. https://dx.doi.org/10.1016/j.carbpol.2020.116364

Harkin, D., & Dunlop, D. (2018). Vascular trauma. *Surgery (Oxford), 36*(6), 306–313.

Heal, C. F., Banks, J. L., Lepper, P. D., Kontopantelis, E., & van Driel, M. L. (2016). Topical antibiotics for preventing surgical site infection in wounds healing by primary intention. *Cochrane Database of Systematic Reviews, 11*(11), CD011426. https://dx.doi.org/10.1002/14651858.CD011426.pub2.PMID: 27819748

Hokuto, D., Nomi, T., Yasuda, S., Kawaguchi, C., Yoshikawa, T., Ishioka, K., . . . Kanehiro, H. (2016). The safety of the early removal of prophylactic drainage after liver resection based solely on predetermined criteria: a propensity score analysis. *HPB, 19*(4), 359–364.

Ito, E., Yoshida, M., Suzuki, N., Imakita, T., Tsutsui, N., Ohdaira, H., . . . Suzuki, Y. (2018). Prophylactic retention suture for surgical site infection: a retrospective cohort study. *Journal of Surgical Research, 221*, 58–63. https://dx.doi.org/10.1016/j.jss.2017.08.012

Jones, V., & Milton, T. (2000). When and how to use adhesive film dressings. *NT Plus – Wound Care (Supp.). Nursing Times, 96*, 3–4.

Kim, B., Sgarioto, M., Hewitt, D., Paver, R., Norman, J., & Fernandez-Penas, P. (2018). Scar outcomes in dermatological surgery. *Australasian Journal of Dermatology, 59*(1), 48–51.

Krpata, D. (2019). Wound closure and management. *Surgical Infections, 20*(2), 135–138. https://dx.doi.org/10.1089/sur.2018.235

LeBlanc, K., Campbell, K. E., Wood, E., & Beeckman D. (2018). Best practice recommendations for prevention and management of skin tears in aged skin: an overview. *Journal of Wound Ostomy and Continence Nursing, 45*(6), 540–542. https://dx.doi.org/10.1097/WON.0000000000000481

Lv, X., Cao Song, C., He, H., Jiang, C., & Youxiang Li, Y. (2017). Transvenous retrograde AVM embolisation: indications, techniques, complications and outcomes. *Interventional Neuroradiology, 23*(5), 504–509. https://dx.doi.org/10.1177/1591019917716817

Marchegiani, G., Perri, G., Pulvirenti, A., Sereni, E., Azzini, A., Malleo, G., . . . Bassi, C. (2018). Non-inferiority of open passive drains compared with closed suction drains in pancreatic surgery outcomes: a prospective observational study. *Surgery, 164*(3), 443–449. https://dx.doi.org/10.1016/j.surg.2018.04.025

McCance, K., & Huether, S. (2019). *Pathophysioloy: the biologic basis for disease in adults and children* (8th ed.). St. Louis, MO: Elsevier.

McCarthy, J. (2015). Sutures, needles and instruments. In J. C. Rothrock & D. R. McEwen (Eds.), *Alexander's care of the patient in surgery* (15th ed., pp. 189–210). St. Louis, MO: Mosby.

McCaughan, D., Sheard, L., Cullum, N., Dumville, J., & Chetter, I. (2018). Patients' perceptions and experiences of living with a surgical wound healing by secondary intention: a qualitative study. *International Journal of Nursing Studies, 77*, 29–38. https://dx.doi.org/https://dx.doi.org/10.1016/j.ijnurstu.2017.09.015

Mirmohammad-Sadeghi, M., Pourazari, P., & Akbari, M. (2017). Comparison consequences of Jackson-Pratt drain versus chest tube after coronary artery bypass grafting: A randomized controlled clinical trial. *Journal of Research in Medical Sciences, 22*(1), 134. https://dx.doi.org/10.4103/jrms.JRMS_739_17

Mohr-Sasson, A., Spira, M., Rahav, R., Manela, D., Schiff, E., Mazaki-Tovi, S., … Sivan, E. (2018). Ovarian reserve after uterine artery embolization in women with morbidly adherent placenta: a cohort study. *PLoS ONE, 13*(11), e0208139. https://dx.doi.org/https://dx.doi.org/10.1371/journal.pone.0208139

Morris, C. (2006). Wound management and dressing essentials. *Wound Essentials, 1*, 178–183.

Myles, P., Smith, J., Forbes, A., Silbert, B., Jayarajah, M., Painter, T., . . . Wallace, S. (2017). Tranexamic acid in patients undergoing coronary-artery surgery. *New England Journal of Medicine, 376*(2), 136–148.

Norman, G., Goh, E. L., Dumville, J. C., Shi, C., Liu, Z., Chiverton, L., … Reid, A. (2020). Negative pressure wound therapy for surgical wounds healing by primary closure. *Cochrane Database of Systematic Reviews, 6*(6), CD009261. https://dx.doi.org/10.1002/14651858.CD009261.pub6. PMID: 32542647

Okhunov, Z., Yoon, R., Lusch, A., Spradling, K., Suarez, M., Kaler, K., . . . Landman, J. (2018). Evaluation and comparison of contemporary energy-based surgical vessel sealing devices. *Journal of Endourology, 32*(4), 329–337. https://dx.doi.org/10.1089/end.2017.0596

Ortega, G., Rhee, D. S., Papandria, D. J., Yang, J., Ibrahim, A. M., Shore, A. D. … Abdullah, F. (2012). An evaluation of surgical site infections by wound classification system using the ACS-NSQIP. *Journal of Surgical Research, 174*(1), 33–38. https://dx.doi.org/10.1016/j.jss.2011.05.056

Park, H., Suk, K., & Park, J. (2018). A case of intraoperative anaphylaxis caused by bovine-derived thrombin. *Allergy, Asthma and Immunology Research, 10*(2), 184–186.

Peker, N., Biler, A., Hortu, İ., & Şendağ, F. (2019). Effectiveness of a one-day laparoscopic suture course. *Journal of Obstetrics and Gynaecology, 39*(7), 981–985. https://dx.doi.org/10.1080/01443615.2019.1584882

Philip, C., Le Mitouard, M., Maillet, L., De Saint-Hilaire, P., Huissoud, C., Cortet, M., & Dubernard, G. (2018). Evaluation of NovaSure® global endometrial ablation in symptomatic adenomyosis: a longitudinal study with a 36 month follow-up. *European Journal of Obstetrics, Gynecology, and Reproductive Biology, 227*, 46–51.

Phillips, N. (2017). *Berry & Kohn's operating room technique* (13th ed.). St. Louis, MO: Elsevier.

Ramirez, M., Deutsch, H., Khanna, N., Cheatem, D., Yang, D., & Kuntze, E. (2018). Floseal only versus in combination in spine surgery: a comparative, retrospective hospital database evaluation of clinical and healthcare resource outcomes. *Hospital Practice, 46*(4), 189–196. https://dx.doi.org/10.1080/21548331.2018.1498279

Ramundo, J. M. (2016). Wound debridement. In R. A. Bryant, & D. P. Nix (Eds.), *Acute and chronic wounds. current management concepts* (5th ed., pp. 295–305). Maryland Heights, MO: Mosby Elsevier.

Royal Australian and New Zealand College of Gynaecologists (RANZCOG). (2017). Management of postpartum hemorrhage (PPH). Retrieved from <https://ranzcog.edu.au/RANZCOG_SITE/media/RANZCOG-MEDIA/Women%27s%20Health/Statement%20and%20guidelines/Clinical-Obstetrics/Management-of-Postpartum-Haemorrhage-(C-Obs-43)-Review-July-2017.pdf?ext=.pdf>.

Sano, K., Kimura, K., Hashimoto, T., & Ozeki, S. (2013). Two-stage tendon sheath reconstruction using sublimis tendon and silicone Penrose drain after severe purulent flexor tenosynovitis: a case report. *Hand, 8*(3), 343–347. https://dx.doi.org/10.1007/s11552-013-9507-8.

Sawada, K., Kawarada, O., & Yasuda, S. (2018). Empirical embolisation for intermittent spontaneous muscle haemorrhage associated with anticoagulation therapy. *Heart Asia, 10*(1), 1–2.

Sheik-Ali, S., & Guets, W. (2018). Absorbable vs non absorbable sutures for wound closure. Systematic review of systematic reviews. *Wound Medicine, 23*, 35–37.

Singh, S., Young, A., & McNaught, C. (2017). The physiology of wound healing. *Surgery (Oxford), 35*(9), 473–477.

Sorg, H., Tilkorn, D., Hager, S., Hauser, J., & Mirastschijski, U. (2017). Skin wound healing: an update on the current knowledge and concepts. *European Surgical Research, 58*(1–2), 81–94. https://dx.doi.org/10.1159/000454919

Stevens, P. (2009). Vacuum-assisted closure of laparotomy wounds: a critical review of the literature. *International Wound Journal, 6*(4), 259–266.

Suarez, S., Conde-Agudelo, A., Borovac-Pinehiro, A., Suarez-Rebling, D., Eckardt, M., Theron, G., & Burke, T. (2020). Uterine balloon tamponade for the treatment of post partum haemorrhage: a systematic review and meta analysis. *American Journal of Obsetrics and Gynecology, 222*, 293e1–52.

Swanson, T. (2014). *Wound management for the advanced practitioner*. Melbourne: IP Communications.

Swapnika, D., Priya, P., Priya, S., & Allirathinam, A. (2018). A comparative study between intramuscular oxytocin and intramuscular methyl ergometrine in the active management of third stage of labour. *International Journal of Reproduction, Contraception, Obstetrics and Gynecology, 7*(5), 1943.

Tacconi, L., Spinelli, R., & Signorelli, F. (2019). Skin glue for wounds closure in brain surgery: our updated experience. *World Neurosurgery, 121*, e940–e946. https://dx.doi.org/10.1016/j.wneu.2018.10.023

Tu, Y., Chang, W., Wu, C., & Sheu, B. (2019). Improved hemostasis with plasma kinetic bipolar sealing device in the vaginal steps of laparoscopic-assisted vaginal hysterectomy. *Taiwanese Journal of Obstetrics and Gynecology, 58*(1), 64–67. https://dx.doi.org/10.1016/j.tjog.2018.11.012

Turrentine, F. E., Giballa, S. B., Shah, P. M., Jones, D. R., Hedrick, T. L., & Friel, C. M. (2015). Solutions to intraoperative wound classification miscoding in a subset of American College of Surgeons National Surgical Quality Improvement Program patients. *American Surgeon, 81*(2), 193–197.

Van Den Heever, T., Barrett, C., Webb, M., Spruyt, M., & Louw, C. (2015). Postoperative internal iliac artery embolisation as salvage therapy for bleeding in an HIV-positive patient with giant cell tumour of bone: case report. *Southern African Journal of Critical Care, 31*(1), 30–31.

Van Tiggelen, H., Alves, P., Ayello, E., Bååth, C., Baranoski, S., Campbell, K., . . . Beeckman, D. (2021). Development and psychometric property testing of a skin tear knowledge assessment instrument (OASES) in 37 countries. *Journal of Advanced Nursing, 77*(3), 1609–1623. https://dx.doi.org/10.1111/jan.14713

Wakelam, O., Dimitriadis, P., & Stephens, J. (2017). The use of FloSeal haemostatic sealant in the management of epistaxis: a prospective clinical study and literature review. *Annals of the Royal College of Surgeons of England, 99*(1), 28. https://dx.doi.org/10.1308/rcsann.2016.0224

Wang, D., Xu, S., Qiu, X., Zhu, C., Li, Z., Wang, Z., . . . Liu, L. (2018). Early usage of Bakri postpartum balloon in the management of postpartum hemorrhage: a large prospective, observational multicenter clinical study in South China. *Journal of Perinatal Medicine, 46*(6), 649–656.

Watanabe, J., Ota, M., Kawamoto, M., Akikazu, Y., Suwa, Y., Suwa, H., . . . Nagahori, K. (2017). A randomized controlled trial of subcutaneous closed-suction Blake drains for the prevention of incisional surgical site infection after colorectal surgery. *Clinical and Molecular Gastroenterology and Surgery, 32*(3), 391–398. https://dx.doi.org/10.1007/s00384-016-2687-2

Webster, J., Liu, Z., Norman, G., Dumville, J. C., Chiverton, L., Scuffham, P., . . . Chaboyer, W. P. (2019). Negative pressure wound therapy for surgical wounds healing by primary closure. *Cochrane Database of Systematic Reviews, 3*(3), CD009261. https://dx.doi.org/10.1002/14651858.CD009261.pub4

Weinberg, L., Hanus, G., Banting, J., Abu-Ssaydeh, D., Spanger, M., Goh, S., & Muralidharan, V. (2017). Preoperative left hepatic lobe devascularisation to minimize perioperative bleeding in a Jehovah's Witness undergoing left hepatectomy. *International Journal of Surgery Case Reports, 36*, 69–73. https://dx.doi.org/10.1016/j.ijscr.2017.05.005

White, W., & Asimus, M. (2014). Assessment and management of non-viable tissue. In T. Swanson, M. Asimus, & W. McGuiness (Eds.), *Wound management for the advanced practitioner* (Ch. 8, pp 170–203). Melbourne: IP Communications.

World Union of Wound Healing Societies (WUWHS). (2016). Consensus document closed surgical incision management: understanding the role of NPWT. Retrieved from <https://www.woundsinternational.com/resources/details/consensus-documents-closed-surgical-incision-management-understanding-the-role-of-npwt-wme>.

World Union of Wound Healing Societies (WUWHS) (2019). Consensus Document: Wound exudate effective assessment and management. Retrieved from <https://www.woundsinternational.com/resources/details/wuwhs-consensus-document-wound-exudate-effective-assessment-and-management>.

Wu, X., Tian, W., Kubilay, N. Z., Ren, J., & Li, J. (2016). Is it necessary to place prophylactically an abdominal drain to prevent surgical site infection in abdominal operations? A systematic meta-review. *Surgical Infections, 17*(6), 730–738.

Xu, M., & Tao, Y. L. (2019). Drainage versus no drainage after laparoscopic cholecystectomy for acute cholecystitis: a meta-analysis. *American Surgeon, 85*(1), 86–91.

Yeates, W. (1962). A new tissue drain. *The Lancet, 280*(7266), 1150. https://dx.doi.org/https://dx.doi.org/10.1016/S0140-6736(62)90905-4

FURTHER READING

Berg, A., Fleischer, S., Kuss, O., Unverzagt, S., & Langer, G. (2012). Timing of dressing removal in the healing of surgical wounds by primary intention: quantitative systematic review protocol. *Journal of Advanced Nursing, 68*(2), 264–270. https://dx.doi.org/10.1111/j.1365-2648.2011.05803.x

Gillespie, B. M., Bull, C., Walker, R., Lin, F., Roberts, S., & Chaboyer, W. (2018). Quality appraisal of clinical guidelines for surgical site infection prevention: a systematic review. *PLoS ONE, 13*(9), e0203354. https://dx.doi.org/10.1371/journal.pone.0203354

Gurusamy, K. S., Allen, V. B., & Samraj, K. (2012). Wound drains after incisional hernia repair. *Cochrane Database of Systematic Reviews, 15*, 2. https://dx.doi.org/10.1002/14651858.CD005570.pub3

Ibrahim, M. I., Moustafa, G. F., Abd Al-Hamid, A. S., & Hussein, M. R. (2014). Superficial incisional surgical site infection rate after cesarean section in obese women: a randomized controlled trial of subcuticular versus interrupted skin suturing. *Archives of Gynecology and Obstetrics, 289*, 981–986.

Mioton, L. M., Jordan, S. W., Hanwright, P. J., Bilimoria, K., & Kim, J. (2013). The relationship between preoperative wound classification and postoperative infection: a multi-institutional analysis of 15,289 patients. *Archives of Plastic Surgery, 40*(5), 522–529. https://dx.doi.org/10.5999/aps.2013.40.5.522

Rothrock, J., & McEwen, D. (Eds.). (2015). *Alexander's care of the patient in surgery* (15th ed.). St. Louis, MO: Elsevier Saunders.

Schulz, G., Ladwig, G., & Wysocki, A. (2005). Extracellular matrix: review of its roles in acute and chronic wounds. Retrieved from <http://www.worldwidewounds.com/2005/august/Schultz/Extrace-Matric-Acute-Chronic-Wounds.html>.

Voigt, J., & Driver, V. R. (2012). Hyaluronic acid derivatives and their healing effect on burns, epithelial surgical wounds, and chronic wounds: a systematic review and meta-analysis of randomized controlled trials. *Wound Repair and Regeneration, 20*, 317–331.

Wang, I., Walker, R., & Gillespie, B. M. (2018). Pressure injury prevention for surgery: results from a prospective, observational study in a tertiary hospital. *Journal of Perioperative Nursing, 31*(3), 25–28. https://dx.doi.org/10.26550/2209-1092.1035

CHAPTER 12

Postanaesthesia Nursing Care

PAULA FORAN • KATHRYN JOHNS

EDITOR: MENNA DAVIES

LEARNING OUTCOMES

- Discuss the design and purpose of the postanaesthesia care unit (PACU)
- Describe the handover process from the anaesthetist to the nurse and the nursing responsibility for accepting the care of a patient
- Explain the initial assessment and management of an immediate postanaesthesia patient and the ongoing assessment and interventions required for safe care
- Discuss common postanaesthesia complications, including the recognition of deteriorating patients and their management
- Discuss an overview of acute pain management of the postanaesthesia patient and describe common pharmacological and non-pharmacological treatments
- Describe the management of special patient populations
- Discuss the discharge criteria for postanaesthesia patients and describe the handover procedure from the PACU to the ward

KEY TERMS

airway	discharge criteria
bronchospasm	handover
complications	laryngospasm
deterioration	pain management

INTRODUCTION

The purpose of the postanaesthesia care unit (PACU) is to monitor and stabilise patients in the immediate postoperative (PO) period. All patients who have undergone anaesthesia and surgery must be closely monitored in the PACU during the immediate PO period; during this time the PACU nurse looks for alterations in vital signs, reporting alterations and initiating corrective treatment when required.

The first documented PACU was set up in Britain in the 1700s following the realisation that, in the immediate PO period, patients were vulnerable (American Society of Peri-Anesthesia Nurses, 2019). By the 1940s, there was a new understanding of the susceptibility of patients when they first recovered from anaesthesia, and not just the surgery. It was, therefore, essential to provide a room close to the theatre where patients could be cared for by specially trained nurses to reduce deaths from respiratory failure immediately after surgery (American Society of Peri-Anesthesia Nurses, 2019). Surgical and anaesthetic techniques have developed enormously since then, but the main focus of patient care in the PACU has remained the same – that is, critical evaluation and stabilisation of patients following surgery, with a strong emphasis on anticipation, prevention and treatment of complications arising from anaesthesia and/or surgery (Foran & Nilsson, 2019; Schick, 2018). Note that the PACU may also be referred to as the postanaesthesia recovery unit (PARU) or recovery room.

This chapter presents the role and function of the PACU and the assessment and management of the postsurgical, postprocedural and postanaesthesia patient. The chapter examines many important complications, including an overview of acute postoperative pain management. Finally, the chapter discusses discharge criteria.

THE ROLE OF THE NURSE AND FUNCTION OF THE PACU

The role of the PACU nurse (for specific details see Chapter 1) is to provide a high standard of expert nursing care to patients in this specialist area until their condition has stabilised to a point where they are considered 'ward ready' or are able to be discharged home in a day surgery setting. The PACU is staffed by nurses who are specially trained to manage and care for patients during this vulnerable period and to promptly summon assistance from expert medical staff (the anaesthetist or surgeon) when required.

In order to anticipate the complications of surgery and anaesthesia, it is essential that the nurse understands what complications are likely for each patient. There are general complications that can occur in all patients; however, each anaesthetic or surgical procedure may have its own unique complications. It is therefore essential that the PACU nurse has knowledge of both general and specific complications associated with anaesthesia and surgical procedures when caring for patients postoperatively.

Many patients present for surgery with several comorbidities, which, combined with the stress of anaesthesia and surgery, can affect their immediate PO management. The PO patient is vulnerable because of altered physiological, psychological and cognitive function. This places patients in a state of reliance on nursing and medical staff to ensure their safety, privacy, dignity and comfort during a phase when they are unable (or inadequately able) to advocate or care for themselves (Sundqvist, Holmefur, Nilsson, & Anderzén-Carlsson, 2016).

PACU DESIGN FEATURES

PACUs are located within operating suites, with the location and design enabling quick and easy access between each operating room (OR) and the PACU to allow surgeons/anaesthetists to respond immediately when summoned to assist in the management of PO complications (Australian and New Zealand College of Anaesthetists [ANZCA], 2020).

Departments outside the operating suite (endoscopy, radiology and cardiac investigation laboratories) and free-standing day surgery units that administer anaesthesia and/or sedation must also have a designated area for safe patient recovery and provide the same level of accessibility and prompt management in patient care as mainstream PACUs (ANZCA, 2020).

The PACU is an unrestricted area – meaning that, although traffic is limited, it still allows ward nurses to collect PO patients and other healthcare workers to enter in their street clothes (Australian College of Perioperative Nurses [ACORN], 2020a). See Chapter 5 for further information on traffic zones.

Figs 12.1 and 12.2 show a PACU and patient bays that may be found in Australia and New Zealand. A PACU should have two bed bays for each operating room (ACORN, 2020a).

PACUs are designed in two stages:
- Stage 1 – patients recovering immediately from anaesthesia
- Stage 2 – patients requiring observation following discharge from Stage 1 or for patients who have undergone their procedures using light sedation or local anaesthesia. The latter patients are returned directly to Stage 2, where they often recover on reclining chairs and remain until deemed ready for discharge home. This may be seen in a day surgery setting (ACORN, 2020a; Burden, 2018; Foran & Hoch, 2020).

Nurses in a PACU must be able to administer medication protocols for management of patient care (such as opioid, antiemetic and naloxone) and it is also recommended that they are Advanced Life Support trained and accredited (ANZCA, 2020). For these reasons the Australian College of Perianaesthesia Nurses (ACPAN) recommends that Stage 1 PACU is staffed by Division 1 registered nurses (RNs) only (ACPAN, 2019).

Each patient bay should be at least 9 square metres, which may be appropriate for simple procedures; however, this may increase to 18 square metres to allow for more-complex patients requiring extra monitoring, X-ray and resuscitation equipment (ANZCA, 2020). Specific provision of extra space for infection prevention may also need consideration (Australian Commission on Safety and Quality in Health Care [ACSQHC/the Commission], 2017a, 2017b; ANZCA, 2020).

Many standards govern the management and care provided within PACUs and include those produced by ACORN, ACPAN, the Perioperative Nurses College of the New Zealand Nurses Organisation (PNC

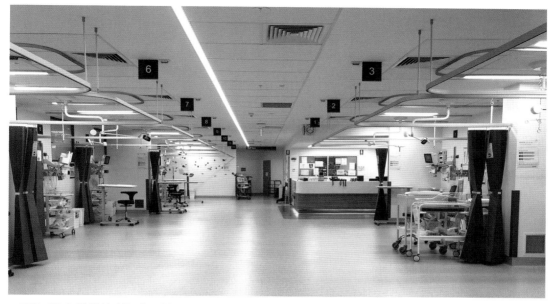

FIG. 12.1 PACU in Werribee Mercy Hospital Post Anaesthetic Care Unit, Victoria, Australia. (Source: Author.)

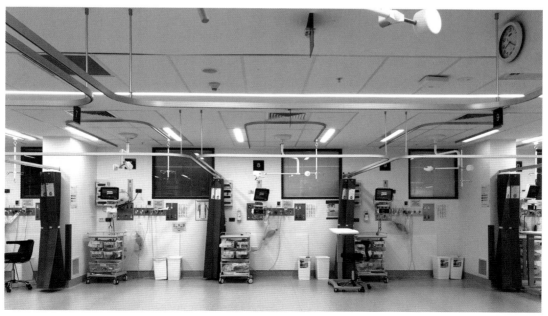

FIG. 12.2 Patient bays in PACU in Werribee Mercy Hospital Post Anaesthetic Care Unit, Victoria, Australia. (Source: Author.)

BOX 12.1
Equipment for all PACUs

All PACUs (including those with only minor surgery) must provide each bed space with:

- oxygen flowmeter and patient oxygen delivery systems that are capable of delivering high concentrations of inspired oxygen to the patient
- suction equipment including a receiver, hand pieces and a range of suction catheters
- pulse oximeter
- equipment for blood pressure measurement, both manual and automatic - including cuffs suitable for all sized patients managed in the facility.

(Source: ANZCA (2020) PS04 Statement on post anaesthetic care unit, p. 4.)

NZNO), ANZCA and the National Safety and Quality Health Service (NSQHS) Standards. The equipment standards for PACUs are in line with the ANZCA Standard PS04 (ANZCA, 2020). In response to several adverse events, including death, one of the reasons for the early updating of ANZCA's statement on the PACU was to include more stringent guidelines on equipment and staffing for all anaesthetising facilities including plastic, dental and day surgery units (ANZCA, 2020).

See Boxes 12.1–12.4 for PACU equipment required.

STAFFING OF THE PACU

Specialist nursing staff who are educated in the care of patients recovering from anaesthesia must always be present in the PACU (ANZCA, 2020). The ratio of RNs needs to be flexible; however, one supernumerary nurse should manage patient flow and staff allocations. At all times (regardless of patient flow), two nurses, one of whom must be a competent postanaesthesia nurse with skills appropriate to the level of patient, are required within the PACU (ACORN 2020b). ACORN standards (2020b) state the staffing requirements in the PACU as follows:

- All patients are observed on a 1:1 basis by an anaesthetist or a registered PACU practitioner until they have regained control of their airway, have stable observation within acceptable limits and are awake and able to communicate purposefully.
- A 2:1 nurse-to-patient ratio (or higher) is often required during the initial reception phase (when a patient requires airway support or assisted ventilation, or is critically ill, unstable or complicated). The additional staff member may be the OR nurse who escorted the patient or the anaesthetist who must stay until the patient is stable.
- A minimum of a 1:2 nurse-to-patient ratio is recommended during the stabilisation phase, where patients are both conscious and haemodynamically stable, with a sedation score of greater than 2.

BOX 12.2
Equipment Within Each PACU Area

Within each PACU area there must be:

- devices available in a ratio of one per two bed spaces, for manual ventilation with oxygen with a minimum of two such devices
- equipment and drugs for airway management including endotracheal intubation. Difficult intubation equipment must be easily accessible
- capnography where there is any possibility that a patient may be intubated or require intubation in the PACU
- ECG monitoring capability
- means of nebulising medications
- emergency and other drugs. Ideally, there should be separate trolleys/packs for specific emergencies. Such emergencies include cardiorespiratory arrest, anaphylaxis, local anaesthesia toxicity and malignant hyperthermia (if triggering agents are used). Such kits

should include approved cognitive aids/management cards

- range of intravenous equipment and fluids and a means of warming those fluids
- ready access to analgesic, anti-nausea and local anaesthetic drugs
- a range of syringes and needles
- a means of measuring body temperature
- equipment for point of care testing of blood glucose and ketones
- a stethoscope
- ready access to a defibrillator
- a handwashing basin
- a written routine for checking equipment and drugs must be established and used regularly.

(Source: ANZCA (2020) PS04 Statement on post anaesthetic care unit, p. 4-5.)

BOX 12.3
Additional Equipment in Facilities Conducting Anaesthesia or Major Surgery

Easy access is required to the following additional equipment in facilities where general anaesthesia, neuraxial or major regional anaesthesia and body cavity or other major surgery is conducted:

- 12-lead electrocardiograph
- end-tidal carbon dioxide monitor
- neuromuscular function monitor
- warming cupboard
- patient-warming devices
- refrigerator for drugs and blood

- procedure light
- basic surgical tray
- blood gas, haemoglobin and electrolyte measurement
- diagnostic imaging services
- apparatus for mechanical ventilation of the lungs and expired carbon dioxide monitoring
- heated humidified high-flow nasal oxygen
- monitors for direct arterial and venous pressure monitoring
- equipment for inserting a urinary catheter.

(Source: ANZCA (2020) PS04 Statement on post anaesthetic care unit, p. 5.)

BOX 12.4
Requirements for Trolleys/Beds

- Have a firm base and mattress which enables effective CPR
- Tilt from one or both ends both head up and head down at least 15 degrees
- Be easy to manoeuvre
- Have efficient and accessible brakes
- Provide for sitting the patient up
- Have secure side rails which must be able to be dropped below the base or be easily removed
- Have provision for maintaining intravenous infusions

(Source: ANZCA (2020) PS04 Statement on post anaesthetic care unit, p. 5-6.)

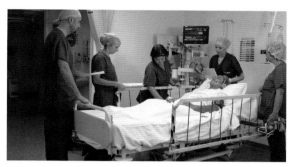

FIG. 12.3 Clinical handover taking place in a PACU. (Source: Flinders Medical Centre, South Australia.)

CLINICAL HANDOVER IN THE PACU

Patients should be transported to the PACU by the anaesthetist and the instrument or circulating nurse (depending on local policy). Patients must be observed continuously during transfer as complications may occur, including apnoea, respiratory obstruction, hypoxaemia leading to hypoxia, and vomiting. The patient's conscious state may vary from awake and alert to semi-conscious or unconscious (with the possibility of an unprotected airway).

A formal clinical **handover** (Fig. 12.3) is provided by the treating anaesthetist to the PACU nurse who is caring for the patient at the time of transfer (Fig. 12.4) (ANZCA, 2013b). It is important for nurses to understand this process, knowing what information needs to be extracted from the clinical handover, as the nurse is taking responsibility for the patient's care (Foran & Nilsson, 2019). In addition, some hospitals stipulate that a nursing handover is carried out by one of the perioperative nurses who participated in the surgical procedure, providing information about the operative process, dressings, drain tubes and any notable intraoperative events; see Fig. 12.5.

PATIENT MANAGEMENT IN THE PACU
Initial patient management

The treating anaesthetist is required to remain with the patient until the PACU nurse assigned to the patient is available to receive handover. In some hospitals, the nurse (instrument/circulating) who has assisted in the patient transfer will remain and accept the handover from the anaesthetist (and hence care of the patient) until a PACU nurse is available. It is important that PACU nurses do not take extra patients until they are able to do so, as these patients may be potentially unstable and require the nurse's full attention (one nurse to one patient) on admission.

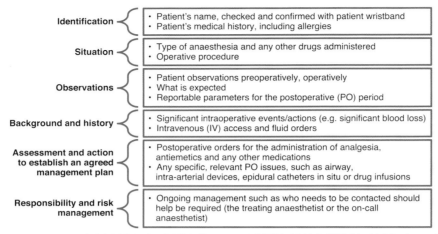

FIG. 12.4 Application of ISOBAR in the PACU. (Sources: ACORN, 2020d; ANZCA, 2013b; Australian Commission for Safety and Quality in Healthcare, 2017b.)

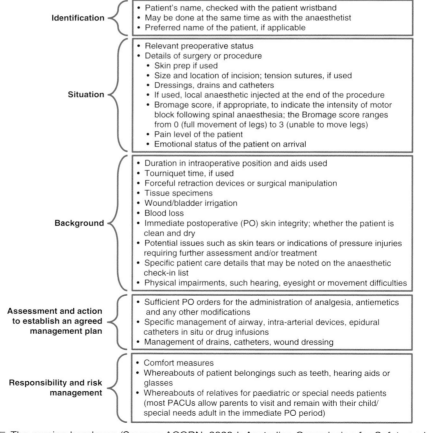

FIG. 12.5 The nursing handover. (Sources ACORN, 2020d; Australian Commission for Safety and Quality in Health Care, 2017b.)

PATIENT SCENARIOS

Mr James Collins is a 78-year-old man who has been admitted for an elective right total knee replacement (TKR). Mr Collins' full history and a brief description of the healthcare setting is provided in the Introduction at the front of the book for readers to review when answering the questions in this unfolding scenario.

SCENARIO 12.1: THE PACU NURSE'S ROLE

Mr Collins enters the PACU escorted by the treating anaesthetist, Dr De Silva, and circulating nurse, RN Rob Cohen, who had been involved in his care. Dr De Silva provides handover to the receiving PACU RN, Jenny Sang, indicating that the patient had been given a spinal anaesthetic with intravenous sedation and a nerve block has been inserted for continuous pain management postoperatively. RN Cohen, the circulating nurse, provides an intraoperative nursing handover, including dressings, drain tubes, venous thromboembolism (VTE) management and intraoperative events including tourniquet time.

Critical Thinking Questions

- What checking procedures need to be undertaken to ensure that the PACU (bays and whole PACU) is ready to accept Mr Collins?
- What are the initial assessments that RN Sang, the PACU nurse, must complete to ensure she has a comprehensive understanding of Mr Collins' condition?
- What are the potential risks specific to the care of Mr Collins? Consider potential complications relating to both anaesthesia and surgery.

Assessment of Airway and Breathing

The PACU nurse makes an initial assessment of the patient's **airway**, breathing and colour. If it is apparent that the patient is unable to maintain their own airway, the nurse must remain with the patient and provide airway support (see Table 12.1 for examples of airway support). A second nurse may assist by assessing and documenting blood pressure (BP), heart rate, respirations, oxygen saturation (S_pO_2), level of consciousness and pain status, all of which are priorities at this time (ACORN, 2020b). A systematic approach to airway assessment follows a 'look, listen and feel'

approach; any untoward findings require immediate action (see Feature box 12.1).

Respirations

In order to accurately measure a patient's respiratory rate, it needs to be taken over one full minute, making this vital sign that is most often neglected in clinical practice, despite the knowledge that the respiratory rate is considered to be the single most important vital sign in deteriorating patients (Foran & Nilsson, 2019). During clinical deterioration, it has also been noted that the respiratory rate has been salient, as it is the first vital sign to change, therefore heralding impending problems in all stages of patient deterioration (Loughlin, Sebat, & Kellett, 2018).

Normal respiratory rates vary enormously between patients, which is why it is essential to have a set of preoperative baseline observations for comparison during the PO period. The normal adult respiratory rate is between 12 and 20 respirations per minute (rpm) (Schick, 2018), commonly 18–20 rpm. The respiratory rate may be taken with a stethoscope at the same time as performing chest auscultation. Auscultation of the chest will allow assessment of the quality and intensity of breath sounds. Any abnormal breath sounds, such as wheezing, gurgling or crackles, that are identified should be documented and reported to the anaesthetist for further management (Schick, 2018).

Anaesthetic agents and analgesics can slow the respiratory rate from the preoperative baseline; however, a respiratory rate of less than 8 or above 30 rpm should activate an immediate emergency response and 'escalation of care' for a deteriorating patient in the PACU. If medical staff members are not immediately available, a medical emergency team (MET) response will be triggered for this level of patient deterioration. Patients who have undergone general anaesthesia are particularly vulnerable as they may be recovering from neuromuscular blockade, have generally been given opioids and are sedated. (See Table 12.1 for further information about respiratory assessment.) Obese patients have specific issues with airway management, as identified in Feature box 12.2.

Patient Observations and Monitoring

Once the initial priorities have been met and the patient is maintaining their own airway, a more thorough assessment can be undertaken using a head-to-toe approach,

TABLE 12.1
Common Immediate Postoperative Respiratory Complications

Complications and Causes	Mechanisms	Manifestations	Interventions
Tongue falling back	Muscular flaccidity associated with decreased consciousness and muscle relaxants	Use of accessory muscles Snoring respirations Decreased air movement	Patient stimulation Jaw thrust Chin lift Artificial airway
Retained thick secretions	Secretion stimulation by anaesthetic agents Dehydration of secretions	Noisy respirations Rhonchi	Humidified O_2 Suctioning Deep breathing and coughing IV hydration IPPV with mucolytic agent Chest physiotherapy
Laryngospasm	Irritation from secretions, endotracheal tube or anaesthetic gases Most likely to occur after removal of endotracheal tube	Inspiratory stridor (crowing on inspiration) Sternal retraction Acute respiratory distress	High-flow O_2 therapy Reassurance Positive-pressure ventilation Possible intubation
Laryngeal oedema	Allergic drug reaction Mechanical irritation from intubation Fluid overload	Barking respirations (like a seal) on expiration	O_2 therapy Antihistamines Corticosteroids Sedatives Possible intubation
Bronchospasm	Increased smooth muscle tone with closure of small airways	Wheezing Dyspnoea Tachypnoea ↓ S_pO_2	O_2 therapy Bronchodilators Humidified O_2 Deep breathing Incentive spirometry Early mobilisation
Atelectasis	Bronchial obstruction caused by secretions or decreased lung volumes	Noisy breath sounds ↓ S_pO_2	CPAP
Aspiration	Inhalation of gastric contents	Bronchospasm Atelectasis Crackles Respiratory distress ↓ S_pO_2	O_2 therapy Chest X-ray Antibiotics ? intubation

CPAP = continuous positive-airway pressure; IPPV = intermittent positive-pressure ventilation.
(Source: Foran, P., & Nilsson, U. (2019). Post-anaesthesia recovery. In L. Aitken, A. Marshall, & W. Chaboyer (Eds.), *Critical care nursing* (4th ed., pp. 909–940). Sydney: Elsevier.)

including wound status, dressings, location of drain tubes and nature and quantity of drainage, presence of catheters, patent cannula or IV fluid therapy in progress and temperature measurement. Assessment of the patient's skin integrity is also important. This initial assessment is known as the ABCDE method: **a**irway, **b**reathing, **c**irculation, **d**ressing/drain tubes plus **e**verything else (e.g. IVs, catheters, temperature); VTE prophylaxis may already be in place and should continue or be initiated in the PACU, as requested by the surgeon/anaesthetist. The patient should be continuously observed by the nurse watching the patient's respirations and colour. In a stable patient, continuous monitoring such as ECG, pulse oximetry and automatic or manual BP readings should be taken throughout the patient's stay and accurate documentation is imperative (ACORN, 2020a). Haemodynamic status is determined via assessment and documentation of vital signs, including:

- ECG, recommended in Stage 1 recovery (Foran, 2020; Schick, 2018)

FEATURE BOX 12.1
Airway Assessment

LOOK

Assessment of the patient's airway includes the following:

- look for misting and demisting of the oxygen mask (or if an laryngeal mask airway is in situ, that the T-piece bag is inflating and deflating), indicating that effective respiration is taking place
- the patient's colour should be pink, indicating that the patient is receiving adequate oxygen
- chest movement should be symmetrical as the chest rises and falls, indicating effective respiration
- the patient should not be using the accessory muscles of respiration, indicating ineffective respiratory effort or possible upper airway obstruction
- the respiratory rate should be normal, not shallow or laboured
- the patient should be conscious and able to respond to commands to take a deep breath
- pulse oximetry should show good oxygen saturation levels. Normal saturation levels are between 97% and 100% (Drain, 2018a); however, it is important to remember that if patients are receiving O_2 this may disguise decreased respiratory function

- it is also important to review the patient's baseline observations and to immediately report to the treating anaesthetist patients who are not meeting the above criteria.

LISTEN

Assessment of the patient's airway includes the following:

- breath sounds should be present but not noisy (e.g. gurgling, snoring). If the patient is making abnormal noises as they breathe, these may indicate an upper airway obstruction, which could be caused by the presence of saliva/vomitus in the oropharynx, by the tongue falling backwards, or by laryngospasm
- a wheeze should not be heard as this indicates a lower airway obstruction (e.g. bronchospasm).

FEEL

Assessment of the patient's airway includes the following:

- place a hand on the patient's chest to assess whether chest movements are symmetrical, indicating effective respiration.

(Source: Schick, 2018.)

FEATURE BOX 12.2
Airway Management of Obese Patients

Airway management in patients who are obese may be difficult and hazardous owing to anatomical features, such as a large tongue and excessive pharyngeal and palatal soft tissue, impairing neck movement and making mask ventilation awkward. There is a direct correlation between the degree of obesity a patient suffers and the risk and rate of pulmonary complications (Clifford, 2018). Functional residual capacity may also decline, particularly if the weight of the chest wall exceeds the closing capacity of the alveoli, leading to a resultant small airway closure, ventilation/perfusion (V/Q) mismatch and subsequent hypoxia (Clifford, 2018).

- easy access to end-tidal carbon dioxide ($ETCO_2$) (ANZCA, 2020)
- arterial oxygen saturation (S_aO_2) level
- respiratory rate and depth
- heart rate
- BP
- temperature
- urine output

- conscious state, using sedation score according to local PACU chart.

Unstable patients require prolonged assessment with intervention and documentation according to the individual's condition (ACSQHC/the Commission, 2017a). Specific observations are undertaken when required, such as a full neurological observations assessment using the Glasgow Coma Scale for neurosurgical patients, those with a head injury or those who have not regained consciousness appropriately; a Modified Bromage Scale for central neural blockade; blood glucose levels for diabetic patients; and vascular observations (colour, warmth, sensation, movement and peripheral return) for all limb surgeries, plastic or vascular surgery patients and patients with plaster casts. Peripheral return is assessed by pushing on the patient's fingertips/toes to decrease vascularity and then observing its return: if it returns very quickly, this is referred to as brisk; if it returns very slowly, this is referred to as sluggish. These observations will also be applied to patients who have had an intraoperative tourniquet applied. In a patient with decreased peripheral circulation, or one who is becoming peripherally shut down, there may be slow or no vascular return and, if so, this must be reported to the appropriate surgical/anaesthetic team.

When receiving PO patients, it is essential that the nurse has a full understanding of the possible complications of each procedure that has been performed (Foran & Nilsson, 2019). Some examples of specific complications include:

- upper airway obstruction following surgery under the muscle layer of the neck such as thyroidectomy, parotid cyst
- water intoxication and/or sodium depletion in surgery that flushes large amounts of saline solution or water under pressure, such as in transurethral resection of the prostate (TURP) and endometrial ablation – hyponatraemia can occur in any procedure where water or glycine is used as an irrigating fluid, as these fluids exit the body taking sodium with them (Dowling & Fyrdenberg, 2016); water intoxication may occur in procedures where any irrigating fluid is absorbed in sufficient amounts to produce systemic manifestations
- specific vascular observations for patients following free-flap surgery such as deep inferior epigastric perforators (DIEP) or transverse rectus abdominis myocutaneous (TRAM) flaps – observing not just for arterial vascularity but also for venous engorgement
- postpartum haemorrhage following lower uterine segment caesarean section (LUSCS) requiring assessment with fundal height measurements (see further information later in the chapter under 'Management of the obstetric patient')
- cervical shock causing a fall in both heart rate and BP in gynaecological patients (Foran & Nilsson, 2019).

Cardiovascular Assessment

PO patients are at risk of developing cardiovascular complications as they may have experienced some degree of blood loss, have been administered anaesthetic medications or have undergone temperature changes that may have altered vascularity (inadvertent hypothermia will cause vasoconstriction that may elevate blood pressure). In addition, a central neural block may have caused vasodilation, with possible drop in blood pressure and/or, in a high block, interference to the body's sympathetic responses, which may cause bradycardia. Conversely, pain may potentially increase heart rate (Foran & Nilsson, 2019).

Cardiovascular complications are commonly seen in the PACU and range from benign ectopic beats to life-threatening haemodynamic collapse (O'Brien, 2018b). When making a cardiovascular assessment, it is important for the nurse to remember and evaluate three vital components of the circulatory system: the heart as a pump, the circulating blood volume and the arteriovenous system (Schick, 2018). This is completed by assessing vital signs such as the ECG, heart rate, BP, skin and peripheral tissue return (e.g. hands and feet) and level of consciousness (Foran & Nilsson, 2019). Together these factors ensure adequate tissue perfusion, which in turn is reliant on a satisfactory cardiac output (Schick, 2018).

ECG

Dysrhythmias can occur as a result of common complications such as hypoxaemia leading to hypoxia, hypercarbia, inadvertent perioperative hypothermia (IPH) or pain (O'Brien, 2018b). Other alterations to ECGs may be caused by acid–base or electrolyte imbalance, cardiac ischaemia (seen in ST segment changes), bladder distension, hypovolaemia or the effects of anaesthetic medications (O'Brien, 2018b).

Recent literature has also highlighted several advantages such as: the detection of asymptomatic cardiac arrhythmias (new-onset atrial fibrillation shown to increase the risk of stroke and myocardial injury after non-cardiac surgery), the saving of precious time in a cardiac arrest, and the additional learning for nurses who consistently observe an ECG trace in the PACU (Foran, 2020).

Hence it is important for vulnerable postanaesthetic patients to be connected to an ECG monitor during Stage 1 recovery to aid in monitoring for the onset of some of these conditions.

Heart rate

Although the use of pulse oximetry or ECG monitoring provides a numerical value for the heart rate, it is essential to palpate the patient's pulse as well, as this gives information not provided by monitoring devices, such as the regularity and strength of the pulse (e.g. thready, bounding). Touching the patient to palpate the pulse also allows an opportunity to assess skin temperature (cool, clammy) and provide reassurance to the patient. It is also important, as with all vital signs, to review the patient's notes to ascertain the preoperative baseline heart rate and whether any anomalies are noted.

Blood pressure

BP is measured using either automatic non-invasive equipment that cycles at least every 5 minutes or manual readings. If the nurse has concerns about a patient's automatic BP reading, a manual reading should be taken to confirm the findings. The patient's preoperative BP readings should be noted to provide a baseline comparison for the PO readings. A BP reading 20% above or below the patient's normal reading may be considered abnormal and corrective measures should be undertaken. Such findings can be attributed to a number of factors such as pain, haemorrhage and alterations to vascularity (Schick, 2018) caused by central neural blockade, hyperthermia or sepsis.

Level of Consciousness

Assessing a patient's emergence from general anaesthesia and awareness of self and surroundings requires close monitoring; it is also an excellent indicator of airway, breathing and cardiac sufficiency, and neurological function (O'Brien, 2018b). The patient's level of consciousness is usually assessed concurrently with airway, breathing and circulation, using verbal or gentle tactile stimulation. It includes determining the patient's:

- orientation and alertness
- ability to follow commands (e.g. 'take a deep breath')
- ability to move all limbs as per preoperative status, where surgery and anaesthetic approach allow (O'Brien, 2018b).

Central Neural Blockade

Central neural blockade or neuraxial anaesthesia is a generic term for epidural, spinal, epidural–spinal or caudal anaesthesia , which blocks pain during a surgical procedure. Many of the medications used in epidural or spinal anaesthesia continue to provide pain relief in the PO period, with local anaesthetic agents having differing durations of action. Local anaesthetic agents with adrenaline (epinephrine) may be given if a longer duration of action is required (Nagelhout, 2018a). Care of the patient following epidural or spinal anaesthesia requires an understanding of the possible complications associated with this type of anaesthesia. These complications are wide ranging, from minor irritations to possibly life-threatening events (Nagelhout, 2018a), and include spinal and epidural haematoma, postdural puncture headache, high spinal block, hypotension, bradycardia, nausea and vomiting, urinary retention and transient neurological symptoms (Nagelhout, 2018a) and local anaesthetic toxicity (see 'Local anaesthetic' later in this chapter).

Patients who have had local anaesthetic blocks must have the anaesthetised area protected, including advising patients with dental blocks not to bite their tongue. In arm blocks, patients must be warned not to lift anaesthetised arms for fear of the arm falling suddenly, resulting in injury. Care must be taken with cot sides and bed rails to prevent jamming the patient's anaesthetised body parts. Care is also required when using warm packs, as sensation is impeded. As well as normal PO observations, continual assessment for possible complications should be maintained including:

- continual assessment with the Bromage Scale
- discussions with the patient regarding the onset of pain or tenderness at the catheter site
- observation of the epidural catheter site for bleeding, swelling or redness
- catheter migration (Nagelhout, 2018a).

Patients who received a spinal block will have a greater motor block than those who received an epidural. This occurs as local anaesthetic is injected directly into the subarachnoid space with cerebrospinal fluid and non-myelinated spinal nerves, providing a denser motor block (Foran & Nilsson, 2019). Caution must be taken when the block appears to have worn off and the patient is about to ambulate, as the patient may have residual motor block. The nurse should establish when walking is required and provide support until full motor function has returned. The Bromage score measures the intensity of motor block and motor function by assessing the patient's ability to move their lower extremities (Anaesthesia UK, 2017). A modified Bromage Scale is:

- Score 1. Complete block (unable to move feet or knees)
- Score 2. Almost complete block (able to move feet only)
- Score 3. Partial block (just able to move knees)
- Score 4. Detectable weakness of hip flexion while supine (full flexion of knees)
- Score 5. No detectable weakness of hip flexion while supine
- Score 6. Able to perform partial knee bend (Anaesthesia UK, 2017).

Temperature Control

Patients require temperature monitoring to commence on arrival to the PACU and every 15 minutes during their stay to initiate management if it is found that inadvertent perioperative hypothermia (IPH) has occurred (ACORN, 2020c). The management will be discussed later in the chapter.

In locations such as the PACU where patients are likely to be haemodynamically unstable, it is vital to obtain an accurate 'core' temperature reading. *Core temperature* refers to the temperature in parts of the body that are protected by thermal regulation to ensure survival in extreme conditions: the cranium, thoracic cavity and abdominal cavity. The core temperature provides important information to guide clinical judgement; for example, a patient who is hypothermic (core temperature below 36°C) (Duff et al., 2018) may, as a consequence, be vasoconstricted – this can elevate the BP even in the presence of hypovolaemia. Similarly, a hyperthermic patient may be vasodilated; this can cause the BP to fall. Due to the connection between temperature and blood pressure, it is vital that normothermia be achieved prior to discharge to ensure accurate blood pressure readings. Tympanic temperature measurement is commonly used in the PACU as it remains a reliable, non-invasive and low-risk reflection of core temperature (Vincent-Lambert, Smith, & Goldstein, 2018).

General Comfort and Safety Measures

Nursing care initiated in the operating suite, such as prevention of VTE with sequential compression devices or arteriovenous foot pump, must continue in the PO phase. In some surgical procedures, these devices may be commenced in the PACU after discussion with the appropriate surgeon. Antiembolism socks/stockings must be correctly fitted.

Psychological care is important, as the patient may be anxious about the outcome of surgery; the presence of a nurse speaking gently, reassuring and reorienting the patient to time and place can be very comforting. Most PACUs allow family members to visit, particularly for paediatric patients or special needs patients, and the presence of a family member or carer can reduce patient anxiety and make the patient feel more secure.

General comfort measures for the patient include:

- position changes
- providing extra pillows
- providing active warming devices if the patient is hypothermic; otherwise, providing a warm blanket as required
- washing off excess skin preparations and providing a face washer for the patient's use
- assisting with range-of-motion exercises
- encouraging deep breathing
- providing mouth care with moistened swabs and ice chips to suck for patients who can tolerate fluids and replacing dentures
- offering toileting – a bottle or a bedpan
- returning the patient's spectacles and/or hearing aid, as appropriate (O'Brien, 2018a).

POSTANAESTHESIA AND POSTSURGICAL COMPLICATIONS

There is a range of **complications** that surgical patients may experience. These are associated with the use of anaesthetic agents, the surgical intervention or patient characteristics, or any combination thereof.

The Deteriorating Patient

Both Australia and New Zealand have produced guidelines to assist healthcare personnel recognise and respond to acute physiological **deterioration** in patients. Measurable physiological abnormalities occur prior to adverse events such as cardiac arrest and death, and early recognition of changes in a patient's condition, followed by prompt and effective treatment, can reduce

mortality (ACSQHC/the Commission, 2017a; Health Quality and Safety Commission New Zealand, 2020). Patient vital signs must be taken accurately, with frequency determined by the patient's condition, and changes must be reported to allow corrective treatment. Surgical adverse events are common and have a substantial impact on both the patient and the wider community (Wain, Kong, Bruce, Laing, & Clarke, 2019).

Airway and Breathing Complications

One of the most common airway complications in the immediate PO period is airway obstruction (O'Brien, 2018b). Altered gas exchange may see early changes in pulse oximetry (decreased S_pO_2) and CO_2 retention (increased end-tidal CO_2) (Schick, 2018). The depressant effects of anaesthesia can mean that PO patients are unable to protect their airway. Additional signs of airway obstruction include increased respiratory effort, use of the accessory muscles of respiration and noisy or abnormal breathing.

See Table 12.1 for a summary of common PO respiratory complications.

Hypoxaemia

Hypoxaemia is an abnormally low concentration of oxygen in arterial blood (Drain, 2018a). All airway and breathing complications are serious in varying degrees as they put the patient at risk of decreased oxygenation and possible hypoxaemia. Hypoxia is evident when the partial pressure of oxygen in arterial blood (P_aO_2) is less than 60 mmHg. This complication can result from an upper airway obstruction (such as obstruction by the tongue or secretions, laryngospasm or subglottic oedema) or a lower airway obstruction (such as bronchospasm or non-cardiogenic pulmonary oedema). Airway obstruction may be caused by a simple problem (such as poor mandibular positioning where the tongue falls back, obstructing the airway) or a more-complex one (such as laryngospasm with no air entry or as a result of hypoventilation) (O'Brien, 2018b). Any of these problems can cause life-threatening hypoxia if not rectified immediately.

Hypoxia (of whatever cause) is a medical emergency; if suspected, the PACU nurse should press the emergency bell and summon medical assistance immediately. Treatment will range from elevating the mandible to providing positive pressure ventilation with a bag and mask, intubation, cricothyroid puncture or, if all else fails, creating a surgical airway (tracheostomy). It is imperative that the nurse is familiar with all of the emergency airway equipment and algorithms that must be followed in a 'can't intubate, can't oxygenate' (CICO) situation. (See Chapter 8, for further information on the management of CICO.)

Obstruction by the tongue

Relaxation of the tongue may occur in patients who have not fully recovered from anaesthetic agents such as opioids, sedatives or muscle relaxants (O'Brien, 2018b). The signs and symptoms of tongue obstruction are noisy, gurgling, choking sounds; irregular respirations; and decreased arterial oxygen saturation readings (less than 90%). In many cases the PACU nurse can open the patient's airway by providing jaw support (if not contraindicated), which can help restore airway patency (Fig. 12.6). However, in some cases an artificial airway may be required to prevent obstruction that occurs when the patient's tongue and epiglottis fall back on the posterior pharyngeal wall. If a patent airway cannot be established, the PACU nurse should call for urgent medical assistance.

Obstruction by secretions/blood

The upper airway can be obstructed by the presence of secretions such as mucus or blood. The signs and symptoms of this complication include noisy, gurgling, choking sounds; coughing; irregular respirations; and decreased oxygen saturation readings – with a pulse oximetry reading of 90% or less indicating hypoxaemia, which can rapidly lead to hypoxia. Management includes:

- gentle suctioning of the mouth and oropharynx using a Yankauer sucker or suction catheter

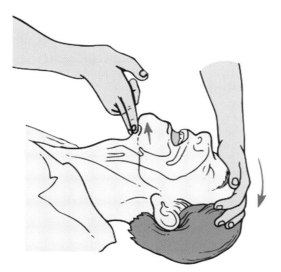

FIG. 12.6 Opening the airway with the head-chin-lift manoeuvre. (Source: Lewis, S. Dirksen, S., Heitkemper, M., & Bucher, L. (2014). *Medical–surgical nursing* (9th ed.). Elsevier. Section 3.)

- repositioning patients on their left side to assist in draining secretions from the mouth and careful monitoring (the left side is the position of choice as it allows the stomach to be dormant and has a lower risk of aspiration).

If hypoxaemia continues, the PACU nurse should call for urgent medical assistance by pressing the emergency bell.

Laryngospasm

Laryngospasm is an involuntary forceful spasm of the laryngeal musculature that is caused by stimulation of the superior laryngeal nerve (Butterworth, 2018a). Although it can occur in patients of any age, it occurs more commonly in young patients and is most common in infants 1–3 months old (Butterworth, 2019a). Laryngospasm can result in either incomplete or complete airway obstruction (Wright, 2018), with the latter fortunately being less common. Laryngospasm may be avoided by extubating the patient either while awake and reversed or while deeply anesthetised and paralysed; both techniques have advocates (Butterworth, 2019a). Extubation during the interval between these two extremes is generally recognised as more hazardous (Butterworth, 2019a). The presence of secretions in the oropharynx may also cause laryngospasm. Closure of the cords in response to these stimuli is a protective reflex but it can become a life-threatening event as the airway is compromised.

Partial closure of the vocal cords results in a crowing-like noise on inspiration, known as an inspiratory stridor. The patient may be awake when this occurs and will show signs of distress as this is a very frightening experience. Signs and symptoms of laryngospasm include:

- inspiratory stridor
- dyspnoea
- distress/sweating
- an upper airway noise heard on auscultation.

As some patients may already have oxygen therapy, these symptoms may or may not include a decrease in oxygen saturation levels.

Initial management by the nurse includes:

- immediately informing the treating anaesthetist or medical staff
- sitting the patient up, as this facilitates better ventilation (provided the patient is not hypotensive and it is not contraindicated by the nature of the surgery)
- giving oxygen by mask, if not already in situ
- gently suctioning the upper airway
- giving the patient explanation and reassurance
- providing airway support, as discussed earlier in this chapter (Wright, 2018).

Laryngospasm is terrifying for an awake patient: reassurance and a calm demeanour from nurses and doctors are of the utmost importance, as patient anxiety can exacerbate this condition. If the oxygen saturation is falling, it is necessary to summon urgent medical assistance. If the above actions are unsuccessful, the following may be required:

- gentle positive-pressure ventilation (place a bag-valve mask with a reservoir bag connected to oxygen firmly over the patient's nose and mouth and gently inflate the bag)
- forward jaw thrust
- IV lignocaine
- if hypoxia develops, paralysis of the patient with IV suxamethonium or rocuronium and use of controlled ventilation (Butterworth, 2019a).

Post-intubation croup/subglottal oedema

Post-intubation croup or subglottal oedema is a complication that occurs later than laryngospasm, but usually appears within 3 hours of extubation (Butterworth, 2019a). It may occur in adults, but is most commonly seen in patients aged 1–4 years and is due to glottic or tracheal oedema, which can be lessened in children with endotracheal tubes without a cuff that allow a slight gas leak at 10–25 cm H_2O, as the tube does not touch the tracheal walls (Butterworth, 2019a). The manufacturers of newer types of cuffed paediatric endotracheal tubes suggest they allow a cuffed tube with reduced tracheal trauma. Signs and symptoms of this PO complication include:

- inspiratory stridor
- chest retractions
- hoarseness
- a croup-like cough
- apprehensiveness
- restless.

As in all respiratory conditions, the PACU nurse should sit the patient up (provided the patient is not hypotensive), provide oxygen and call for medical assistance.

Bronchospasm

Bronchospasm is a lower airway obstruction, characterised by spasmodic smooth muscle contraction that causes narrowing of the bronchi and bronchioles (O'Brien, 2018b). It is more common for bronchospasm to occur in patients with a pre-existing pulmonary illness such as asthma or chronic obstructive pulmonary disease, but it may also develop in healthy patients in the presence of allergy, anaphylaxis or pulmonary aspiration. If a patient without a pre-existing pulmonary condition develops bronchospasm, the underlying cause may be an allergy or pulmonary aspiration, so this should raise a level of suspicion that one of these situations may have occurred. Signs and symptoms of bronchospasm include:

- coughing
- distinct wheeze upon auscultation
- noisy shallow respirations
- chest retractions
- use of the accessory muscles of breathing
- prolonged expiratory phase of respiration
- hypertension
- tachycardia.

Nursing care includes sitting the patient up (if they are not hypotensive), providing oxygen, calling for medical assistance and reassuring the patient. Initial management will include removing the identified cause if possible (O'Brien, 2018b), with treatment depending on the cause, specific symptoms and severity of the bronchospasm. The PACU nurse should carry out instructions from the medical staff, which may include giving the patient humidified oxygen and administering a beta$_2$-adrenergic agonist (O'Brien, 2018b). In severe cases, intubation and intermittent positive-pressure ventilation may be required, and antihistamines, antibiotics and steroids may also be considered (O'Brien, 2018b).

Inadequate reversal of muscle relaxants

Initial airway assessment may reveal that a patient is not moving an adequate tidal volume, has weak breathing and shallow respirations. This can be an indication that the muscle relaxants have not been adequately reversed. These patients may exhibit dyspnoea and paroxysmal breathing (forward to backward abdominal breathing) and may be distressed. Treatment will depend on the severity of the symptoms and may include providing oxygen therapy, sitting the patient up (if they are not hypotensive), assessing the CO_2 and O_2 saturations and reassuring the patient. In compromised patients the anaesthetist must be summoned and further reversal drugs may be given (O'Brien, 2018b).

Hypoventilation

Hypoventilation may occur in the PO period owing to the effects of sedation, opioids, residual anaesthetic agents or neuromuscular-blocking agents and thoracic or abdominal incisions causing pain (O'Brien, 2018b). Symptoms include a decreased respiratory rate, shallow respirations and an increase in end-tidal CO_2. The PACU nurse should provide oxygen and call for medical assistance. Treatment includes identifying the cause (e.g. pain, narcosis); management will depend on the causative factor (O'Brien, 2018b).

PATIENT SCENARIOS

SCENARIO 12.2: PATIENT DETERIORATION

On arrival in the PACU, Mr Collins had an S_pO_2 of 95% on room air. After 10 minutes in the PACU, RN Sang notes a drop in his S_pO_2 from 95% to 90%.

Critical Thinking Questions

- What interventions must RN Sang now undertake?
- What would you identify as being a potential cause of this situation?
- What is the significance of a drop in S_pO_2 in relation to the patient's partial pressure of oxygen?
- What ongoing pain assessment and pain management should RN Sang undertake for Mr Collins?

General Complications

Postoperative nausea and vomiting

Postoperative nausea and vomiting (PONV) is most undesirable and the most common PO complication seen in the PACU (Peterson, 2018). All immediate PO patients with emesis are at risk of aspiration as they may also have a decreased state of consciousness and obtunded airway reflexes. PONV can be prevented by:

- avoiding hypotension
- consider ongoing oxygen therapy
- treating pain
- avoiding sudden movement.

Generally nausea precedes vomiting; in this case the PACU nurse should provide the patient with oxygen and administer an antiemetic (O'Brien, 2018b). The patient must be observed by a PACU colleague while the medications are being accessed. If an antiemetic has not been prescribed, the anaesthetist should be contacted so that this can be addressed. If vomiting occurs, the PACU nurse should swiftly place the unconscious or semi-conscious patient in a left lateral position (taking into consideration the type of surgical procedure performed). Suction must be ready for the nurse to remove any gastric aspirate from the mouth and oropharynx. The fully awake patient with a satisfactory BP and gag reflex may be sat upright by the nurse and provided with an emesis bag. A vomiting patient must never be left alone.

Common pharmacological agents for the management of nausea and vomiting include serotonin receptor blockers (ondansetron) and dopamine receptor blockers (droperidol). Alternative non-pharmacological measures such as pressure point therapy may be useful in patients who have received medication and still feel nauseated.

Inadvertent perioperative hypothermia (IPH)

IPH has been associated with increased mortality and morbidity among elective surgical patients (Akers et al., 2019). It is essential to rewarm hypothermic patients prior to discharge from the PACU (temperature at discharge should be 36°C). Active warming devices such as forced-air convection warmers have been shown to be the most effective, both in financial saving to the health-care facility and in prevention of known complications for the patients (Conway et al., 2019). See Chapters 8 and 9 for further information on the management of IPH.

Hypotension

Hypotension in the immediate PO period is a common occurrence and may be due to a number of factors including untreated dehydration, blood loss, vasodilation causing pooling of blood in the extremities and anaesthetic agents or opioids. As the patient recovers from surgery and the BP returns to normal, a rise in BP may cause resected tissue to ooze blood. Often, the patient's natural haemostatic mechanisms will control the bleeding, but occasionally haemorrhage will occur. Active bleeding may be seen through a wound dressing or in drains. It may also occur insidiously or be hidden, for example in the uterus after LUSCS surgery, resulting in the patient exhibiting the signs and symptoms of hypovolaemic shock. Careful assessment by the PACU nurse of the patient's wound, drains and catheters, and fundal height in LUSCS patients, is essential, as is the frequent monitoring of vital signs.

Sustained hypotension or untreated hypotension can lead to the development of shock in relation to blood loss or an altered vascularity that occurs secondary to sympathetic blockade and vasodilation after regional anaesthesia.

Shock

Shock is a condition of circulatory impairment leading to inadequate vital organ perfusion and oxygen delivery with life-threatening cellular dysfunction (Myrna, 2018). Shock is characterised by a decrease in BP (a 20%–30% decrease from the patient's baseline) and an increase in heart rate, and it is not an uncommon occurrence in PO patients (O'Brien, 2018b). This is because surgical patients may have had significant blood loss leading to hypovolaemic shock, or may have had misdistribution of circulation from vasodilation due to central neural blockade (Foran & Nilsson, 2019).

In caring for the patient suffering from shock, the PACU nurse should lie the patient flat with the legs elevated and provide supplemental oxygen (if not already in use). The nurse should call for medical assistance and check the patient's peripheral return at the fingernail beds to assess whether peripheral shutdown has occurred, suggesting compensation (Foran & Nilsson, 2019). Depending on the type and cause of shock, medical management may include fluid resuscitation therapy; in the case of misdistribution of circulation from an epidural or spinal injection of local anaesthetic, medications such as metaraminol (a potent sympathomimetic agent) may be used to provide some vasoconstriction to increase the BP (Foran & Nilsson, 2019). If haemorrhage is the cause, resuscitation of the patient is commenced. Unresolved haemorrhage may require the patient to be returned to the operating room to find the cause of the bleeding and to initiate surgical haemostasis.

Hypertension

Hypertension may be pre-existing in some patients, or it may be indicative of a patient who has pain or anxiety. It is vital for the PACU nurse to compare PO observations with the patient's baseline observations. If the patient's BP is more than 20% higher than the baseline readings, the nurse should obtain medical advice.

Hyperthermia

Possible causes of hyperthermia in perioperative patients include a pre-existing febrile state (where infection was present preoperatively, such as in an appendicectomy), malignant hyperthermia, thyroid crisis, a blood transfusion reaction, overheating in infants and neurological damage post head injury or neurosurgery. The PACU nurse should investigate the cause of hyperthermia; treatment will include leaving only a sheet to cover the patient and applying a cool face wash to the patient's forehead (being cautious not to induce shivering as this increases temperature). If the cause of the hyperthermia is known, the PACU nurse will give antipyretic agents as ordered and continue to monitor the temperature every 5 minutes to ensure that the patient does not become hypothermic. In severe cases such as a septic shower (which is the sudden systemic influx of pathogens) or malignant hyperthermia, when the temperature is close to the human critical thermal maximum of 41.6°C, the nurse must immediately contact anaesthetic/surgical team staff and place ice packs on the axilla and groin. (See Chapter 8 for further information on malignant hyperthermia.)

Urinary retention

The inability to void, namely urinary retention, is a common PO complication which may potentially cause bladder overdistension (Foran & Nilsson, 2019). Central neural blockage, block detrusor contraction and bladder sensation during general anaesthesia may cause bladder atony by interfering with autonomic regulation of detrusor tone (Foran & Nilsson, 2019). Adding to this problem, sedative hypnotics and volatile anaesthetics may also suppress detrusor contraction, and in turn the micturition reflex (Foran & Nilsson, 2019). Ultrasound bladder scan is a non-invasive, safe method of measuring bladder volume (Foran & Nilsson, 2019). The gold standard of treatment for bladder distension (volume >500 mL) is catheterisation, and can be either intermittent, where the catheter is removed after bladder emptying, or indwelling (Foran & Nilsson, 2019).

High spinal/epidural block

The PACU nurse should assess dermatomes after spinal and epidural anaesthesia to identify the exaggerated dermatome spread that can occur. Signs and symptoms may include dyspnoea, numbness or weakness in the upper extremities, nausea (which often precedes hypotension) and bradycardia (Butterworth, 2019b).

A high block may also cause blocking of the cardiac sympathetic fibres originating from T1 to T4, which in turn can cause loss of chronotropic and inotropic drive and a fall in cardiac output, leading to hypotension and bradycardia. In this instance, medical assistance must be summoned immediately.

Emergence delirium

Emergence delirium is seen in the immediate recovery period. It is defined as an acute alteration in cognition, characterised by fluctuating consciousness and attention deficit (Read, Maani, & Blackwell, 2017). In its mild form, an awake patient may exhibit disorientation, restlessness, irrational conversations and inappropriate behaviour, and this is often referred to as emergence excitement (O'Brien, 2018b). Patients with emergence delirium, in addition to the symptoms just discussed, may also have hallucinations, hypersensitivity to external stimuli and hyperactivity, with the patient often screaming and thrashing (O'Brien, 2018b). Emergence delirium is a serious PO complication, raising safety concerns for both the patient and the staff; hence prevention of injury is vital in both groups (O'Brien, 2018b).

Children have a higher incidence of emergence delirium than adults. Adults who have received certain medications including ketamine, droperidol, opioids, benzodiazepines, scopolamine, atropine or large doses of metoclopramide are also susceptible. In addition, patients who have suffered a recent tragedy or bereavement, patients with severe preoperative anxiety and patients with a history of drug dependency or psychiatric illness are more likely to suffer emergence delirium (O'Brien, 2018b). The patient's eyes will look glazed and they will appear not to have any response to verbal dialogue. Speaking to the patient in a raised voice tends to worsen the situation. Calm, confident reassurance by the PACU nurse is advised. Emergence delirium may last about 20 minutes, with the patient eventually falling back to sleep and waking with no recollection of the incident.

Initial management of the patient with emergence delirium by the PACU nurse involves:

- ensuring the patient's safety and calling for assistance
- ruling out hypoxia and hypoglycaemia
- treating the cause, if known
- considering sedation
- importantly, protecting these vulnerable patients from accidental self-injury (O'Brien, 2018b).

If the nurse knows that a patient is prone to emergence delirium, preparations can be made for the patient's safe recovery by obtaining padded cot or bed bumpers to prevent injury and by ensuring that security staff are available in the case of a strong adult. See Chapter 5 for further information about staff safety.

Aspiration pneumonitis

Aspiration pneumonitis is severe inflammation of the lungs caused by the aspiration of gastric contents (Boulette, 2018). Preoperative patient fasting is aimed at minimising the risk of aspiration. Pregnant women, those with gastro-oesophageal reflux disease, and obese and non-fasting patients are all at increased risk of aspiration pneumonitis (O'Brien, 2018b).

Clinical progression after aspiration varies widely, from no symptoms to very mild symptoms, bronchopneumonia and possibly development of acute pulmonary oedema. The severity is determined by several factors including the aspirate pH, the quantity of aspirate and the presence of solid particles. Symptoms include tachypnoea, tachycardia, cough and possible bronchospasm (O'Brien, 2018b). While this condition may be dramatic on onset, it can also be insidious in nature. Bronchospasm that occurs in a healthy patient should raise the PACU nurse's suspicion of a possible aspiration (Foran & Nilsson, 2019).

MANAGEMENT OF PAIN IN THE PACU

One of the greatest challenges that face PACU nurses daily is the provision of effective pain relief (Foran & Hoch, 2020). There are over 313 million surgical procedures performed every year worldwide (Weiser et al., 2016) and, despite evidence-based recommendations, the availability of myriad analgesic medications and sound pain management guidelines, the undertreatment of postoperative pain remains a significant problem (Foran & Hoch, 2020; Ulatowska, Brzeźniak, Głowacka, & Bączyk, 2018).

In up to 22% of cases of persistent unresolved postoperative pain, pathways may be set up that lead to development of chronic pain (Stuit & O'Sullivan, 2017), which, in the worst-case scenario, may last a lifetime (Pasero, 2018).

For these reasons, PACU nurses need to ensure their patients receive the highest-quality pain management by fully understanding the PO pain management guidelines that exist in their specific healthcare facility. Nurses as patient advocates must contact medical staff to review patients with unresolved or difficult to manage pain. This includes:

- unexpected levels of pain
- pain that is not responding to analgesics
- sudden increased pain scores, which may signal development of an underlying complication (ANZCA, 2013a).

In any of these situations, medical staff must be alerted.

The most appropriate environment to manage and control a patient's initial pain is while still in the PACU, where the nursing ratios are one to one (during pain protocol) – this makes it easier to provide IV analgesics and seek advice from the anaesthetist if pain relief is not being achieved – rather than on the ward, where patient-to-nurse ratios are lower, making it more difficult to treat severe or unmanageable pain effectively.

Physiology of Pain

Pain is a subjective experience which involves complex physiological and emotional responses. The physiological response is the perception of pain, nociception, which occurs when trauma is experienced – for example, when a surgical skin incision is made (Fig. 12.7).

Injury to the tissue initiates a cascade of mediators (e.g. prostaglandins, bradykinin) which assist in the transmission of pain signals via afferent fibres to the spinal cord, where it is processed in the dorsal horn. Neurotransmitters released from the afferent fibres bind with nearby cells to either inhibit or activate the cells, producing a reaction to pain.

Endogenous opioids can block the effects of the neurotransmitters, and therapeutic approaches to target

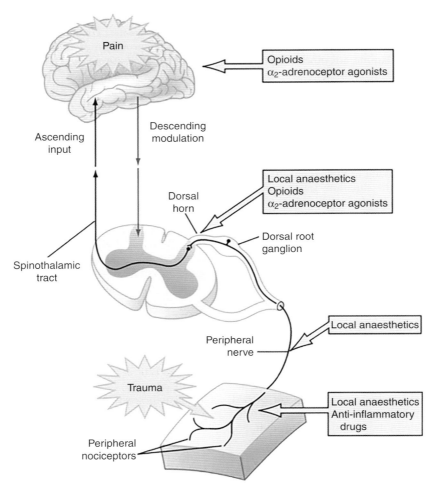

FIG. 12.7 Pain pathway. (Source: https://aneskey.com/wp-content/uploads/2016/05/B9781437727920000439_ f043-006-9781437727920.jpg.)

pain transmission include the use of opioid analgesia (e.g. morphine) (Schoenwald, Palomano, & Fillman, 2020).

From the dorsal horn, the pain stimuli travel to the brain via the afferent pathways in the spinothalamic tract to the thalamus and somatosensory cortex, where the site and type of stimuli (e.g. pain, temperature, pressure) are interpreted, resulting in motor, sensory and emotional responses (Schoenwald et al., 2020). The following sections discuss how these responses can be assessed and managed using both pharmacological and non-pharmacological strategies.

Pain Assessment and Management

Pain assessment and **pain management** can be difficult in the emergence phase of anaesthesia, owing to the impaired conscious state of patients and their difficulty communicating their perception of pain to the nurse. In addition, normal haemodynamic responses to pain, such as tachycardia and hypertension, may be depressed because of the ongoing effects of the anaesthesia (Pasero, 2018). Doses of analgesia must be titrated to the individual patient and are dependent on the patient's age, tolerance to analgesics, pain level, sedation score and medical history (Pasero, 2018). Patients who present with a drug dependency may require much larger doses of analgesia and may be greatly advantaged by assistance from an acute pain service.

As pain differs in patients and is subjective, it is essential to use an assessment tool to measure a patient's pain level. One assessment tool that is commonly used

Numerical rating scale

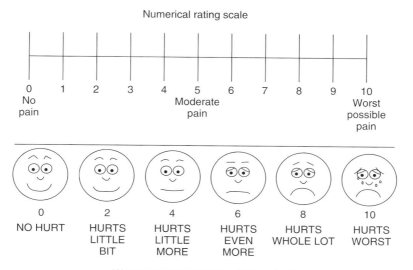

FIG. 12.8 Visual scales for assessing pain. (Source: Odom-Forren, J. (Ed.). (2018). *Drain's perianesthesia nursing: a critical care approach* (7th ed.). St Louis, MO: Elsevier.)

in the PACU is the verbal analogue score (VAS), which assesses pain severity on a scale of 0 to 10, with 0 being no pain and 10 being the worst pain imaginable. By inviting patients to quantify their pain level numerically, the VAS enables the nurse to assess whether analgesic medications are required or have been effective for the individual patient. For children or those who may otherwise be unable to communicate their pain (e.g. cognitively impaired patients), the Wong–Baker FACES Pain Rating Scale can be used; see Fig. 12.8.

Pharmacological interventions

Table 12.2 gives a summary of commonly used analgesic drugs.

Pain is a complex phenomenon and, as there are different mechanisms that cause pain, using one method to relieve pain may not be adequate (Pasero, 2018). The gold standard of PO pain relief encompasses multimodal analgesia where combinations of analgesics with differing underlying mechanisms not only provide greater pain relief, but also allow lower doses of the individual medications (Pasero, 2018). Analgesic medications may include paracetamol, opioids, non-steroidal anti-inflammatory drugs (NSAIDs) and local anaesthetics, as well as adjuvant agents including gabapentinoids such as gabapentin (originally developed as an antiepileptic treatment, but also very effective in treating chronic neuropathic pain), clonidine and selected

antidepressants and anticonvulsants. Non-pharmacological therapies must be considered, but only as complementary to pharmacological therapies (ANZCA, 2013a).

Opioid analgesics

Opioid analgesics provide a rapid onset of pain relief, and first-line opioids include morphine and fentanyl (Drain, 2018b; Pasero, 2018). Titrating IV opioids in the immediate PO period requires a delicate balance between relieving acute pain and avoiding oversedation. Many PACUs use a pain protocol in the form of an algorithm (flow chart) to enable the PACU nurse to administer the prescribed analgesics by means of intermittent IV bolus doses of opioids (e.g. morphine or fentanyl) while concurrently assessing the patient for signs of respiratory depression or sedation. Standard pain protocols for adult patients require older patients to receive smaller opioid doses owing to their reduced tolerance and increased susceptibility to side effects, particularly respiratory depression and sedation (Pasero, 2018). In the event of increasing sedation or respiratory depression, the PACU nurse must summon medical staff such as the treating anaesthetist. An opioid antagonist such as naloxone may need to be administered by the PACU nurse to reverse these serious adverse effects (Pasero, 2018).

Morphine. Morphine remains one of the most commonly used IV opioid analgesics for acute PO pain in the PACU. It has a slower onset and peak but longer

TABLE 12.2
Commonly Used Analgesic Drugs

GENERAL OPIOID CONSIDERATIONS

The following considerations are applicable to all opioid analgesic medications.

Mode of Action:

Morphine, fentanyl, oxycodone and codeine all attach to μ-opioid receptors in the CNS, inhibiting the transmission of the pain impulses.
Tapendatol and tramadol have a similar mode of action and also inhibit noradrenaline reuptake.

Precautions/Special Populations

Where possible, avoid concurrent use of sedative-causing agents such as benzodiazepines, antipsychotic agents and sedating antihistamines.
Patients with the following conditions require greater monitoring during opioid administration as they are at great risk of developing adverse effects:
  • increased BMI
  • sleep apnoea
  • increased intracranial pressure
  • head injury
  • renal impairment
  • hepatic impairment
  • significant pre-existing respiratory disease
  • older >70–75 years

Adverse Effects

Respiratory: Respiratory depression, bronchospasm
Cardiovascular: Postural hypotension, bradycardia, vasodilation and hypotension (more common with IV administration)
Neurological: Confusion, sedation, delirium, cough suppression, euphoria, dysphoria, miosis and impaired cognition
Dermatological: Urticaria, pruritis, sweating, flushing
Gastrointestinal: Nausea, vomiting, decreased gastric motility and emptying, anorexia, increased antral tone, prolonged large bowel transit time, constipation, decreased anal sphincter tone
Musculoskeletal: Myoclonus (sudden and involuntary muscle jerking and spasm)
Urinary: Urinary retention, increased difficulty in micturition, increased external sphincter tone, increased detrusor muscle tone

OPIOID	Onset	Duration	Dosage	Precaution/Special Considerations/Adverse Effects
Morphine	5–10 min, peaks 15–30 min (IV route)	3–4 h (IV route) Controlled-release preparation 12 and 24 h (MS contin)	0.5–2 mg initial dose and then titrate to pain and sedation score (recommended dose for acute pain in adults and children >50 kg) 0.5 mg Initial dose for patients >70 years	Recommended initial does 0.5 mg for patients >70 years
Fentanyl	3–5 min, peaks 10–15 min (IV route)	2–40 min (IV route)	There is significant variance in the recommended dosage The route of administration, indication for use and the age of the patient greatly impact on the required dosage It is recommended to be guided by hospital protocols	Bradyarrhythmia may be exacerbated Safe for use in renal failure Often indicated as an adjunct to general anaesthesia or epidural Observe for rash, erythema, bradycardia
Oxycodone	15–30 min (0.25–0.5 h) for peak effects post IV administration	4-hourly	IV: 0.5–2 mg then titrate to pain and sedation score 0.5 mg initial dose for patients >70 years Oral: 5–15 mg	Avoid in patients with severe hepatic and renal impairment Initial dose to be decreased if creatinine clearance is <30 mL/min Oral preparation not to be used in the presence of swallowing disorders Tablets can become highly viscous in water and can swell Choking, difficulty swallowing, regurgitation and gagging have been reported Tablets to be swallowed whole

TABLE 12.2
Commonly Used Analgesic Drugs—cont'd

OPIOID	Onset	Duration	Dosage	Precaution/Special Considerations/Adverse Effects
Codeine	Usually given in combination with paracetamol, absorbed rapidly reaching peak effects at 30–60 min	3–4 h	Adults: 30–60 mg up to a maximum of 240 mg daily Child >12 years: 0.5–1 mg per kg (max single dose 60 mg) up to a maximum of 240 mg daily	Contraindicated in breastfeeding mothers, children <12 years and patients <18 undergoing tonsillectomy or adenoidectomy
Tapentadol	30 min onset and peaks at 1.25 h post administration	4–6 h Controlled-release 12 h	Oral: 50–100 mg Initial dose 50 mg, 2nd 50 mg dose can be administered 1 h post initial dose	Avoid concurrent use with SSRIs as this increases the risk of serotonin syndrome
Tramadol	1 h, peaks 2–4 h (oral route) IV route produces a more rapid onset and peaks at 45 min	3–6 h	IV and IM 50–100 mg (max 600 mg daily and 300 mg daily for patients >75) Oral 50–100 mg (max 400 mg daily and for patients >75 300 mg)	Use of tramadol in conjunction with SSRIs can cause serotonin toxicity Avoid use of controlled preparation: • in people >75 • in the presence of constipation • in those with hepatic and renal impairment May cause nausea, sweating, dizziness and sedation

GENERAL NSAID CONSIDERATIONS

The following considerations are applicable to all NSAID analgesic medications.

Mode of Action

Kertorolac is a non-selective COX-1 and COX-2 inhibitor
Parocoxib and celecoxib are selective COX-2 inhibitors

Precautions/Special Populations

Risk of renal failure is increased when NSAIDs (non-selective and selective) are used concurrently with diuretics, angiotensin II receptor blockers or angiotensin connecting enzyme inhibitors
The use of NSAIDs is contraindicated for any patient with pre-existing renal impairment, cirrhosis, heart failure and cardiovascular disease

Adverse Effects

Cardiovascular: Hypertension, fluid retention, increased risk of myocardial infarction, increased risk of stroke, increased risk of cardiovascular death
Gastrointestinal: Increase in upper abdominal pain, increased risk of ulcer formation (peptic, oesophageal and within the mucosa of the small bowel), increased risk of gastrointestinal bleeding, increased risk of gastric erosion
Renal: Increased risk of renal impairment

Continued

TABLE 12.2
Commonly Used Analgesic Drugs—cont'd

NSAID	Onset	Duration	Dosage	Precaution/Special Considerations/Adverse Effects
Ketorolac	Peak effects at 50 min post a 30 mg dose	IV/IM: 4–6 h Oral: 6–8 h	IV/IM: 10 mg initial dose, 10–30 mg 4–6 h (max daily dose 60 mg) Oral: 10 mg 6–8 h (max daily dose 30–40 mg) Consider reduced dose for patients with mild renal impairment, <50 kg, or >65 years	IV injection should be administered over 15 s May cause sweating, itching, pain at injection site, purpura
Paracoxib	Onset 7–14 min and peaks at 2 h	6–24 h	IV/IM: 40 mg single dose, 20 mg for patients with moderate hepatic renal impairment and women <50 kg and >65 years	
Celecoxib	Peaks effects at 2–3 h for fasting patients Non-fasting patients peak effects at 4–6 h	12–24 h	400 mg single dose (day of surgery) 200 mg daily or BD (up to a maximum of 5 days post op then cease) Recommended to reduce dose by half for patients with moderate hepatic impairment	Avoid use in patients who have allergies to sulfonamides Avoid use in severe hepatic impairment Reduced dose is indicated for use in patients with mild hepatic impairment

NON-OPIOID ANALGESICS

Mode of Action

Panadol's action is not fully determined, but is believed to inhibit prostaglandin synthesis and the serotonergic pathway

Panadol	IV: 5–10 min onset and peaks at 1 h post administration Oral: 10 min onset and peaks at 60 min post administration	4–6 h	IV: 1 g with maximum daily dose of 4 g (patients >50 kg) 15 mg per kg with maximum dose of 60 mg per kg per day (patients <50 kg) Oral: 0.5–1 g max daily dose 4 g	Pre-existing liver disease IV infusion should be over at least 15 min Decreased BMI

COX = cyclo-oxygenase; NSAID = non-steroidal anti-inflammatory drug; SSRI = selective serotonin reuptake inhibitor.
(Sources: Colwell, 2018; Australian Medicines Handbook, 2019; eTG complete therapeutic guidelines, 2019; MIMS online data version, 2019.)

duration of action compared with other first-line opioids such as fentanyl (Pasero, 2018).

Fentanyl. Fentanyl has a fast onset, within 3–5 minutes; however, it has a shorter duration of action than morphine. Given intravenously, its analgesic properties are 80 to 125 times more potent than morphine. Note that the dose is in micrograms (μg), not milligrams (mg) (Pasero, 2018). (See Chapter 3 for a report on the death of Paul Lau from a postoperative medication error involving fentanyl.)

Targin. Oral prolonged-release oxycodone/naloxone, a controlled-release tablet containing a combination of oxycodone–hydrochloride and the opioid antagonist naloxone hydrochloridedihydrate, is gaining in popularity (Manassero, Fanelli, Ugues, Bailo, & Dalmasso, 2018). Research box 12.1 contains more information.

Tramadol. Tramadol is an atypical centrally acting analgesic owing to its combined effects as an opioid agonist and a serotonin and noradrenaline (norepinephrine) reuptake inhibitor. Tramadol causes significantly less respiratory depression and less impairment to gastrointestinal motor function at equivalent analgesic doses compared with morphine. While it has been

RESEARCH BOX 12.1
Oral Prolonged-release Oxycodone/naloxone

Two different randomised clinical trials of oral versus intravenous opioids compared pain levels after cardiac surgery and knee replacement surgery. In cardiac surgical patients, results showed that doses of oral oxycodone/naloxone were significantly lower compared with IV morphine (in the presence of similar pain scores), revealing promising results for this oral opioid even in painful PO procedures (Ruetzler et al., 2014). Similar results were found by Manassero and colleagues (2018), who revealed that in the immediate PO period after total knee replacement, the patients receiving oral prolonged-release oxycodone/naloxone experienced the same to better pain control than those receiving morphine IV, with a similar degree of PO nausea and vomiting (Manassero et al., 2018).

known for some time that tramadol is a contributing factor in the development of PO delirium, there is now evidence from Stephens and colleagues (2015) that there is a drug interaction between tramadol and ondansetron (an antiemetic) in the early PO period that decreases the effectiveness of tramadol.

Tapentadol. Tapentadol is a centrally acting opioid analgesic that binds to the μ-opioid receptor and is a noradrenaline-reuptake inhibitor. In contrast to tramadol, it has no relevant functional serotonin-reuptake inhibition and no active metabolites. Taken orally, it has been shown to have analgesic effects similar to those of oxycodone (Australian Medicines Handbook, 2020).

Pethidine. Pethidine (meperidine) is a synthetic opioid with decreasing usage noted worldwide, owing to multiple disadvantages compared with other opioids (Schug, Palmer, Scott, Halliwell, & Trinca, 2016). Its use is strongly ill-advised in the acute setting because of strong links with dependency (Australian Medicines Handbook, 2020).

Non-steroidal anti-inflammatory drugs (NSAIDS). The term 'non-steroidal anti-inflammatory drugs' refers to a range of drugs that includes coxibs (COX-1 and COX-2 inhibitors) (Bryant, Knights, Darroch, & Rowland, 2019). NSAIDs have analgesic, anti-inflammatory and antipyretic effects and are effective for a variety of acute pain states. NSAIDs may produce renal, gastrointestinal and some platelet-related adverse effects, which precludes their use in some surgical patients. The coxibs available at present include celecoxib, etoricoxib and parecoxib, the injectable precursor of valdecoxib. Coxibs offer the potential for effective

analgesia with fewer side effects than other classes of NSAIDs (Bryant et al., 2019).

Diclofenac. Diclofenac is a NSAID that is useful for pain relief following pelvic gynaecological surgery, insertion of ureteric stents and ureteric colic. It is absorbed rapidly by the gut and has a half-life of 1–2 hours (Bryant et al., 2019).

Ibuprofen. Ibuprofen has the least number of side effects of the NSAIDs and is an effective analgesic but a weaker anti-inflammatory. It is known to be useful for pain relief following dental extractions and laparoscopy (Bryant et al., 2019).

Ketamine. The principal effect of ketamine is as an antihyperalgesic, antiallodynic and antitolerance agent, not as a primary analgesic. Its main role is as an adjuvant in the treatment of pain associated with central sensitisation, such as in severe acute pain, neuropathic pain and opioid-resistant pain. It is also known to reduce the incidence of chronic postsurgical pain and to attenuate opioid-induced tolerance and hyperalgesia (Tizani, 2017).

Paracetamol. Paracetamol is an important and well-tolerated analgesic used in PO pain management. It has been found to have a significant opioid-sparing effect when used in multimodal approaches to pain management. It can be given orally preoperatively and is rapidly absorbed via the gastrointestinal route. Intravenous administration is frequently used for patients postoperatively (Bryant et al., 2019).

Serotonin syndrome

Certain medications used in acute pain relief, such as pethidine, tramadol, antidepressants, monoamine oxidase inhibitors and tapentadol, when given with selective serotonin reuptake inhibitors (SSRIs) (e.g. fluoxetine [Prozac]) may result in the release of excessive amounts of serotonin, causing *serotonin syndrome* (Nagelhout, 2018b). This condition is a rare but potentially life-threatening condition and may present within minutes up to 24 hours after initial injection. It is characterised by neurological changes such as confusion, agitation, neuromuscular excitement and autonomic stimulation (tachycardia, hypertension and ventricular extrasystoles) (Nagelhout, 2018b). Treatment includes ceasing the causative agents, treating individual symptoms and possibly administration of serotonin antagonists such as methysergide and cyproheptadine (Nagelhout, 2018b).

Codeine in children

The American Food and Drug Administration (FDA) recommends avoiding use of codeine in children, particularly after tonsillectomy and adenoidectomy for obstructive sleep apnoea, owing to the possible risk of respiratory depression (Hoefner-Notz, 2018).

Patient-controlled analgesia

The major goal of patient-controlled analgesia (PCA) is to avoid the peaks and troughs of analgesia by enabling patients to administer their own analgesia as they need it, in order to control their pain (Pasero, 2018). Patients are able to anticipate activities such as coughing or movement that are associated with increased pain and provide themselves with an opioid bolus in advance. The PCA device is programmed to a predetermined maximum dose as a bolus and there is a lockout period after each bolus to prevent overdose. PCA devices are programmed based on the patient's needs and the pharmacokinetics of the drug being administered (Pasero, 2018). PCA works effectively if commenced when the patient is pain free or has a manageable level of pain. To facilitate this, the PACU nurse administers a bolus dose of opioid analgesia prior to commencing PCA. If possible, the use of PCA should be discussed with patients preoperatively to educate them in the operation of the device. Other patient-controlled local anaesthetic devices such as patient-controlled epidural analgesia (PCEA) and continuous wound catheters delivering local anaesthesia are also available in some healthcare facilities.

Local anaesthetic

A variety of local anaesthetic blocks and infiltration may be given to assist in PO pain management. These range from simple infiltration of the local anaesthetic into the surgical incision site, to arm blocks, femoral blocks and transversus abdominis plane (TAP) blocks. These may form part of the multimodal approach. The PACU nurse should observe for any signs of local anaesthetic toxicity following a possible overdose of the local anaesthetic drugs. Life-threatening circulatory collapse, convulsions, agitation and loss of consciousness may result, requiring immediate resuscitation measures to support circulation and breathing. The administration of lipid emulsion (Intralipid) is also recommended as a treatment for local toxicity (Association of Anaesthetists of Great Britain and Ireland [AAGBI], 2020; Australian and New Zealand Anaesthetic Allergy Group [ANZAAG], 2016). (See Chapter 8 for further information.)

Non-pharmacological pain management

In addition to pharmacological measures, common non-pharmacological pain relief measures may include elevation of the affected body part where applicable, appropriate temperature management, patient positioning so as not to put stress on the surgical incision, breathing exercises and distraction strategies such as music therapy (Lang & Makic, 2020).

Acute pain service

Most large training hospitals have an acute pain service (APS), which is generally run from the Department of Anaesthesia (Pasero, 2018). This service provides an excellent resource for the management of patients' pain and for ongoing staff education. In some hospitals, anaesthetic or PACU nurses may be included in the APS, which provides these nurses with a great opportunity for professional development as well as increasing pain services for patients.

SPECIAL POPULATIONS
Management of Patients With Diabetes Mellitus

The universal goals of care for a patient with diabetes mellitus in the PO period are to stabilise vital signs, promote would healing and correct fluid and electrolyte imbalances (Wagner, 2018). The PACU nurse regularly checks blood sugar levels and urine for evidence of glycosuria while also monitoring fluids and electrolytes. The stresses imposed by surgery and anaesthesia cause imbalances that may require active management to return blood sugar levels to within the normal range. Patients may require dextrose infusions for hypoglycaemia or insulin infusions on a sliding scale during the perioperative period, depending on their blood sugar results, as well as IV fluids to treat dehydration. Hyperglycaemia and coma may be difficult to ascertain in an unconscious patient, making regular blood sugar monitoring a vital component of the overall diabetic patient care.

Management of the Obstetric Patient

Pregnant patients may present for surgery unrelated to their pregnancy, such as carpel tunnel repair or laparoscopic cholecystectomy. Conversely, many other surgeries are pregnancy related, such as cervical cerclage (to maintain a pregnancy in cervical insufficiency) or a delivery such as caesarean section (classic or lower uterine) (Wilner, 2018).

However, the most common obstetric patient to be seen in the PACU is the LUSCS patient. In addition to the normal PO observations, blood loss must be checked with each set of observations by assessing the per-vaginal (PV) loss and by assessing the fundal height (Wilner, 2018). The perineal pad may have a moderate amount of lochia rubra (PV loss), but if there are two or more saturated pads in the first hour this would be considered excessive, or if active bleeding was noted (trickling), then haemorrhage would be suspected. The fundus is the top of the uterus and, as part of routine observations, should be gently palpated to check its height in relation to the umbilicus and firmness (indicating that the uterus has contracted following delivery). In cases where there is active bleeding from the uterus, fundal height would rise and the uterus would feel soft (often termed 'boggy'). Any of these signs, together with active PV loss, may indicate possible postpartum haemorrhage requiring urgent assessment by the obstetrician. Checking the fundal height will be uncomfortable for the patient, as it will be close to the incision site, and the reason for undertaking the check must be explained to the patient. The procedure should be carried out by nurses who have had education in the assessment of postpartum patients.

Careful BP readings must also be taken, with particular attention to hypertension, which may be a sign of pre-eclampsia – a condition unique to pregnancy and characterised by high blood pressure, fluid retention and proteinuria. In severe cases, the condition can lead to eclampsia and seizures, which can compromise the health of both mother and baby. The condition is usually relieved by delivery of the baby, but pre-eclampsia can continue immediately post delivery, requiring careful observations of the mother's blood pressure together with noting any complaints of headaches or visual disturbances. The occurrence of these signs and symptoms requires urgent medical assessment (Agency for Clinical Innovation [ACI], 2019).

Management of the Paediatric Patient

Caring for paediatric patients requires experience, expertise and an understanding of the uniqueness of this population. As this population covers such a wide range of ages, sizes and developmental stages, meeting the needs of this diverse group can present a huge challenge to perioperative nurses.

The smaller the child, the smaller the airway – making very young children and babies vulnerable to airway obstruction, laryngospasm and post-extubation croup (Butterworth, 2019a). (See the information earlier in the chapter on management of laryngospasm.) This can be even more problematic when the surgical site and airway are shared, as in ear, nose and throat (ENT) surgery, which is the most common surgical specialty for the paediatric group. Very careful respiratory observations and constant monitoring of pulse oximetry are essential. Loss of a patent airway in a child is a medical emergency and the PACU nurse must immediately press the emergency bell.

Cardiovascular status may be even more important in children than in adults because they do not have the same physiological reserves (Hoefner-Notz, 2018). Blood loss must be carefully observed, and if active bleeding occurs this should be accurately measured. The PACU nurse must summon the assistance of the treating anaesthetist and/or the surgical team, and the BP should be taken. Heart rates are very important in this population and bradycardia in a child may be very serious, as it reveals a decreased cardiac output, so medical help should be immediately summoned.

Paediatric patients require support from their parents and carers alike. Parental presence may assist nursing staff too, as parents can distinguish normal from abnormal behaviours and make children feel safer. Including parents/carers in handover procedures will make them feel involved in their child's care and also allow the opportunity to ask questions.

Having an environment conducive to children is also desirable, as it may be more familiar to them. This means having dedicated bays for their recovery, with protected side rails available on beds and cots and child-friendly pictures on the wall, as well as allowing younger children to have a toy or security blanket with them (Hoefner-Notz, 2018).

Care of the Older Patient

Care of older patients may be complicated in the PO period as they often have comorbidities. These may include, but are not limited to, cardiac conditions, hypertension, respiratory conditions, osteoarthritis, decreased vision, decreased hearing, fluid and electrolyte imbalance, dementia and diabetes. To treat many of these conditions, the patient commonly takes both prescribed and non-prescribed medications.

Ageing alters pharmacokinetics, affecting the liberation, absorption, distribution, metabolism and excretion of medications (Gendron, 2018). Recovery from anaesthesia may be prolonged in older patients, and an understanding of specific medications and careful administration is required. Some medications may be titrated in smaller doses, such as seen in opioid administration.

Older patients should have their hearing aids, dentures and spectacles available for use during the PO period to aid in situational awareness. PO cognitive dysfunction has been reported to be 10% higher in older patients (Alalawi & Yasmeen, 2018) and may manifest itself immediately after surgery. Although potentially reversible, cognitive dysfunction may last up to 6 months, so any alteration in cognition must be reported so that a full assessment can be made.

The PACU nurse should note the older patient's pressure injury risk assessment score and reassess skin integrity in the immediate PO period. Older patients are particularly vulnerable to developing pressure injuries, as their skin may be paper-thin and they often have bony prominences (see Chapter 9 for further information). Movement may be impeded because of arthritis, so careful movement is required when positioning or repositioning the patient. The PACU nurse should take into account the length of time the patient has been on the operating table and the position required for the surgery. These factors may cause PO discomfort for the patient.

Care of the Obese Patient

Nursing care of obese patients includes compassion (as they are often embarrassed by their body image), careful respiratory assessment, O_2 therapy and positioning. If the patient has a normal BP, it is best practice to nurse the patient sitting up to reduce the weight of the chest wall from impeding ventilation. By sitting up, the weight of the chest wall is redistributed, allowing greater tidal volume. If the patient is hypotensive (requiring lying flat), a discussion with the anaesthetist is required to assess which problem is worse; however, the 'banana' position (head up and feet up) may be employed. It is essential to provide support for positioning to ensure that an upright sitting position is maintained. If the patient is edentulous, replace the teeth, as these will assist in upper airway support (Clifford, 2018). (See Feature box 12.2 and Chapters 7, 8 and 9 for further information about care of the obese patient.)

Obesity is also recognised as a common risk factor for obstructive sleep apnoea (OSA), which is characterised by repeated obstruction of the upper airway during sleep that leads to intermittent hypoxaemia and disturbed sleeping patterns (Hyun-Joon, Seung-Hak, Sung-Wan, Su-Jung, & Young-Guk, 2020). Patients who suffer from OSA are believed to have a greater risk of respiratory complications following general anaesthesia; however, patients may present in the PACU unaware of their pre-existing condition (Setaro, Reinsel, & Brun, 2019). Nurses must be particularly watchful for these symptoms in the obese patient.

PATIENT SCENARIOS

SCENARIO 12.3: PATIENT DETERIORATION (CONTINUED)

Mr Collins has been in the PACU for 45 minutes and he continues to display periods of apnoea with declining oxygen saturation levels while on room air.

Critical Thinking Questions

- What is the continued management of this situation?
- What may be the cause of apnoeic periods and what are the implications of the situation if not treated effectively with appropriate follow-up?
- What interventions should be undertaken to optimise Mr Collins' outcome?

Other Special Populations

Other special populations who may require additional nursing care or special carer considerations may include:

- fathers/partners/support persons of women following childbirth
- children and patients with intellectual disabilities, who may require a family member/familiar carer

- patients requesting gender segregation for religious/cultural reasons
- traumatised or distressed patients
- gender-diverse patients
- patient with known infectious diseases
- patients who may require radiation safety protocols applied.

DISCHARGE PLANNING

Planning for a patient discharge occurs through the entire perioperative process, ensuring ongoing education and understanding of the procedure and possible complications while allowing the patient to resume greater self-care during this progression (Foran & Hoch, 2020). This is particularly relevant in day surgery settings, when patients are provided with both verbal and written PO instructions and medications if required (ACSQHC/the Commission, 2017b; ANZCA, 2018).

Discharge Criteria

A **discharge criteria** system is used by nurses to determine when a patient is 'ward ready' or can be discharged home from Stage 2 PACU. Several scoring systems are available to assess patients being discharged to the ward, such as

---

FEATURE BOX 12.3
A Patient-focused Discharge Criteria System

CONSCIOUS STATE

- The patient must be conscious and able to respond appropriately to verbal stimuli.

RESPIRATORY FUNCTION

- The patient must be able to protect their airway.
- The patient has a cough reflex.
- The respiratory rate must be greater than 12 breaths per minute.
- Oxygen saturation may be assessed by trialling the patient on room air for at least 10 minutes prior to discharge. If the S_pO_2 is less than 94% on room air in an otherwise healthy patient, the PACU nurse should discuss with medical staff prior to discharge.

CARDIOVASCULAR FUNCTION

- Vital signs need to be within normal limits, referring to the patient's baseline observations.
- Heart rate and BP should be within 20% of baseline values.
- If this is not met but the patient is otherwise stable, the patient may be discharged only after consultation with the anaesthetist and the variance written on the patient's PO orders.

TEMPERATURE

- The patient's core temperature should be between 36°C and 37°C.

PAIN

- Pain management continues until the patient is pain free, has pain at a manageable level or the vital signs indicate that it is inappropriate to continue, such as seen in a respiratory rate of less than 12 breaths per minute.

NAUSEA AND VOMITING

- Nausea always needs to be treated. Patients with persistent nausea may be returned to the ward on oxygen after liaison with the anaesthetist and appropriate treatment ordered.

WOUND CARE

- There should be no excessive drainage from wound sites or drain tubes.
- Ooze through dressings must be marked and the time and date noted.
- Drain tube bottles are to be labelled with the amount, date and time.
- The fundal height in post-LUSCS patients should be equal to or less than the level of the umbilicus.

INTRAVENOUS LINES

- IV bags need to have an IV label completed and attached.
- IV bungs that are left in situ need to be flushed with saline prior to discharge to the ward; this should be noted on the patient's record.

SPECIFIC OBSERVATIONS

- Specialised observations may be required, such as neurological observations or vascular observations, and these must be within normal limits.

PATIENT COMFORT

- The patient needs to be in a position of comfort in a clean, dry bed.

DOCUMENTATION

- Nursing documentation must be completed contemporaneously and legibly in ink.
- Medical staff should have written up appropriate notes and orders – for example, orders for IV fluids, pain relief, antiemetics and specific medications such as antibiotics and PO orders.
- If a score system is used to detect deterioration of patients in the ward areas, the last set of patient observations should be transcribed onto the ward chart and a score calculated prior to discharge. This provides a baseline for the ward nurses and alerts the PACU staff if the patient is still not 'ward ready'. It is not appropriate to send a patient to the ward when their observations are at, or very close to, triggering a medical emergency team call (Foran & Nilsson, 2019).

LUSCS = lower uterine segment caesarean section.

---

the Aldrete numerical scoring system and the Postanaesthesia Discharge Scoring System (PADSS) (Foran & Nilsson, 2019). Some healthcare providers prefer a patient-focused approach, whereby the patient must meet all discharge criteria prior to being transferred to the ward or Stage 2 PACU. Discharge criteria may differ between PACUs, depending on the level of the expertise of the ward nurse and the type of surgery performed. Feature box 12.3 is an example of a patient-focused approach.

Prior to discharge from Stage 2 PACU in day surgery units, the patient will need to have met the discharge criteria for ambulatory care patients (Feature box 12.4),

FEATURE BOX 12.4
Discharge Criteria for Ambulatory (Day) Care Patients

- Stable vital signs for at least 1 hour
- Oriented in time, place and person
- Adequate pain control
- Minimal nausea, vomiting or dizziness
- Adequate oral hydration
- Minimal bleeding or wound drainage
- Able to pass urine
- A responsible carer is available to accompany and transport the patient home

- Discharge authorised by an appropriate member of staff
- Suitable analgesia provided
- Written and verbal instructions given (to patient and carer)
- Any required teaching completed (for patient and carer)
- The patient's readiness for discharge is confirmed

(Sources: ACORN, 2020d; Australian and New Zealand College of Anaesthetists, 2020.)

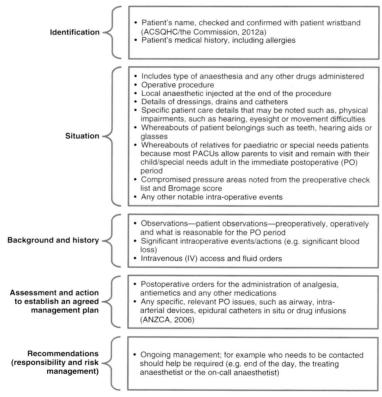

Identification
- Patient's name, checked and confirmed with patient wristband (ACSQHC/the Commission, 2012a)
- Patient's medical history, including allergies

Situation
- Includes type of anaesthesia and any other drugs administered
- Operative procedure
- Local anaesthetic injected at the end of the procedure
- Details of dressings, drains and catheters
- Specific patient care details that may be noted such as, physical impairments, such as hearing, eyesight or movement difficulties
- Whereabouts of patient belongings such as teeth, hearing aids or glasses
- Whereabouts of relatives for paediatric or special needs patients because most PACUs allow parents to visit and remain with their child/special needs adult in the immediate postoperative (PO) period
- Compromised pressure areas noted from the preoperative check list and Bromage score
- Any other notable intra-operative events

Background and history
- Observations—patient observations—preoperatively, operatively and what is reasonable for the PO period
- Significant intraoperative events/actions (e.g. significant blood loss)
- Intravenous (IV) access and fluid orders

Assessment and action to establish an agreed management plan
- Postoperative orders for the administration of analgesia, antiemetics and any other medications
- Any specific, relevant PO issues, such as airway, intra-arterial devices, epidural catheters in situ or drug infusions (ANZCA, 2006)

Recommendations (responsibility and risk management)
- Ongoing management; for example who needs to be contacted should help be required (e.g. end of the day, the treating anaesthetist or the on-call anaesthetist)

FIG. 12.9 ISBAR handover requirements in the PACU. (Sources: ACORN, 2020d; Australian Commission for Safety and Quality in Health Care, 2017b.)

including that they have a person to transport them home. Day surgery patients will usually receive a phone call by a nurse on the day following surgery to check that their recovery is progressing and to answer any questions (ACORN, 2020d; ANZCA, 2018).

PATIENT HANDOVER FROM PACU NURSE TO WARD NURSE

When handing patients over to the ward staff, the ISBAR tool is again used (ACSQHC/the Commission, 2017b). Fig. 12.9 outlines the ISBAR handover requirements.

PATIENT SCENARIOS

SCENARIO 12.4: POSTOPERATIVE CLINICAL HANDOVER

Mr Collins' recovery has progressed well and RN Sang is preparing to hand his care over to the ward nurse, RN Markham.

Critical Thinking Questions

- What are RN Sang's main considerations when preparing to discharge Mr Collins from the PACU?
- Using the ISBAR tool, describe the key points that RN Sang will include in her clinical handover of Mr Collins to RN Markham.

CONCLUSION

This chapter has outlined the purpose and role of the PACU, the handover procedure from the OR to the PACU nurse, the ABCDE of recovery, the management of important complications, an overview of pain management, the management of specific populations and discharge criteria. The knowledge presented enables the PACU nurse to provide patients with a safe recovery from both anaesthesia and surgery, to monitor the patient's vital signs, manage pain, anticipate complications and provide comfort and reassurance.

RESOURCES

American Association of Nurse Anesthetists
https://www.aana.com
American Society of PeriAnesthesia Nurses
https://www.aspan.org
Association for Perioperative Practice
https://www.afpp.org.uk/home
Australian and New Zealand College of Anaesthetists
https://www.anzca.edu.au
Australian College of Perianaesthesia Nurses
https://www.acpan.edu.au
Australian College of Perioperative Nurses
https://www.acorn.org.au
Australian Day Surgery Nurses Association (ADSNA)
http://adsna.info
British Anaesthetic & Recovery Nurses Association
https://www.barna.co.uk
Day Hospitals Australia
https://www.dayhospitalsaustralia.net.au
International Association for the Study of Pain
https://www.iasp-pain.org
International Federation of Nurse Anesthetists
https://www.aana.com

Perioperative Nursing College of the New Zealand Nurses Organisation
https://www.pnc.org.nz

REFERENCES

Agency for Clinical Innovation (ACI). (2019). Pre eclampsia. Retrieved from <https://www.aci.health.nsw.gov.au/networks/icnsw/patients-and-families/patient-conditions/pre-eclampsia>.

Akers, J., Dupnick, A., Hillman, E., Bauer, A., Kinker, L., & Hagedorn Wonder, A. (2019). Inadvertent perioperative hypothermia risks and postoperative complications: a retrospective study. *AORN Journal*, 109(6), 741–747. https://dx.doi.org/10.1002/aorn.12696

Alalawi, R., & Yasmeen, N. (2018). Postoperative cognitive dysfunction in the elderly: a review comparing the effects of Desflurane and Sevflurane. *Journal of Perianesthesia Nursing*, 33(5), 732–740. https://dx.doi.org/10.1016/j.jopan.2017.04.009

American Society of Peri-Anesthesia Nurses. (2019). ASPAN's history timeline. Retrieved from <https://www.aspan.org/About-Us/History/History-Timeline>.

Anaesthesia UK. (2017). Bromage Score. Retrieved from <https://www.frca.co.uk/article.aspx?articleid=100316>.

Association of Anaesthetists of Great Britain and Ireland [AAGBI]. (2020). Management of severe local anaesthetic toxicity. Retrieved from <https://anaesthetists.org/Portals/0/PDFs/Guidelines%20PDFs/Guideline_management_severe_local_anaesthetic_toxicity_v2_2010_final.pdf?ver=2018-07-11-163755-240&ver=2018-07-11-163755-240>.

Australian and New Zealand Anaesthetic Allergy Group (ANZAAG). (2016). Anaphylaxis management guidelines. Retrieved from <http://www.anzaag.com/Mgmt%20Resources.aspx>.

Australian and New Zealand College of Anaesthetists (ANZCA). (2013a). PS41 Guidelines on acute pain management. Retrieved from <https://www.anzca.edu.au/getattachment/558316c5-ea93-457c-b51f-d57556b0ffa7/PS41-Guideline-on-acute-pain-management>.

Australian and New Zealand College of Anaesthetists (ANZCA). (2013b). PS53 Statement on the handover responsibilities of the anaesthetist. Retrieved from <https://www.anzca.edu.au/getattachment/021e4205-af5a-415d-815d-b16be1fe8b62/PS15-Guideline-for-the-perioperative-care-of-patients-selected-for-day-stay-procedures>.

Australian and New Zealand College of Anaesthetists (ANZCA). (2018). PS15 Guidelines for the perioperative care of patients selected for day stay procedures. Retrieved from <https://www.anzca.edu.au/getattachment/021e4205-af5a-415d-815d-b16be1fe8b62/PS15-Guideline-for-the-perioperative-care-of-patients-selected-for-day-stay-procedures>.

Australian and New Zealand College of Anaesthetists (ANZCA). (2020). PS04 Statement on the post-anaesthesia care unit (pilot). Retrieved from <https://www.anzca.edu.au/safety-advocacy/standards-of-practice/policies,-statements,-and-guidelines>.

Australian College of PeriAnaesthesia Nurses (ACPAN) (2019). Professional Standards for Perianaesthesia Nursing. Retrieved from <https://acpan.edu.au/pdfs/standards/acpan-professional-standards-v1.pdf>.

Australian College of Perioperative Nurses (ACORN). (2020a). Managing the post anaesthetic care unit. In *ACORN standards for perioperative nurses in Australia* (16th ed., Vol. 2). Adelaide: Author.

Australian College of Perioperative Nurses (ACORN). (2020b). Staffing for safety. In *ACORN standards for Perioperative Nurses in Australia* (16th ed., Vol. 2). Adelaide: Author.

Australian College of Perioperative Nurses (ACORN). (2020c). Hypothermia. In *ACORN standards for perioperative nurses in Australia* (16th ed., Vol. 2). Adelaide: Author.

Australian College of Perioperative Nurses (ACORN). (2020d). Post anaesthesia care unit nurse. In *ACORN standards for perioperative nurses in Australia* (16th ed., Vol. 2). Adelaide: Author.

Australian Commission on Safety and Quality in Health Care (ACSQHC/the Commission). (2017a). *National consensus statement: essential elements for recognising & responding to acute physiological deterioration* (2nd ed.). Sydney: Author.

Australian Commission on Safety and Quality in Health Care (ACSQHC/the Commission). (2017b). *Guide for day procedure services.* Sydney: Author.

Australian Medicines Handbook. (2020). *Australian medicines handbook.* Adelaide: Author.

Boulette, E. (2018). Care of the pregnant patient. In J. Odom-Forren (Ed.), *Drain's perianesthesia nursing: a critical care approach* (7th ed., pp. 744–752). St. Louis, MO: Elsevier.

Bryant, B., Knights, K., Darroch, S., & Rowland, A. (2019). *Pharmacology for health professions* (5th ed.). Sydney: Elsevier.

Burden, N. (2018). Care of the ambulatory surgical patient. In J. Odom-Forren (Ed.), *Drain's perianesthesia nursing: a critical care approach* (7th ed., pp. 664–676). St. Louis, MO: Elsevier.

Butterworth, J. (2018a). Pediatric anesthesia. In J. Butterworth, D. Mackey, & J. Wasnick (Eds.), *Morgan & Mikhail's clinical anesthesiology* (6th ed., pp. 897–929). New York: McGraw-Hill.

Butterworth, J. (2018b). Spinal, epidural and caudal blocks. In J. Butterworth, D. Mackey, & J. Wasnick (Eds.), *Morgan & Mikhail's clinical anesthesiology* (6th ed., pp. 959–996). New York: McGraw-Hill.

Clifford, T. (2018). Care of the patient undergoing bariatric surgery. In J. Odom-Forren (Ed.), *Drain's perianesthesia nursing: a critical care approach* (7th ed., pp. 656–663). St. Louis, MO: Elsevier.

Colwell, A. (2018). Pain management. In J. Odom-Forren (Ed.), *Drain's perianesthesia nursing: a critical care approach* (7th ed., 431–455). St. Louis, MO: Elsevier.

Conway, A., Gow, J., Ralph, N., Duff, J., Edward, K., Alexander, K., & Bräuerm, A. (2019). Implementing a thermal care bundle for inadvertent perioperative hypothermia: a cost-effectiveness analysis. *International Journal of Nursing Studies, 97*, 21–27. https://dx.doi.org/ 10.1016/j.ijnurstu.2019.04.017

Dowling, C., & Fyrdenberg, M. (2016). Urogenital problems. In J. Smith, J. Fox, A. Saunder, & M. Kon Yii (Eds.), *Hunt & Marshall's clinical problems in surgery* (pp. 323–344). Sydney: Elsevier.

Drain, C. B. (2018a). The respiratory system. In J. Odom-Forren (Ed.), *Drain's perianesthesia nursing: a critical care approach* (7th ed., pp. 155–188). St. Louis, MO: Elsevier.

Drain, C. B. (2018b). Opioid intravenous anesthetics. In J. Odom-Forren (Ed.), *Drain's perianesthesia nursing: a critical care approach* (7th ed., pp. 284–296). St. Louis, MO: Elsevier.

Duff, J., Walker, K., Edward, K. L., Ralph, N., Giandinoto, J. A., Alexander, K., . . . Stephenson, J. (2018). Effect of a thermal care bundle on the prevention, detection and treatment of perioperative inadvertent hypothermia. *Journal of Clinical Nursing, 27*(5–6), 1239–1249. https://dx.doi.org/10.1111/jocn.14171

Foran, P. (2020). ECG for all patients in the PACU: some say why? I say why not? *Journal of Perianaesthesia Journal, 33*(2), e26–28. https://dx.doi.org/10.26550/2209-1092.1087

Foran, P., & Hoch, C. (2020). Postoperative care. In D. Brown, H. Edwards, T. Buckley, & R. Aitken (Eds.), *Lewis's medical-surgical nursing ANZ* (5th ed., pp. 387–412). Sydney: Elsevier

Foran, P., & Nilsson, U. (2019). Post-anaesthesia recovery. In L. Aitken, A. Marshall, & W. Chaboyer (Eds.), *Critical care nursing* (4th ed., pp. 909–940). Sydney: Elsevier.

Gendron, T. (2018). Care of the older patient. In J. Odom-Forren (Ed.), *Drain's perianesthesia nursing: a critical care approach* (7th ed., pp. 733–743). St. Louis, MO: Elsevier.

Health Quality and Safety Commission New Zealand. (2020). Patient deterioration: recognition and response. Retrieved from <https://www.hqsc.govt.nz/our-programmes/patient deterioration/workstreams/recognition-and-response-systems/>.

Hoefner-Notz, R. (2018). Care of the pediatric patient. In J. Odom-Forren (Ed.), *Drain's perianesthesia nursing: a critical care approach* (7th ed., pp. 707–732). St. Louis, MO: Elsevier.

Hyun-Joon, A., Seung-Hak, B., Sung-Wan, K., Su-Jung, K., & Young-Guk, P. (2020). Clustering-based characterization of clinical phenotypes in obstructive sleep apnoea using severity, obesity, and craniofacial pattern. *European Journal of Orthodontics, 42*(1), 93–100. https://dx.doi.org/ 10.1093/ejo/cjz041

Lang, C., & Makic, M. (2020). Managing postoperative pain: rethinking adjuvant therapies. *Journal of Perianesthesia Nursing, 35*(2), 212–214.

Loughlin, P., Sebat, F., & Kellett, J. (2018). Respiratory rate: the forgotten vital sign – make it count! *The Joint Commission Journal on Quality and Patient Safety, 44*, 494–499. https://dx.doi.org/10.1016/j.jcjq.2018.04.014

Manassero, A., Fanelli, A., Ugues, S., Bailo, C., & Dalmasso, S. (2018). Oral prolonged-release oxycodone/naloxone offers equivalent analgesia to intravenous morphine patient-controlled analgesia after total knee replacement. A randomized controlled trial. *Minerva Anestesiologica, 84*(9), 1016–1023. https://dx.doi.org/10.23736/S0375-9393.18.12297-8

Myrna, E. (2018). Care of the shock trauma patient. In J. Odom-Forren (Ed.), *Drain's perianesthesia nursing: a critical care approach* (7th ed., pp. 774–797). St. Louis, MO: Elsevier.

Nagelhout, J. (2018a). Regional anesthesia. In J. Odom-Forren (Ed.), *Drain's perianesthesia nursing: a critical care approach* (7th ed., pp. 329–344). St. Louis, MO: Elsevier.

Nagelhout, J. (2018b). Additional drugs of interest. In J. Nagelhout & E. Sass (Eds.), *Nurse anesthesia* (6th ed., CH. 14). St. Louis, MO: Elsevier.

O'Brien, D. (2018a). Postanesthesia care complications. In J. Odom-Forren (Ed.), *Drain's perianesthesia nursing: a critical care approach* (7th ed., pp. 398–416). St. Louis, MO: Elsevier.

O'Brien, D. (2018b). Patient education and care of the postanesthesia patient. In J. Odom-Forren (Ed.), *Drain's perianesthesia nursing: a critical care approach* (7th ed., pp. 385–397). St. Louis, MO: Elsevier.

Odom-Forren, J. (Ed.). (2018). *Drain's perianesthesia nursing: a critical care approach* (7th ed.). St Louis, MO: Elsevier.

Pasero, C. (2018). Pain management. In J. Odom-Forren (Ed.), *Drain's perianesthesia nursing: a critical care approach* (7th ed., pp. 431–455). St. Louis, MO: Elsevier.

Peterson, C. R. (2018). The hepatobiliary and gastrointestinal system In J. Odom-Forren (Ed.), *Drain's perianesthesia nursing: a critical care approach* (7th ed., pp. 221–227). St. Louis, MO: Elsevier.

Read, M., Maani, C., & Blackwell, S. (2017). Dexmedetomidine as a rescue therapy for emergence delirium in adults: a case series. *A & A Case Reports, 9*(1), 20–23. https://dx.doi.org/10.1213/xaa.0000000000000510

Ruetzler, K., Blome, C., Nabecker, S., Makarova, N., Fischer, H., Rinoesl, H., & Koinig, H. (2014). A randomised trial of oral versus intravenous opioids for treatment of pain after cardiac surgery. *Journal of Anesthesia, 28*(4), 580–586. https://dx.doi.org/10.1007/s00540-013-1770-x

Schick, L. (2018). Assessment and monitoring of the perianesthesia patient. In J. Odom-Forren (Ed.), *Drain's perianesthesia nursing: a critical care approach* (7th ed., pp. 357–384). St. Louis, MO: Elsevier.

Schoenwald, A., Palomano, R., & Fillman, M. (2020). Pain management. In D. Brown, H. Edwards, T. Buckley, & R. Aitken (Eds.), *Lewis's medical-surgical nursing ANZ.* (5th ed., pp. 84–116). Sydney: Elsevier.

Schug, S., Palmer, G. M., Scott, D. A., Halliwell, R., & Trinca, J. (2016). Acute pain management: scientific evidence, fourth edition, 2015. *Medical Journal of Australia, 204*(8), 315–317. https://dx.doi.org/10.5694/mja16.00133

Setaro, J., Reinsel, R., & Brun, D. (2019). Preoperative screening for obstructive sleep apnea and outcomes in PACU. *Journal of Perianesthesia Nursing, 34*(1), 66–73. https://dx.doi.org/10.1016/j.jopan.2017.10.005

Stephens, A. J., Woodman, R. J., & Owen, H. (2015). The effect of ondansetron on the efficacy of postoperative tramadol: a systematic review and meta-analysis of a drug interaction. *Anaesthesia, 70,* 209–218. https://dx.doi.org/10.1111/anae.12948

Stuit, D., & O'Sullivan, C. (2017). Ketamine as part of a multimodal approach to postoperative pain management. *American Association of Nurse Anesthetists Journal, 85*(5), 369–374.

Sundqvist, A. S., Nilsson, U., Holmefur, M., & Anderzén-Carlsson, A. (2016). Perioperative patient advocacy: an integrative review. *Journal of Perianethesia Nursing, 31*(5), 422–433. https://dx.doi.org/10.1016/j.jopan.2014.12.001

Tizani, A. (2017). *Harvard's nursing guide to drugs* (10th ed.). Sydney: Elsevier.

Ulatowska, A., Brzeźniak, H., Głowacka, A., & Bączyk, G. (2018). Evaluation of postoperative pain in patients treated surgically. *Polish Nursing, 70,* 358–364. http://dx.doi.org/10.20883/pielpol.2018.44

Vincent-Lambert, C., Smith, C., & Goldstein, L. (2018). Hypothermia in trauma patients arriving at an emergency department by ambulance in Johannesburg, South Africa: a prospective study. *Pan African Medical Journal, 31,* 136. doi: 10.11604/pamj.2018.31.136.13615

Wagner, V. (2018). Care of the patient with chronic disorders. In J. Odom-Forren (Ed.), *Drain's perianesthesia nursing: a critical care approach* (7th ed., pp. 690–706). St. Louis, MO: Elsevier.

Wain, H., Kong, V., Bruce, J., Laing, G., & Clarke, D. (2019). Analysis of surgical adverse events at a major university hospital in South Africa. *World Journal of Surgery, 43*(9), 2117–2122. https://dx.doi.org/10.1007/s00268-019-05008-9

Weiser, T., Haynes, A., Molina, G., Lipsitz, S., Esquivel, M., Uribe-Leitz, T., & Gawande, A. (2016). Size and distribution of the global volume of surgery in 2012. *Bulletin of the World Health Organization, 94,* 201. https://dx.dxi.org/10.2471/BLT.15.159293

Wilner, W. (2018). Care of the obstetric and gynecologic surgical patient. In J. Odom-Forren (Ed.), *Drain's perianesthesia nursing: a critical care approach* (7th ed., pp. 624–636). St. Louis: Elsevier.

Wright, S. (2018). Assessment and management of the airway. In J. Odom-Forren (Ed.), *Drain's perianesthesia nursing: a critical care approach* (7th ed., pp. 417–430). St. Louis, MO: Elsevier.

FURTHER READING

Edwin, N., & Hicks, L. (2019). Pharmacogenetics of postoperative nausea and vomiting. *Journal of Perianesthesia Nursing, 34*(6), 1088–1105. https://dx.doi.org/10.1016/j.jopan.2019.03.007

Foran, P. (2020). ECG for all patients in the PACU: some say why? I say why not? *Journal of Perioperative Nursing, 33*(2), e26–28. https://dx.doi.org/10.26550/2209-1092.1087

Granum, M., Kaasby, K., Skou, S., & Grønkjær, M. (2019). Preventing inadvertent hypothermia in patients undergoing major spinal surgery: a nonrandomized controlled study of two different methods of preoperative and intraoperative warming, *Journal of Perianesthesia Nursing, 34*(5), 999–1005. https://dx.doi.org/10.1016/j.jopan.2019.03.004

Gurka, M., Filipp, S., & DeBoer, M. (2018). Geographical variation in the prevalence of obesity, metabolic syndrome, and diabetes among US adults. *Nutrition and Diabetes, 8*(1), 1–8. Retrieved from <https://www.researchgate.net/publication/323881600>. https://dx.doi.org/10.1038/s41387-018-0024-2

Harper, N. J. N., Cook, T. M., Garcez, T., Farmer, L., Floss, K., Marinho, S., . . . Macguire, N. (2018). Anaesthesia, surgery, and life-threatening allergic reactions: epidemiology and clinical features of perioperative anaphylaxis in the 6th National Audit Project (NAP6). *British Journal of Anaesthesia, 121*(1), 159–171. https://dx.doi.org/10.1016/j.bja.2018.04.014

Kellett, J., & Sebat, F. (2017). Make vital signs great again – a call for action. *European Journal of Internal Medicine, 45*, 13–19. Retrieved from <https://pubmed.ncbi.nlm.nih.gov/28941841/>. https://dx.doi.org/10.1016/j.ejim.2017.09.018

Malignant Hyperthermia Group, Australia & New Zealand (MH ANZ). (2018). Malignant hyperthermia resource kit. Retrieved from <http://malignanthyperthermia.org.au/wp-content/uploads/2018/09/MALIGNANT-HYPERTHERMIA-RESOURCE-KIT-2018.pdf>.

Wardhan, R., & Chelly, J. (2017). Recent advances in acute pain management: understanding the mechanisms of acute pain, the prescription of opioids, and the role of multimodal pain therapy. *F1000Research, 6*, 2065. https://dx.doi.org/10.12688/f1000research.12286.1.

CHAPTER 13

Perioperative Practice in Non-traditional Environments

BRIGID M. GILLESPIE • SALLY SUTHERLAND-FRASER • MENNA DAVIES
• BEN LOCKWOOD
EDITOR: BRIGID M. GILLESPIE

LEARNING OUTCOMES

- Identify and describe issues in relation to perioperative practice in rural and remote settings
- Discuss cultural safety and cultural competence in relation to perioperative practice in non-traditional environments such as rural and remote areas
- Outline considerations that perioperative nurses need to be aware of when practising in humanitarian and military contexts
- Discuss the differences between extended practice and advanced practice roles applied to the perioperative context
- Discuss different aspects of the nurse educator and nurse researcher roles

KEY TERMS

cultural safety

disaster zones

extended and advanced practice roles

humanitarian settings

humanitarian work

military settings

nurse researchers

perioperative nurse educators

rural and remote settings

INTRODUCTION

The traditional operating room (OR) suite is no longer the primary site for surgical interventions or diagnostic procedures, and a range of hospital departments, as well as freestanding facilities, are now well established 'perioperative environments'. Perioperative practice extends beyond these now commonplace, conventional clinical environments. Perioperative nurses practise in rural and remote areas within Australia and New Zealand. They also provide humanitarian assistance and serve in the armed forces, delivering clinical care to patients and their military colleagues when required. Non-traditional perioperative roles are also enacted in extended and advanced practice specialties, including educating and training the next generation of perioperative nurses as clinical educators and researchers. While the context of practice is vastly different from the traditional 'metropolitan' settings with which many of us are familiar, the principles of perioperative care remain unchanged.

In this final chapter, we consider how the principles of perioperative care outlined in earlier chapters can be applied in non-traditional settings. Throughout the chapter, we provide a patient scenario based on one of the case studies used throughout the book, include snippets of research and pose questions to provoke critical thinking in context. The chapter is divided into three major sections. We will discuss perioperative practice relative to: (i) **rural and remote settings**, (ii) **humanitarian settings** and **military settings**, and (iii) the context of **extended and advanced practice**, education and research roles.

Consider the scenario below as you read this chapter. Revisit this scenario and critical thinking questions posed throughout the chapter based on your knowledge, experience and new understandings you develop through reading this chapter.

PATIENT SCENARIOS

SCENARIO 13.1: CULTURAL SAFETY AND CULTURAL COMPETENCE

Mrs Patricia Peterson, a 42-year-old Indigenous woman, has returned home to her rural community after having an emergency laparoscopic cholecystectomy in a regional hospital. Mrs Peterson's full history and a brief description of the healthcare setting is provided in the Introduction to this book for readers to review when answering the questions in this unfolding scenario.

Mrs Peterson attends a follow-up appointment at her local hospital outpatients department with registered nurse (RN) Anne Fuller, who assesses her in relation to her postoperative recovery. During this appointment, RN Fuller focuses on providing Mrs Peterson with postoperative education on wound incision care, diet, exercise and resuming daily activates.

During the consultation, RN Fuller asks Mrs Peterson a series of questions about her postoperative recovery including operative site care, diabetes care and medications management.

Critical Thinking Questions

Consider some of the potential questions RN Fuller might ask Mrs Peterson during her visit to the outpatients clinic.

- What strategies could RN Fuller use to promote cultural safety in this situation?
- How would RN Fuller know that Mrs Peterson understands the information given to her in relation to postoperative education?

RURAL AND REMOTE SETTINGS

It is important to develop policies aimed at meeting the needs of various groups within the community and to identify ways to remove the barriers for accessing healthcare, such as differing concepts of health and illness. These may be culturally based and so affect the understanding of causation, treatment and impact of compliance. Indigenous people, socioeconomically disadvantaged people and those living in rural and remote areas are groups of special interest because of their high incidence of health problems compared with the remainder of the population (Australian Department of Health Authority [ADHA], 2013; Australian Institute of Health and Welfare [AIHW], 2018; New Zealand Ministry of Health [NZMH], 2014a). Further, many Indigenous Australians and New Zealanders have other unique issues related to accessing healthcare (AIHW, 2018; NZMH, 2014a). Communication and language barriers, together with the remoteness of some communities, additionally hinder access to allied health or pharmaceutical treatment regimens. The failure to fully meet these health needs contravenes the National Guidelines (Australian Commission on Safety and Quality in Health Care [ACSQHC/the Commission], 2019), which address the requirement for equitable access for all consumers.

Despite the increase in the implementation of telehealth initiatives in rural and remote Indigenous communities (Robinson, 2018), not all Australians have equal access to elective surgery (or other interventions). Similarly, Māori and Pacific Islander peoples in New Zealand have greater unmet healthcare needs. These are explored in Feature box 13.1.

Cultural Safety and Awareness

In Chapters 1 and 7, you were first introduced to the concept of 'cultural safety', which is founded on participation, protection and partnership between patients and their healthcare providers (Richardson & Williams, 2007). A key premise of **cultural safety** is the recognition of the uniqueness of the individual and knowing that each person carries their cultural identity. Hence, culturally competent healthcare providers respect patients' health beliefs, understand the biophysical context in which patients experience illness and work in partnership to plan care (Chun, Deptula, Morihara, & Jackson, 2014). This involves designing healthcare services that are responsive to the needs of different patient populations. Feature box 13.2 provides an example of cultural safety in the context of Indigenous health.

FEATURE BOX 13.1
Indigenous, Māori and Pacific Islander Peoples: Rates of Surgical Interventions

Indigenous Australians have a lower rate of access to procedures compared with non-Indigenous Australians with the same condition (ADHA, 2013). Additionally, they spend more time on the waiting list before accessing surgery compared with other Australians. This is for most performed procedures but is particularly marked for cataract extraction and total knee replacement surgeries. For the latter procedure, 23% of Indigenous patients waited more than a year for surgery (AIHW, 2013), which is twice the rate for non-Indigenous Australians.

In New Zealand, Māori and Pacific Islanders report higher levels of unmet need for healthcare, although increased access to elective surgery and concomitant reduction in waiting times has been reported (NZMH, 2014a). However, limited participation was reported in a bowel cancer screening pilot study being conducted in the Waitemata District Health Board region.

In both countries, these outcomes are deemed to be the result of low literacy rates and environmental barriers (failure to receive testing kits) (ADHA, 2013; NZMH, 2014b, 2014c).

FEATURE BOX 13.2
Cultural Safety – Cultural Circumcision

Cultural safety should be at the forefront of a female nurse's mind when conducting a preoperative assessment on an Aboriginal male patient about to have a cultural circumcision. If a male nurse is unavailable in the first instance, then the female nurse should always ask the patient or escort if it is acceptable for them to be conducting the assessment because in some Aboriginal cultures it is inappropriate for women to be involved in 'men's business'. If the patient declines to be assessed by a female, then a male perioperative nurse or Aboriginal Health Practitioner should be sought to complete the assessment.

Rhiannon Robinson RN, BN Grad Cert.Periop, Katherine, Northern Territory

FEATURE BOX 13.3
'The Bus' – New Zealand's Novel Approach to Providing Surgical Services to Rural Communities

The MHS unit, colloquially referred to as 'The Bus', travels through the rural communities of both islands, making more than 25 stops during a 5-week cycle. On arrival at one of these designated stops, 'The Bus', which has a well-equipped operating room (OR), is located close to a medical centre or hospital so that power can be sourced from the host facility (although back-up generators are on board the bus, if required). Medical and nursing staff are sourced locally, and are organised in advance by MHS staff.

Patient access to this service is the same as in bigger population centres – via general practitioner (GP) referral to specialist surgeon/proceduralist and subsequent inclusion on a waiting list. In due course, pre-booked procedures are organised with the patient. Over 300 types of procedures are provided across the following specialties:

- general surgery
- gynaecology
- orthopaedic
- dental surgery
- plastic surgery
- endoscopy.

A key feature of this service is to provide educational opportunities to rural health professionals. Initially focused on skills training for nurses to support them working in the OR and recovery areas, this program has developed to provide a wider range of education sessions to ensure that rural health professionals maintain their individual professional competencies.

(Source: Mobile Health Solutions. (2019). *Day surgery for rural NZ.* https://mobilehealth.co.nz/.)

New Zealand has developed a novel way of providing ambulatory care to rural patients following the closure of many small local hospitals. Mobile Health Solutions (MHS) is a privately owned company which works in partnership with the Ministry of Health, District Health Boards and other health providers to deliver perioperative services to the doorstep of 25 rural communities. MHS aims to provide effective, efficient surgical care with a patient-centred focus which eliminates the need for patients to travel great distances for their procedures and keeps them close to their support networks. Since the inception of this service 20 years ago, over 25,800 elective day surgery procedures have been completed (MHS, 2019). This is approach highlighted in Feature box 13.3.

Multiculturalism and Cultural Diversity in the Workplace

So far in this chapter, we have covered aspects of cultural safety and diversity that apply to at-risk populations in rural and remote areas. Multiculturalism has become the norm in the healthcare workforce in many developed countries, mostly because of immigration (Australian College of Perioperative Nurses, 2020;

Clayton, Isaacs, & Ellender, 2016). However, how is cultural diversity managed in the workplace? The perioperative environment is characterised by technology, clinical efficiency and interdisciplinary teamwork (Gillespie et al., 2018). Therefore, communication is pivotal and even more so when working with other disciplines as part of the perioperative team. Further, when team members belong to different multicultural backgrounds, each with their own unique style, background and training, there is a potential for breakdowns in communication (Clayton et al., 2016). Research box 13.1 summarises the findings of a qualitative study that described perioperative nurses' experiences in a multicultural work setting.

The scope for perioperative nurses to practise in various clinical roles across diverse contexts and cultures is boundless. As you progress through this chapter, you will undoubtedly appreciate the importance of being culturally aware when practising in rural, remote and humanitarian contexts. Feature box 13.4 presents a narrative based on one perioperative nurse's personal journey while working in an under-resourced and isolated region of the world.

RESEARCH BOX 13.1
Perioperative Nurses' Experiences Working in a Multicultural Work Setting

Clayton and colleagues (2014) conducted an interpretive phenomenological study to explore the lived experiences of perioperative nurses in a multicultural operating room suite in Melbourne.

Fourteen nurses working in different perioperative roles were interviewed.

Thematic findings revealed three themes that described difficulties in communication in relation to patient care, working atmosphere, and social integration.

The authors concluded that catering to the needs of patients from linguistically diverse backgrounds is a challenge. Developing strategies to improve communication and building camaraderie may improve communications.

(Source: Clayton, J., Isaacs, A. N., & Ellender, I. (2016). Perioperative nurses' experiences of communication in a multicultural operating theatre: a qualitative study. *International Journal of Nursing Studies*, 54, 7–15. https://dx.doi.org/10.1016/j.ijnurstu.2014.02.014.)

FEATURE BOX 13.4
Perioperative Nursing in Pacific Island Countries, a Personal Journey

My first visit to the Solomon Islands (SI) was in 2010. I travelled from Sydney with two nursing colleagues – my manager and another colleague from the emergency department (ED). We were invited by the SI government to undertake an external review of the nursing services in the ED and operating rooms (ORs).

At the time, I knew very little about the Pacific and could not accurately name or place many of the neighbouring islands. I searched the internet for a map to get my bearings. I also searched for information about the experiences of the outsider.

I was acutely aware of my ignorance. As a perioperative nurse, I was confident as a district clinical nurse consultant, with 20 plus years of experience as a perioperative nurse clinician and educator. My ignorance related to the context of this assignment: How much did I know about the SI people, their language and culture? What did I know about SI history and politics? What could I expect of the SI economy, especially in relation to healthcare expenditure and health outcomes? What standards of nursing care could I expect to observe in SI? Was I already making judgements based on experiences from my career working within a highly regarded and well-resourced health system and living in a wealthy country? My searches led me to

colleagues who had worked in the Pacific region; they reinforced the importance of asking such questions prior to leaving Australian shores.

However, my real learning only started when I was 'in-country', listening to the SI nurses, observing them in their workplace and spending my days with them as they attended to their patients and daily routines. The broad judgements I might once have made about the SI nurses' standards and their practices were now more reliably informed by my direct observations. These observations shaped my burgeoning understanding of SI culture and values.

The limitations of an ageing infrastructure and lack of equipment and resources were factors beyond the SI nurses' control. Each day, these limitations defined the context and boundaries of care and influenced teams' performance. Yet, even in such circumstances, where standards, infrastructure or resources fell short of those in my own workplace, I could not fault the hands-on care and nurturing that the SI nurses showed for each patient.

In the decade since this formative experience with SI nurses, I have continued to learn about healthcare delivery and nursing practice in Pacific Island Countries (PICs) as an independent consultant. I have sought out opportunities to return as an educator and advisor and have been fortunate

FEATURE BOX 13.4
Perioperative Nursing in Pacific Island Countries, a Personal Journey—cont'd

to work as a volunteer with perioperative colleagues, travelling to Vanuatu and SI through organisations such as Orthopaedic Outreach and the Royal Australasian College of Surgeons (RACS) Pacific Island Programs (PIP). I have also been fortunate to collaborate with colleagues and Pacific-based organisations, notably the Pacific Community, on a wide range of educational endeavours related to perioperative nursing, with the benefit of further travel to many more PICs. This ongoing collaboration includes perioperative managers and clinical nurses from 14 nations stretching almost 8000 kilometres across the Pacific Ocean.

With the support of the Australian College of Perioperative Nurses (ACORN), this collaboration produced the first Pacific standards for perioperative nursing and a matching set of observational tools to audit the nurses' compliance with the standards (Davies et al., 2017; Davies, Sutherland-Fraser,

Taoi, & Williams, 2016). The development of these standards and tools was informed by the cultural beliefs and values of PIC peoples. They reflect the best practices for working within resource-limited PICs.

From the foundations of cultural safety and practice development (Brockback & McGill, 2006; ICN, 2013; Shah, Nodell, Montano, Behrens, & Zundt, 2011), I worked one-on-one with perioperative nurses, once again 'in-country', to develop a local mentor program for PICs (Sutherland-Fraser, 2018). A growing sense of self-determination and collective identity has enabled the PIC nurses to establish the Pacific Island Operating Room Nurses Association (PI-ORNA) and strengthen their autonomy (see more information about this in Chapter 1).

Sally Sutherland-Fraser, RN, MEd, FACORN, MNSWOTA, MACN

PATIENT SCENARIOS

SCENARIO 13.2: CULTURAL COMPETENCE

Critical Thinking Questions

- Do perioperative nurses have the time to be culturally competent and manage diversity? Provide a rationale for your answer.
- What contextual factors in rural and remote settings help and/or hinder cultural competence?

Rural Perioperative Team Training Programs in Rural and Remote Areas

Rural and remote healthcare facilities face additional challenges in recruiting and retaining nurses. Financial constraints limit the ability of small facilities to compete with their urban-based counterparts, which offer more-flexible working hours and continuing education and upskilling opportunities. Shortages of qualified perioperative nurses, anaesthetists and surgeons in these small rural and remote communities affects patients' access to safe and sustainable healthcare services. Perioperative nurses practising in these locations are also required to be 'generalists', practising safely across a broad range of skill sets and varied medical and surgical specialties with limited access to education and training. The Department of Health in Queensland prioritised the need to provide perioperative nurses working in rural and remote areas with additional training. Feature box 13.5 describes this initiative, which has been implemented since 2017.

FEATURE BOX 13.5
Rural Perioperative Team Training Program

PROGRAM AIM

The *Rural Perioperative Team Training Program* is a multifaceted, multidisciplinary team training program that has been developed to support clinicians to deliver and maintain safe, sustainable service delivery in rural and remote Queensland.

The scenario-based education and training program consists of technical and non-technical skills with a focus on team communication.

PROGRAM BENEFITS

The Rural Perioperative Team Training Program aims to promote:

- improved patient safety/patient outcomes
- improved performance
- better understanding and appreciation of individual roles and responsibilities
- improved communication and culture
- improved staff satisfaction
- delivery of high-quality healthcare.

(Source: Centre of Clinical Excellence. (2019). Rural Perioperative Team Training Program. https://clinicalexcellence.qld.gov.au/improvement-exchange/rural-perioperative-team-training-program.)

HUMANITARIAN AND MILITARY SETTINGS AND THE IMPACT OF PANDEMICS
Humanitarian Work and Natural Disasters

The Centre for Research on the Epidemiology of Disasters defines a disaster as *'a situation or event that overwhelms local capacity, necessitating a request at the national or international level for external assistance; an unforeseen and often sudden event that causes great damage, destruction and human suffering'* (Guha-Sapir, Hoyois, & Below, 2016, p. 103). These events can be either natural or manmade, the former caused by cyclones, earthquakes or floods, while the latter are caused by deliberate human action or negligence (e.g. armed conflicts, industrial and nuclear incidents, fires) (Centurion, Crestani, Dominguez, Caluwaerts, & Benedetti, 2018). All inhabited areas around the world are vulnerable to natural disasters, but the toll on victims varies depending on disaster preparedness and development in each country. Low- and middle-income countries (LMICs) are especially exposed to the negative impacts of such natural events.

LMICs have limited resources to manage natural disasters (Haverkamp et al., 2018; Merchant et al., 2015). The lack of human and material resources because of geographical isolation, a chronically fragile healthcare system and political instability reduces their ability to recover in the aftermath of a natural disaster (Centurion et al., 2018; Haverkamp et al., 2018). In the aftermath, the population needs swell, placing more pressure on already fractured infrastructures.

The burden of injuries is immense; hence the availability of prompt and qualified surgical care is critical (Centurion et al., 2018). The concentration of unmet need is highest in LMICs. The poorest third of the world population represents only around 4% of all performed surgical procedures (Meara et al., 2015; Rose et al., 2015). As such, providing surgical care after a natural disaster becomes more critical because the usual burden of surgical and obstetric conditions is added to the need to provide urgent surgical care (Centurion et al., 2018).

For nearly 50 years, international non-governmental, non-profit and humanitarian medical organisations such as the International Red Cross and Médecins Sans Frontières (also known as 'Doctors Without Borders') have provided surgical care to vulnerable populations (Centurion et al., 2018; Haverkamp et al., 2018). Surgical care in the aftermath of natural disasters in LMICs is often provided by international medical teams assembled for a specified period (Merchant et al., 2015). International teams of surgeons, anaesthetists, instrument nurses and ward nurses are deployed for specific periods of time. The surgical team may not have been exposed to certain procedures (not undertaken in their daily practice), situations or conditions but their skills are transferrable to the context. There will also invariably be differences in the availability of certain drugs, biomedical equipment and devices, and other resources and consumables that surgical teams may ordinarily take for granted (Centurion et al., 2018). Other contextual factors that surgical teams have to manage every day are the variation in water quality and quantity, unreliable electricity, inadequate waste disposal resources, infection prevention and control measures, the disposal of corpses and climatic conditions of such austere environments (Centurion et al., 2018; Haverkamp et al., 2018). Feature box 13.6 illustrates one perioperative nurse's reflections on working as a volunteer in a developing country.

Preparation is essential and team members require between 2 and 5 years of clinical experience in their disciplines/field (Haverkamp et al., 2018). Prior to deployment, these surgical teams participate in disaster preparedness programs including advanced trauma life support training. Research box 13.2 highlights the results of a survey of healthcare professionals who have been deployed in **disaster zones**.

Undertaking volunteer work in developing countries requires thorough preparation from a cultural, physical and psychological perspective. While having some knowledge about the cultural context is essential, it is often impossible for perioperative nurse volunteers to have comprehensive knowledge of what to expect if they have not had any previous experience working in resource-limited contexts. Feature box 13.7 describes the experience of a seasoned perioperative nurse (and volunteer) during her deployment to the Philippines with the Australian Medical Assistant Team (AusMAT) (Rogers, 2016). AusMAT teams are self-sufficient, multidisciplinary units comprising doctors, nurses, paramedics, firefighters, pharmacists, radiographers and environmental health workers from around Australia and New Zealand.

The challenges that prevail in **humanitarian work** are similar to those faced by surgical teams in the armed forces, perhaps with the exception of the threat of gunfire and the brutality of injuries treated, which in war zones can be more horrific and confronting (Agazio, 2010).

Military Settings

Over the past 80 to 100 years, the focus of military health services in the Australian and New Zealand

FEATURE BOX 13.6
Working as a Volunteer

BRIEFING FOR VOLUNTEERS

Stepping outside your comfort zone can be an enjoyable and rewarding experience, and if the opportunity arises, I recommend that you consider working as a volunteer in a developing country.

If you are considering working as a volunteer, ensure you are well prepared before you travel. All volunteers will have a pre-trip health check and will need to update their immunisations that are appropriate to the destination (e.g. malaria prophylaxis). It is advisable to take your own scrubs and theatre shoes.

Many medical and volunteer organisations in Australia provide international volunteer health services to developing countries. Most volunteer organisations will cover airfares and accommodation; you will volunteer your time and expertise. The following skills and experiences are desirable:

* relevant professional experience and expertise
* teamwork, tolerance and cross-cultural understanding
* management and organisational development skills
* willingness and ability to train others
* ability to cope with stressful and challenging situations
* ability to work with limited clinical resources
* experience leading a team
* flexibility to adapt to rapid changes in circumstances
* experience travelling overseas, especially in developing countries.

There are many contextual nuances in cross-cultural healthcare. It is important to respect the people and community you are working with, to be flexible and to be willing to change your goals to suit the situation on the ground. Ensure that you observe local customs and strive to build successful working relationships and friendships with your hosts.

Do not panic if things do not happen quickly. In most developing countries, the lifestyle is at a much more leisurely pace. Many patients will travel for kilometres to see the surgical team, and are happy to sit and wait without complaint.

If possible, have a family member or an interpreter present when the patient is being consented for procedures. Some patients will want to please and, as a sign of respect, will readily nod indicating they understand. But, often, patients will not have understood the information. Also, they may not be able to comply with post-operative treatments because of cultural or religious beliefs.

Be mindful that equipment is a precious commodity, so avoid making modifications. Check that all necessary equipment is present and working before starting a case. The availability of instruments varies, but they are generally old and fatigued. Most organisations will supply enough consumables required for each trip. Confirm prior to departure that arrangements are made for the return of equipment taken with the team; do not spontaneously donate equipment.

The wards are usually very busy, so it is essential to liaise with host medical teams before treatment decisions are made for complex cases. Many hospitals do not have high-dependency or intensive care units. There are limited pathology services available, and some hospitals have no blood donation services; if blood is required, a relative will donate.

We take so much for granted working in our everyday clinical contexts with ready access to equipment and resources. Working as a volunteer in a developing country makes you appreciate what you may otherwise take for granted working in a state-of-the-art operating room facility.

Lesley Stewart, RN, RM, CPON, FACORN

RESEARCH BOX 13.2
Preparedness for Deployment to Disaster Zones

Haverkamp and colleagues (2018) conducted a cross-sectional survey of 284 healthcare professionals who had been deployed to disaster zones to provide surgical care.

Survey items included questions related to pre-deployment training, deployment experiences, self-perceived preparedness and the personal impact of deployment. Survey items used a response scale of '1 very unprepared' to '5 more than sufficient'.

'The survey response rate was 54% (153/284). Respondents rated their self-perceived preparedness as 4/5 (more than sufficient), and for paediatric trauma, 3/5.

Higher rates of self-perceived preparedness were found in respondents who had previously been deployed, or who had attended at least one master class ($p < 0.05$). Additional training was requested most frequently for paediatrics (65/150), fracture surgery (46/150) and burns treatment (45/150). Over 75% of respondents identified the need for debriefing with colleagues.

Study authors concluded that participants perceived that they were sufficiently prepared for deployment.

(Source: Haverkamp, F. J. C., Veen, H., Hoencamp, R., Muhrbeck, M., von Schreb, J., Wladis, A., & Tan, E. (2018). Prepared for mission? A survey of medical personnel training needs within the International Committee of the Red Cross. *World Journal of Surgery, 42*(11), 3493–3500. https://dx.doi.org/10.1007/s00268-018-4651-5.)

FEATURE BOX 13.7
AusMAT Deployment to Tacloban

OPERATION PHILIPPINES

In November 2013, the Philippines was struck by Typhoon Haiyan, killing 6193 people and injuring around 28,000 others. The Philippines government had requested medical assistance to help cope with the high numbers of casualties.

I received a call asking whether I was available for deployment. After the work I had done in establishing our surgical unit and disaster training, I was keen to contribute to this effort.

Two days following our arrival in Tacloban, the Philippines, we set up our base in an airfield and opened our hospital, known as Camp Kookaburra. Most of our patients sustained injuries because of the typhoon. These wounds included fractures and soft-tissue injuries.

Initially, few patients presented for surgery, fearing that their limbs would be amputated. But, once patients were aware that the team's focus was on saving their limbs, our field hospital was inundated! We performed 17 to 20 cases per day and were responsible for sterilising and processing equipment. We often did not finish our day's work until well into the night.

Resources were limited and improvising became the 'new normal'. While we had a good inventory of surgical instruments, the numbers of consumables we were able to travel with was limited. Despite the shortage of resources, we never compromised patient care.

We made clinical and resource decisions based on the needs of each individual case.

Although we performed surgeries in a tent, we adhered to the same clinical and ethical principles as we would if practising at home. During our 4-week deployment, our dedicated team:

- treated 2735 patient presentations
- performed 238 operations
- managed 541 occupied bed days
- coordinated 60 patient transfers
- witnessed 9 deaths
- delivered 3 babies.

Our patients were truly amazing; despite losing everything including family members, they had such high praise for our medical team. If given the opportunity, I would do it again in a heartbeat.

(Source: Paraphrased by Brigid Gillespie based on Rogers, W. (2016). AusMAT deployment to Tacloban. *Journal of Perioperative Nursing*, *29*(2), 38–41.)

---

defence forces has been to prepare for combat (Australian Defence Force [ADF], 2020; Sheard, Huntington, & Gilmour, 2020). However, federal government agencies in both Australia and New Zealand now require the ADF and New Zealand Defence Force (NZDF) to be equipped and trained for peacekeeping and humanitarian assistance, as well as for war. This shift in focus has been driven by global political changes, including the changes in governments' strategic intent (ADF, 2020). Indeed, supporting those who have been affected by disaster – whether natural or manmade – is essential to preserving peace, security and stability in today's world (Rivers & Gordon, 2017). Military nursing officers serving in the air force, the army and the navy have had a long and proud history of providing support and aid during and following disasters.

Military nursing officers work in a variety of environments, and carry out roles not only as civilian RNs, but also as military officers (Blaz, Woodson, & Sheehy, 2013; Rivers & Gordon, 2017). An important role that a military nursing officer undertakes is as a member of multidisciplinary, and often international, trauma/resuscitation/surgical teams. These teams play a vital role in the delivery of frontline care to members of their military, allied

defence force personnel and civilians during times of conflict, disaster and humanitarian situations (Conlon, Wiechula, & Garlick, 2019). Australia's military nurses practise in hostile, remote and dangerous environments, for often-unspecified periods in war-torn regions of Southeast Asia (e.g. East Timor, Bali, Afghanistan) (Conlon et al., 2019). They are tasked with the burden of undertaking their military duties alongside ensuring the safety of their patients, themselves and their medical equipment when deployed in areas of conflict (Agazio, 2010; Dierkes, 2011). When deployed, military nurses often endure harsh conditions, being forced to 'improvise' owing to a lack of medical equipment, resources and supplies (Agazio, 2010). Research box 13.3 provides a glimpse into the experiences of military nursing officers from the Australian perspective.

Clearly, austere environments pose significant challenges for the nurses who must work in those settings. In the field, military nurses must find ways to mitigate the effects of equipment failures and the often-limited electric power; dust, sand, and other environmental contaminants; patient transport limitations; and continued threats of direct and indirect fire (Blaz et al., 2013; Rivers & Gordon, 2017). In both humanitarian and wartime

---

RESEARCH BOX 13.3
The Lived Experiences of Military Nursing Officers

A hermeneutical phenomenological study by Conlon and colleagues (2019) aimed to gain an in-depth understanding of the lived experiences of nursing officers when deployed as members of military trauma teams.

This study, undertaken in Australia, used in-depth interviews with six nurse participants who were serving as commissioned officers in the ADF. Thematic analysis was used to analyse the textual data and identify common themes.

Through the analysis, the following themes emerged: telling their stories; the role – who we are and what we do; the environment – it is so different; training – will it ever fully prepare you; working in teams – there's no 'I' in team; and leadership – will the real leader please stand up!

The study authors concluded that the experiences described by these Australian military nurses are rarely voiced outside of military circles. Participants often experienced tension between their dual roles as nurses and defence force officers. Unlike their civilian counterparts, these nursing officers could not go home at the end of their shifts.

(Source: Conlon, L., Wiechula, R., & Garlick, A. (2019). Hermeneutic phenomenological study of military nursing officers. *Nursing Research, 68*(4), 267–274.)

FEATURE BOX 13.8
One Nurse's Journey in the Australian Defence Force

Registered Nurse Sharon Bown spent 16 years in the Royal Australian Air Force (RAAF) as a nursing officer.

During her RAAF service, she was deployed on three tours of duty. Sharon served in East Timor and Afghanistan, and was commander of the RAAF Base Townsville Health Centre from 2008 to 2011. She was also the commander of the surgical/critical care team deployed in Afghanistan in 2008.

As a nursing officer, Sharon was exposed to myriad situations not experienced in civilian life: from teaching East Timorese orphans to learn English, to attending to wounded coalition soldiers choppered from the Afghan desert into her surgical unit.

Sharon was critically injured in a near-fatal helicopter crash in East Timor and sustained serious physical injuries including a spinal injury, fuel burns and a shattered jaw. Despite these serious injuries, Sharon fought her way back to health to command an RAAF health unit in Afghanistan.

While Sharon's military service was distinguished and inspirational, it came at the cost of her mental and physical health. Sharon developed post-traumatic stress disorder and, in 2015, was discharged from the RAAF on medical grounds, having been deemed unfit to continue military service (Bown, 2016).

Since leaving the ADF, Sharon has been appointed to a high-profile role on the council of the Australian War Memorial. She is also undertaking a Bachelor of Psychological Science degree, pursuing her interest in exploring the effects of military service.

(Source: Bown, S. (2016). *One woman's war and peace: a nurse's journey in the Royal Australian Air Force*. Sydney: Exilse Publishing.)

---

missions, military nurses often assume greater responsibilities, performing more autonomously while caring for highly complex patients with polytrauma injuries (Agazio, 2010). The negative impacts of witnessing human suffering during deployment have an indelible impact on the military nurses whose role it is to provide support (Rivers & Gordon, 2017). In some cases, such experiences can trigger long-lasting psychological distress. Feature box 13.8 highlights one young nurse's journey as an officer in the ADF.

The Impact of Pandemics

A pandemic is defined as the 'worldwide spread of a new disease' (World Health Organization [WHO], 2010). Pandemics such as a COVID-19 (a novel coronavirus) have had unprecedented and profound impacts on the way we live and work. For perioperative nurses working on the frontline, this pandemic has not only altered the ways in which they deliver clinical care but has also meant that many have had to be redeployed into other frontline roles – for instance, PACU nurses having to be upskilled and/or retrained to practise in ICU settings.

Pandemic Response in Perioperative Services

During a pandemic, such as the global health emergency caused by SARS-CoV2 and COVID-19, healthcare services need to have robust strategies to manage patient care, ensure staff safety and guarantee that material resource supply chains are adequate (Brethauer et al., 2020; Krishnamoorthy et al., 2020; Wong et al., 2020a, 2020b).

To facilitate access to critical and intensive care beds in healthcare services for the increased patient influx caused by a pandemic, a state of emergency may be declared; this may be administrated by local government, police or military services. The impact on perioperative services is a reduction or cessation of non-essential (elective) surgery and a requirement to perform only urgent or critical emergency surgery. This frees capacity in critical and intensive care beds, with access potentially required to recovery units for overflow of ventilated patients (De Simone et al., 2020; Krishnamoorthy, Bartz & Raghunathan, 2020; Wong et al., 2020a).

Pandemics involving respiratory infection (such as COVID-19) may require specialised techniques for aerosol-generating procedures (AGPs) such as intubation, ventilation, extubation, high-speed drilling, and oral and thoracic surgery (Meng et al., 2020; Wong et al., 2020b). This often necessitates a rapid change of practice involving intensive staff consultation, review, training and simulation to ensure effective patient care and staff safety. Clinical spaces where AGPs occur may require negative-pressure air flow, which may demand air conditioning and engineering work. Such containment measures and changes to work flows reduce the risk of transmission to staff and patients (Wong et al., 2020b).

A major consideration during a pandemic is the supply of personal protective equipment (PPE) and hand hygiene products. As seen during the COVID-19 pandemic, global shortages of PPE and essential products caused many critical services to make do, with suboptimal practices such as extended mask usage, recycling of PPE and inadequate hand hygiene facilities, which may have contributed to the burden of the pandemic (National Institute for Occupational Safety and Health [NIOSH], 2020; WHO 2020). Healthcare services and the manufacturing supply chains that support them need to ensure that adequate supply is maintained via judicious resource management strategies.

Undoubtedly, pandemic responses affect all aspects of healthcare, particularly emergency, critical care and perioperative services. Adequate preparation involves consideration of many different areas, controls and phases of the pandemic, and in perioperative services the interests and safety of staff and patients are paramount.

PERIOPERATIVE ROLES IN EXTENDED AND ADVANCED PRACTICE, EDUCATION AND RESEARCH

Extended and Advanced Practice Roles

The Nursing and Midwifery Board of Australia (NMBA) (2018) defines advanced practice as a *'continuum along which nurses develop their professional knowledge, judgement and skills to a higher level of capability (or demonstrated)'* (https://www.nursingmidwiferyboard.gov.au/Codes-Guidelines-Statements/FAQ/fact-sheet-advanced-nursing-practice-and-specialty-areas.aspx). Practising at an advanced level means that nurses are practising at their

'top of license' – that is, to the boundaries of their scope of practice (Duff, 2019). However, advanced practice should not be confused with the nurse practitioner role, which is governed by legislation and government regulations. Arguably, the lack of clarity in the definition of scope of practice itself has made it challenging to describe and operationalise what scope of practice includes for nurses working at an advanced practice level (Birks, Davis, Smithson, & Cant, 2016).

The NMBA defines scope of practice as *'the full spectrum of roles, functions, responsibilities, activities and decision-making capacity that individuals within that profession are educated, competent and authorised to perform'* (https://www.nursingmidwiferyboard.gov.au/Codes-Guidelines-Statements/Frameworks.aspx) (NMBA, 2019). Historically, factors that have shaped nurses' scope of practice include the local context, the needs of their patients, their level of education and competence, and policy requirements (Birks et al., 2016). As such, scope of practice is not clearly delineated, and needs to be assessed based on the individual context, on a case-by-case basis (Duff, 2019). However, the boundaries between scope of advanced practice and extended practice are sometimes blurred, and often debatable (Birks et al., 2016).

In Australia, extended (or expanded) scope of practice for RNs is embedded in the nurse practitioner role, underpinned by an established regulatory safety framework (Australian Nursing and Midwifery Federation [ANMF], 2019). Thus extended practice includes expertise beyond what is currently recognised by the nursing profession (Duff, 2019). An example of an extended practice is the registered nurse endoscopist role (as described in Chapter 1). RNs wanting to extend their scope of practice need to follow the nurse practitioner pathway to endorsement regulated by the NMBA. However, given the minimal national regulation of extended and advanced practice roles in Australia, identifying elements that enable nurses to be utilised at optimum capacity is important for understanding factors that enable them to take up extended practice roles. Research box 13.4 presents the result of a national survey describing the barriers and enablers to role extension.

Clearly, organisational context contributes to shaping nurses' scope of practice, but it is also important to recognise the impact that global trends have had on shaping and redefining perioperative roles. Over the past few decades, in countries such as the UK and the US, there has been a steady rise in the number of non-nursing personnel in the OR (Gillespie & Pearson, 2013) – for instance, non-nursing personnel working in instrument and anaesthetic assistant roles. Following

> **RESEARCH BOX 13.4**
> **Barriers and Enablers to Nursing Role Expansion: a Cross-sectional Survey**
>
> A national survey of nurses was conducted by Birks and colleagues (2019) to describe the barriers and enablers to RNs extending their scope of practice. The sampling frame included nurses who were members of peak professional organisations, and the survey was administered electronically via email and social media.
>
> Of the 1874 surveys that were returned, 1205 (64.3%) were useable as they provided responses to at least 80% of the questions.
>
> Nurse respondents reported that poor professional and organisational support, role ambiguity, a lack of remuneration and a lack of clear guidelines were barriers to role extension.
>
> Enablers to role expansion reported by respondents included professional satisfaction, potential for career advancement and the desire to meet the healthcare organisation's needs.
>
> The authors concluded that professional and regulatory bodies, health educators, healthcare organisations and employers all play an important role in extension of nursing scope beyond geographical or social need.

(Source: Birks, M., Davis, J., Smithson, J., & Lindsay, D. (2019). Enablers and barriers to registered nurses expanding their scope of practice in Australia: a cross-sectional study. *Policy, Politics, and Nursing Practice*, *20*(3), 145–152. https://dx.doi.org/10.1177/1527154419864176.)

> **RESEARCH BOX 13.5**
> **Enacting the Role of the Non-medical Surgical Assistant, a Literature Review**
>
> Hains, Strand and Turner (2017) undertook a narrative literature review to describe differences in how the role of the non-medical surgical assistant (NMSA) is defined and enacted across the US, Canada, the UK and New Zealand. These countries were comparable to the Australian context because they shared similar standards in relation to clinical practice and healthcare.
>
> Review methods included systematic database searches using search terms, including the grey literature. Another source of information for this review involved contacting NMSAs, using snowball-sampling methods to identify additional contacts from the US, Canada, the UK and New Zealand.
>
> The findings of the review suggested that, across these four countries, the term NMSA was synonymous with other terms such as first surgical assistant, registered nurse first assistant, perioperative nurse surgeon's assistant and nurse practitioner, depending on the country and its regulatory requirements.
>
> In addition, the ways in which these roles were enacted across these countries differed in relation to education requirements and having a standardised curriculum, title protection, national regulation, assessment and diagnostics, the ability to order investigations and prescribing rights.
>
> These authors concluded that the role of NMSA requires education at Master's level, a standardised curriculum and national regulation – all of which are essential for autonomous practice (Hains et al., 2017).

(Source: Hains, T., Strand, H., & Turner, C. (2017). A selected international appraisal of the role of the non-medical surgical assistant. *Journal of Perioperative Nursing, 30*(2), 37–42.)

this trend, healthcare organisations in both the public and private sectors around Australia have increasingly included anaesthetic technicians to support the anaesthetist. Clearly, we must ensure a continued nursing presence in the OR (Gillespie & Pearson, 2013) but, rather than lament role erosion, we should be focusing on developing and embracing emerging perioperative roles. The challenge for the perioperative specialty in moving forward is to develop a standardised nomenclature and curriculum to better enable implementation of these extended roles. In Research box 13.5, the results of a literature review that described the ways the first surgical assistant role was operationalised across countries are presented.

In Australia, the role of the perioperative nurse surgical assistant (PNSA) was first introduced in 2001 (Brennan, 2001). Most PNSAs work in the private sector; however, perioperative nurses with PNSA qualifications but without nurse practitioner qualifications are unable to access the Medical Benefits Schedule (MBS). Hence they are not eligible to get a Medicare provider number to claim against procedure item numbers (Smith, Hains, & Mannion, 2016). This is important for perioperative nurses who practise in these extended roles in the private sector, where MBS item numbers are used to bill patients for procedures (Yang & Hains, 2017).

Undoubtedly, organisational context drives changes in nursing roles and scope of practice (Smith et al., 2016). A case in point illustrates perfectly the need to provide a service. Senior nurses at the Sunshine Coast Private Hospital (SCPH) explored the potential for using PNSA-qualified perioperative nurses for public lists undertaken at the SCPH (Smith et al., 2016). Reasons identified for deciding to use PNSAs for public operating lists on the private campus included the following:

- uncertainty related to staffing of medical registrars and residents to provide support for operating lists

- previous positive experiences with PNSAs in the private sector
- support from surgeons who had previous experience working with PNSAs
- differences in remuneration between private and public sectors.

The introduction of the PNSA role at the SCPH facility was evaluated following the trial period: surgeons and perioperative nurses were surveyed about their experience in working with the PNSAs (Smith et al., 2016). The results of the staff surveys indicated that PNSAs were perceived as being skilled, knowledgeable, helpful and supportive. Role extension offers new and exciting possibilities for perioperative registered nurses wanting a challenge that is rewarding, both professionally and personally. Feature box 13.9 details one nurse's journey to becoming a nurse practitioner.

FEATURE BOX 13.9
One Nurses' Journey to Becoming a Nurse Practitioner

Nurse practitioner and current Chief Executive Officer of the Australian College of Perioperative Nurses, Rebecca East, reflects on her journey to becoming a nurse practitioner (NP).

In 2011, Rebecca commenced studies in a Graduate Certificate program as a perioperative student through Deakin University. Rebecca enjoyed the week-long introductory program so much that she then enrolled in a Graduate Diploma of Perioperative Nursing. Rebecca had been inspired to continue her studies and complete her Master's in perioperative nursing: *'My passion grew as my love for the perioperative world blossomed.'*

After several conversations with colleagues, Rebecca applied to undertake another Master of Nursing program as an NP. After 2 years of study and juggling the commitments of family life, Rebecca had successfully completed her Master's NP qualification.

She is currently practising in Victoria at the Bendigo Orthopaedic and Sports Medicine Clinic, and works across a variety of roles, ranging from preoperative education to providing intraoperative assistance to undertaking postoperative reviews. She also acts as a primary referrer to other specialties, triages referrals and coordinates the everyday running of the clinic.

Importantly, as an NP, Rebecca can provide care that traverses the patient's care continuum.

(Source: East, R. (2015). Becoming a perioperative nurse practitioner: my journey. *Journal of Perioperative Nursing, 28*(3), 49.)

Perioperative Education – Past, Present and the Virtual Future

In Australia, hospital-based general nursing training programs prevailed until the mid 1980s. These certificate level programs required nursing students to undertake 4–6 weeks of 'on-the-job' clinical practice in the perioperative environment. This clinical exposure to the OR inspired many nurses to follow a perioperative career after completing their three- or four-year general nursing certificate.

However, following the gradual transfer of preregistration nurse education to the tertiary sector, starting in the late 1980s, perioperative nursing was viewed by many universities as a specialised area, and therefore of limited value in a generalist, undergraduate program. This led to a dramatic decrease in the numbers of nursing students exposed to the perioperative environment. Perioperative nursing leaders across the state and national associations expressed concerns about the continuation of a nursing presence in the OR: without nursing students having clinical exposure to the specialty during their Bachelor's program, the recruitment of future generations of perioperative nurses was in jeopardy. It was clear that giving undergraduate nursing students the opportunity to witness surgical procedures provides students with valuable experience to develop their surgical nursing practice and aseptic technique, and would provide them with other transferable nursing skills and knowledge.

Across many of the states of Australia, perioperative associations and senior perioperative clinicians lobbied at both government and tertiary levels for the inclusion of a perioperative clinical practicum in the undergraduate program. Their determination and tenacity paid off, with undergraduate clinical perioperative experience being re-instated in many Bachelor of Nursing curricula around the country. The recruitment of **perioperative nurse educators** was key to the success of clinical placements in perioperative departments. To cater (once again) for nursing student placements in the OR, it was vital that hospitals assemble education teams to provide undergraduate nursing students with structured learning experiences. In addition to providing undergraduate students with clinical placements, many hospitals have developed new graduate transition-to-practice programs, providing novice perioperative nurses with an opportunity to segue into postgraduate studies.

The role of a nurse educator and/or clinical nurse educator brings with it great responsibility. Educators are role models and must have current knowledge of clinical practice and professional standards and policies, and be able to develop contemporary resources that extend perioperative nursing students' critical thinking skills. In addition, they require patience, good communication and unwavering discipline to maintain their own standards of practice, and must be above reproach, always 'doing the right thing'. Perioperative nurse educators must sometimes manage instances of poor practice, which increases the potential for conflict with fellow staff members. Assertiveness combined with evidence-based knowledge is required to resolve these situations.

The clinical area is only one environment where educators practise. The tertiary sector provides perioperative nurses with the opportunity to develop clinical and theoretical programs at undergraduate and postgraduate levels, pursue research and assist in shaping the next generation of perioperative nurses. Some perioperative nurses have conjoint appointments, giving them 'the best of both worlds' – a foot in the clinical area with a local hospital combined with an academic appointment.

The virtual classroom and innovative simulation environments are technological advances that have revolutionised the way in which healthcare professionals, including perioperative nurses, are educated. The opportunity to practise key technical and non-technical skills using simulation, in particular teamwork with the whole surgical team, have become powerful tools in reducing the risks of adverse events or patients. Feature box 13.10 outlines the history of the first perioperative nursing course delivered in distance mode.

Perioperative Nurse Researchers

Perhaps research is not the first alternative role many perioperative nurses would consider as a career path. **Nurse researchers** identify research questions in collaboration with clinicians and health consumers, design and conduct scientific studies, collect and analyse data, supervise and mentor research students, and disseminate their findings. Nurse researchers collaborate with experts in other healthcare disciplines such as medicine, nutrition, pharmacy, psychology and beyond to engineering, human factors and science, to name a few. These collaborations are important to better address vexing research questions of clinical importance and relevance to health consumers.

Much of what we do in perioperative nursing is still based on practices that are steeped in history and tradition rather than being based on robust evidence (Duff, 2020). While clinical care that is founded on evidence-based practice is the gold standard, many practices in the OR do not reflect this. Even when evidence is available, it is not always applied in practice (Duff, 2020).

FEATURE BOX 13.10
Perioperative Education – From a Distance

In 1991, the NSW College of Nursing (now the Australian College of Nursing) took the bold step of conducting the first postgraduate perioperative nursing course by distance learning. Despite the success of face-to-face perioperative courses conducted in many large metropolitan hospitals, the NSW Operating Theatre Association voiced concerns that perioperative nurses working in rural areas were missing opportunities to study their specialty. For nurses in rural areas to complete a course, it meant leaving home, work and family to study in Sydney. While many did so, it was challenging, and the College met that challenge.

The College, under the leadership of Executive Director, Judith Cornell, an eminent perioperative nurse who was instrumental in the formation of ACORN, took up the challenge of developing a program that could be completed through distance learning. It was an ambitious plan and was met with a great deal of scepticism: many perioperative nurses did not believe that such a practical specialty could be delivered through distance mode. The course was presented using printed course materials. Virtual classroom streaming, videos and online courses, common today, were still some years away, and email communication was not always available for the students in isolated rural areas.

The course, funded through the NSW Health Department, was a great success, particularly with the target audience of rural perioperative nurses. Feedback from students who completed the early course offerings was highly positive. Many students said that it had transformed their practice and their lives in general, giving many their first experience of study since their initial general nurse's training. These courses also inspired many perioperative nursing students to continue tertiary studies.

Word of the success of the first courses spread to other states/territories and soon fee-paying students from across Australia enrolled. From these early print-heavy courses, the course has been refined many times in conjunction with students, who are now enjoying the benefits of all that technology can offer with a fully online course. The course is seen as the forerunner of similar postgraduate courses now offered by many universities across Australia.

Menna Davies MHlth Sc, RN, FACORN
Perioperative Course Coordinator,
NSW College of Nursing, 1990–2000

As long ago as 2008, in a letter to the Editor of the *Journal of Perioperative Nursing*, Gillespie and Hamlin identified the need for perioperative nurses to generate new knowledge to advance their specialty to improve and build on current practice. Unfortunately, not a lot has

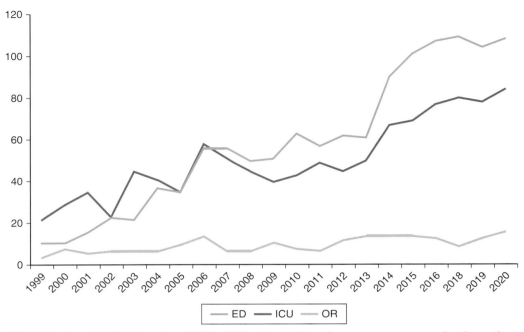

FIG. 13.1 Annual publications from 1999 to 2020 related to intensive care, emergency and perioperative nursing, represented by the green line (labelled as 'OR'). (Source: Duff, J. (2020). The imperative to build research capacity and promote evidence-based practice in Australian perioperative nurses. *Journal of Perioperative Nursing*, *33*(2), e1–e11. https://dx.doi.org/10.26550/2209-1092.1086.)

changed in the intervening years since the publication of that letter. Crucially, compared with other specialties such as intensive care and emergency nursing, perioperative nursing is lagging in terms of research generation and dissemination (Duff, 2020). Fig. 13.1 shows, from the past 20 years, the numbers of annual publications per year over of perioperative nursing compared with other high-acuity specialties of emergency and intensive care nursing.

So, why would perioperative nurses want to pursue a research career? Perioperative nurse researchers are uniquely positioned to influence the thinking (and practices) of other perioperative nurses. Nurse researchers often travel and live in places they have never been to before, collaborate with stellar researchers from other backgrounds and cultures, and mentor the next generation of nurse researchers. Strengthening research capacity in our specialty will help to build a strong evidence base to demonstrate 'what we do and why it is beneficial' to patients (Duff, 2020). In doing so as nurse researchers, we contribute to maintaining a continued nursing presence in the OR.

What is the career path to becoming a nurse researcher? The career path begins with a keen interest in nursing research. Completing studies in research at

either undergraduate Honours or postgraduate Master's level gives budding researchers the beginning skills to undertake a small, discrete research project. Successful completion of a research degree may even lead to enrolment in a PhD or professional doctorate. If you are interested in pursuing a research career, seek out some successful perioperative nurse researchers who have trodden this path. They will be able to offer some sage advice in how to go about this.

CONCLUSION

In this chapter, we have discussed key considerations around working in rural and remote settings in relation to cultural safety and cultural competence. We have briefly explored what it means to work in a multicultural workforce and have identified some of the challenges of practising in humanitarian and military settings. We have also described the profound changes to perioperative health services delivery. Finally, we have discussed advanced and extended practice, nurse education and nurse researcher roles. We hope that this chapter has inspired you as a perioperative nurse to consider working in non-traditional environments and roles. The nurses' experiences you have read in the chapter feature boxes demonstrate that there are many diverse and rewarding career pathways for the perioperative nurse. The only limits are those you impose on yourself.

ACKNOWLEDGEMENTS

We acknowledge the contributions of Dr Lois Hamlin and Lyn Rapley, who were co-authors of Chapter 13 in the second edition of this textbook.

RESOURCES

The following list is an example of the many professional organisations and charities which provide perioperative nurses with opportunities to work or volunteer in healthcare services of low- and middle-income countries (LMICs):
Australian College of Perioperative Nursing (ACORN)
https://www.acorn.org.au/grants – awards-and-scholarships
Australian Defence Force (ADF)
https://www.defencejobs.gov.au/jobs/reserves/air-force/nurse
Australian Volunteers
https://www.australianvolunteers.com/about-us/
Interplast
https://www.interplast.org.au/get-involved/work-or-volunteer-with-us/
Mercy Ships Australia
https://mercyships.org.au/volunteer/
Royal Australasian College of Surgeons (RACS) Global Health
https://www.surgeons.org/for-the-public/racs-global-health/

REFERENCES

Agazio, J. (2010). Army nursing practice challenges in humanitarian and wartime missions. *International Journal of Nursing Practice, 16*(2), 166–175. https://dx.doi.org/10.1111/j.1440-172X.2010.01826.x

Australian College of Perioperative Nurses (ACORN). (2020). *ACORN standards for perioperative nursing in Australia* (16th ed., Vol. 2). Cultural diversity. Adelaide: Author.

Australian Commission on Saftey and Quality in Health Care (ACSQHC/the Commission). (2019). *AS18/04: Advice on the applicability of Aboriginal and Torres Strait Islander specific actions*. Sydney: Author. Retrieved from <https://www.safetyandquality.gov.au/sites/default/files/2020-05/Advisory%20AS1804%20-%20Advice%20on%20the%20applicability%20of%20Aboriginal%20and%20Torres%20Strait%20Islander%20specific%20actions.pdf>.

Australian Defence Force. (2020). Capability. Retrieved from <https://news.defence.gov.au/capability>.

Australian Department of Health Authority (ADHA). (2013). National Aboriginal and Torres Strait Islander health plan 2013–2023. Retrieved from <https://www1.health.gov.au/internet/main/publishing.nsf/content/B92E980680486C3BCA257BF0001BAF01/$File/health-plan.pdf>.

Australian Institute of Health and Welfare (AIHW). (2013). *Australian hospital statistics, 2012–13. Elective surgery waiting times.* Retrieved from <www.aihw.gov.au/publication-detail/?id = 60129544692>.

Australian Institute of Health and Welfare (AIHW). (2018). *Australia's health 2018.* Australia's health series no. 16. AUS 221. Canberra: Author. Retrieved from <https://www.aihw.gov.au/reports/australias-health/australias-health-2018/contents/table-of-contents>.

Australian Nursing and Midwifery Federation (ANMF). (2019). Is it advanced or expanded practice? Retrieved from <https://www.anmf.org.au/pages/professionaljuly- 2014>.

Birks, M., Davis, J., Smithson, J., & Cant, R. (2016). Registered nurse scope of practice in Australia: an integrative review of the literature. *Contemorary Nurse, 52*(5), 522–543.

Birks, M., Davis, J., Smithson, J., & Lindsay, D. (2019). Enablers and barriers to registered nurses expanding their scope of practice in Australia: a cross-sectional study. *Policy, Politics, & Nursing Practice, 20*(3), 145–152. https://dx.doi.org/10.1177/1527154419864176

Blaz, D. A., Woodson, J., & Sheehy, S. (2013). The emerging role of combat nursing: The ultimate emergency nursing challenge. *Journal of Emergency Nursing, 39*(6), 602–609. https://dx.doi.org/10.1016/j.jen.2013.09.001

Bown, S. (2016). *One woman's war and peace: a nurse's journey in the Royal Australian Air Force.* Sydney: Exilse Publishing.

Brennan, B. (2001). The registered nurse as a first surgical assistant: the 'downunder' experience. *Seminars in Perioperative Nursing, 10*(2), 108–114.

Brethauer, S. A., Poulose, B. K., Needleman, B. J., Sims, C., Arnold, M., Washburn, K., … Pawlik, T. M. (2020). Redesigning a department of surgery during the COVID-19 pandemic. *Journal of Gastrointestinal Surgery, 24*(8), 1852-1859. doi:10.1007/s11605-020-04608-4.

Brockbank, A., & McGill, I. (2006). *Facilitating reflective learning through mentoring and coaching.* London: Kogan Page Ltd.

Centre of Clinical Excellence. (2019). Rural Perioperative Team Training Program. Retrieved from <https://clinicalexcellence.qld.gov.au/improvement-exchange/rural-perioperative-team-training-program>.

Centurion, M. T., Crestani, R., Dominguez, L., Caluwaerts, A., & Benedetti, G. (2018). Surgery with limited resources in natural disasters: what is the minimum standard of care? *Current Trauma Reports, 4*(2), 89–95.

Chun, M. B., Deptula, P., Morihara, S., & Jackson, D. S. (2014). The refinement of a cultural standardized patient examination for a general surgery residency program. *Journal of Surgical Education, 71*(3), 398–404. https://dx.doi.org/10.1016/j.jsurg.2013.10.005

Clayton, J., Isaacs, A. N., & Ellender, I. (2016). Perioperative nurses' experiences of communication in a multicultural operating theatre: a qualitative study. *International Journal of Nursing Studies, 54*, 7–15. https://dx.doi.org/10.1016/j.ijnurstu.2014.02.014

Conlon, L., Wiechula, R., & Garlick, A. (2019). Hermeneutic phenomenological study of military nursing officers. *Nursing Research, 68*(4), 267–274.

Davies, M., Sutherland-Fraser, S., Taoi, M.H. & Williams, C. (2016). Developing standards in Pacific Island countries: the Pacific perioperative practice bundle (Part 1). [online]. *Journal of Perioperative Nursing in Australia, 29*(2), 42–47.

Davies, M., Sutherland-Fraser, S., Mamea, N., Raddie, N., & Taoi, M.H. (2017). Implementing standards in Pacific Island countries: the Pacific perioperative practice bundle (Part 2). [online]. *Journal of Perioperative Nursing in Australia, 30*(1), 41–48.

De Simone, B., Chouillard, E., Di Saverio, S., Pagani, L., Sartelli, M., Biffl, W. L., … Catena, F. (2020). Emergency surgery during the COVID-19 pandemic: what you need to know for practice. *Annals of the Royal College of Surgeons of England, 102*(5), 323–332. https://dx.doi.org/10.1308/rcsann.2020.0097

Dierkes, D. (2011). Deployment to Afghanistan: perioperative nursing outside the comfort zone. *AORN Journal, 94*(3), 271–278. https://dx.doi.org/10.1016/j.aorn.2011.01.015

Duff, J. (2019). See one, do one, teach one: advanced perioperative nursing practice in Australia. *Journal of Perioperative Nursing, 32*(4), 3.

Duff, J. (2020). The imperative to build research capacity and promote evidence-based practice in Australian perioperative nurses. *Journal of Perioperative Nursing, 33*(2), e1–e11. https://dx.doi.org/https://doi.org/10.26550/2209-1092.1086

East, R. (2015). Becoming a perioperative nurse practitioner: my journey. *Journal of Perioperative Nursing, 28*(3), 49.

Gillespie, B., & Hamlin, L. (2008). Where to publish – the impact factor. *Journal of Perioperative Nursing, 21*(4), 5–6.

Gillespie, B., & Pearson, E. (2013). Perceptions of self-competence in theatre nurses and operating department practitioners. *Journal of Perioperative Nursing, 26*(1), 29–34.

Gillespie, B. M., Harbeck, E. L., Lavin, J., Hamilton, K., Gardiner, T., Withers, T. K., & Marshall, A. P. (2018). Evaluation of a patient safety programme on Surgical Safety Checklist Compliance: a prospective longitudinal study. *BMJ Open Quality, 7*(3), e000362. https://dx.doi.org/10.1136/bmjoq-2018-000362

Guha-Sapir, D., Hoyois, P., & Below, R. (2016). Annual disaster statistical review 2015: the numbers and trends. Retrieved from <http://www.cred.be/sites/default/files/ADSR_2015.pdf>.

Hains, T., Strand, H., & Turner, C. (2017). A selected international appraisal of the role of the non-medical surgical assistant. *Journal of Perioperative Nursing, 30*(2), 37–42.

Haverkamp, F. J. C., Veen, H., Hoencamp, R., Muhrbeck, M., von Schreeb, J., Wladis, A., & Tan, E. (2018). Prepared for mission? A survey of medical personnel training needs within the International Committee of the Red Cross. *World Journal of Surgery, 42*(11), 3493–3500. https://dx.doi.org/10.1007/s00268-018-4651-5

International Council of Nurses (ICN). (2013). Position statement: cultural and linguistic competence. ICN: Geneva. Retrieved from <https://www.icn.ch/nursing-policy/position-statements>

Krishnamoorthy, V., Bartz, R., & Raghunathan, K. (2020). Rational perioperative utilisation and management during the COVID-19 pandemic. *British Journal of Anaesthesia, 125*(2), e248–e251. https://dx.doi.org/10.1016/j.bja

Meara, J. G., Leather, A. J., Hagander, L., Alkire, B. C., Alonso, N., Ameh, E. A., . . . Yip, W. (2015). Global surgery 2030: evidence and solutions for achieving health, welfare, and economic development. *Lancet, 386*(9993), 569–624. https://dx.doi.org/10.1016/s0140-6736(15)60160-x

Meng, L., Qiu, H., Wan, L., Ai, Y., Xue, Z., Guo, Q., … Xiong, L. (2020). Intubation and ventilation amid the COVID-19 outbreak: Wuhan's experience. *Anesthesiology, 132*(6), 1317–1332. https://dx.doi.org/10.1097/ALN.0000000000003296

Merchant, A., Hendel, S., Shockley, R., Schlesinger, J., Vansell, H., & McQueen, K. (2015). Evaluating progress in the global surgical crisis: contrasting access to emergency and essential surgery and safe anesthesia around the world. *World Journal of Surgery, 39*, 2630–2635.

Mobile Health Solutions (MHS). (2019). *Day surgery for rural NZ.* Retrieved from <https://mobilehealth.co.nz/>.

National Institute for Occupational Safety and Health (NIOSH). (2020). The physiological burden of prolonged PPE use on healthcare workers during long shifts [science blog]. Retrieved from <https://blogs.cdc.gov/niosh-science-blog/2020/06/10/ppe-burden/>.

New Zealand Ministry of Health (NZMW). (2014a). Annual report for the year ended 30 June 2014. Retrieved from <http://www.health.govt.nz/publication/annual-report-year-ended-30-june-2014>.

New Zealand Ministry of Health (NZMW). (2014b). Evaluation of the bowel screening pilot follow-up provider survey. Retrieved from <https://www.health.govt.nzfinal-followup-bsp-provider-survey-150414>.

New Zealand Ministry of Health (NZMW). (2014c). Revised draft evaluation of the bowel screening pilot 2013 immersion visit. Retrieved from <https://www.health.govt.nzbps-immersion-visit-report150414>.

Nursing and Midwifery Board of Australia (NMBA). (2018). Fact sheet: Advanced nursing practice and specialty areas within nursing. Retrieved from <https://www.nursingmidwifery-board.gov.au/Codes-Guidelines-Statements/FAQ/fact-sheet-advanced-nursing-practice-and-specialty-areas.aspx>.

Nursing and Midwifery Board of Australia (NMBA). (2019). Decision-making framework. Retrieved from <https://www.nursingmidwiferyboard.gov.au/Codes-Guidelines-Statements/FAQ/fact-sheet-advanced-nursing-practice-and-specialty-areas.aspx>.

Richardson, S., & Williams, T. (2007). Why is cultural safety essential in health care? *Medicine & Law, 26*(4), 699–707. Retrieved from <https://www.ncbi.nlm.nih.gov/pubmed/18284111>.

Rivers, F., & Gordon, S. (2017). Military nurse deployments: similarities, differences, and resulting issues. *Nursing Outlook, 65*(Suppl. 5), S100–S108. https://dx.doi.org/10.1016/j.outlook.2017.07.006

Robinson, R. (2018). The evolution of perioperative telehealth in Katherine, Northern Territory, Australia. *Journal of Perioperative Nursing, 31*(3), 47.

Rogers, W. (2016). AusMAT deployment to Tacloban. *Journal of Perioperative Nursing, 29*(2), 38–41.

Rose, J., Weiser, T., Hider, P., Wilson, L., Gruen, R., & Bickler, S. (2015). Estimated need for surgery worldwide based on prevalence of diseases: a modelling strategy for the WHO Global Health Estimate. *Lancet, 3*(S2), S13–S20.

Shah, S.K., Nodell, B., Montano, S.M., Behrens, C., & Zundt, J.R. (2011). Clinical research and global health: Mentoring the next generation of health care students. *Global Public Health*, 6(3), 234–246. https://dx.doi.org/10.1080/174416 92.2010.49424

Sheard, M., Huntington, A., & Gilmour, J. (2020). Nursing services in the New Zealand Defence Force: a review after 100 years. *Journal of Military and Veterans' Health*, 24(1), 6–11. Retrieved from <https://jmvh.org/article/nursing-services-in-the-new-zealand-defence-force-a-review-after-100-years/>.

Smith, C., Hains, T., & Mannion, N. (2016). An opportunity taken: Sunshine Coast University Private Hospital's perioperative nurse surgeon's assistant experience. *Journal of Perioperative Nursing*, 29(3), 23.

Sutherland-Fraser, S. (2018). Transforming practice through mentoring: a coming of age case study (unpublished conference paper). Inaugural ACORN / ASIORNA International Conference, Adelaide, May 2018.

Wong, J., Goh, Q. Y., Tan, Z., Lie, S. A., Tay, Y. C., Ng, S. Y., & Soh, C. R. (2020a). Preparing for a COVID-19 pandemic: a review of operating room outbreak response measures in a large tertiary hospital in Singapore. *Canadian Journal of Anaesthesia*, 67(6), 732–745. https://dx.doi.org/10.1007/s12630-020-01620-9.

Wong, W. Y, Kong, Y. C, See, J. J., Kan, R. K. C., Lim, M. P. P., Chen, Q., … Ong, S. (2020b). Anaesthetic management of patients with COVID-19: infection prevention and control measures in the operating theatre. *British Journal of Anaesthesia*, 125(2), e239-e241. https://dx.doi.org/10.1016/j.bja.2020.04.014.

World Health Organization (WHO). (2010). What is a pandemic? Retrieved from <https://www.who.int/csr/disease/swineflu/frequently_asked_questions/pandemic/en/>.

World Health Organization (WHO). (2020). Shortage of personal protective equipment endangering health workers worldwide. Retrieved from <https://www.who.int/news/item/03-03-2020-shortage-of-personal-protective-equipment-endangering-health-workers-worldwide>.

Yang, L., & Hains, T. (2017). The plight of the perioperative nurse practitioner in Australia. *Australian Nursing and Midwifery Journal*, 24(10), 36.

FURTHER READING

Blaz, D. A., Woodson, J., & Sheehy, S. (2013). The emerging role of combat nursing: the ultimate emergency nursing challenge. *Journal of Emergency Nursing*, 39(6), 602–609. https://dx.doi.org/10.1016/j.jen.2013.09.001

Boutonnet, M., Pasquier, P., Raynaud, L., Vitiello, L., Bancarel, J., Coste, S., . . . Ausset, S. (2017). Ten years of en route critical care training. *Air Medical Journal*, 36(2), 62–66. https://dx.doi.org/10.1016/j.amj.2016.12.004

Cai, Y. L., Ju, J. T., Liu, W. B., Zhang, J. (2018). Military trauma and surgical procedures in conflict area: a review for the utilization of forward surgical team. *Military Medical*, 183(3–4), e97–e106. https://dx.doi.org/10.1093/milmed/usx048

Centurion, M. T., Crestani, R., Dominguez, L., Caluwaerts, A., & Benedetti, G. (2018). Surgery with limited resources in natural disasters: what is the minimum standard of care? *Current Trauma Reports*, 4(2), 89–95. https://dx.doi.org/10.1007/s40719-018-0124-4

Robinson, R. (2018). The evolution of perioperative telehealth in Katherine, Northern Territory, Australia. *Journal of Perioperative Nursing*, 31(3), 47. Retrieved from <https://search.informit.com.au/documentSummary;dn=9444980 70647959;res=IELHEA>.

Glossary

Ablation Amputation, excision of any part of the body or removal of a growth or harmful substance.

Accountability Nurses and midwives must be prepared to answer to others, such as healthcare consumers, the relevant national nursing and midwifery regulatory authority, their employer and the public for their decisions, actions and behaviours, and the responsibilities that are inherent in their roles. Accountability cannot be delegated. Registered nurses or midwives who delegate an activity to another person are accountable not only for the delegation decision, but also for monitoring the standard of performance of the activity by the other person and for evaluating the outcomes of the delegation.

Accreditation Public recognition by a healthcare accreditation body of the achievement of accreditation standards by a healthcare organisation, demonstrated through an independent external peer assessment of that organisation's level of performance in relation to the standards.

Advance health directive (AHD) Also known as a living will, a document that expresses a patient's preferences regarding end-of-life issues. An AHD becomes effective only when an individual loses the capacity to make those choices themselves.

Adverse event An incident in which unintended harm results to a person receiving healthcare.

Advocacy Speaking or intervening on behalf of another. Nurses act as patients' advocates when the latter are unable to do so owing to their physical or mental condition.

Air handling Refers collectively to the systems and processes within Australian healthcare facilities which control air flow, air filtration, pressure gradients and ventilation, as well as air conditioning, temperature and humidity. The term appears in the Australian Health Facilities Guidelines.

Ambulatory procedures/care Also known as day surgery. Usually refers to the care of patients on a day-only basis. However, it also encompasses extended day-only (EDO) and other variously titled, high-volume, short-stay (HVSS) models of care (MOC).

Anaerobic Absence of oxygen.

Anaesthetic assistant A member of the perioperative team who assists the anaesthetist in the anaesthetic management of the patient. The assistant may be a nurse or a technician who must be educated and competent in the range of anaesthetic procedures carried out within the local healthcare facility in order to provide safe and effective support to both the anaesthetist and the patient.

Analgesia Absence of pain in response to a stimulus that would normally produce pain.

Angiography Injection of contrast medium into an artery and subsequent radiological examination; used to determine the patency of an artery and collateral circulation.

Angioplasty Reconstitution or recanalisation of a blood vessel; may involve balloon dilation, mechanical stripping of intima, forceful injection of fibrinolytics or placement of a stent.

Apnoea Complete absence of breathing.

Arrhythmia Any deviation other than the normal pattern of the heartbeat.

Asepsis Absence of pathogenic microorganisms on living tissue.

Aseptic field Refers to the area around the surgical site that has been prepared by cleansing with an antimicrobial agent and draping, separating it from the rest of the patient's body. The aseptic field also includes all furniture covered with drapes, such as the instrument table and the surgical team who are gowned and gloved.

Aseptic technique Any healthcare procedure in which added precautions are taken to prevent contamination of a patient, an object or an area by microorganisms. See also *standard aseptic technique* and *surgical aseptic technique*.

Atraumatic Pertaining to therapies or therapeutic instruments and devices (e.g. needles) that are unlikely to cause tissue damage.

Autonomy The ethical principle of self-determination and independence.

Basic life support (BLS) Emergency treatment of a victim of cardiac or respiratory arrest through cardiopulmonary resuscitation and emergency cardiac care.

Bougie A long, thin flexible rod that can be passed through an endotracheal tube (ETT) to enable the tube to be moulded to a shape that can be guided through the laryngeal opening.

Bradycardia A pulse rate less than 50 beats per minute.

Bronchospasm An excessive and prolonged contraction of the smooth muscle of the bronchi and bronchioles, resulting in acute narrowing and obstruction of the respiratory airway. Contractions may be localised or general and may be caused by irritation (e.g. secretions, airway equipment or pulmonary aspiration) or injury to the respiratory mucosa, infections, allergies, drug hypersensitivity or the rapid introduction of volatile anaesthetic agents. Bronchospasm is the chief characteristic of asthma and bronchitis, and is managed by increasing the level of inhalational anaesthesia, bronchodilators (e.g. salbutamol) and other drugs (e.g. steroids, ketamine or adrenaline) or by repositioning the endotracheal tube in anaesthetised patients.

Capnography Graphical representation of expired carbon dioxide (CO_2), often termed end-tidal CO_2. An adaptor placed in the breathing circuit during general anaesthesia collects CO_2, which is then analysed and displayed as a waveform on a monitor. Measurement assists in early detection of technical catastrophes (e.g. oesophageal intubation) or changes in the patient's respiratory, circulatory or metabolic condition.

Cardiac arrest The cessation of cardiac mechanical activity with the absence of a detectable pulse, unresponsiveness and apnoea (or agonal respirations).

Cardiac catheterisation Insertion of a catheter into a large vein or artery (in the arm or leg), which, in the case of venous cannulation, is then directed into the superior vena cava and the right atrium, or following arterial cannulation is threaded into the proximal aorta and left ventricle. As the catheter tip passes through the chambers and vessels of the heart, the blood pressure is monitored and blood samples may be taken. Injection of contrast medium aids in examination of cardiac structures and heart motion. The procedure accurately identifies congenital heart disease, tricuspid stenosis and valvular incompetence.

Cardioversion The attempt to restore the heart's normal sinus rhythm via an electric shock delivered by a defibrillator either internally or externally. Application of the shock is synchronised to the QRS complex.

Central nerve block Administration of local anaesthetic drugs into the subarachnoid or epidural space, which blocks nerves as they exit the spinal cord and causes large areas of the lower body to lose sensation (hence, the term *block*).

CICO A term used in anaesthetic practice which stands for 'can't intubate, can't oxygenate'. It is a term used to describe a failure to deliver oxygen as a result of upper airway obstruction (at or above the immediate subglottic region) which persists despite all reasonable airway rescue manoeuvres at or above this level, termed 'supraglottic rescue'.

Clinical decision making The cognitive processes and strategies that nurses use when utilising data to make clinical decisions regarding patient assessment and care.

Clinical governance This is the main vehicle by which healthcare organisations are held accountable for ensuring high standards of healthcare (including dealing with poor professional performance), for continuously improving the quality of their services, and for creating and maintaining an environment in which clinical excellence can flourish.

Clinical pathway A document outlining a standardised, evidence-based, multidisciplinary and cost-effective management plan that identifies an appropriate sequence of clinical interventions, associated timelines and milestones, and expected outcomes for a homogeneous patient group.

Clinical practice guidelines (CPGs) Statements and patient care recommendations based on the best available evidence (e.g. systematic reviews) for specific clinical circumstances that assist practitioners in their day-to-day practice. Clinical practice guidelines provide a basis for the evaluation of care and the allocation of resources.

Closed wound suction Any of several techniques for draining potentially harmful fluids (e.g. blood, pus, serosanguineous fluid or tissue secretions) from surgical wounds. Postoperative drainage aids the healing process by removing dead space and helping to draw healing tissues together. Closed wound suction devices usually consist of disposable transparent containers attached to suction tubes and portable suction pumps.

Coagulopathy A pathological condition that affects the ability of the blood to coagulate.

Code of conduct A collection of standards and rules of behaviour.

Code of rights In New Zealand, the Health and Disability Commissioner Act 1994 and subsequent amendment incorporate the code of health and disability services consumers' rights (Code of Rights), which is wide and extends to any person or organisation providing a health service to the public. The code of rights also covers all health professionals and one of its obligations is to take reasonable action in the circumstances to give effect to the rights and comply with the duties.

Cognitive impairment Deficiency in the ability to think, perceive, reason or remember that may result in the loss of ability to attend to one's activities of daily living.

Compartment syndrome A pathological condition caused by the progressive development of arterial compression and consequent reduction of blood supply to the extremities. Clinical manifestations include swelling, restriction of movement, brown urine, myoglobinuria, vascular compromise and severe pain or lack of sensation. Treatment includes elevation, removal of restrictive dressings or casts and, potentially, surgical decompression (often in the form of a fasciotomy, to relieve the pressure).

Competence Combination of skills, knowledge, attitudes, values and abilities that underpins effective and/or superior performance in a profession/occupational area.

Complementary therapies Treatments not considered part of mainstream Western medicine and that are generally used as an adjunct to standard medical treatments. These include massage, relaxation techniques, osteopathy, acupuncture, chiropractic, aromatherapy, meditation and naturopathy. Complementary and mainstream medicine combined is known as *integrative medicine*.

Compliant Refers to the ease with which lungs can be inflated; compliant lungs are more readily inflated than incompliant lungs.

Computed tomography (CT) An imaging procedure that makes use of computer-processed combinations of many X-ray images taken from different angles to produce cross-sectional (tomographic) images (virtual 'slices') of specific areas of a scanned object, enabling the user to see inside the object without cutting it.

Confidentiality The non-disclosure of information about a person unless consented to by that person, or an authorised person, or under statutory authority or in the public interest under strict conditions. Preserving confidentiality of patient information is a primary duty of healthcare professionals and is included in codes of ethics and health legislation.

Conscious sedation A drug-induced depression of consciousness during which patients are able to respond purposefully to verbal commands or light tactile stimulation. Conscious sedation can be achieved by a wide variety of drugs including propofol and may accompany local anaesthesia. All conscious sedation techniques should provide a margin of safety that is wide enough to render loss of consciousness unlikely.

Core temperature The temperature of the deep structures of the body, such as the liver.

Cricoid pressure *See Sellick's manoeuvre.*

Cultural safety The provision of effective healthcare to persons of dissimilar cultures, respecting difference and ensuring that care is not diminishing, demeaning or disempowering. Cultural safety encompasses not only ethnicity or origin but also age, gender, disability, sexual identity, socioeconomic status, spiritual beliefs and migrant experience.

Culture A set of learned values, beliefs, customs and behaviour that is shared by a group of interacting individuals.

Dead space Air or empty space between layers of tissue or beneath wound edges that have been approximated.

Debride To remove dirt, foreign objects, damaged tissue and cellular debris from a wound or burn so as to prevent infection and promote healing. In treating a wound, debridement is the first step in cleansing; it allows thorough examination of the extent of the injury.

Defibrillation The application of a controlled electrical shock to the victim's chest in order to terminate a life-threatening cardiac rhythm.

Electronic health record (EHR)/electronic medical record (EMR) An individual patient's medical record in digital format. EHR systems coordinate the storage and retrieval of individual records with the aid of computers. EHRs/EMRs are usually accessed on a computer, often over a network that comprises records from many locations and/or sources. A variety of types of healthcare-related information may be stored and accessed in this way. EHRs/EMRs may also be personally controlled. Integrated EHRs are increasingly seen as the way to achieve quality and continuity in treatment, to fill the gaps in public health research and to contain costs; however, such systems have created many concerns about privacy.

Electrosurgical unit (ESU) (diathermy machine) A system that generates a high-frequency electrical current, which creates heat in body tissue, resulting in coagulation or desiccation of tissue. This provides haemostasis and a bloodless field during a surgical procedure. There are two main types: monopolar and bipolar. Use of the former requires placement of a patient return electrode (diathermy plate/pad) on/under the patient's body, away from the operative site.

Emotional intelligence The ability to understand and manage one's own emotions and those of others. This quality gives individuals a variety of skills, such as the ability to manage relationships, navigate social networks, and influence and even inspire others.

Endogenous Originating from within the body or produced from internal causes.

Endoscope An illuminated optic instrument for visualising the interior of a body cavity or organ. It may be rigid or flexible, and is introduced through a natural orifice or inserted via an incision. Fibreoptic endoscopes have great flexibility and can reach previously inaccessible areas.

Endoscopy Visualisation of the interior of organs and cavities of the body with an endoscope. The gastrointestinal tract, hepatobiliary system, pancreatic ducts, renal system, upper and lower airways and female reproductive system can all be examined, and cytological and histological samples collected. Some conditions can also be treated via an endoscopic procedure.

Endotracheal tube (ETT) A large-bore, disposable catheter made of silicone or PVC tubing that is inserted through the mouth or nose and into the trachea to the point above the bifurcation of the trachea. It is used to deliver anaesthetic gases and oxygen directly into the trachea through the vocal cords. ETTs may have a single or a double lumen (for lung surgery). Adult-sized ETTs have a cuff at their distal end, which when inflated with air seals off the trachea, permitting positive-pressure ventilation and decreasing the risk of aspiration.

Epidural anaesthesia/analgesia A type of central nerve block in which a local anaesthetic drug is injected via a fine catheter into the epidural space surrounding the dural membrane, which contains cerebrospinal fluid and spinal nerves. The catheter lies between the dura mater and the ligamentum flavum at the L3–4 or L5–6 level. An epidural injection can be used to facilitate surgery of the lower half of the body and/or provide prolonged postoperative analgesia.

Error A generic term encompassing all of those occasions in which a planned sequence of mental or physical activities failed to achieve its intended outcome and when the failure cannot be attributed to the intervention of some chance agency.

Eschar Black necrotic tissue or scab that results from trauma, such as thermal or chemical burns, infection or ulcerating skin disease.

Ethical Right or morally acceptable.

Ethics The study of morals and values (including ideals of autonomy, beneficence and justice).

Evaluation and Quality Improvement Program (EQuIP 6) The Australian Council on Healthcare Standards' framework to improve the quality and safety of healthcare. It comprises a 4-year continuous quality assessment and improvement accreditation program for healthcare organisations that supports excellence in consumer/patient care and services.

Evidence-based nursing The conscientious, explicit and judicious use of theory-derived, research-based information in making decisions about care delivery to individuals or groups of patients.

Exogenous Originating outside of the body or an organ of the body, or produced from external causes.

5 moments of hand hygiene Part of the World Health Organization's global program, 'Save Lives Clean Your Hands', launched in 2009. The program identifies each occasion when hand hygiene should be performed, that is (1) before touching a patient, (2) before commencing a procedure, (3) after a procedure or body fluid risk exposure, (4) after touching a patient, and (5) after touching a patient's surroundings.

General anaesthesia A reversible, unconscious state characterised by amnesia, loss of sensation, analgesia and suppression of reflexes.

Haemodynamic monitoring Measurement of pressure, flow and oxygenation within the cardiovascular system.

Haemostasis Termination of bleeding by mechanical or chemical means or by the coagulation processes of the body, which comprise vasoconstriction, platelet aggregation and thrombin and fibrin synthesis.

Hazard Something which has the potential to cause harm to a person.

Health policy A statement of a decision regarding a goal in healthcare and a plan to achieve that goal (e.g. to prevent an epidemic, a program for inoculating a population is developed and implemented).

Healthcare-associated infection (HAI) Also known as nosocomial infection or hospital-acquired infection. Infection acquired during the course of receiving healthcare. Common causative agents include *Candida albicans*, *Escherichia coli*, *Pseudomonas*, *Staphylococcus aureus*, *Staphylococcus epidermidis*, and hepatitis viruses.

High-flow nasal oxygen (HFNO) Oxygen delivered at a high flow via cannulae to preoxygenate the patient prior to airway management and also during sedation. HFNO therapy consists of a warmed, humidified oxygen/air mixture delivered at flow rates of up to 70 L/min by purpose-built nasal cannulae.

Human factors The interrelationships of people to their environment and to each other that need to be considered to optimise performance and assure safety. In healthcare settings these range from the design of tools such as medical devices, services and systems to the working environment and working practices such as tasks, roles and team behaviours.

Iatrogenic harm Harm that has been produced inadvertently by a member of the healthcare team or by medical or surgical treatment, tests or diagnostic procedures.

Inadvertent perioperative hypothermia (IPH) A common but preventable complication of perioperative procedures that is associated with poor outcomes for patients. IPH should be distinguished from the deliberate induction of hypothermia for medical reasons. During the first 30–40 minutes of anaesthesia, a patient's temperature can drop below 35.0°C. Reasons for this include loss of the behavioural response to cold, impairment of thermoregulatory heat-preserving mechanisms under general or regional anaesthesia, anaesthesia-induced peripheral vasodilation (with associated heat loss) and the patient getting cold while waiting for surgery. Current practice is to initiate active warming measures if the patient's temperature drops below 36.0°C.

Incident An event or a circumstance that could have led, or did lead, to unintended and/or unnecessary harm to a person and/or to a complaint, loss or damage.

Indigenous Respectfully refers here to Aboriginal and Torres Strait Islander peoples as the sovereign people of this land and acknowledges the diverse languages and rich cultures. The term 'First Nations' also recognises Aboriginal and Torres Strait Islander peoples as separate and unique sovereign nations. 'First Nations' is widely used in Canada and other countries.

Infection Invasion of the body by pathogenic microorganisms that reproduce and multiply, causing disease by local cellular injury, secretion of a toxin or antigen–antibody reaction to the host.

Infection prevention The policies and procedures of a hospital or other health facility to minimise the risk of spreading healthcare-associated or community-acquired infections to patients or members of staff.

Inflammation The normal response of connective tissue and blood vessels to sublethal irritation or injury. Inflammation may be acute or chronic, the timescale relating to the nature of the injurious stimulus. The cardinal signs of inflammation are redness, heat, swelling and pain, often accompanied by loss of function.

Informed consent Authorisation obtained from a patient to perform a specific test or procedure. The concept of informed consent is a composite of (1) the person's consent to a procedure (or participation in a research study), and (2) the nature and extent of information that must be provided in order for the person's decision to be adequately informed. A broad indication of the nature and risks of the procedure is sufficient to defeat an action in trespass, assuming that the other requirements of a valid consent are met, including voluntariness and competence of the patient.

Intraoperative Pertaining to the period during a surgical procedure.

Justice That which concerns fairness or equity, often divided into three parts: (1) procedural justice, concerned with fair methods of making decisions and settling disputes; (2) distributive justice, concerned with fair distribution of the benefits and burdens of society; and (3) corrective justice, concerned with correcting wrongs and harms through compensation or retribution.

Laparoscopy Examination of the abdominal cavity and viscera using a laparoscope (viewing tube) inserted through one or more small incisions in the abdominal wall, usually around the umbilicus. Laparoscopic surgery can be diagnostic or therapeutic (e.g. laparoscopic cholecystectomy and removal of the gallbladder via the laparoscopic incisions). It is a form of minimally invasive surgery (MIS).

Laryngeal mask airway (LMA) Also called a supraglottic device. The device is used for maintaining a patent airway during general anaesthesia without tracheal intubation. It consists of a tube connected to an oval-shaped inflatable cuff which is positioned above (supra) the glottis and seals the larynx. See supraglottic device.

Laryngospasm Spasmodic closure of the larynx. It may be caused by local irritation, such as the presence of secretions, airway equipment or pulmonary aspiration in the back of the pharynx, resulting in partial or complete spasm of the vocal cords and an inability to breathe effectively. Partial laryngospasm may be characterised by a 'crowing' sound made on inspiration. However, in total laryngospasm no sound is made, as no air moves into or out of the lungs; ineffective respiratory effort will be noted in chest movement.

Laser An acronym for 'light amplification by stimulated emission of radiation'. The energy generated by laser equipment can be used to destroy or refashion tissue and fix it in place. Laser beams can be harmful to the eyes of personnel activating and assisting with procedures, so protective goggles must be worn.

Latex allergy Anaphylactic hypersensitivity to the soluble proteins in latex, most often seen in patients sensitised by repeated exposure to latex. Reactions range from irritant dermatitis and eczema to anaphylactic collapse.

Local anaesthesia Direct administration of an agent (e.g. lignocaine) to tissues to induce the absence of pain sensation in that part of the body. Local anaesthetics do not depress consciousness.

Magnetic resonance imaging (MRI) A scanning technique that exposes the body to a strong magnetic field and uses the electromagnetic signals emitted by the body to form an image of soft tissue and cells.

Malignant hyperthermia A rare, life-threatening, genetic hypermetabolic condition characterised by severe hyperthermia and rigidity of the skeletal muscles triggered by inhalational anaesthetics and the muscle relaxant succinylcholine. Treatment involves the use of dantrolene sodium injection, administration of 100% oxygen, removal of triggering agents, immediate cooling, cessation of surgery and correction of acidosis and hyperkalaemia.

Māori The Indigenous people of New Zealand; they comprise about 10% of the country's population.

Massive transfusion protocol (MTP)/critical bleeding protocol A resource, usually in the form of a template, developed to assist the healthcare team in clinical decision making when managing a patient with critical bleeding, requiring the infusion of large volumes of blood products.

Medical device-related pressure injuries Medical devices have the potential to cause localised damage to the patient's skin and/or underlying soft tissue, usually over a bony prominence. Such medical devices include, but may not be limited to, airways, catheters, drains, IV lines, masks, nasal prongs, sequential compression devices and tourniquets as well as discarded items such as caps from needles, etc.

Microorganism Any living organism that can be seen only under a microscope. Microorganisms may be pathogenic and include bacteria, algae, protozoa, fungi (cellular), viruses and prions (acellular).

Minimally invasive surgery (MIS) Also known as minimal access surgery (MAS). Surgery undertaken with only a small incision or no incision at all, such as through a cannula with a laparoscope or an endoscope.

National Standards The National Safety and Quality Health Service (NSQHS) standards were developed by the Australian Commission on Safety and Quality in Health Care (ACSQHC) to drive the implementation of safety and quality systems and improve the quality of healthcare in Australia. The 10 NSQHS standards provide a nationally consistent statement about the level of care that consumers can expect from health service organisations.

Near miss An unplanned event that did not result in injury, illness or damage but that had the potential to do so.

Negative-pressure wound therapy (NPWT) A method of removing excess exudate and infection from a wound so as to promote healing in acute or chronic wounds. The therapy involves controlled application of subatmospheric pressure to the wound bed using a sealed wound dressing connected to a vacuum pump.

Negligence A legal term defined as 'causing damage unintentionally but carelessly'. A court will determine negligence based on reasonable foreseeability that the damage might have been possible, the existence of a duty of care to the person damaged, a breach in that duty could be demonstrated and that damages were indeed experienced by the victim.

Neuraxial block A collective term for spinal and epidural anaesthesia.

Neutral zone (hands-free zone) A predetermined location on the surgical aseptic field, agreed upon by the surgical team, where sharps are placed in puncture-proof containers for transfer to and from the team during surgery. This safety strategy prevents two team members simultaneously touching sharps, reducing the risk of sharps injury.

Never events Also termed *sentinel events* in Australasia. A term coined in the early 2000s and used in the UK and the USA to signify adverse events that are unambiguous (clearly identifiable and measurable), serious (resulting in death or significant disability) and usually preventable.

Notification A concern raised about a registered health practitioner's or student's professional behaviour or clinical practice, also known as a complaint. Notifications can be made by individuals or organisations to the Australian Health Practitioner Regulation Agency (AHPRA), which manages notifications in partnership with national Nursing and Midwifery Board of Australia (NMBA) and state/territory boards. Notifications may result in disciplinary action being taken against the health professional. See also *Professional misconduct* and *Unprofessional conduct*.

Open disclosure Explaining to a patient/relative/carer the facts and circumstances surrounding an adverse event. It is not an admission of liability, but rather an opportunity to express regret, provide information on potential consequences, explain steps to manage the event and prevent recurrence.

Operating room (OR) Refers to the room in which surgery or surgical procedures are performed. Also known as the operating theatre.

Operating suite Refers collectively to the department with a suite of rooms where a surgery or surgical procedure is performed. It includes numerous patient care areas such as holding bays, anaesthetic rooms, scrub bays, operating rooms or theatres as well as the postanaesthesia care unit. It also includes staff areas such as reception, offices, staff tearooms and storage areas. Also known as the perioperative department or perioperative suite.

Pacific Islander peoples Refers to people from the island groups of Micronesia, Melanesia and Polynesia. Despite often being grouped together, populations from these regions are heterogeneous, with diverse cultures, languages and religions.

Pandemic A disease that spreads over multiple countries or continents.

Patient-controlled analgesia (PCA) A drug delivery system that dispenses an intravascular dose of a narcotic analgesic when the patient pushes a switch on an electric cord. The device consists of a computerised pump with a chamber holding a syringe of drug. The patient administers a dose of narcotic when the need for pain relief arises. A lockout interval automatically inactivates the system if the patient tries to increase the amount of narcotic within a preset period.

Patient journey Begins as early as the prehospital patient assessment and includes the period of hospitalisation and surgical intervention, through to discharge home for recovery and rehabilitation in the community.

Personal information Information by which individuals or collectives can be identified. This is defined in the Privacy Act 1988 (Cth) as information or an opinion (including information or an opinion forming part of a database), whether true or not, and whether recorded in a material form or not, about an individual whose identity is apparent, or can reasonably be ascertained, from the information or opinion.

Personal protective equipment (PPE) A range of equipment, such as gloves, eye protection, masks and plastic aprons, used to protect healthcare staff from infectious organisms.

Point of care testing (PoCT) Point of care testing is when pathology assessment or tests are conducted close to the point of patient care. This sometimes occurs in procedure rooms or the operating room (e.g. breast specimen X-ray) and has the advantage of rapid delivery of test results, ensuring timely or immediate intervention and treatment.

Policy A principle or guideline that governs an activity and that employees or members of an institution or organisation are expected to follow.

Postoperative Pertaining to the period of time after surgery. It begins with the patient's emergence from anaesthesia and continues throughout the time required for the acute effects of the anaesthetic and the surgery or procedure to abate.

Preoperative Pertaining to the period before a surgical procedure. Commonly the preoperative period begins with the first preparation of the patient for surgery or other procedure and ends with the induction of anaesthesia in the operating suite.

Pressure injury A localised injury to the skin and/or underlying tissue, usually over a bony prominence or related to a medical or other device. The injury may be due to unrelieved pressure, friction and/or shearing or moisture (or a combination of more than one factor).

Primary intention healing Wound healing that occurs when a surgical incision or clean laceration is closed primarily with sutures, Steri-strips, or tissue adhesive.

Privacy Control over the extent, timing and circumstances of sharing oneself (physically, behaviourally or intellectually) with others. Implies a zone of exclusivity, where individuals and collectives are free from the scrutiny of others.

Procedural sedation and/or analgesia Implies that the patient is in a state of drug-induced tolerance of uncomfortable or painful diagnostic or interventional medical, dental or surgical procedures. Lack of memory of distressing events and/or analgesia may be the desired outcome, but lack of response to painful stimulation is not assured.

Professional misconduct Conduct by a health practitioner that is substantially below the standard reasonably expected of a registered health practitioner of an equivalent level of training or experience.

Professional practice standard The standard of health professional care as determined by groups within the particular profession.

Pulse oximeter A device that measures the amount of saturated haemoglobin in the tissue capillaries. A beam of light is transmitted through the tissue to a receiver. This non-invasive method of measuring the saturated haemoglobin is a useful screening tool for determining basic respiratory function. A clip-like probe is usually placed on the patient's finger, toe or earlobe. As the amount of saturated haemoglobin alters the wavelengths of the transmitted light, analysis of the received light is translated into a percentage of oxygen saturation (S_pO_2) of the blood, which is displayed on a monitoring device. A reading of 95% or above is considered a satisfactory value.

Quality improvement Evaluation of services provided, with the results achieved compared with accepted standards. Any deficiencies noted or identified serve to prompt recommendations for improvement.

Rapid sequence induction (or intubation) A method of protecting the airway during induction of anaesthesia in patients at risk of aspiration of gastric contents. This is achieved by minimising the time between loss of consciousness and intubation, and by applying cricoid pressure.

Regional anaesthesia Anaesthesia provided by injection of a local anaesthetic drug to block a group of sensory nerve fibres. Types of regional anaesthesia include axillary, brachial plexus, caudal, epidural, pudendal, intercostal, paracervical and spinal anaesthesia.

Respect for persons Has two fundamental aspects: (1) respect for the autonomy of those individuals who are capable of making informed choices and respect for their capacity for self-determination; and (2) the protection of persons with impaired or diminished autonomy (i.e. those individuals who are incompetent or whose voluntary capacity is compromised).

Reusable medical device Any medical device, for example, surgical instruments, endoscopes, anaesthetic equipment etc., which has been deemed by the manufacturer as suitable for reprocessing and which can subsequently be reused on patients.

Risk The chance that any hazard will cause actual harm to a person. It is measured in terms of consequences and likelihood.

Risk management A function of administration of a hospital or other health facility directed towards identification, evaluation and correction of potential risks leading to injury of patients, staff members or visitors and resulting in property loss or damage.

Robotic surgery Remote, computer-assisted telemanipulators developed for use in surgery to overcome some of the limitations associated with laparoscopic equipment. The advanced technology incorporates sophisticated mechanical equipment, which is used to hold and manoeuvre endoscopic instrumentation during minimally invasive surgery (MIS). The surgeon can control robotic devices remotely.

Root cause analysis A systematic approach whereby factors that contributed to an incident are identified and recommendations to prevent recurrence are generated. In the healthcare setting, a team of unbiased experts may be called on to investigate how and why an error occurred by looking more at the system problems that emerged than at individual negligence.

Scope of practice (SOP) The full spectrum of roles, functions, responsibilities, activities and decision-making capacity that individuals within a profession are educated, competent and authorised to perform.

Secondary intention healing Wound healing that occurs when the sides of the wound are not opposed (joined together); therefore healing occurs from the bottom of the wound upwards, resulting in scar formation.

Sellick's manoeuvre A technique used to reduce the risk of aspiration of gastric contents during induction of general anaesthesia. The cricoid cartilage is pushed against the body of the sixth cervical vertebra, occluding the upper end of the oesophagus and preventing passive regurgitation. The technique cannot stop active vomiting. Cricoid pressure is applied immediately after injection of anaesthesia and before tracheal intubation, and as part of a rapid sequence intubation. Regurgitated gastric contents entering the lungs can result in a condition known as Mendelson's syndrome.

Sentinel events Also called *never events* in the UK and the USA. Rare, adverse events leading to serious patient harm or death which are specifically caused by healthcare rather than the patient's underlying condition or illness.

Sepsis Infection or contamination.

Sepsis-induced hypotension A systolic blood pressure <90 mmHg or a reduction of >40 mmHg from baseline in the absence of other causes of hypotension.

Septic shock A form of shock that occurs in septicaemia when endotoxins or exotoxins are released from certain bacteria into the bloodstream. The toxins cause profound hypotension.

Severity assessment code (SAC) A numerical score applied to an incident based on the type of incident, its likelihood of recurrence and its consequence. A matrix is used to stratify the actual and/or potential risk associated with an incident. There are four SAC ratings, ranging from SAC1 (extreme risk) to SAC4 (low risk).

Situation awareness An ability to identify and process many pieces of information from within the environment and act accordingly. Situation awareness requires the ability to watch, listen and understand cues, and anticipate what may happen next. Team members (e.g. those who comprise the surgical team) need to be aware of the big picture, rather than focusing only on a particular task. To achieve this, individuals take in data from their senses, interpret the data and make predictions about what will happen in the future. Situation awareness relies on good teamwork and communication.

Skill mix The relative mix of skilled and experienced staff in a team. For example, in the operating suite there may be experienced, qualified registered nurses (RNs) and enrolled nurses (ENs), less-experienced RNs and ENs, newly graduated/qualified RNs/ENs and various technical, ancillary and other non-nursing personnel. A poor skill mix has a higher proportion of staff with lower-order qualifications and less experience; conversely, a good skill mix has a higher proportion of experienced and qualified staff.

Social media The online and mobile tools that individuals and groups use to share opinions, information, experiences, images and video or audio clips; they include websites and apps used for social networking.

Standard aseptic technique Practised in perioperative and proceduralist settings for procedures that are simple, of short duration and involve only a few key parts (syringe hub or cannula) or sites (entry point to patient, e.g. vein which will require cleaning with antiseptic solution). Key parts and sites must be identified and protected from contact with unsterile items. For standard aseptic technique, the aseptic field is termed 'general', usually requiring non-sterile gloves, e.g. insertion of IV cannulae or injection into an IV line/port. Perioperative nurses may use standard aseptic techniques when inserting an IV or changing a dressing in PACU.

Standard precautions A range of strategies designed to reduce the transmission of microorganisms from both recognised and unrecognised sources – for example, use of safe work practices and protective barriers (e.g. personal protective equipment). Standard precautions apply to blood, all body secretions (except sweat), non-intact skin and mucous membranes (including the eyes).

Stent A scaffolding device inserted into a vessel or passageway to keep it open and prevent closure. Stents can be bare metals or coated with drug-eluting substances.

Sterile Absence of all forms of microbial life.

Sterilisation The processes used to eliminate or destroy all forms of microbial life from equipment and surgical instru-ments, to prepare them for use during a surgical procedure. Methods to achieve sterilisation include the use of steam, ethylene oxide, dry heat, gamma radiation, peracetic acid and gas plasma. *Note* Sterilised items remain sterile only for as long as they remain inside unopened, uncompromised sterile packaging. In the operating room, sterile items are removed from their sterile packaging and are aseptically introduced into the surgical field, where they remain for the duration of the procedure. During that time, these items are exposed to the constant presence of airborne pathogens from the operating room environment and can no longer be considered sterile, even if not used. Therefore, they are considered aseptic, meaning free from additional pathogenic microorganisms.

Supraglottic device A device for securing the airway during anaesthesia which is positioned above the glottis and does not pass through the vocal cords. An example is a laryngeal mask airway (LMA).

Surgical aseptic technique Required when procedures are more complex and longer in duration, involving numerous key parts and key sites. The most obvious examples are surgical procedures where the instrument nurse and surgical team are involved. Anaesthetic nurses will also be required to set up a surgical aseptic field when the anaestheist is inserting invasive monitoring or a spinal anaesthetic. For surgical aseptic technique, the aseptic field is termed 'critical' and requires the use of sterile drapes, instruments and equipment; additionally, all members of the surgical team must wear a sterile gown and gloves.

Surgical plume Plume generated during tissue ablation or disruption while using energy-based devices such as electrosurgical equipment, radiofrequency devices, ultrasonic shears or lasers. This plume has been shown to contain toxins, carcinogens and viruses. The use of surgical plume evacuation units is recommended to protect the surgical team from inhaling the smoke plume.

Surgical/professional conscience A surgical/professional conscience is an individual's professional honesty and inner morality system, which allows no compromise in practice whether a breach occurs within the team or when working alone.

Surgical site infection (SSI) An infection caused by the introduction of pathogenic microorganisms into a wound during or following a surgical procedure. Most commonly caused by staphylococcal, streptococcal, enterococcal or pneumococcal bacteria, with *Staphylococcus aureus* being the most frequently identified organism in SSIs.

Telophase symbol Telophase is the last stage of cell division. A white telophase symbol is used as a visual warning on cytotoxic substances and is also used on purple-coloured cytotoxic waste containers.

Tertiary intention healing Also known as delayed primary closure; occurs when wounds are initially left open after debridement of all non-viable tissue. Wound edges may be sutured closed following a period of open observation, when the wound appears clean and there is evidence of good tissue viability and perfusion.

Tidal volume The volume of air that is moved into or out of the lungs with each breath.

Transmission-based precautions Safeguards designed for patients who are known or suspected to be infected with highly transmissible or epidemiologically important pathogens, for which additional precautions beyond standard precautions are needed to interrupt transmission in hospitals. There are three types of transmission-based precautions: airborne precautions, droplet precautions and contact precautions. They may be combined for diseases that have multiple routes of transmission and, either singly or in combination, are used in addition to standard precautions.

Transoesophageal echocardiography (TOE) An examination that uses a probe with an ultrasound transducer at the tip. As the probe passes through the oesophagus, it sends back clear images of the size of the heart as well as movement of the walls, valvular abnormalities, endocarditis vegetation and possible sources of thrombi.

Ultrasound imaging The use of high-frequency sound, usually greater than 1 MHz, to image internal structures. Unlike radiological examination, ultrasound does not use ionising radiation.

Unethical Wrong or morally unacceptable.

Unprofessional conduct Professional conduct that is of a lower standard than that which might reasonably be expected of the health practitioner by the public or the practitioner's professional peers. Less serious than professional misconduct.

Utilitarian Ethical theory that presupposes an action is right if it achieves the greatest good for the greatest number of people.

Venous thromboembolism (VTE) A condition that involves the development of venous thrombosis and subsequent pulmonary embolus (PE). VTE is a mostly preventable surgical complication, yet remains a significant cause of postoperative morbidity and mortality in the form of chronic venous insufficiency, recurrent thromboembolism and post-thrombotic syndrome.

Voluntary Free of coercion, duress or undue inducement.

World Health Organization Surgical Safety Checklist (WHO SCC) A tool developed by WHO to reduce the occurrence of unnecessary surgical deaths and avoidable complications. The aim of the SSC is to standardise and reinforce accepted safety practices (such as 'Time Out' prior to commencement of surgery) and improve communication and teamwork among members of the surgical team – activities known to improve patient safety.

Index